Galen: An Anthology

Galen: An Anthology

Edited and translated by

P. N. SINGER

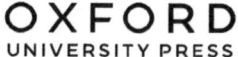
OXFORD
UNIVERSITY PRESS

OXFORD
UNIVERSITY PRESS

Oxford University Press is a department of the University of Oxford.
It furthers the University's objective of excellence in research, scholarship,
and education by publishing worldwide. Oxford is a registered trade mark of
Oxford University Press in the UK and in certain other countries.

Published in the United States of America by Oxford University Press
198 Madison Avenue, New York, NY 10016, United States of America.

Preassigned Control Number is on file at the Library of Congress

ISBN 9780190641399 (hbk)
ISBN 9780190641405 (pbk)

Printed by Sheridan Books, Inc., United States of America

Contents

Acknowledgements

I have benefited from the advice, mentorship, intellectual input and correction of many—too many to acknowledge all individually—in the near forty years of intermittent devotion to Galenic studies that have culminated in this volume.

But I must mention a few.

Geoffrey Lloyd provided the initial inspiration for my study of ancient science, as well as the specific suggestion of a Ph.D. on Galen, and shaped my early understanding of and approach to that study. I am grateful, for a variety of forms of information, guidance and support, moral and intellectual, during those years, to: the late and much missed Paola Manuli and Mario Vegetti; David Sedley, Thomas Rütten and Kostas Valakas; and, in more recent years, to: Sean Coughlin, Catharine Edwards, Christopher Gill, Harold Tarrant, David Leith, Orly Lewis, Lucia Raggetti and the dearly missed Piero Tassinari.

Philip van der Eijk and the financial support of the Wellcome Trust enabled me to return to Galenic research after a long break from it in 2009, and so to extend and improve my translations.

Ralph Rosen provided—albeit in a somewhat indirect and unorthodox manner—the immediate impetus to the project of a revised version of my 1997 Oxford World's Classics volume, from which the present book eventually took shape. He also provided much intellectual stimulation and support besides.

At Oxford University Press, I should like to thank Stefan Vranka for his support of the project; the production and editorial team; and especially the copy-editor, Tim Beck, for his patient, perceptive and meticulous audit of the typescript.

A much older debt, of which I am increasingly conscious, is to my excellent classics teachers at the City of London School: Charles Wright, Harry Lee-Uff, John Hazel, John Carroll, Richard England, Timothy Reader and—last but very far from least—Denis Moore. I remember their dedication, encouragement and teaching very fondly, and without it I would never have come near any such study as that represented by this book.

Tamsyn Barton has been a source of moral support, intellectual stimulation and a great deal more, at various points from my graduate days onwards.

My most abiding and profound gratitude is to my parents, Jean Singer and Konrad Singer, who encouraged my studies and tolerated its unpredictabilities, and who gave me my first intellectual stimulation, as well as their constant support.

Translator's Note

The texts presented in this volume have been selected with a view to giving the reader a broad overview of Galen's writings in as wide a range of areas as possible. The order in which they are presented is thematic rather than either chronological or based on Galen's own classifications; the aim is to introduce the author's life, medical work and scientific and philosophical theories in a logical and accessible manner.

The book began life as a revised and expanded edition of the earlier *Galen: Selected Works*, which appeared in the Oxford World's Classics series in 1997, offering the first-ever English-language version of several of the author's most important writings, in an accessible collection. But both revision and expansion developed in such a way as to make this in effect a wholly new book.

It is distinguished from its predecessor not just by its much larger scale, but in particular by the inclusion, alongside complete treatises, of substantial extracts from longer ones. The treatises translated in the previous volume were predominantly short works, either introductory or summative in nature or with a focus on philosophical, literary or biographical themes. The present volume adds to such works substantial excerpts from Galen's most important writings on anatomical demonstration and psychological theory (*The Doctrines of Hippocrates and Plato*), element theory (*The Elements according to Hippocrates*), the nature of clinical practice and disease diagnosis (*Prognosis, Affected Places*) and pharmacology (*Simple Drugs*), as well as short indicative excerpts from his monumental works on anatomy (*Anatomical Procedures*) and the structures and physiology of the human body (*The Function of the Parts*) and from his magnum opus on healthy lifestyles (*Health*).

Last but my no means least, I have included two texts that were discovered in a manuscript in a Greek library in 2005,[1] and thus not available at the time of the previous publication (*Freedom from Distress, My Own Doctrines*), and also two other short but important works on the nature of medical knowledge (*The Best Method of Instruction* and *Sects for Beginners*). I have also removed one, *Thrasybulus*, and reduced another, *Mixtures*, to excerpted form.[2]

Three of the works published—either in full or in excerpts—here appeared not only in the original 1997 volume but also more recently in the ongoing

---

[1] See the headnote to *Freedom from Distress*, below.
[2] These texts are now available in the Cambridge Galen Translations series (see also next note), in Singer 2023 and Singer and van der Eijk 2018 respectively.

Cambridge Galen Translations series, which since 2013 has offered translations of individual Galenic treatises, with extensive introductions and annotation, in a much more scholarly and specialized format.[3] In those cases, the translation printed here is neither the same as that of the original book nor as that of the Cambridge edition, but is a further revision that aims to retain much of the immediacy of the former while taking account of subsequent corrections and of further thinking (my own and others') on these texts. *Freedom from Distress* also appeared in the first volume of that series, though not in my translation; here too a new translation is presented, in this case taking account of the very substantial body of research that has taken place on that work, even since 2013.

Finally, I have thoroughly revised all the translations that were already present in the earlier volume, in the interests of greater accuracy, and incorporating the results of the latest scholarship and research. My own translation technique has also evolved somewhat in the intervening decades, evincing a stricter commitment to consistency, especially in the rendition of technical terms, and a tendency to somewhat closer adherence to the Greek syntax. Both these developments are reflected in the present volume—without, it is hoped, a severe loss of readability or accessibility.

There has been, it is scarcely an exaggeration to say, an explosion of Galenic studies since I first dipped a tentative toe in those waters nearly four decades ago, and much has changed in the scholarly landscape since 1997. However, no equivalent or replacement to *Galen: Selected Works* has appeared in the intervening years. The present revised and expanded—and much delayed— version is designed to perform the same introductory function as the original and to have the same value as a study and research resource, while offering a wider range of the most important texts, and also taking advantage of much of that body of recent scholarship—in short, to be still more useful than its predecessor.

The volume is also furnished with a chronology, a bibliography and an explanatory list of the major persons mentioned in the texts.

---

[3] These are *The Soul's Dependence on the Body* and *Affections and Errors*, in Singer 2013, and *Mixtures* (appearing here in excerpts) in Singer and van der Eijk 2018.

Introduction

Galen, alongside his hero Hippocrates, is the most important and historically influential medical author of Graeco-Roman antiquity. Unlike Hippocrates, however—a shadowy figure about whom little can be said with certainty[1]—Galen is a clearly identifiable historical person with a distinctive voice and intellectual identity, from whose pen we possess more than 120 extant works, and whose scientific work and career can be traced in detail. He synthesized and adapted the medical theories of his predecessors (including 'Hippocrates'), and on their basis developed his own distinctive models of human psychology, physiology, health, disease, pharmacology and clinical practice, which he defended vigorously against his opponents. He was also an energetic researcher and active physician, insisting on the crucial importance of empirical observation, especially in anatomy, in pharmacology and in the clinical context. From a modern perspective, the validity of his observations will seem in many cases dubious, and his model of empirical research flawed and limited. Central to his project, however, was the ambition to found medical knowledge on repeated observation of the phenomena and on rational argumentation and analysis; and these aims are articulated, with great power and sophistication, in a wide range of empirical and therapeutic contexts.

As an author, moreover, he provides us—as a function of his huge range of interests and his discursive, digressive style—with a wealth of insights, not just into the discipline and practice of medicine in the Graeco-Roman world, but also into a wide variety of aspects of cultural, intellectual, scientific and everyday life.

At some point in the generations after his death his work and his theories and his teachings came to eclipse those of his contemporaries and predecessors; and they conditioned medical instruction and medical practice—both as a model to follow and one to react against—in a variety of historical and geographical contexts, from the fourth until at least the eighteenth century, in Europe, the Near East and beyond. He is also one of the most voluminous authors of antiquity, in terms of writings which have been preserved—a fact clearly related to that posthumous success.

---

[1] A disparate group of texts came to be assembled gradually under the name Hippocrates at various points in antiquity, and has come down to us as the 'Hippocratic corpus'. Modern scholarship has increasingly highlighted the heterogeneous nature of these texts and the impossibility of attributing any with certainty to a historical Hippocrates. Essential in deconstructing the traditional view of Hippocrates remains Smith 1979; see also van der Eijk 2015. Yet the perception of him as 'father of medicine', and of his work as somehow distinctive from the rest of Greek medicine, survives stubbornly in the popular—and often even in the academic—imagination.

Life and Work

Galen (*Galēnos*) was born into a rich family in the Greek-speaking elite of Pergamum in the Roman province of Asia (now Bergama in Turkey) in AD 129.[2] His father, who Galen hints was an architect, has been tentatively identified with one Aelius Nicon, known from Pergamene inscriptions of the period. From him Galen received an early education in mathematics and geometry, before being sent, from the age of 14, to attend the lectures of philosophers belonging to each of main philosophic schools, and from the age of 16 also to study medicine, his first teacher being Satyrus, a student of Quintus. Galen thus began early in life that joint engagement with philosophy and medicine which would inform his later career and intellectual project. Precisely what was the initial motivation or stimulus for this direction of study must remain unknowable; Galen claims that it was due to 'clear dreams' experienced by his father. It seems surely significant, at least, that Pergamum was at this time a considerable intellectual and cultural centre—a status that had been reinforced by a recent building and renovation programme under the emperor Hadrian—and in particular a centre for medical teaching and healing. Here the close proximity of the Asclepieion—the healing sanctuary of the god Asclepius, to which patients came to receive healing through dreams or through the advice of priests—may also be relevant. Although it is not clear what contact Galen had with the Asclepieion, or how closely medical teaching and practice there were connected with those of the city itself, its presence undoubtedly enhanced the status of Pergamum as a medical centre. And the relationship between the temple medicine practised there and the 'rational medicine' of Galen and his teachers seems, contrary to what we might expect, to have been one of mutual respect rather than of hostility.[3]

The paedagogic route on which Galen now embarked was one through which he entered into the elite world of literate, philosophically informed medicine—a pursuit involving long years of study, including, alongside more obviously practical elements, both the analysis of a wide range of texts and the acquisition of sophisticated logical, rhetorical and dialectical skills. A form of medicine, then, which was worlds apart from that of the many artisan practitioners—surgeons, druggists and other non-literate doctors—who also practised in the ancient Mediterranean. And Galen vigorously and

---

[2] Nearly all that we know of Galen's life comes from his own account of it in various autobiographical passages in his writings (several of which appear in this volume); there are no contemporary mentions of him in other sources. For modern accounts of his biography see Mattern 2008, 2013; Boudon-Millot 2007 (introduction), 2012; Nutton 2020.

[3] It seems that Galen at some point met Aelius Aristides, a distinguished literary figure of the period who spent many months at the Asclepieion, of which he gives a vivid account in his writings. On Galen's relationship with Pergamum see Singer 2019a.

repeatedly champions his own philosophical and 'Hippocratic' approach—the long years of dedicated study, the high ethical standards, the need not just for close observation but also for precise distinctions and acute logical analysis enabling the physician to reason about causes in nature and about diseases and their appropriate treatment, whereby medicine itself becomes an art (*technē*) which belongs at the noblest and intellectually highest level. (For such exaltation of the medical art see especially *An Exhortation to Study the Arts* and *The Best Doctor is also a Philosopher*.)

After the death of his father, in 148, Galen embarked on a study tour which was to last until 157. He travelled first to Smyrna, where he studied with the doctor Pelops, as well as with the Platonist philosopher Albinus; then to Corinth and Alexandria, apparently in search of the anatomical teacher Numisianus or his writings. It seems that he stayed for about four years in Alexandria, still at that time the main centre for the study of anatomy. It was at Alexandria, surely, that, alongside the extensive study of anatomy, he developed his deep interest and expertise in the texts of 'Hippocrates'—literary scholarship in general, and Hippocratic scholarship in particular, being prominent amongst the city's specialisms.

On his return to Pergamum at the age of 28, he was given the position of official doctor to the city's gladiators, a position in the gift of the high priest, and renewed several times over the next four years. He claims to have had great success in the role, no gladiator ever dying under his care, and that this was in part the result of his existing anatomical knowledge—which was then further enhanced by the occasional observation of deep wounds sustained by the gladiators.

In 162, at the age of 33, Galen arrived for the first time in Rome, where he stayed until 166, establishing his career through a number of high-profile public debates and anatomical, including vivisectional, demonstrations on animals, and through networking in the higher echelons of Roman society, where he claims to have made a great impression also with a series of spectacularly successful predictions and cures (as recounted especially in *Prognosis*). In 166, as the Antonine Plague first hit Rome in the aftermath of the Parthian War, he returned to Pergamum, but was summoned to Italy by imperial command in 168. Avoiding the fate of joining the imperial army on campaign, he was instead installed in Rome as court physician with responsibility for the young prince Commodus, and with plenty of time to write; the ensuing years saw the completion of a substantial body of his most important works. On the emperor's return in 176 Galen continued his service in the imperial household, now directly for the emperor, and he probably continued to do so through the subsequent reigns of Commodus and Septimius Severus (although some scholars have speculated that the reign of the former may have occasioned a temporary retreat from public life).

A dramatic event took place towards the end of Commodus' reign, which had a serious effect upon Galen: the fire that swept through the area of the Roman forum in 192, destroying many buildings, including imperial libraries and Galen's own personal storeroom, where he kept a wide range of items of great value, in particular manuscripts of both his own and others' writings. The events—as well as the traumatic nature of the previous years, those of Commodus' reign—are recounted in *Freedom from Distress*, presented as a work of ethical philosophy but incidentally functioning as a fascinating document of both autobiography and contemporary history.

He continued to work and write until at least the late 190s; and while it is difficult to date his works, even relatively to each other, with any accuracy, it seems that both pharmacology (or drug recipes) and Hippocratic commentary—in both of which areas he wrote very voluminously—were to a considerable extent the focus of this later phase of his life. The date of his death is unknown: neither the traditional one of 199 nor that of 216 which has largely supplanted it in more recent scholarship is based on any very reliable evidence.

Position in History: Predecessors and Afterlife

While Galen's historical influence is enormous, the originality of his contribution is difficult to assess. This is partly related to the situation mentioned at the outset: we possess Galen's writings in abundance, but we lack, with few exceptions, the writings of his contemporaries and more recent predecessors, some of whose theories and observations were clearly of great importance in the development of his own. Galen exacerbates this problem through his own 'classicizing' approach. That is to say, he tends ideologically always to advert to the greats of the classical Greek world of five hundred years or more before his own time—the 'ancients' (*palaioi*), most notably Hippocrates and Plato, and to a lesser extent Aristotle. These are the authorities whom he claims to respect and follow (albeit not uncritically), while he obscures or passes over his indebtedness to the 'more recent' (*neōteroi*) doctors, which seems in many areas to have been more significant. Thus, it is highly likely that—to give just a few examples—he was strongly indebted to Herophilus and Archigenes in his theory of diagnosis through the pulse; to Athenaeus of Attalia in his theory of elements and disease; and to Erasistratus in areas of his physiology. These are all obscure figures to us, known only from fragments, in many cases fragments constituted by quotations in Galen's own works; worse than that, they are figures against whom Galen is frequently polemicizing at the moment that he gives those quotations. The nature of their influence has to be gathered in spite of the paucity of the sources, and by reading between the lines of that polemic. Such are the complexities of the textual transmission of ancient medical writing, and of its interpretation.

In anatomy, his influences and the nature of his contribution are clearer. Here he gives a detailed account of his teachers and of the previous writings which he studied, and also of his departures from their accounts, based on his own observations. The crucial figures were all students of Marinus, an anatomist of a couple of generations before Galen's time, and/or of Marinus' student Quintus. Galen studied this existing body of knowledge intensively, and took it as the basis for his own anatomical research. (See here both *My Own Books* and *Anatomical Procedures*.)

In pharmacology, too, Galen tells us a lot about his predecessors; a large part of his work in this area, the *Compound Drugs*, consists substantially of recipes taken, and often quoted verbatim, from previous sources, representing a body of knowledge going back, in some cases, hundreds of years; and predecessors are mentioned in *Simple Drugs* too.

His most frequently acknowledged predecessors, however, remain Hippocrates and Plato. But their influence upon Galen is not a straightforward one. In both cases he is highly selective in the texts on which he focuses, and arguably distortive in his interpretation of them; and in the former case—where the question of authorship of individual works was already highly contentious—the extent of his tendency to read his own views back into the Hippocratic text is such that from a modern scholarly perspective he seems almost to be creating Hippocrates in his own image. Both the selection of texts to be taken as 'Hippocratic'— central amongst them *The Nature of the Human Being*, the *Epidemics* and the *Prognostic*—and the interpretation of the first of those works, in particular, as congruent with Galen's own views, are contentious to say the least.[4]

The synthesis that Galen produces on the basis of these sources, and indeed the very project of reconciling Hippocratic with Platonic (and other philosophical) views—as shown most spectacularly in *The Doctrines of Hippocrates and Plato*—are intellectually ambitious and argumentatively impressive. Central to this synthesis are Galen's element theory, on the one hand, and his physiology of the three central organs, brain, heart and liver, with their respective systems of nerves, arteries and veins, on the other, which he presents as a restatement of Plato's tripartite theory of the soul (rational, spirited, desiderative).

In all these areas—medical–clinical, anatomical, pharmacological, physiological–theoretical—Galen is in different ways drawing on previous authors, some of whom he acknowledges more clearly than others. In all cases, however, it seems that he produces his own interpretation and his own refinements of the previous theories or observations, aiming to incorporate or synthesize them within his own overall model, or models, of explanation.

To turn to his afterlife. While the early stages of the process by which Galen came to dominate, and then largely to eclipse, other medical authorities is not clear, by AD 500 we find a corpus of his work already established in the medical

---

[4] See in this volume *The Elements according to Hippocrates*.

curriculum at Alexandria; and we also find his work in use in Latin translation in Ravenna about a century later. His writings were excerpted (though not in this case to the exclusion of other authors) in the medical handbooks of the so-called 'encyclopaedists' of the Byzantine world, Oribasius of Pergamum, Alexander of Tralles, Paul of Aegina and Aëtius of Amida, between the fourth and the seventh century; and his work continued to exert influence, though certainly not always without resistance, in the Greek-speaking east. A crucial further development was the interest in Galen, alongside other Greek scientific authors, at the Abbasid court of Baghdad in the eighth to the tenth century, leading to the translation into Syriac and then Arabic of a large number of his works, and their subsequent influence in the Arabic-speaking or Islamicate world and in geographical areas influenced by it—ranging from mediaeval Spain, through north Africa and the Near East to the Indian subcontinent, where some version of Galenism still survives in the form of the so-called 'Unani' medicine, and even to eastern Asia. Galen's influence in the Latin-speaking west, meanwhile, began in earnest with the translation of some of his works, as well as of Arabic compilations based on his work, from Arabic into Latin by Constantine the African at Monte Cassino in Italy in the eleventh century. These translations were used at the medical school of Salerno, where there also originated, largely on their basis, a first version of the so-called *Articella*. This was a compilation of medical texts, mainly Hippocratic and Galenic, which underwent many revisions but in some form was adopted in the medical curriculum of most European universities, up until the sixteenth century.

Knowledge of Galen's work in the west was enhanced and extended by further translations, both from Arabic, especially by Gerard of Cremona in the twelfth century—who also translated works by Arabic authors with a strong Galenic influence, most notably the *Canon* of Avicenna, which came to play a major role in mediaeval university teaching—and then directly from Greek, most notably by Burgundio of Pisa, also in the twelfth century, and by Niccolò of Reggio in the fourteenth.

The sixteenth century saw an increasing number of available Latin translations, now also in print, as well as the first Greek edition of Galen's works, the Aldine, in 1525; and Galen's work continued not just to dominate medical education but to be a focus of and stimulus to Humanist intellectual debates. It seems that, contrary to the view often promulgated in popular or simplified histories of medicine, the existence of more accurate and fuller texts of Galen's works actually went hand in hand with a renewed interest in direct anatomical observation, rather than the latter pursuit supplanting the former. The human body and the classical text, according to this Humanist anatomical approach, must both, jointly, be the object of close analysis and observation, in a process which will correct the anatomical errors of the past. Even Vesalius, who famously noted discrepancies between Galen's text and the observed reality, took himself to be working within a Galenic framework and adjusting, not overturning, the Galenic model; and Galen's works continued to be central to anatomical teaching at universities well beyond that.

Scientific developments from the seventeenth to the nineteenth century saw the gradual removal of Galen from this central role in providing medical education and representing accepted medical knowledge. From this point onward interest in Galen will be largely scholarly and historical, although there are also philosophers and physicians, from the nineteenth to the early twentieth century, who see in him an important and admirable model, in terms of his scientific methodology, his ethics, or his broader approach to the nature of the human organism and its environment.

Philosophy and Scientific Explanation

As we have seen, philosophical training and philosophical texts were a central element of Galen's formation. This underlies his work in two crucial senses.[5] One is that he regards certain branches of philosophy, most notably logic and ethics, as valuable, if not essential, studies in their own right, quite independently of their medical relevance. For example, he wrote voluminously on logic and on the method of demonstration, including a large number of commentaries on the logical works of Aristotle and other predecessors, though this body of work is almost entirely lost. The other is that philosophy provides him with the intellectual model and language with which he seeks explanations in the scientific field. Galen has a clear view of what constitutes true scientific knowledge (*epistēmē*); this must be based on scientific demonstration (*epistēmonikē apodeixis*). The starting-points of such demonstrations must be truths evident either to reason or to sense perception; and the arguments proceeding from them must be logically rigorous. Mathematics and geometry provide the ideal model to be followed in a demonstration.[6] Of course, how well or consistently Galen lives up to—or is able to live up to—these standards in his own work is a pertinent question; a prominent case in point would be the arguments by which Galen purports to 'demonstrate' the veracity of his version of element theory. But the theoretical model of scientific method is a compelling one, and one that has attracted contemporary philosophical interest.

---

[5] For a fuller overview of the significance of philosophy in Galen see Singer 2016/2021.

[6] For Galen's account of demonstration, and of different epistemic grades of argument, see *The Doctrines of Hippocrates and Plato* II.3, pp. 242–4 below; for mathematical or geometrical proof as a model *Affections and Errors* I.8, p. 474, II.3–5, pp. 483–4 and 488–90.

It is also true, importantly, that Galen acknowledges the necessity of allowing different levels of epistemic certainty in different domains of analysis or activity: the prediction of the course of a disease, for example, or a suggested course of exercise or drug dosage, will not admit of the same degree of certainty as the proof that the source of the nerves is in the brain. In such contexts we must rather make a preliminary best estimate (*stochasmos*), which will be subject to adjustment or revision in the light of further evidence or experience.

The relationship between theory (*logos*) and the results of observation or experience (*peira*) is, indeed, another major philosophical theme that underlies Galen's medical methodology. Here he is responding to a rivalry which existed between contemporary medical sects, as laid out in detail in *Sects for Beginners*. On the one hand there are the Dogmatists or Rationalists (essentially, anyone with an underlying theory of what causes diseases and of the internal workings of the body), on the other the Empirics (*empeirikoi*), who refrain from theoretical pronouncements and work only on the basis of experience, or 'what has worked in the past'. Galen here steers a middle course. Relying on experience is infinitely preferable to ignoring its results, and will in many cases get you to the right answer without any need for theoretical speculation; and it is certainly better than working with a theory of how the body works which is simply wrong—as do, for example, his perennial *bêtes noires*, the Methodists, who have a hopelessly reductive and mistaken model of disease causation, as well as of treatment.[7] But there are cases where failure to make a valid deduction or inference, based on experience but also on anatomical or physiological knowledge, about the disease causation—e.g. where a disease has its original cause in a different part of the body from that where the symptoms are manifest—will lead you astray.

We then have a further analysis of disease aetiology, whereby it is broken down into antecedent (*prokatarktikos*) and preceding (*proēgoumenos*) causes. The latter correspond to the internal factors or bodily dispositions which explain why the former, external (e.g. environmental) influences do not have the same effects on all individuals.

There is also another mode of causal analysis, of great importance to Galen's overall world view, but of more relevance to theoretical study or analysis than to the practice of medicine. For Galen, a scientific description of any part of the human body, or indeed of any organism in the natural world, must centrally include an account of that part's purposive relationship to its function. The only sensible explanation, in his view, for the structures observed in anatomy is that they have been designed precisely and specifically for the purpose for which they are intended; indeed, anatomy can be regarded as a kind of religious practice—the true 'mystery religion', devoid of the obfuscation and ritual that exists in actual

---

[7] On his interactions with and view of this group see *Prognosis* and *Sects for Beginners*.

religions. In this context his constant target is that group of thinkers—the Atomists and the followers of Asclepiades—who believe that the random motions of particles could have given rise to the complex and perfectly functioning organisms that we observe, as well as to those, like Erasistratus, who favour a mechanistic over a teleological account of the operations of the organs of the body.

Here, while he is agnostic about the details, the higher-level metaphysics or theology, his belief in the fundamental notion that the biological world, and the human organism in particular, is governed by intelligence, is absolute. He expounds these views eloquently, and aims to substantiate them by reference to the actual internal structures seen in anatomy, throughout his magnum opus *The Function of the Parts of the Human Body*.

At the same time, there is a strongly materialist or physicalist aspect to his scientific explanations, seen most vividly in *The Soul's Dependence on the Body*; here the focus is on a 'bottom-up' explanation of not only bodily but also mental or 'soul' phenomena: all can be understood, causally, in terms of the particular mixture (*krasis*) of the elements (earth, air, fire, water) or qualities (hot, cold, wet, dry) in the body or organ in question; this corresponds to Galen's general model of analysis of the composition of bodies in the universe quite generally. Whether the apparent tension between the teleological and the 'bottom-up' model of explanation is resolved has been a matter of debate; at any rate Galen himself seems to perceive some tension between the two.[8]

Ethics and the Soul

We mentioned above that there are certain branches of philosophy that Galen regards as valuable in their own right, and to be pursued independently of any interest in medicine. One of these—in a sense the most important, as it affects one's everyday life and one's possibility of happiness—is that of ethics. Galen wrote a considerable number of short treatises in this area, participating in a discourse which was prominent in Roman imperial times, that of practical ethics, sometimes also defined as 'the therapy of the soul'.[9] Ethical or emotional wellbeing, which is understood as in many ways parallel to, but nevertheless distinct from, bodily wellbeing, essentially consists in the health or correct state of the soul or psyche (*psuchē*). It should be understood here that, while the conventional translation 'soul' has been preserved, the Greek word in itself has no 'spiritual' or other-worldly connotations. At the most fundamental level, to

---

[8] As suggested, for example by a couple of passages in *Mixtures*; see I.8, pp. 208–9 and II.6, p. 215 below.

[9] The two surviving ones, *Freedom from Distress* and *Affections and Errors of the Soul*, are translated in this volume; passages of the longer *The Doctrines of Hippocrates and Plato* are relevant to this discourse too.

say that we have a *psuchē* is simply to say that we carry out the functions of perception, voluntary motion, cognition and so on. (In a broader sense, even plants can be said to have a soul, which is just to say that they have an internal principle of self-maintenance which, for example, 'knows' what nutrition to take from the soil; in a narrower sense, meanwhile, *psuchē* can also be used to refer more specifically to the domains that we would call the mental and emotional.)

In this discourse, Galen again presents himself as fundamentally Platonic in his analysis: crucial to a correct approach to the problem of living well—of eliminating error and troublesome emotional disturbance ('affection' or passion, *pathos*) is to understand the fundamental distinction between the rational and non-rational parts of the soul; and, within the latter, the further important distinction between the 'spirited' or irascible (*thumoeides*) and desiderative or appetitive (*epithumētikon*), which correspond respectively to the competitive urge and to the drive to fulfil the appetites for food and sex. Alongside this theoretical analysis, Galen offers a range of types of practical advice, most drawn from the existing 'practical ethics' discourse—such as gradual habituation, daily self-assessment, the enlisting of external advice—to improve one's ethical or emotional state.

Galen's Medical Model and Curriculum

A striking feature of Galen's work is that he aimed to classify and organize his own writings thematically into a kind of medical curriculum or correct order. (There is an apparent irony or paradox in this ambition, since he also frequently makes the claim that he initially intended none of his works for an audience beyond intimate friends, students and associates, and only reluctantly agreed to prepare his works for such dissemination.) This order, laid out in *My Own Books* and in *The Order of My Own Books*, can be understood both in paedagogic terms—certain specific treatises follow on from others in the course of study—and also in conceptual or logical terms—there is a thematic dependence of one body of knowledge upon the other. The following is a brief summary, roughly following the order Galen lays out in those books, of the main areas of medical knowledge within this system.

Anatomy and Physiology

Anatomy is fundamental for Galen and underlies much of his work. His commitment to anatomy is crucial to his enterprise, and his achievements in it, drawing on those of predecessors, are impressive. He was limited in Rome to the dissection of animal specimens, amongst which he most frequently used Barbary apes, although it seems that the inspection of human specimens, at least skeletons, was still possible in Alexandria. This limitation which led to some important misconceptions, for example his focus on the 'retiform plexus', to which indeed he ascribes considerable physiological importance (see *The Doctrines of Hippocrates and Plato*, n. 58); he also famously hypothesized the existence of certain structures not visible to the naked eye. But the commitment to direct anatomical observation is central and pervasive in his work; and he wrote extensively about both the practical techniques of dissection and the detailed findings of anatomy, giving detailed and accurate descriptions of many structures in the body.[10] (The present volume is able to give only a glimpse of this aspect of Galen's work, which however is covered extensively in existing translations and publications.) The findings of anatomy are vital for Galen from two points of view. The first, which we have noted, is the more theoretical or abstract one: a knowledge of anatomy gives you some sense of the intelligence which informs the universe, and is an antidote against the nonsensical explanations of physical and biological processes offered by Atomists or mechanists. The second is more practical. Here what is crucial is that the study of anatomy is intimately linked to that of physiology or function (*chreia*). Galen classifies a whole series of his treatises—essentially those on physiology—as having as their subject 'the activities and functions of the parts made apparent in anatomy',[11] and to learn about these activities and functions is precisely the practical point of the discipline. This, then, will have important benefits for disease diagnosis: an understanding of the internal functioning of the parts of the body will help us understand also what their malfunctioning may entail, and is thus of major clinical relevance.

Central to that physiology (as laid out especially in *The Doctrines of Hippocrates and Plato*) is the model of the three central organs, brain, heart and liver, each with its corresponding system—the nerves, the arteries and the veins respectively. The brain is responsible for cognition and also (through the nerves) for perception and voluntary motion; the heart and the arteries for the maintenance of vital function; the liver and the veins for the nutrition of the body. The function of the liver and the veins is thus further connected to that of the stomach in the digestive process, which is understood in terms of 'coction' or cooking (*pepsis*) of the foodstuffs taken in, in such a way that they are turned into blood, or to an appropriate mixture of blood and the other 'fluids' (or humours, *chumoi*), from which the various tissues of the body are made. The heart and arteries, meanwhile, have a crucial interaction with the

---

[10] See *My Own Books*, ch. 4, pp. 25–9 below; and the extracts from *Anatomical Procedures* in this volume.

[11] *My Own Books*, ch. 5, p. 29 below.

lungs, from which they receive 'breath' (*pneuma*); the 'vital breath' (*pneuma zōtikon*) which moves through the arteries, along with the blood, somehow assists in regulation of the body's vital function, while a part of it is also transformed into the 'soul breath' (*pneuma psuchikon*) which exists in the ventricles of the brain and moves through the nerves, or at least as far as the parts of these nearest to the brain, transmitting the impulses responsible for sensation and muscular motion.

The Composition of the Human Body; Health and Disease

In accordance with the model of element or quality theory, the human body itself, and each of its individual parts, are constituted by some mixture of the hot, the cold, the wet and the dry (the scheme is laid out both in *The Elements according to Hippocrates* and in *Mixtures*). Meanwhile the digestive process, which replenishes the body and ideally maintains it as it is, may give rise to excesses or imbalances in one direction or another, depending on the precise nature of the foodstuffs taken. Such imbalances may also be brought about by such external factors as the quality of the air, the ambient temperature, physical exercise and emotional disturbances of various kinds, which also affect the bodily mixture.[12] In more detail, such imbalances in the body, especially those arising from foodstuffs, are understood in terms of the fluids (or humours, *chumoi*), which, in addition to blood, are phlegm, yellow bile and black bile. These last three are essentially residues or by-products of digestion, the excesses of which must be eliminated. In states of health one attempts to keep the body as close as possible to the state of heat, cold, etc., that it currently enjoys, by an appropriate diet and lifestyle; equally, small adjustments can also be made through changes to diet and exercise.

Greater departures from the normal state will ultimately lead to states which are defined in terms of actual disease. Thus, excessive cold and moisture, which are also associated with excessive phlegm, tends to lead to one particular kind of fever (the 'quotidian', which is also associated with winter), while excessive heat and dryness, associated with yellow bile, may lead to the 'tertian' fever; and so on. One sees that there is an interplay of environmental factors with fundamental qualities and fluids and also that there is a continuum between states of good balance, through states of suboptimal balance, to states of bad balance, which will ultimately lead to the presence of a definable disease entity.

---

[12] See *Health* I.2–3, pp. 320–2 below for the basic theoretical model; more broadly, the work gives the detail on such lifestyle and diet prescriptions for different bodily conditions; specifically on the effect of emotional or 'soul' factors on bodily health, see *Health* I.8, p. 323 below.

Diagnosis, Prognosis and Therapy

When, then, we move from the domain of approximate balance or imbalance of the qualities to actual disease, we require a robust diagnostic and therapeutic model to deal with this. For purposes of diagnosis (and of prognosis, which in the ancient world went hand in hand with and indeed had more salience than diagnosis), the physician must train himself to recognize a range of signs or symptoms, including bodily complexion, the nature of the substances excreted and, very prominently, the pulse. As well as writing an important commentary on the *Prognostic* of 'Hippocrates', Galen wrote voluminously on the pulse, which in his theoretical model admits of a bewildering range of variables, all of which the aspiring doctor should learn to distinguish.[13] It will also be relevant in many cases to enquire into the patient's recent habits and lifestyle.

Fever (*puretos*) has a particular prominence in the ancient medical discourse (historically, in terms of retrospective diagnosis, much of what is classified under this heading has been analysed as malaria). And again the ancient discourse, Galen's in particular, recognizes a remarkable range of variables—especially when one admits the possibility that a patient may be suffering from more than one of these periodically recurrent fevers simultaneously.[14] There is—as with the variables in the pulse—a systematicity and neatness here that again takes us far from modern perceptions. Fevers are typically analysed in terms of a four-phase progress: inception, growth, maturity and decline, and divided into the broad categories of quotidian (recurring every day), tertian (recurring every other day), quartan (recurring every three days) and hectic (more or less constant). This is bound up with the well-known notion of the 'crisis' (*krisis*): recurrent fevers reach a peak or paroxysm (*paroxusmos*) in a regular and predictable way, and this is a key or 'critical' moment in terms of the course of the disease in one direction or another, and also in terms of treatment (typically one avoids giving food until after this moment has passed).

Severely aberrant states of mixture, or diseases, may require treatment by stronger methods, beyond diet, exercise and lifestyle. These stronger methods usually consist either in the administering of drug preparations, on the one hand, or in venesection, on the other. Both are employed to remove imbalances of fluids: specific drugs have the capacity to draw to themselves and thus

---

[13] See in this volume *The Pulse for Beginners*; and note also the relevance of the pulse for diagnosis and prognosis in *Prognosis*. The range of variables which Galen discusses in the longer treatises seem completely fantastic from a contemporary perspective; on the other hand, the parallel has been made with traditional Chinese medicine, which recognizes and practically employs many variables not known to modern western medicine. Scepticism may be somewhat allayed by considering how much more may be discernible by human touch in an age which has not come to be wholly reliant on mechanical or electronic instruments.

[14] See *Prognosis*, ch. 3, pp. 51–2 below: the patient is described as suffering from three quartan fevers.

remove specific fluids, while venesection by removing blood simultaneously removes any fluid present in excess, because such fluids were understood to be contained in the venous blood in particular.

Among the other important specific disease states—again understood ultimately in terms of qualitative imbalance, but with further ramifications depending on the precise place in the body and the course of the disease—are phrenitis, melancholy and hysteria.[15]

There are also, of course, particular conditions for which surgery is required, and Galen describes a number of such manual interventions, including the couching of cataracts, the treatment of fractures and the reduction of intestines following a deep wound that has led to their prolapse, and the subsequent suturing of the stomach. In each case he gives considerable detail, though it is unclear and perhaps doubtful that he would have carried out such procedures himself, probably rather supervising the procedure but relying for the manual operation on one of the artisan surgical specialists that existed in the Graeco-Roman world.

Pharmacology

Galen wrote three very voluminous treatises of pharmacology, as well as some shorter ones, both addressing theoretical questions of the nature and variety of forms of efficacy of drugs and listing in detail both individual 'simples' (that is, individual plant, mineral or animal substances used in treatments) and 'compounds' (that is, recipes). By his own account he also possessed a substantial personal collection of both *materia medica* and recipes; and it seems that he expended considerable energy, throughout his life, in the gathering of both recipes and substances, from all over the known world.[16] In the course of his pharmacological writings he also gives us striking and informative insights into the range of recent contemporary practices in this area, detailing, alongside the work of practitioners whom he respects and draws upon, the magically or astrologically based treatises of some, and the use of disgusting or illegal bodily substances, as well as of poisons, by others—all of which he rejects.

We have seen above how the use of such drugs (*pharmaka*) fits into the overall picture of Galenic medicine: one has recourse to drugs to correct the balance

---

[15] The diagnostic model as given in *Affected Places* strongly emphasizes the importance of taking account of the internal structures and processes in the body in a disease aetiology. The specific diseases mentioned here are also discussed at length in that work.

[16] For his discussion of the theoretical issues, and a taste of his list of simples, see the extracts from *Simple Drugs* in this volume. For his account of his own collections (and their loss) see *Freedom from Distress*. Elsewhere Galen recounts his personal efforts to procure substances in places as far flung as Syria Palaestina (possibly in the area of the Dead Sea) and Lemnos; and he mentions a wide variety of other provenances throughout his works on drugs.

of the body when the milder method of treatment through diet and lifestyle is not sufficient; and some of these drugs, the 'purgative' or 'cleansing' drugs, act through a *specific* capacity that they have to draw off one of the fluids—yellow bile, black bile or phlegm.

The case of such specific drug capacities is for Galen an interesting one, occasioning one of his distinctively open-ended analyses, or admissions of ignorance. In accordance with the overall reductionist model of the hot, the cold, the wet and the dry, of which all physical things are some mixture, drugs too—or most drugs—can be analysed in terms of their relevant capacities: they either heat, cool, moisten or dry (or some combination of these), and these effects can in some sense be quantified: a particular drug may have two degrees of heating and one of drying, for example (on a scale of one to four). When, however, one comes to more complex of *specific* capacities—for example that of purging a particular fluid from the body, but also the capacities of many poisons—that simple analysis seems inadequate. Here, Galen sees the need for a different model, and speaks in terms of the drug acting *in virtue of its whole substance*. We might from a contemporary perspective translate this into talk of emergent properties—the drug, though composed like everything else of some mixture of the fundamental qualities—has some property which cannot be analysed in terms of those components. And it is notable, here, that similar language is indeed used in the context of the soul: some texts suggest that here, too, what is in play is a 'specificity of the whole substance', that is an emergent property which cannot be analysed, or at least not readily understood, in terms of bodily mixture.[17]

Another way of looking at this is to say that Galen is at this point abandoning explanation; in some of his texts the statement that a drug acts 'through its whole substance' seems equivalent to the statement that its action was unpredictable and inexplicable.[18] This approach perhaps dovetails with the perception already made about the focus on drugs and drug recipes in Galen's later life; it seems that both the later books of *Simple Drugs* and much of the *Compound Drugs* belong to this later phase, and that in it Galen is more concerned with assembling and cataloguing information on the effects of various substances and recipes than he is in trying to make those effects fit his neat explanatory scheme.

Galen in the Literary and Intellectual Culture of His Time

Much has been written in recent years about Galen's rhetorical and literary qualities and profile, his role within the socio-intellectual culture sometimes

---

[17] See *My Own Doctrines*, ch. 14, pp. 108–9 below.
[18] See *Simple Drugs* V.1, p. 416, VI.1.1, pp. 420–1, XI.24, pp. 426–7, and for analysis Singer 2020.

referred to as the 'Second Sophistic'.[19] Galen enjoyed the highest-level kind of elite education available in the Graeco-Roman world, which started with Greek language and grammar (alongside in his case mathematics) and proceeded to imbue the pupil with a comprehensive knowledge of Greek literary classics, as well as literary analysis and rhetorical technique.

And he exemplifies that culture to an extraordinary degree, not only showing off his knowledge of the vast array of Greek classics from which he quotes, from Homer and Hesiod, through the lyric poets and Euripides to the comedians, and including the prose writers Xenophon and Thucydides, and more recent writers such as Plutarch—all this, of course, alongside the philosophical classics, Plato, Aristotle and the early Stoics, and the various previous medical authors with whom he is conversant—but even writing specific works on rhetorical, linguistic, literary and lexical matters.[20]

But the other central aspect of the 'Second Sophistic' is, as its name suggests, the use of this literary knowledge and the argumentative techniques learnt for rhetorical ends. This was a culture in which careers could be made in oratory, and success in a variety of elite contexts depended crucially on how one performed in public debate, argument and speech-making. We have already seen how Galen's early career in Rome was built partly on his success in such public contexts, both lecturing or debating and performing anatomical demonstrations; and his skill in such rhetorical or argumentative techniques—in arguing on the basis of texts, and formulating polemical arguments against specific opponents or in support of a set thesis—is well exemplified by some of the texts in this volume, most notably *The Doctrines of Hippocrates of Plato* and *The Soul's Dependence on the Body*.

Some scholars tend to resist any analysis in literary or rhetorical terms, as undermining the seriousness of Galen's views or arguments in either philosophy or medicine. But such analysis surely highlights a very prominent feature of Galen's writing, and tells us a great deal about the way in which he operated within his society. Moreover, to say that an author expresses himself rhetorically, gears his argument in a particular way for particular purposes, or indulges in spectacular (sometimes, from a modern perspective, absurd) attempts to assemble the most diverse authorities in support of his view is not in any way to deny the seriousness with which that author holds the view in question. Nor is it to deny the seriousness and credibility of the underlying argumentative strategy thus deployed—although it may tend to cast doubt on the extent to which all the arguments deployed can be taken as *equally* credible or intellectually convincing. Crucial to note here is that Galen himself acknowledges the

[19] See especially Mattern 2008; Gill, Whitmarsh and Wilkins 2009; Salas 2020.
[20] See *My Own Books*, ch. 20, p. 40 below. Unfortunately none of these works survives.

existence of different kinds of arguments of different epistemic status, and does not claim to be operating always at the highest level, that of scientific demonstration. Indeed, there are occasions where he openly states that a particular argument was produced in a competitive spirit or to defeat such-and-such an opponent.[21]

It is true that the use of more rhetorical modes of argument, whereby much more time and effort is expended on the destruction of an opponent than on the positive advancing of one's own view, may lead to some unclarity in detail about what that positive view is; this is indeed sometimes undoubtedly the case with Galen, and gives rise to interpretive problems. To give just a few examples: it is quite difficult to know *with precision* what he takes to be the physiological role of psychic breath (*pneuma zōtikon*); he seems to be unclear, or to waver, as to *precisely* what is happening, at the lowest level, in the mixture that gives rise to basic substances; and his ultimate view on the nature or definition of the soul is avowedly uncertain. He argues in *The Soul's Dependence on the Body* both for the position that the soul is dependent on bodily mixture and for the position that the soul is best understood as *being* a bodily mixture; and the relationship between the position of that text and his view of the soul–body relationship in other texts is not clear, or at least not explicitly clarified. All this in spite of the fact that he is very clear, in each case, about the errors his intellectual opponents make by not adopting his own views.

It should be understood that medicine was a highly competitive business in the ancient world, and that success in argument or debate—including sometimes debate at the patient's bedside!—constituted one pathway towards success in it. In the absence of established institutions that awarded degrees or confirmed who was fit to practise, and in a culture where public debate and rhetorical skill were highly valued, were indeed closely enmeshed in many aspects of professional life, the ability to deploy such skills to bring about a positive reception of one's work by an audience was a crucial part of one's armoury; and Galen deploys them to great effect, as it were combining the expertise of a 'Second Sophistic' operator with those of a practising physician and medical— and philosophical—theorist. In keeping with this activity, Galen's aims are, as indeed he frequently points out, largely practical, and while there are crucially important theoretical points at issue between him and his opponents, there are others—those 'not necessary either for the curing of disease... or for the purposes of ethical, practical... philosophy'—where a degree of vagueness or uncertainty may be allowed. Galen indeed presents his own distinctive account of the different possible degrees of epistemic certainty that belong to different

---

[21] See e.g. the reference to a book composed 'in the context of the rivalry of a particular moment' in *My Own Books*, ch. 1, p. 21 below.

areas of enquiry, in what is sometimes called his 'philosophical testament', *My Own Doctrines*.[22]

A final aspect of Galen's literary activity should be mentioned, since it constitutes a very large part of his output: his work as commentator. Galen in fact wrote commentaries on a large range of both medical and philosophical works, although only those on Hippocrates have survived in anything other than fragmentary form. And, just as we suggested, in the context of the 'Second Sophistic', that Galen should be seen as putting his rhetorical skills and training to the service of his activity as a practising physician, so too here: Galen is not *just* drawing on an Alexandrian training in philology and textual analysis, engaging in those activities in the same way as any other Alexandria-trained scholar; rather he is putting those activities, in a unique way, to the service of his specific scientific project.

Quite *how* unique were his activity and approach in this area, is a difficult question to answer. Philological work on Hippocratic, as on other ancient, texts, work undertaken from the perspective of a purely antiquarian or scholarly interest in the author, had, it seemed, gone on at Alexandria for generations. That is, one could work on the text of Hippocrates—and consider among other things questions of authenticity of attribution—as one might on any other text, without any investment in the view that this was a uniquely important medical author, let alone one relevant to the contemporary medical discourse; and it seems scholars had done just that. The perception of Hippocrates as an authority figure—as one who had come closer to the truth in medical matters than any, or at least than most, who had followed him, if only one could get past the obscurity and the brevity of expression to uncover what he was truly saying—seems to have been a much more recent one. Until at least late Hellenistic times he would appear in a list of ancient medical authors and their theories as just one author amongst many: such is the case in the text known as the *Anonymus Londinensis*.

And, though that newer perception of Hippocrates was certainly not confined to Galen—it is clear that in his time some people fought over Hippocratic authority as in different times and places people would over biblical authority—it is also true that it was far from universally shared. Martianus the Erasistratean, and the Methodists in general, are just two examples of those opponents of Galen who reject Hippocratic authority altogether, rather than try to enlist it on their side; and to them one can add, presumably, the countless artisan physicians for whom any text-based study was simply irrelevant to their practice. Against this, it seems that a number of Empiric doctors claimed Hippocrates as theirs.

---

[22] *My Own Doctrines*, chs. 14–15, pp. 108–11 below.

Here we are hampered by our lack of evidence for Galen's contemporaries or immediate predecessors in Hippocratic commentary: Galen is operating in the context of a specific intellectual community, but we unfortunately know very little about that community. Most of what we know of them comes from his own brief remarks in the context of his approval or (more often) rejection of their interpretations. Nor is Galen's own activity easy to summarize or pin down. His approach, as already mentioned, has been characterized as 'creating Hippocrates in his own image'; but in fact his methodology is more complex and nuanced than that. On the one hand, he makes a distinction between the practice of simply explaining or clarifying the work of an author and that of arguing for its correctness, and claims that he himself uses the criteria of historical plausibility (e.g. of a particular lexical item or verbal form) to establish authenticity of a text, rather than his own agreement or disagreement. On the other, it seems undeniable that the choices he has made in deciding which texts to regard as canonical is at a fundamental level connected with his assumption that Hippocrates is generally correct (and therefore in agreement with his own views).

The end product of this engagement, at any rate, is a body of texts which constitute a remarkable case study in ancient techniques of scholarly argument and textual analysis; and at the same time a body of texts in which he develops or elaborates his own views on a range of medical and even philosophical matters, sometimes in ways that are unique within his corpus.[23]

Whatever the truth about Galen's lost contemporaries, Galen's own work, here too, is in a sense a synthesis. And, as with the extraordinary project, in *The Doctrines of Hippocrates and Plato*, of reconciling a range of disparate authorities and using them as the basis from which to argue for his own distinctive scientific position, so here too, we are tempted to think, we are looking at an intellectual enterprise which is unique within the ancient world. Both enterprises, of course, might possibly seem less unique if we possessed more of the work of Galen's contemporaries or immediate predecessors—the note of scholarly caution should always be sounded—but in any case both *are* remarkable scholarly and scientific enterprises, and ones which arise from the peculiar literary and intellectual culture of Galen's time.

---

[23] For example, in one passage in his commentary on book VI of the *Epidemics* he presents a formulation on the nature of the substance of the soul which is subtly different from that found anywhere else; and in another, extended, passage from the same work he takes a brief mention of the patient's 'opinion' (*gnōmē*) in the Hippocratic text as a springboard from which to launch into a range of case histories of persons whose anxiety or other mental fixation caused severe physical consequences.

Summary

Galen has been a controversial figure in modern times, largely despised, when not simply ignored, in intellectual history and the history of medicine; often still blamed, on the grounds of his outdated medical theories, his 'dogmatism', or certain errors in his anatomical observations, for having 'held up the course of scientific progress'. Perhaps at last such anachronistic and unhistorical perceptions can be put to one side, and Galen can be assessed for his achievements and his work as understood within their own historical context, and for his distinctive intellectual aims: an attempt—however flawed and imperfectly executed—to build medical knowledge on the twin pillars of reason and empirical observation, alongside a hugely ambitious project of collecting, synthesizing and analysing the existing knowledge of his time, in areas as diverse as logic, causal analysis, psychology, ethics, anatomy, diet and pharmacology.

In the context of that project, he brought forward a range of arguments on the nature of science and the relationship of theory and observation, and on the nature and limits of scientific knowledge, that are still worthy of our attention; he encouraged and stimulated the practice of empirical research and in particular the practice of dissection and the teaching of anatomy; and he made contributions to practical ethics, and observations on the relationship of emotional or mental states to bodily health, and on our understanding of the relationship of mind and body, which are, at the very least, distinctive and arresting. Alongside that, he presents us, through the sheer variety of his work and his writing in a range of contexts, with perhaps the richest insight into ancient everyday life, and into Graeco-Roman intellectual culture, of any author whose work has survived to us. And he remains, of course, a figure of enormous historical importance, in an extraordinarily wide range of historical and geographical contexts. For all these reasons his work deserves the attention, not just of classical scholars and historians of medicine and science, but of anyone interested in the ancient world, or in cross-cultural conceptions of health, disease, mind, body and human nature.

Further Reading

For Galen's actual texts see the Note on Texts, Editions and Online Resources.

The following is a guide to the most important recent monographs and collections of essays on Galen, arranged thematically. Full references for the works here mentioned appear in the Bibliography.

Collections of essays, general

Haase and Temporini 1994; Hankinson 2008; Gill, Whitmarsh and Wilkins 2009; Singer and Rosen 2024.

Collections of essays on philosophical themes

Barnes, Jouanna and Barras 2003; Adamson, Hansberger and Wilberding 2014; Hankinson and Havrda 2022.

Biography, clinical work and socio-intellectual context

Barton 1994; Mattern 2008; Boudon-Millot 2012; Mattern 2013; Nutton 2020.

Anatomy and physiology

Singer 1956; May 1968; Debru 1996; Rocca 2003; Salas 2020.

Philosophy and psychology

Tieleman 1996; Gill 2010; Singer 2013; Singer 2016/2021; Devinant 2020; Vinkestejn 2022.

Legacy and reception

Bouras-Vallianatos and Zipser 2019; Das 2020.

Chronology

120s[1]   Major redevelopment and renovation of the city of Pergamum, an intellectual hub within Roman Asia as well as the seat of the healing sanctuary of Asclepius (Asclepieion), under the emperor Hadrian. Galen's father (possibly Aelius Nicon) is an architect and prominent member of the city's elite.

129   Galen (*Galēnos*)[2] is born at Pergamum (August/September). From an early age he is given training in mathematics and geometry by his father.

143   He begins to attend the lectures of philosophers at Pergamum, including representatives of each of the major philosophical schools: Stoic, Platonist, Aristotelian and Epicurean.

145–8   Galen pursues the study of medicine in conjunction with that of philosophy. His first teachers are Satyrus and Pelops, both belonging to the school of the earlier anatomist Quintus. To this period belong his first writings, including *The Dissection of the Womb* and *Medical Experience*.

148   Death of Galen's father. Galen travels to Smyrna, following his teacher Pelops, and here studies also with the Platonist Albinus. At Smyrna he writes some anatomical works based on the teaching of Pelops.

148–57   Formative period of travel and study. Galen moves from Smyrna to Corinth (*c.* 151), then to Alexandria (*c.* 153), in search of the best anatomical teachers and texts. The longest period is spent in Alexandria, the main centre for both the study of anatomy and the scholarly discipline of Hippocratic commentary.

157   Galen returns to Pergamum, where he is given a public appointment as physician to the gladiators—an appointment which is renewed several times over the next four years.

162–6   First stay in Rome. Galen participates in public debates and in anatomical—including vivisectional—demonstrations on animals, and develops his profile as a physician through a number of spectacularly successful diagnoses and cures of elite Roman citizens, amongst them members of the imperial family. He provokes the animosity of other elite doctors, and develops an especially

---

[1] It should be noted that the events of Galen's life are mainly attested only by Galen's own writings, with little or no independent confirmation; also that it is often impossible to assign clear dates to his works, which were revised at different times throughout his life. The dates given represent best guesses, and in many cases correspond to the date of final writing-up of a work previously given in oral or draft form.

[2] On Galen's name, and in particular whether he also bore a family name or *nomen gentilicium* (either the traditionally ascribed Claudius or Aelius), which would imply his possession of Roman citizenship, see Nutton 2015.

strong rivalry with the prominent Methodist school of practitioners. He writes the first six books of *The Doctrines of Hippocrates and Plato* and the first book of *The Function of the Parts of the Human Body*, both ostensibly for Flavius Boethus, a distinguished senator and amateur of philosophy and medicine; also *Sects for Beginners*, *The Pulse for Beginners*, and a number of other works, especially of anatomy.

166   Outbreak of plague at Rome, due to infection brought to Rome by troops returning from campaign in Parthia. Galen returns to Pergamum, either to escape the plague or for other personal reasons.

168/9   Galen is summoned back to Italy, to serve under the emperors Marcus Aurelius and Lucius Verus on their military campaign in Germany. Both in the course of this journey from Asia to Rome and subsequently, Galen undertakes travel to source rare items of *materia medica*. On arrival in Italy he succeeds in persuading Marcus to release him from duty with the army; he goes to Rome for the second time, where he is attached to the imperial household.

169–76   Galen 'collects together and brings into permanent form' the results of his medical studies, research and experience thus far; to this period belong many of his major works, including *The Elements according to Hippocrates*; *Mixtures*; *Natural Capacities*; *Semen*; *The Function of Breathing*; the remaining books of *The Function of the Parts of the Human Body* (II–XVII) and of *The Doctrines of Hippocrates and Plato* (VII–IX); the four major treatises on the pulse; the first part of his major pharmacological work, *Simple Drugs* (books I–VIII) and of the clinical magnum opus *The Therapeutic Method* (books I–VI); the shorter *The Therapeutic Method to Glaucon*; *Crises*; *Critical Days*; *Fulness*; *The Distinct Types of Fever*; a number of other works concerning the classification and diagnosis of diseases and clinical practice; and possibly the first of the Hippocratic commentaries, at least in their preliminary versions. (At this and other periods he also writes a large number of works now lost to us, especially the foundational logical treatise *Demonstration* and commentaries on a wide range of previous medical and philosophical authors.) Galen consolidates his status as chief doctor in the imperial household. According to his own account, he has now given up public debates and demonstrations, relying rather on his clinical success with patients.

176   Marcus Aurelius returns to Rome (an occasion which possibly gives rise to the composition of Galen's self-publicizing work, *Prognosis*).

176–80   Galen continues to serve the imperial household, especially the emperor Marcus Aurelius, for whom he regularly prepares the famous theriac drug; he also continues to write commentaries on Hippocratic works.

180   Death of Marcus Aurelius; accession of Commodus.

180–92   Reign of Commodus, notorious as a reign of terror. Galen perhaps retreats from court life, spending more time in Campania, where he owns a property. To this period probably belong a number of further Hippocratic commentaries and *The Order of My Own Books*.

192	Fire destroys many of the buildings in the area of the Roman Forum, including libraries and Galen's own storeroom, containing valuable medical instruments, items of *materia medica* and manuscripts, both of Galen's own works and of others'; the losses are recorded in *Freedom from Distress*, probably composed shortly afterwards. Death of the emperor Commodus.
193	Accession of Septimius Severus.
193–	Last phase of Galen's life. He continues to serve as imperial physician.

The precise dating of Galen's works from 176 onward is difficult. Most of the Hippocratic commentaries belong to this broad period, but are difficult to date within it. Some, such as that on the sixth book of Hippocrates' *Epidemics*, were clearly written after 193, as was the important clinical work *Affected Places*, and the philosophically reflective treatises *The Shaping of the Embryo*, *The Art of Medicine*, and *My Own Doctrines*. The completion of *The Therapeutic Method* (books VII–XIV) and of *Simple Drugs* (IX–XI) also belong to this last phase of Galen's life, as does the composition, at least in their final form, of the other main pharmacological works, *The Composition of Drugs according to Kind*, *The Composition of Drugs according to Places* and *Antidotes*, and of *My Own Books*. The major works on diet and on healthy lifestyle, *The Properties of Foodstuffs* and *Health*, probably also date to this last period, or at least to the late 180s or early 190s, although they have traditionally been dated earlier.[3] *The Soul's Dependence on the Body* has traditionally been considered one of Galen's very last works, but without any solid evidence.

c. 200 (?)[4]	Galen dies, probably at Rome.
4th–7th centuries	

Galen's writings excerpted by Greek medical authors (the 'encyclopaedists' Oribasius, Aëtius, Paul and Alexander).

5th century

First evidence for major role of Galen in medical education, at Alexandria, where the treatises are anthologized to form a sixteen-book curriculum.

5th/6th century

First substantial project of translation of Galen's works, into Syriac, by Sergius (also based at Alexandria); translation and paedagogic use of his works also in Latin, at Ravenna.

---

[3] See now Singer 2023, 68–79.

[4] In contemporary scholarship the traditional date of 199 for Galen's death has been supplanted by that of 216. The later date, derived from an isolated remark in an Arabic text which arguably relays information from a sixth-century philosopher at Alexandria, may possibly be better grounded than the former, which appears in a tenth-century Byzantine encyclopaedia; but neither can be regarded as in any way reliable.

8th/9th century

Large number of Galen's works translated into Arabic, especially by Ḥunayn ibn Isḥāq and his workshop at Baghdad. From this point onward, through further transmissions and translations, Galen will play a major role in medicine in the Islamicate world and beyond, including in southern Spain, in Mediterranean Jewish communities, in Persia and in south Asia.

9th–12th centuries

Critical engagement with Galen's philosophy and medicine by intellectuals and physicians in Islamicate world, including Abū Bakr al-Rāzī (Rhazes), al-Ghazālī, ʿAlī ibn Riḍwān, and ibn-Sinā (Avicenna), whose *Canon of Medicine* (*c.* 1012) contains much Galenic material.

11th–12th centuries

Translations of Galen's works into Latin from Arabic, by Constantine the African in Italy and Gerard of Cremona in Spain; the latter also translates Arabic compendia, in particular Avicenna's *Canon*. Creation at Salerno of the *Articella*, a collection of medical texts based largely on Constantine's translations; this, alongside the *Canon*, will play a dominant role in medical university education in Europe until the sixteenth century.

12th–14th centuries

Translation of large number of Galen's works into Latin from Greek, especially by Burgundio of Pisa and Niccolò of Reggio.

15th–16th centuries

Humanist interest in Galen's writings from both philosophical and medical perspectives; new Latin translations and use of improved texts in university teaching. Twenty-two editions of Galen's 'Opera Omnia' are printed in Latin between 1490 and 1625; the first Greek edition appears in 1525. Vesalius and other humanists use Galen's anatomical works as basis for anatomy and dissection, while also developing critical approach.

17th–19th centuries

Galen maintains strong influence in university teaching and medical practice, in Europe and beyond.

19th century

Galenic medicine finally superseded as theoretical model, though use of Galenically based lifestyle or dietary prescriptions or *materia medica* survives longer, especially through practice of 'Unani' medicine in central and southern Asia.

20th–21st centuries

Development of scholarly-historical interest in Galen, considered both as a source for the history of medicine and ancient culture and as a serious figure in the history of philosophy.

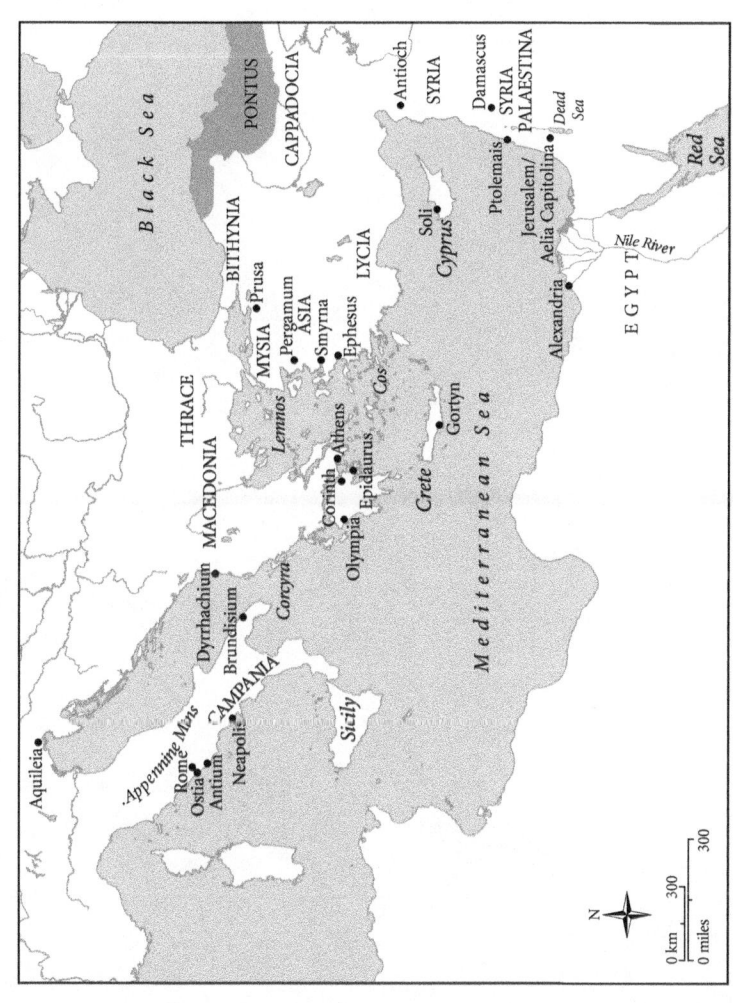

Map 1. The Mediterranean world in Galen's time. Drawn by Wendy Giminski; from S. Mattern, *The Prince of Medicine: Galen in the Roman Empire*; reproduced by permission of Oxford University Press.

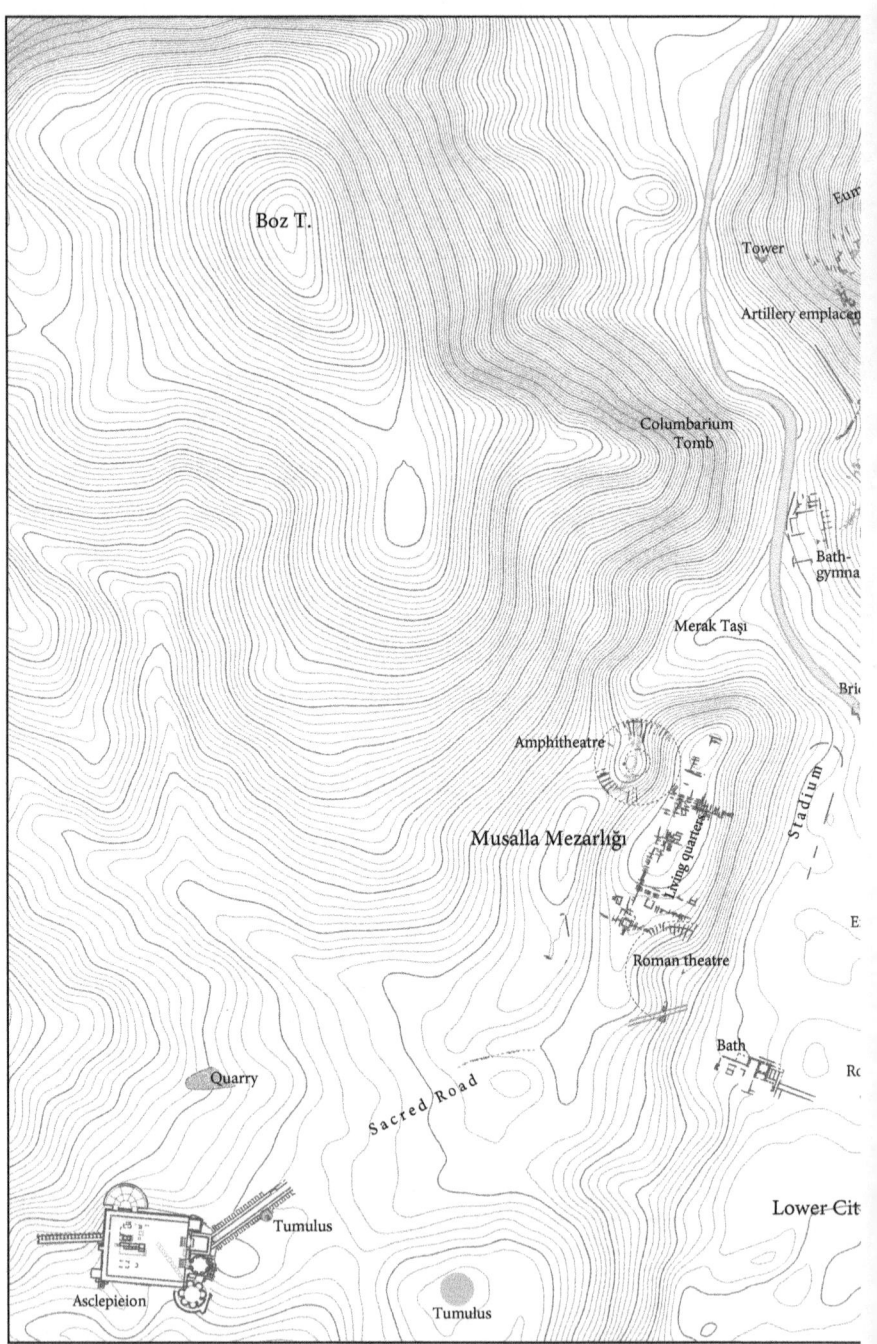

Map 2. The ancient city of Pergamum and surrounding area, including the Asclepieion. Reproduced by permission of the Deutsches Archäologisches Institut, Istanbul. Digitale Karte von Pergamon 1.1 (DAI 2020).

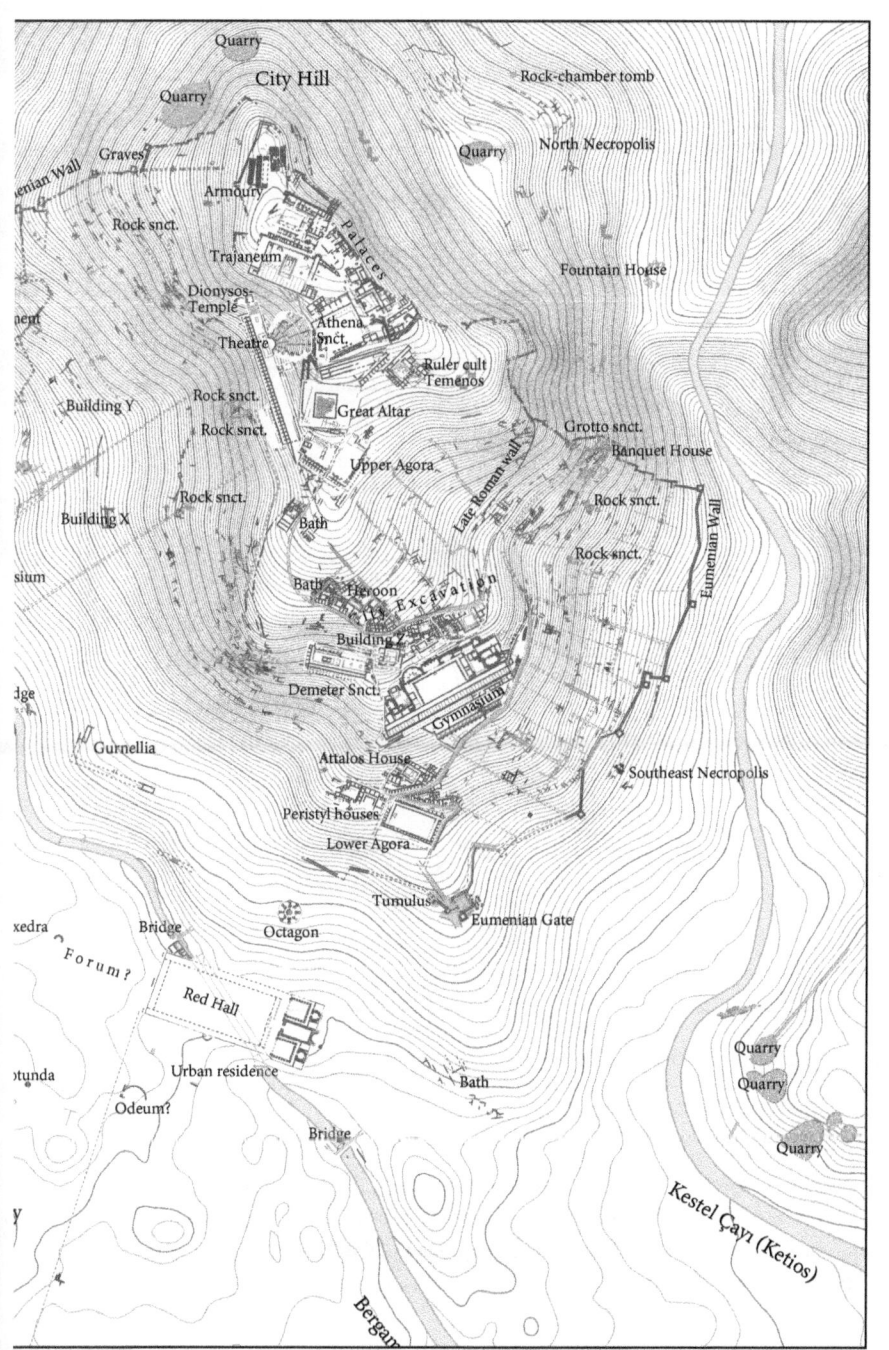

Quarry

City Hill

Quarry

Rock-chamber tomb

Quarry

North Necropolis

Graves

Armoury

Rock snct.

Trajaneum

Palaces

Fountain House

Dionysos-
Temple

Athena
Snct.

Theatre

Ruler cult
Temenos

Building Y

Rock snct.

Great Altar

Grotto snct.

Rock snct.

Upper Agora

Banquet House

Rock snct.

Building X

Rock snct.

Bath

Rock snct.

Rock snct.

Bath

Heroon

Excavation

Building Z

Gymnasium

Demeter Snct.

Gurnellia

Attalos House

Southeast Necropolis

Peristyl houses

Lower Agora

Tumulus

Bridge

Eumenian Gate

xedra

Forum?

Octagon

Red Hall

otunda

Urban residence

Bath

Odeum?

Bridge

Kestel Çayı (Ketios)

Bergama

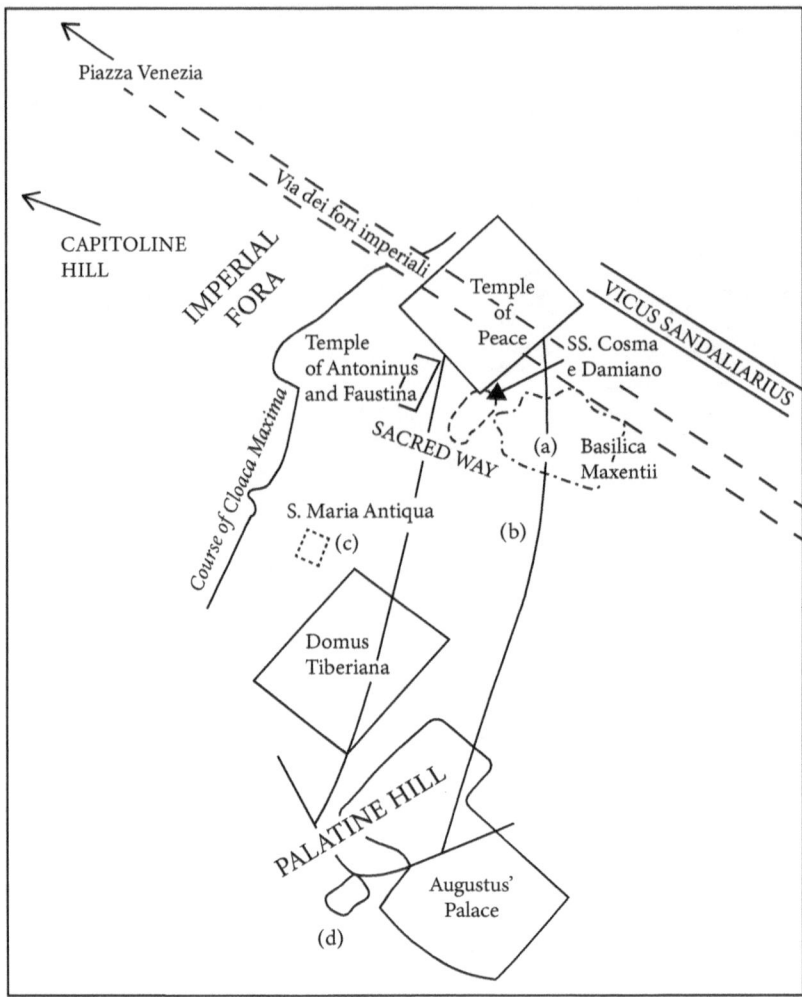

Piazza Venezia

Via dei fori imperiali

CAPITOLINE
HILL

IMPERIAL FORA

Temple
of
Peace

VICUS SANDALIARIUS

Temple
of Antoninus
and Faustina

SS. Cosma
e Damiano

Course of Cloaca Maxima

SACRED WAY

(a)   Basilica
       Maxentii

S. Maria Antiqua

(b)

☐ (c)

Domus
Tiberiana

PALATINE HILL

Augustus'
Palace

(d)

Legend
(a) Horrea Piperataria (Spice Market), possible site of Galen's storeroom
(b) Horrea Vespasiani, possible site of Galen's storeroom
(c) Possible site of library of Domus Tiberiana
(d) Double library at Temple of Apollo

Map 3. The centre of imperial Rome, showing the course of the fire of AD 192 and the locations of Galen's storeroom and Rome's libraries. From P. N. Singer (ed.), *Galen: Psychological Writings*; reproduced by permission of Cambridge University Press.

Note on Texts, Editions
and Online Resources

With a few exceptions, the Greek text of all Galen's works appears (along with Latin translation) in the edition of K. G. Kühn (1821–33), which is still used for reference purposes.

The position of each text within Kühn's edition, where this is available, has been given at the beginning of each of the following translations, and Kühn page numbers given in the margins throughout.

Where a more recent and scholarly edition of the Greek text exists, this has been mentioned at the outset, and the text of the most recent edition has in general been followed in the translation. (Full bibliographical details of editions are given in the Bibliography.) Significant departures from either Kühn or the modern edition have been mentioned in notes. For longer works abridged or excerpted here, a reference has also been given to complete English translations published elsewhere.

The volumes of Kühn's edition of Galen's works are freely available to download on the Biu Santé website: https://www.biusante.parisdescartes.fr/histoire/medica/resultats/index.php?tout=galien%20kühn&op=OU&statut=charge&fille=o&cotemere=45674.

The editions of the Corpus Medicorum Graecorum are freely available to consult on their website: https://cmg.bbaw.de/epubl/online/editionen.html.

I

LIFE, BOOKS AND MEDICAL CAREER

Freedom from Distress

This short but fascinating text was fortuitously discovered in 2005 by a young French scholar, Antoine Pietrobelli, in a manuscript that had been overlooked in a library in Thessaloniki.[1]

The work, framed as a response to a letter from an unknown friend from Galen's youth, was written in the aftermath of a great fire that consumed many of the imperial buildings in the area of the Forum at Rome, along with the depositories of a number of private individuals, including Galen, in AD 192, and of the death of the notorious emperor Commodus at the end of the same year. It opens a remarkable window into Galen's career, everyday life and personal attitudes, and into ancient medical and intellectual life more broadly. In particular, it offers unique insights into surgical and pharmacological practices, as well as into the nature of books—their production, editing and copying—and libraries in the ancient world.

The text also forms part of Galen's distinctive and original contribution to the discourse of practical ethics and the 'therapy of the soul'.

Greek title: Περὶ ἀλυπίας (*Peri alupias*)
Kühn: not present
Editions: Boudon-Millot, Jouanna and Pietrobelli 2010 (with French translation); Garofalo and Lami 2012 (with Italian translation); Polemis and Xenophontos 2023

1.[2] I have received your letter, in which you ask me to reveal to you what training, arguments or doctrines prepared me in such a way that I never become distressed. As you remark, you yourself personally witnessed my loss, during

---

[1] The manuscript, Vlatadon 14, also contains fuller versions than were previously available of three other works included in this volume: *My Own Books*, *The Order of My Own Books* and *My Own Doctrines*; but for the present text it is the only extant manuscript. The treatise has attracted a huge amount of scholarly interest since its discovery, for the historical and archaeological questions it sheds light on, for the ethical views it puts forward and their relationship with the Graeco-Roman ethical tradition, and in terms of the philological challenges it presents. The text as transmitted in the manuscript is vitiated by many errors and is in parts lacunose or difficult to read. A wide range of conjectures and emendations, as well as interpretations of particular passages, have been put forward by scholars. Alongside the editions mentioned, see especially Manetti 2012; Nutton in Singer 2013; Petit 2019 (in which Singer 2019c contains my own analysis of some of the most difficult cruces and Singer 2019d a discussion of the work's ethical standpoint). The edition of Polemis and Xenophontos appeared after the present translation was completed and could not be systematically taken into account; but it seems that their interpretations do not differ in many points from those represented in the version given here.

[2] Unlike the other works in this volume, this text has no chapter numbers, these being an innovation of early modern editors, and not part of Galen's original writing. Both the section numbers and the page numbers given here are those of the French edition, which have been adopted for convenience of reference.

one fierce outbreak of the long-running plague,[3] of a number of household staff, amounting to almost all those that I had at Rome. You had heard, too, that I had three or four times previously suffered something similar, in terms of very large financial losses. 2. You say that you observed that I was not moved even for a moment by those losses; but that what happened to me this time, whereby all the goods that I had in storage in the depositories by the Sacred Way were destroyed in the Great Fire, went far beyond all that. 3. You understood the extent and value of items in question; and yet you heard from ⏐ an eye-witness that I was in no way grieved, but maintained my serenity and went about my usual activities as before. 4. What amazed you particularly was not so much that I was seen to bear without distress the loss, in that fire, of silver, gold, silver plate, and many financial papers that had been deposited there, but also that of a great number of works that I had composed here, along with a very large collection of drugs, both simple and composite, and a wide range of instruments. 5. Some of these were medical instruments of a more usual kind, which, as I said before, I could hope to replace; but there were also some of my own invention, where the model had been shaped in wax by my own hand and then given to a bronze-smith to replicate, and these cannot be replaced without a great investment of time and effort.

6. The same applies to those books—both works of the classical authors and my own compositions—which I had corrected by hand; and also to those substances known as antidotes, ⏐ of which, as you say, you are aware that I had a very large stock. That of theriac,[4] in particular, extended to eighty pounds by weight; and the quantity of cinnamon was greater than what you would find in the warehouses of all the traders put together; and I had plentiful stocks of other rare commodities too. 7. You say that you also heard how the scholar Philides[5] wasted away with depression and distress, and died, after his books were burnt in the Fire; others, too, went around for a long period dressed in black, emaciated, and with pale yellow complexions, like mourners.

8. For of course people had stored their most valuable possessions in the depositories by the Sacred Way, confident that they were safe from fire. Their confidence arose from the facts that the buildings had no wood in their

---

[3] Galen refers to the so-called Antonine Plague, which had its first outbreak at Rome in 166 (see also *My Own Books*, ch. 1 with n. 14), but probably continued to flare up again periodically over the next three decades.

[4] A well-known drug preparation, for which there were a number of recipes, involving a wide range of ingredients, including the viper flesh from which it derives its name (*thēriakon* = 'of a wild animal'), and sometimes opium. The original recipe was attributed to Andromachus, court doctor to the emperor Nero in the previous century. While its original purpose was as an antidote or prophylactic against poison, it enjoyed popularity in elite circles—including with the emperor Marcus Aurelius—for its broader supposed health benefits; and one of Galen's particular duties at court was that of preparing the theriac for him. See also *Prognosis*, ch. 3 and ch. 11, pp. 54 and 61 below.

[5] 'Scholar' translates *grammatikos*; see *My Own Books*, n. 4; *An Exhortation to Study the Arts*, n. 7; and *My Own Doctrines*, n. 4. The form of the scholar's name is uncertain.

construction, even in the doors, that there were no private houses in the imme-diate proximity, and that—because the documents of four imperial procurators were kept in that place—they were under constant military guard. 9. Indeed, those of us who rented depository space in that particular area paid a premium for this and placed our belongings there without any concern.[6]

10. There was one particular additional circumstance in my case: I was about to leave for Campania,[7] and had placed in the depository all the instruments, drugs and books (as well as quite few items of silver) that were normally in my own house, for safe-keeping I during my absence. So all these had been packed 5 up there too, and were destroyed along with the other valuables.

You say that you have heard of all these circumstances but would like to get a more reliable account of them from me. 11. What you find really remarkable is that I did not succumb to grief even when afflicted by all these kinds of loss; and I must say that you write no more than the truth. On hearing the news, in Campania, that all these things had been destroyed, I bore it very easily, with-out being moved even slightly. 12a. Back in Rome, I had to do without every-thing one needs when one wants to sort something out quickly [...][8] and was aware of the problem, as I am to this day, finding myself constantly in want of this or that book, instrument or drug.

12b. In fact, you are not even aware of the worst aspect of the loss of these books, which is that there is now no hope of getting hold of them again, since all the libraries on the Palatine were destroyed on that same day. 13. It is impos-sible to find copies of those rare books of which no copy had been deposited anywhere else; and so too of certain works which, though not in themselves particularly rare, were valuable because of the accuracy of that particular ver-sion of the text: the Callinian, Attician or Pedoukinian manuscripts, the Aristarchan ones I (the two Homers), Panaetius' text of Plato, and many other 6 such works, which contained the actual writing of those men who had either composed, or transcribed, the work in each case. For there were also in those collections the original autographs by many scholars, of works by the classical orators, doctors and philosophers.[9]

---

[6] Galen's storeroom was probably either in the Horrea Piperataria or in the Horrea Vespasiani: these were large warehouses, situated on either side of the Sacred Way (Via Sacra), within which private individuals could rent storage space. The former was also the location of Rome's main spice market. See Map 3.

[7] Galen had a second home outside Rome in Campania, probably in the Bay of Naples, a popular retreat for elite Romans; it is possible that he was by this time in semi-retirement there. See further n. 23 below.

[8] There is a lacuna at this point. Another possible interpretation is: 'I quickly became aware of the problem.'

[9] The text here is difficult: there is doubt both as to the identity of some of the persons referred to and as to whether Galen is really talking of actual autograph manuscripts (*autographa*) as opposed to simply copies (*antigrapha*), and if so whether autograph works of the authors in question or of particular scholars. My translation adopts this last solution, which seems the most plausible.

14. In addition to all this, I also on that day lost manuscripts which I had corrected and completely cleaned up; these were works which were unclear in their expression and full of errors of transcription, and where I had decided to produce in effect my own edition. In these cases I had annotated the text carefully in the interests of achieving complete accuracy, so that there were neither superfluous nor missing words; but also to achieve the same in relation to conventional marks of notation: the single or double *paragraphē*, or the *korōnis*[10] between books of a work, and of course the point and comma, which as you know are of such great importance in unclear texts that the reader who pays attention to them may be able to do without a commentator.

15. Such was the case with the texts of Theophrastus, Aristotle, Eudemus, Clytus and Phaenias,[11] with most of those of Chrysippus,[12] and with all the ancient doctors. 16. But what will distress you most is | that, beyond the books described in the so-called Catalogues,[13] I had found some others, both in the Palatine libraries and in those in Antium, which were clearly authentic works of the author whose name they bore, being similar both in language and in ideas. Amongst these were the works of Theophrastus, and especially his books on scientific knowledge. 17. Now, his works on plants, explicated in two long treatises, everyone has, but that of Aristotle was found by me in a book immediately following on from that one, and was transcribed; it is now lost. In the same manner, too, many works of Theophrastus and of certain other ancient authors, which were not mentioned in the Catalogues, as well as some which were mentioned there but were evidently not those works. I found many works in this category in the libraries on the Palatine—and I also prepared others in Antium.

18. The situation now, however, is that the books on the Palatine were lost on the same day as our own books: the Fire laid waste not only the depositories by

Callinus and Atticus are elsewhere mentioned as well-known scribes or literary editors, the latter (who may or may not be the same as Cicero's famous friend) by Galen himself. Aristarchus, librarian at the Library of Alexandria in the third–second century BC, produced renowned editions of Homer's *Iliad* and *Odyssey*.

[10] The *korōnis* was a manuscript figure indicating the end of a book, or sometimes a sequence of poems; the *paragraphē* was a line, single or double, used for smaller divisions within the text.

[11] All the characters mentioned here alongside Aristotle were philosophers in the Aristotelian tradition.

[12] Galen's interest in texts by Chrysippus is particularly striking in view of his close engagement, and fierce criticism, of the philosopher elsewhere: see *The Doctrines of Hippocrates and Plato*, passim.

[13] The Catalogues (*Pinakes*) were lists, originally written and displayed on tablets, of the holdings of the imperial libraries. The correct interpretation of this sentence, as well as of the rest of both this and the next paragraph, is much disputed. In particular, the reference to a library at Antium—the location of an imperial summer palace—is uncertain: 'Antium', at the three places where it occurs, represents an emendation of the actual manuscript reading, which I have adopted. In favour of the emendation is that it seems to make best sense of three otherwise obscure expressions in the Greek; against it is that Galen nowhere else mentions the library at Antium. Also disputed is the precise identity and relationship of the works by Aristotle and Theophrastus here mentioned.

the Sacred Way but also, before these, those in the sanctuary of the Temple of Peace, and finally those on the Palatine [|] and in the Tiberian House, as it is 8 known—for here too there was a library filled with a wide range of books. Those in Antium, on the other hand, were already close to destruction when I first came to Rome. 19. This was a result of the negligence of a succession of individuals in charge of them. At that earlier time, then, the manuscripts in that collection gave me a lot of trouble in transcription; now, however, they are completely useless and cannot even be unravelled because the papyrus has been glued together by mould. For that place is damp and enclosed, and very humid in the summer.

20. Perhaps, too, you will be distressed at the loss of my treatise on Attic words, and on everyday things and the terms for them. As you know, this was in two parts, one covering Old Comedy, the other the prose writers (though it happened that a copy of the latter part had already been sent to Campania). In fact, if the Fire at Rome had happened two months later, copies of all our treatises would already have reached Campania.

21. For everything intended for distribution had had two copies made already, apart from those which were to remain in Rome; my friends back in Pergamum were asking [|] to have all my treatises sent to them so that they could 9 place them in a public library—just as certain other individuals in other cities had already done with many of my works—and I had decided to have copies of them all in Campania too.[14]

22. So, then, as I have said, all my works had been produced in two copies, in addition to those that were to remain in Rome. 23a. Now, the fire occurred at the end of winter, and my plan was that at the beginning of summer I would send to Campania both those copies which were to be kept there and those which I intended to send to Asia once the Etesian Winds had arrived. 23b. But Fortune ambushed me, depriving me of many of my own books, but most particularly the lexical treatise that I had written, based on terms selected from the whole corpus of Old Comedy. 24a. As you know, Didymus had already written an explanation of the everyday words, as well as of all the rare ones, in fifty books; and I had produced an abridged version of these books in six thousand lines. 24b. I believed that such an edition would be useful for rhetors and scholars, and indeed for anyone wishing to follow Attic usage, or indeed (25) to [understand

---

[14] The procedure Galen describes in relation to his own works is apparently one whereby the original versions of works intended for distribution were stored in a lock-up in Rome, before being periodically copied, in which process two copies were taken, one for his own personal library in Campania and one for circulation via friends by means of being deposited in a library, presumably at Pergamum itself. Works could also, of course, be copied separately by or for friends (as also described in *My Own Books*). The works of his own which Galen lost without hope of recovery were those which had not yet been copied in either of these ways, as well as a number of more informal works or notes never intended for circulation. The passage is also noteworthy as being apparently the only place where Galen clearly admits his own direct agency in the process of *ekdosis* or distribution of his own works.

terms] of great importance in practical contexts. An example was furnished just
10   recently, when a doctor who enjoys a high reputation at Rome stated | that groats
were not yet in use in the time of Hippocrates, and that this was the reason that
in *Regimen in Acute Diseases* he recommends barley-gruel above all other cereals;
if, the argument ran, groats had been known in the Greek world at the time, he
would not have recommended anything else in preference to them.

26. Now, in the work on health called *Regimen*, in particular, which some say
to be by Hippocrates, others by Philistion, still others by Aristo[15]—all authors of
great antiquity—the term groats is indeed found, as it is also in the comic writers
of classical times. 27. *Abudokoma* and *aburtakē*, as well as whatever else was
unclear to the reader, were defined in our treatise—terms of which Didymus
had already given a very good explanation—and also rice-wheat, chickling, bitter vetch and groats; and, indeed, all the other cereals, vegetables, harvest fruits,
grape-pressed wine, 'seconds' wine, bushy olives, fruits, herbs, animals, instruments, utensils, equipment and all everyday things and terms. 28. The accounts
of such terms taken from Comedy had not yet been transferred to Campania,
whereas by a stroke of fortune those taken from prose writers had; the latter run
to forty-eight large books, some of which will perhaps need to be split into two,
since they contain more than four thousand lines of hexameter length.[16]

29. None of these losses grieved me, although the works were of great extent,
11   valuable and difficult to replace; | nor did that of my notes,[17] which were of two
kinds. Some were so well formed that they could be of use to others too, while
others were only for my own use, though having the same mnemonic function
as the former. 30. Then there was the very large number of synopses summarizing the chief points of many medical and philosophical works; but even the loss
of these did not distress me.

31. What might there be, you ask, still worse than all those things thus far
mentioned—something which might yet have the power to cause distress? Well,

---

[15] The work mentioned here is the Hippocratic *Regimen*, though confusingly referred to here in
the same words that may also refer to the *Regimen in Health* (that is, the third section of *The Nature
of the Human Being*), which however Galen considers—unlike *Regimen*—to be essentially
Hippocratic in content. The reference to groats (*chondroi*) is in chapter 9 of the *Regimen*. It seems
that beyond the present reference nothing is known of this Aristo, who is clearly not to be confused
with Aristo of Chios.

[16] Galen alludes to a division into 'books' which will naturally take place once a text reaches such
a length as to be unmanageable on one scroll. The number of books mentioned here seems very large
but is perhaps partially explained by the format of the work, involving a large number of quoted
extracts from the works in question. The dactylic hexameter, the six-foot line of classical epic poetry,
could be used as a standard measure for lines of prose works. Hexameter lines vary in length between
thirteen and seventeen syllables; it seems that Galen regards sixteen syllables as the standard or average length of a prose line. See also *The Doctrines of Hippocrates and Plato* VIII.1, with n. 59.

[17] 'Notes' translates *hupomnēmata*, the literal sense of which is related to memory: they are a
form of writing done to assist recollection, e.g. lecture notes, notes on a text, or notes to use while
giving an oral presentation. (The word is, however, sometimes used by Galen to refer to his writings
more generally.) See also *My Own Books*, nn. 25 and 47.

I shall tell you. I was convinced that I had a more remarkable collection of pharmacological recipes than anyone else in the Roman Empire, partly as a result of chance and partly through my own efforts. 32. A double good fortune had furnished me with these. First, there was a rich man in my home country, who was so interested in the knowledge of valuable drugs that he sometimes bought recipes for more than a hundred gold pieces. The fellow was so devoted to this pursuit that he was able to buy not only those most highly prized, in terms of their substance,[18] by each of the present-day practitioners, but also those of previous generations of practitioners.

33. The recipes of all these drugs I had been preserved, with the utmost care, 12 on two stitched parchments,[19] which were then given to me, quite spontaneously, by one of his heirs, with whom I happened to be very friendly.

34. This, then, was my first stroke of good fortune with regard to the provision of drugs; the second was as follows. When I first arrived in Rome, in my thirty-third year, I met a fellow-citizen and fellow-student of mine, Teuthras by name, who had obtained the similar collection of the doctor Eumenes,[20] another Pergamene and the greatest enthusiast in this area within the whole medical profession.

35. These recipes had been gathered from the whole of the civilized world, in the course of various trips abroad, after which he remained in Rome until his death. Teuthras died in the first outbreak of the Plague and had left it to me shortly after that first arrival in Rome. 36. On the basis of these resources, I used to be able to obtain any remarkable drug[21] that someone might have without difficulty: I would offer two or three similar ones in return.

37. Not only, then, were all these parchments destroyed in the fire—and even this I considered a small matter—but so too was my treatise, composed with great attention to detail, on the *Composition of Drugs*, in which I described my own method of composition I of the most well-regarded drugs. Only a few drug 13 recipes were preserved because they had already been given to my students.

[18] Some scholars have suggested that one should read 'within Asia' in place of the phrase 'in terms of their substance'.

[19] It seems that Galen is here speaking of a simple version, or forerunner, of the parchment codex—what would later develop into the bound book. Some scholars take the phrase in question, 'folded *diphthera*', to refer simply to a leather wallet in which the recipes were kept, presumably on separate pieces of parchment or papyrus: the term *diphthera* can mean both wallet and parchment. But *diphthera* was in use as a general word for a 'book'—the physical substrate on which something is written—from early times, as attested by Herodotus; it would thus seem odd for Galen to use it, in the context of a discussion of texts, to refer to something other than that. Moreover *ptuktos*, 'folded', was also used from early times to describe the object on which a message was written, even if this was a tablet—which was presumably hinged through some form of stitching.

[20] Or possibly 'Eudemus', a doctor from Pergamum whom Galen mentions on several other occasions. If 'Eumenes' is correct, the person is otherwise unknown.

[21] Although 'drug' is the literal translation, it seems clear from the context that the reference here is to drug *recipes*. (Both actual drug preparations and recipes for them are regarded as valuable commodities in this text, and there is perhaps some elision of the two categories.)

38. So, perhaps you will say that you now desire even more earnestly to understand how, in spite of losing such a great variety of goods, any single one of which losses would have been extremely distressing to other people, I was not grieved as certain individuals were, but accepted what had happened quite easily. 39. I shall give you a twofold answer. The first part belongs to a type of account which you will remember, since you have heard them on many occasions; but let me remind you again now.

The philosopher Aristippus was not content with an economical lifestyle; indeed, he used every day to give large sums of money to the most attractive courtesans of the day[22] to spend on extremely lavish feasts, even though he himself went short in many respects. 40. One day he was walking up to the city from Peiraeus—for he used to make not just short but even long journeys on foot—when he noticed that his servant was struggling with his load, which was a sack full of gold. He instructed him to empty out a sufficient quantity of it that the rest would be easy for him to carry. 41. The same rationale led to the following behaviour on his part. Aristippus possessed four plots of agricultural
14 land | in his home country; but as a result of some circumstance that arose he lost one of them and was left with three. 42. One of his fellow-citizens came up to commiserate with him over the loss. Aristippus laughed. 'Why should you commiserate with me for having three plots of land, each of them equal in extent to your single plot of land? Should I not rather commiserate with you?'

With these words he gave an excellent exemplification of something that I have said very frequently. One should not focus on something that one has lost. Indeed, one should reflect on how it is that someone who has inherited three plots of land from his father finds it difficult to endure the sight of one owning thirty. 43. Or how, even if he has thirty, he looks to someone else who has fifty; or if he has that number, to one who has seventy—and so on up to someone who has more than a hundred. In this way, he gradually reaches the point of desiring everything, and so is in perpetual poverty, since that desire is not fulfilled. 44. The person whose attention is not on how many pieces of land
15 someone else possesses but on the sufficiency of his own | to his personal needs will bear the loss of any which are superfluous without trouble. 45. One who possesses only one piece of land and then loses it is left completely without means and might reasonably be grieved; but a person who loses one of four is placed in the same position as one who originally had three, so that it is not such a great achievement if he suffers no distress at being left with that number. For a person who has never possessed a single piece of land to bear his poverty without distress, as Crates did—that is a significant achievement; and still more so if he does not have a home either, like Diogenes.

---

[22] Or possibly: 'to the most devoted of his companions.'

46. It was no extraordinary deed on my part, then, to remain completely without grief at these material losses. What was left to me was always far more than sufficient. 47. Indeed, one should rather pity the man with an annual income of 100,000 drachmas and outgoings of 10,000, if he is distressed at the loss of 30,000; what would be natural would be for such a person not even to be grieved if he lost 90,000 each year, since the remaining 10,000 are sufficient to sustain him. 48. It is the insatiability of such people which has caused us to regard with amazement those who are in fact not doing anything amazing. If anything, we should be amazed at individuals who lose everything and are still not grieved at all, like Zeno of Citium, who is supposed to have said, on hearing of a shipwreck | in which he had lost all his property: 'Thank you, 16 Fortune, for driving me into the Stoa and the philosopher's cloak!'

49. It was not, then, such an enormous achievement on my part to consider all sorts of material loss as a small thing—or, for that matter, to have the same attitude to my position at the imperial court, which, indeed, I not only did not desire in the first place, but actually attempted to resist on a number of different occasions, although I was dragged into it by the dictates of Fortune.[23] 50a. Nor was it a great accomplishment not to share the madness of many who have grown old in the imperial court. 50b. The loss of all my drugs, however, of all my books and of my most valuable drug recipes, as well as the editions related to them, and then on top of that the loss of many other treatises, the production of any one of which represented my serious, lifelong devotion to labour—not to have been distressed by this was, indeed, noble and a sign of something approaching highmindedness.[24]

51. And the first factor in bringing me to this state you know yourself, since we were brought up and educated together; then, there was a further contribution from my experience of what happened at Rome. 52. For, as you well know, the observation of political events is also a great educator, reminding us of the workings of | Fortune.[25] In this context, the words given by Euripides to Theseus 17 are especially true; consider them and you will learn:

> So from a wise man once I learnt
> A constant habit of imagined grief:
> To set before myself exile from home,
> Untimely death, and other paths of woe.

[23] The sentence may possibly hint that Galen had actually retired—or been dismissed—from the court under Commodus; see also n. 7 above.

[24] *Megalopsuchia*, literally 'greatness of soul', sometimes translated (through its Latin calque) 'magnanimity'. The word has an Aristotelian heritage, though it is used also by other ethical authors: the main connotation is that of a state of mind in which one is able to regard certain events or experiences as beneath one's notice.

[25] The manuscript reading is *technē*, 'Art' or 'Skill' (which was regarded as in some ways the opposite of *tuchē*, 'Fortune'); but the emendation seems necessary.

> If then some such expected harm befalls,
> It will not stab my soul all unawares.[26]

53. The wise man constantly reminds himself of all that it is possible that he may suffer; and even one who is not wise, if he is not actually living the life of a beast of the field, is somehow aroused by everyday events to some understanding of the nature of human affairs.

54. I believe that you are convinced, as I am, that there have been fewer atrocities committed in all previous human history, to judge from the accounts of its chroniclers, than were recently committed by Commodus within the few years of his reign. The result was that I, too, as I observed each of these atrocities, on a daily basis, schooled my imagination to entertain the loss of all that I possessed, and to the (55) expectation that I might—like others who had done nothing wrong—be punished by exile to a desert island. One who expects both exile and the loss of everything, and has prepared himself to endure those things, is not going to be distressed at some partial loss, wherein all his other possessions remain intact. 56. Having found by experience that those words of Euripides are truer than any others, I exhort you to train the imaginative faculty in your soul for practically every possible turn of Fortune.

57. Such an outcome, however, is only possible in one who is naturally well fitted for courage, as well as having had the advantage of the best education; and in my case good fortune provided this—as indeed you, who were educated alongside me, are well aware. 58. The character of my father was such that every time I remember him I feel an improvement in my soul. No other human being had such a complete reverence for justice and self-restraint; he was like this by nature, without the input of philosophical arguments. 59. He did not frequent philosophers in youth; rather, he had been trained by his father—my grandfather—in both virtue and architecture, in which disciplines he himself was pre-eminent. My father said that both his father and indeed his grandfather had led a similar life to his own; the former had been an architect and the latter a surveyor. 60. You may surely suppose, then, that I, too, was endowed with a similar nature to that of my forebears and that it is as a result of this that I have acquired the character that I have. But one should also consider that it is through having had the same education as them that I have a similar state of the soul.

61. I know that my father attached little importance to human affairs; and I have exactly the same attitude, especially now in my old age. 62. Those who lead lives of the greatest pleasure he considered to be no better than the dogs[27] that one sees being taken round Rome by their owners, who offer their services to females

---

[26] The passage, though it appears in other texts too (including elsewhere in Galen; see n. 31 below) as a quotation of moral value, comes from an unknown play of Euripides.

[27] The manuscript reads *oiōnōn* (birds); both *onōn* (asses) and *kunōn* (dogs) have been suggested as emendations.

for a fee. Nor, however, did he praise those who despise such pleasures but are content with experiencing no pain or distress of soul: his firm conviction was that the good was something greater | and better than that, and that it had its own 20 proper nature, which could not be circumscribed by the notion of mere absence of pain or distress.[28] Now, if one wishes to move away from those concepts and hold that the good is knowledge of things divine and human, I see that human beings have a very small share in that knowledge. If, however, our knowledge in that area is very small, it is evident that we do not have a precise knowledge of all other matters. 64. One who does not have an overall knowledge of things human and divine cannot have such knowledge in individual cases either, nor will he be able to choose and avoid things on the basis of scientific understanding.

For this reason I took it that political activity, and the attempt to plan things for the benefit of human beings, were difficult; and I also observed that people were not at all benefited by the serious efforts of decent people. 65. Constantly nurturing myself in this form of reasoning, I do not attach great importance to any of these matters. I would, then, hardly consider medical instruments, drugs, books, reputation or wealth to be of any great value. What mental disturbance will someone experience at such losses, or as a result of them, if he considers all such things to be of small value? 66. Continual disturbance and distress are the consequence of the view that such deprivation is the deprivation of something great, by contrast with the opposite attitude of constant contempt for such things.

67. Indeed, I did not simply declare all those things mentioned to be | unim- 21 portant, but devoted considerable attention to the subject, as you will know from a study of each of my writings in this area; even so, however, I did not regard these writings as some huge accomplishment, but rather as things composed in the manner of a diversion.

68. Some think that the state of 'non-disturbance' is the good; but such a state, I am sure, is not endurable either to me or to any other human being—or even to animals; for I observe that all have the wish to be active, both in body and in soul. But I have addressed this point in many other works, especially those against Epicurus.

69. I believe, then, that I have given you a complete response to your question regarding the absence of distress; yet I feel that I should also add one further point. 70. You perhaps believe that I make the assertion, in accordance with the assurance of some philosophers that no wise man can ever suffer distress, that I myself am similarly immune—especially since you say that you have never seen me suffer distress.

71. Well, I do not know whether there is anyone so wise as to be completely immune from suffering, but I am clear about my own case: I take no account of

---

[28] Implied here—and made more explicit below—is an attack on the Epicurean approach, which characterized human happiness as *ataraxia*, freedom from emotional disturbance.

material loss, provided that it stops short of total deprivation and exile to a
22   desert island; ⏐ similarly with bodily suffering: my claim to take no account of it
would not extend to the Bull of Phalaris.[29] 72a. The laying-waste of my country
would distress me, too, as would the punishment of a friend by a tyrant, and
other such circumstances. 72b. I pray to the gods that none of these things
befalls me; and it is because no such thing has yet befallen me that you have
observed me free from grief. 73. Indeed, I wonder at Musonius, who is supposed to have been in the habit of saying: 'O Zeus, send me a challenging
circumstance!'[30] On the contrary, my constant prayer is: 'O Zeus, do not send
me any circumstance which has the capacity to grieve me!'

74. My prayer would also be the same with respect to the health of my body.
My hope is that it may remain constantly healthy, rather than that I may show
my fortitude after suffering some serious injury to my head. I think it right to
train my imagination in the expectation of any setback, so as to be able to
endure it reasonably well, but I would not pray for anything to happen to me of
the sort that might have the capacity to cause me distress. 75. I perceive that
I have a precise awareness of the nature of my own condition, as regards both
body and soul; I would therefore not wish to be affected by an external factor of
such magnitude as would destroy my health, nor by some circumstance too
strong for the condition of my soul. 76. This is not to say that I do not concern
myself about the excellence of that condition: I attempt, to the best of my abil-
23   ity, to endue them with sufficient strength ⏐ that they may have the capacity to
withstand those things which distress them. Indeed, even if I have no hope that
my body will acquire the vigour of Heracles, nor my soul that which some say
the wise possess, I nonetheless consider it the better course not willingly to
omit any possible training. 77. I have a very high regard for those words that
Theseus says on behalf of Euripides,[31] in those words:

> So from a wise man once I learnt
> A constant habit of imagined grief:
> To set before myself exile from home,
> Untimely death, and other paths of woe.
> If then some such expected harm befalls,
> It will not stab my soul all unawares.

[29] Phalaris was a Sicilian tyrant who is said to have tortured and killed his victims by shutting
them in a hollow bronze bull, while a flame was lit beneath; Epicurus, who, in common with the
Stoics, believed that the wise man is indifferent to pain, claimed that such a man would be happy
'even inside the Bull of Phalaris'.

[30] Or possibly (giving the quotation in a form attested elsewhere, by Epictetus): 'send me whatever circumstance you wish!'

[31] The phrase 'on behalf of' (if the text is correct here) is interesting for the literary-critical view
it suggests, namely that Euripides is using this character as a mouthpiece for his views.

78a. Indeed, I consider such training the only protection against terrible events. 78b. I am not myself impervious to them all; indeed, it is for this reason that I always say to my associates | —since I am not one to proclaim my ability to 24 perform actions which I have not demonstrated in practice—that I disregard material losses, so long as I am left with sufficient that I suffer neither hunger nor cold, and that I disregard physical pain, so long as I am still able to converse with a friend and follow the words of a book that is read to me. 79a. Very serious pain deprives us of these capacities; and in such cases one has to be satisfied if one is able to show fortitude.

79b. What I have written elsewhere on the absence of distress I consider superfluous to mention to you; I know that you have always been content, as a result of both your nature and your education, with an economical lifestyle, in terms of both food and clothing, and that you exercise complete self-restraint in relation to sexual desires. It is those who are slaves to such desires who find themselves compelled to use more and more money. 80. If they are not rich, they cry and groan night and day, | and lie awake for whole nights on end try- 25 ing to work out how to find the resources to fulfil their desires. They howl if they fail to do so; but if they do succeed they are still unsatisfied, and they sink into that most miserable form of life which is attended by insatiable desires. 81. Who, then, are those who do not suffer distress in the same way as the majority of people? The answer is: those who have only a moderate level of attachment to honour, wealth, reputation or political power. Anyone who is excessively attached to these necessarily ends up leading the most wretched of lives: first, he has no understanding whatever of the identity of the virtue of the soul; secondly, the vices of his soul increase and he suffers constant distress, unable to reach the target which he has set himself.

82. The greatest desires are unfulfillable by virtue of their very scope; thus, no person in a normal condition could possibly rely on them, nor on a person who did rely on them. 83. Experience, on the other hand, is a good guide even in the area of the unexpected. I once had the temerity to question an extremely rich man—he possessed seven million drachmas or more—who neither shared any of his wealth with others nor himself took anything from it. His response was that, just as we preserve all parts of our own bodies, so we should preserve each one of our possessions. | 26

84. I was astonished at this individual's response. On my departure from him, I dictated (in my usual manner) the small book on *The Miserly Rich*;[32] and this too I have sent you.

---

[32] The work, in common with the vast majority of Galen's short works on ethical themes (see *My Own Books*, ch. 15, pp. 38–9 below), does not survive.

My Own Books

Galen's two autobiographical—or as they are sometimes known, 'auto-bibliographical'—treatises, *My Own Books* and *The Order of My Own Books*, are unique documents within the corpus of ancient literature. They offer the modern reader a vivid and multi-faceted insight, not only into Galen's own biography and view of his own works, but also into the literary, medical, scholarly and intellectual life of the period much more broadly.

The two works probably belong to the 190s, with *The Order of My Own Books* apparently written first, since it refers forward both to the other text and to a number of works mentioned in it (e.g. most of the Hippocratic commentaries) as not yet written. However, *The Order of My Own Books* also mentions some works not included in the other work, and the likelihood that a process of revision or updating took place makes it difficult to talk of single date for either of them (or, therefore, to draw chronological conclusions about other works on the basis of their inclusion or non-inclusion within them).

In spite of the difference in title, *My Own Books* is as much about the 'order' of his works as the other, shorter, text. Both are centrally concerned with the overall structure and intellectual coherence of Galen's literary œuvre—with the way in which his works, or at least a core set of them, can be followed as a curriculum of medical study. In spite of some differences in presentation, that order can essentially be summarized as follows. Logical training is a primary requirement for all intellectual or scientific pursuits. The aspiring doctor should follow such training with the study of anatomy (ch. 4 of *My Own Books*), followed by that of the functions of the parts of the body (ch. 5); then the physical composition of human bodies, the fundamental nature of health and disease and the different varieties of the latter (ch. 6); then the therapeutic or clinical method itself (ch. 7); there follows a more specialized focus on diagnosis and prognosis (ch. 8). The study of drugs may be either incorporated with the material of ch. 6, or treated as a separate specialism.

That core thematic structure of *My Own Books* sits alongside a biographical one (occupying chs. 1–3), and partially overlapping with it in content. Here Galen gives some account of his own intellectual development and career, as well as explaining differences between his works which arise from the particular context of their composition, or intended reader. He also makes the claim—a paradoxical one given the above careful construction of his own corpus, as scholars have noted—that his original intention was not to publish any of his works, but that his own project of publication arose from the fact that many of his works had already reach 'the hands of many', against his wishes. The nature of 'publication' in the ancient world should be understood here, which is rather a process of distribution of a work by means of a single hand-written copy at a time. A work might have a formal recipient or dedicatee, as many of Galen's do, but might also be copied repeatedly, with or without the author's or dedicatee's consent. The author's own role in this process of distribution is not always clear, and in Galen's case almost always either mentioned obliquely or directly denied; but see *Freedom from Distress*, n. 14.

A third aspect of the structure of *My Own Books*, finally, is the listing of a series of specialized works in different areas which stand outside the above core curriculum. This includes his very substantial body of Hippocratic commentaries (ch. 9); a range of works discussing the views of other medical authors (chs. 10–13); a large number of works on logic (ch. 14); a series of treatises on individual topics in ethics (ch. 15); works on philosophers (chs. 16–19); and a number of discussions of matters of vocabulary or linguistic usage (ch. 20). With the exception of the Hippocratic commentaries and a few of the ethical works, the works in these categories have overwhelmingly not survived. To some extent these losses may be related to the fire of 192 (on which see *Freedom from Distress*), although the relationship between the works actually listed in chs. 10–20 below and those 'for his own exercise' which he mentions as lost in the fire is unclear. It seems odd to continue to list in a definitive catalogue works which one knows or believes to be permanently lost (although Galen does seem sometimes to do this). On the whole a better explanation of the gaps in survival of Galen's works is probably provided by the way in which different works were used, and especially their perceived value in the generations succeeding Galen's death.

The text available to us has been considerably improved by the discovery of the Vlatadon 14 manuscript,[1] which among other things supplies a substantial passage completely missing from the only other Greek MS. This additional material also resulted in a new numbering of the chapters; where a different chapter number existed in previous editions, this has been given in [ ] after the actual chapter number. There are, further, some words and phrases missing in both Greek manuscripts but supplied from the Arabic version, also consulted by Boudon-Millot; these are indicated by < >.

Greek title: Περὶ τῶν ἰδίων βιβλίων (*Peri tōn idiōn bibliōn*)
Kühn: XIX.8–48
Editions: Müller 1891; Boudon-Millot 2007 (with French translation)

Preface

The validity of your advice regarding the cataloguing of the books of my own   XIX.8 composition, my dearest Bassus, has been proved by events. I was recently in the Sandaliarium, the area of Rome with the largest concentration of booksellers, where I witnessed a dispute as to whether a certain book for sale was by me or someone else.[2] The book bore the inscription: 'Galen, the doctor'.[3] Someone had

---

[1] See *Freedom from Distress*, n. 1.

[2] The Sandaliarium, or Vicus Sandaliarius, was a shopping area adjoining the Forum on its northeastern side, originally named for its concentration of shoe-makers; see Map 3. Bassus is mentioned in a couple of other places by Galen as an associate or student, but his precise identity is uncertain.

[3] The author's name as well as the title of the work formed part of the full title or 'inscription' (*epigraphē*) of an ancient book. It has been suggested that the text should read rather 'Galen's "Doctor"', this being apparently the title of a work falsely attributed to him, and the mention of the

bought the book under the impression that it was one of mine; someone else—a
9 man of letters—struck by the odd form of the title, desired to know I the book's
subject. On reading the first two lines he immediately threw aside the work, saying simply: 'This is not Galen's diction—the inscription is false.' Now, the man in
question had been trained in the fundamental education which Greek children
always used to be given, from the earliest stage, by scholars and orators.[4] Many
of those who embark upon medicine or philosophy these days cannot even read
properly, yet they frequent those who would teach them the greatest and most
beautiful fields of human study—those taught by philosophy and medicine.

Now, this kind of laziness had begun many years ago, when I was still a youth,
but it had not at that time reached the extreme state it has now. It is for this reason, and also because my books have been subjected to all sorts of mutilation at
the hands of many—people who in various countries pass them off[5] as their
own, with various cuts, additions and modifications—that I decided it would be
best, first to explain the reason for these mutilations, and secondly to give an
10 account of I the actual subject of each of my genuine works. Well, as for the fact
of my books being passed off by many people under their own name, my dearest
Bassus, you know the reason yourself: it is that they were given without inscription to friends or pupils, having been composed with no thought for distribution,[6]
but simply at the request of those individuals, who had desired a written record
of lectures they had heard. Now, some of these individuals then died, and their
successors who came into possession of these writings liked them, and began to
pass them off as their own, while others <were shameless enough to sell copies of
the works> themselves, <swindling people who were in need of them; still others
made copies of the books, one after another, altering them in the process and
using them to enhance their own reputation; others, finally,> having been given
works by those who possessed them, took these to their own countries, and, each
corrupting the texts in their own malign way, used them as the basis for their
public presentations.[7] All these people were eventually found out, and many of
those who then recovered the works affixed my name to them. They then discovered

author's name in the genitive being more usual in such 'inscriptions'; on the other hand, this oddity
may be precisely what the man of letters was initially surprised by.
  [4] The terms are *grammatikos* and *rhētōr*, which could also be translated 'teachers of grammar'
and 'teachers of rhetoric'; both were involved at successive stages of the traditional Greek education;
see also the title to ch. 20 below, *An Exhortation*, n. 7 and *My Own Doctrines*, n. 4.
  [5] The verb (*anagignōskein*) literally means simply to read; it presumably refers here to a public
reading of a work, or possibly more broadly to the use of it for a lecture, in either case with the pre-
tence that the work is one's own.
  [6] *Ekdosis*, literally 'giving out', and often translated 'publication'. I have preferred the translation
'distribution', to reflect more clearly the nature of ancient practices in this area, based as they were
on individual acts of presentation, lending or borrowing, or of copying, rather than on any form of
mass production.
  [7] *Epideixis*: the term refers to a public lecture or demonstration involving verbal exposition and
also in some cases practical, anatomical display.

discrepancies between these and copies in the possession of other individuals, and so brought them to me with the request that I correct them.

Since, then, as I have stated above, they were written not for distribution but to fit the particular level and needs of those who had requested them, it follows naturally that some of them are rather extended, while others are compressed; and that their manner of exposition, and indeed the actual theoretical content, vary in their completeness. Those works which were written for beginners ǀ would, 11 quite obviously, be neither complete nor absolutely precise in their teaching. That was not their requirement—nor would such individuals have been able to learn all the material in such a precise manner, without first reaching a certain basic level in the fundamentals. Some of my predecessors would give such works the title of *Outlines*, others *Sketches*, or *Introductions, Synopses* or *Guides*. I simply gave them to my pupils without any such inscription, and it is for that reason that when they later fell into other hands, they were given a number of different titles by different persons. Those which were sent back to me by various persons for correction I decided to inscribe with the title 'for beginners'; and it is with these works that I shall begin.

1. Works composed during the first stay in Rome

I myself did not possess copies of all those works which I had dictated to young men at the beginning of their studies, or in some cases presented to friends at their request. When, however, I came to Rome for the second time and they were, as I have mentioned, sent ǀ to me for correction, I took possession of them 12 and affixed titles <including the words 'for beginners'. Amongst these works that came into my possession was that on the subject of *Sects> for Beginners*: this should be the first book to be read by those who wish to learn the art of medicine. This work teaches one the differences between the different classes of sect (I say 'different classes of sect' because there are more specific differences which the initiate may learn later on in his studies).

The names of the three sects are by now pretty universally known (Dogmatic or Rationalist; Empiric; and Methodist); the individual peculiarities of each, and their differences from each other, are set out in that book. Works also dictated 'for beginners' were that on *Bones* and that on *The Pulse*; and there were also two introductory books given to a Platonist friend during this stay, one containing the anatomy of the veins and arteries, the other that of the nerves; and, for another friend, and *Outline of Empiricism*.[8]

---

[8] This work is not extant in Greek but survives in the Latin translation of Niccolò da Reggio (as *Subfiguratio empirica*).

13   None of these works was in my possession until | I came to Rome for the
second time and received copies from other people. There were other works
written for friends at that same period, of which I did keep copies, because they
had been fully worked up and completed. Among these are the two books of
Causes of Breathing and the four on *The Voice*, which were addressed to a man
of consular rank named Boethus, a practitioner of Aristotelian philosophy. To
him were also addressed the volumes on *Hippocrates' Anatomy* and, subsequently, those on *Erasistratus' Anatomy*.[9] These were written in a more combative spirit on account of one Martianus[10]—two of whose works on anatomy
survive to this day in the possession of many people. Martianus enjoyed a great
reputation at this time; and he was a remarkably malicious and adversarial personality, in spite of his more than seventy years. He had heard very high praise
of a public lecture I had given on a set question of anatomy,[11] and of my teachings on that occasion, from all who had followed them; and so he asked one of
my friends to which sect I belonged. My response was that I regarded those
who declared themselves 'Hippocrateans', 'Erasistrateans', 'Praxagoreans' and so
on as slaves; that I personally took whatever was good from each. He then
14 asked | which of the ancients I most admired. <Learning that I favoured
Hippocrates, he stated that Hippocrates was in his view of no value in the study
of anatomy,> declaring rather the greatness of Erasistratus in all areas of the
art, but especially in this. So it was because of him that I wrote the six books of
Hippocrates' Anatomy and the three of *Erasistratus' Anatomy* in this rather
combative vein.

On another occasion, too, I was speaking in public on the books of the
ancient doctors, and the topic set before me was Erasistratus' work on *The
Bringing-Up of Blood*. A stilus was placed in the book in the customary manner, and as it pointed to that part of the book in which he rejects the use of
venesection, I spoke at some length against Erasistratus, in order to discomfort Martianus, who claimed to be an Erasistratean. Well, this speech got a
very good response; and a friend of mine who was hostile to Martianus begged
me to dictate what I had said, to a person he would send to me who was
trained in a form of shorthand writing, so that, if he had suddenly to leave

---

[9] For Boethus and his patronage of Galen, see *Prognosis*, esp. ch. 2, p. 51 below, and *Anatomical
Procedures* I.1, pp. 65–6 below. *Causes of Breathing* survives in Greek, though in a version which
may be only a summary of the original; *The Voice* survives in fragmentary form; the two works on
the anatomy of Hippocrates and Erasistratus have not survived.
[10] For this figure, one of the most prominent writers on anatomy, and followers of Erasistratus,
in Galen's time at Rome (and for the different forms of his name), see also *Prognosis*, ch. 3 with n. 4.
[11] The word here translated as 'set question', *problēma*, refers to a topic set for public debate in a
competitive arena: the relative skill and accomplishment of different speakers would be gauged by
the requirement to speak on a subject set by someone else, or sometimes by means of a random
process: see next paragraph. *Problēma* has etymological connotations of something 'placed before
one', 'placed in one's way'; it also has a more technical sense in Aristotle's analysis of arguments.

Rome for his home city, he would be able to use it against Martianus during examinations of patients.[12]

What, then, was my surprise, when I subsequently returned to Rome on my second visit, at the summons of the emperors, | to find that, while the friend who had taken the book in this way had died, the book itself, composed in the context of the rivalry of a particular moment, during a public refutation, was now in the possession of a large number of people. What is more, I had done this while I was still quite young—in my thirty-fourth year.

From that moment[13] I decided to give no more public lectures or demonstrations, since I had now achieved a success in treating the sick which was beyond anything that one might have hoped for. For I was well aware of the philistines who cannot bear to hear a doctor praised without dismissing him as a 'word-doctor'. In the hope of avoiding their malicious slanders, I resolved to say nothing more than was absolutely necessary, even at the patient's bedside; to refrain from lecturing before large crowds as I had previously; and to perform no public displays. Rather, my practice of the art alone would suffice to indicate the level of my understanding.

I then remained in Rome a further three years, until the outbreak of the great plague, at which I immediately left the city in haste for my homeland,[14] since no one, <to my knowledge, had been able to find a powerful enough medicine to combat this scourge, which spread everywhere before being extinguished>. To this period too belongs the composition, at the behest of Boethus, of the first six books of *The Doctrines of Hippocrates and Plato* and the | first one of *The Function of the Parts of the Body*. Boethus left Rome before me, with these works in his possession. His destination was Syria Palaestina, where he was to be governor, and where he also died. Therefore I completed both these treatises after a considerable passage of time: on return to my home city I encountered a number of hindrances, which I will relate in due course.

15

16

---

[12] The reference here is to the public and competitive aspect of actual patient examinations, which is indeed seen very clearly in *Prognosis* (see especially chs. 3, 11 and 13). The story is recounted also in another text (*Venesection, against the Erasistrateans at Rome*, ch. 1), where it is specified that the friend was Teuthras.

[13] That is to say, presumably, from a moment after his return to Rome and discovery of this situation, not from the moment of the original public dispute with Martianus. We must then take the beginning of the next paragraph as returning us to the original narrative frame—that of his career during the first stay, 162–6—after the digression of the previous two paragraphs into his experiences on return in 169.

[14] The Antonine Plague, which first broke out in Italy in 166, as the result of a virus brought back by troops returning from the war with the Parthian Empire (in modern-day Iraq and Iran). It is interesting to compare the rather different account of the motivations for his return given by Galen in *Prognosis*, ch. 9, p. 59 below, and tempting to conclude that he is giving a more straightforward and honest account of those motivations here than there.

2. Books of my composition which were given
to me by certain parties on my return home

So I returned from Rome to my native city after the completion of my thirty-seventh year;[15] and there three books were given to me by certain parties which had been written before my departure from Pergamum, when I had gone to Smyrna on account of the doctor Pelops and Albinus the Platonist.[16] One was a tiny work on *The Dissection of the Womb*; another, also quite short, on *Diagnosis of Complaints of the Eyes*; the third a work of some length on *Medical Experience*.[17] The first of these had been given to a certain midwife, the second to a young man who treated eyes. The origin of the third was a two-day debate between Pelops and Philip the Empiric, in which the former aimed to show that the art of medicine could not be constituted through experience alone, and the latter that it could.[18] | I transcribed the arguments that were given on both sides, laying them out in order as an exercise for myself; and I have no idea how this work came to leave my possession without my knowledge.

During my period in Smyrna I wrote three more books, on *The Motion of the Chest and Lungs*,[19] as a favour to a fellow-student. This man was planning to return home after his study tour, and the book was written for his use in practice, on the basis of which he would be able to perform some kind of anatomical display. In the intervening time, however, the young man died. The books remained in the possession of certain other individuals, and it was suspected that the content was mine. Then somebody added his own preface and tried to pass them off as his own; but he was found out. I added a passage to the end of the third of these books, covering my own subsequent discoveries; for what I had written in the three books were the doctrines of my teacher Pelops, with whom I was studying in Smyrna at the time.

---

[15] Part of this journey, which seems to have taken place between the summer of 166 and the early part of 167, is recounted in detail in *Affections and Errors of the Soul* I.4.

[16] Galen refers to the 'study tour' on which he embarked after the death of his father in 148, which took him first to Smyrna and subsequently to Corinth and Alexandria. The public debate he goes on to mention was apparently the occasion of his first meeting Pelops, who was a pupil of Numisianus, in turn a pupil of Quintus, whom Galen regarded as an especial authority in anatomy.

[17] The first of the three works mentioned survives, and is Galen's only extant work in Greek from his youth in Pergamum; the second does not survive, while *Medical Experience* is extant in Syriac-Arabic translation and in Latin.

[18] For the notion of the 'constitution' of the art, and for the Empiricist position, see *Sects for Beginners*, esp. ch. 2, with nn. 4 and 8.

[19] The work has not survived.

3. The books written after these[20]

On return from Rome, then, I established myself in my home city, and returned to my habitual pursuits; but there immediately arrived from Aquileia a summons under the imperial seal. For the emperors had decided to lead an attack on the Germans, after spending the winter there. | So I was forced to travel.   18 I had hopes, however, of being excused; for I had heard that the older of the two emperors was a reasonable man, understanding, gentle and kind. (I refer to the one whose original name was Verus, but who changed to Antoninus[21] on being appointed successor by the Antoninus who ruled after Hadrian; at the same time he gave the name of Verus to Lucius, whom he made his co-ruler.)

On my arrival in Aquileia, there was an outbreak of the plague which caused destruction on a scale previously unknown. The emperors immediately fled to Rome with a small force of men; for the rest of us, survival was a matter of great difficulty, over a long period. The majority, in fact, died, the effects of the plague being compounded by the fact that all this was taking place in the middle of winter. Lucius himself departed this world on the way back to Rome, and Antoninus [Marcus Aurelius] performed the ceremony of deification. After this he concentrated on his campaign against the Germans, and was extremely keen to take me with him. But he was prevailed upon to release me on hearing [from me] of the contrary instructions of his | personal patron god Asclepius—whose   19 servant I, too, declared myself, ever since he saved me from a fatal condition, involving a swelling.[22] The emperor bowed to the wishes of the god, and commanded me to await his own return; for he was hopeful of conducting the war to a speedy resolution. He then set off, leaving behind his son Commodus, at that time still a small child, with instructions to his carers to endeavour to preserve him in a state of health, but to employ my services if ever he fell ill.

During this time, then, I collected together and brought into permanent form both what I had learned from my teachers and what I had discovered myself. I was still engaged in research in some areas, and I also wrote down a lot that I had that was relevant to those enquiries, training myself in many set questions of medicine and philosophy. But most of this material was lost in the great fire in which the Temple of Peace was consumed along with many other

---

[20] The chapter heading is missing except in the Vlatadon MS and the Arabic version; so the contents of this chapter were hitherto classified as a continuation of ch. 2.

[21] The older emperor is Marcus Aurelius (reigned 161–80), on whose relations with Galen see further *Prognosis*. The 'Antoninus who ruled after Hadrian' is his predecessor Antoninus Pius (138–61), who adopted both Marcus and Lucius Verus as his heirs. The date in question is 168/9.

[22] Galen apparently refers to this illness in more detail in *Good and Bad Humoral Fluid*, ch. 1 (VI.757 K.), where he describes an episode, around the age of 20, when he suffered a swelling 'in the region where the liver touches the diaphragm'. There he attributes his deliverance to his resolve to abstain from fruits, not to any divine intervention, but we may perhaps take it that he believed himself in taking that resolve to be acting on the instructions of the god.

buildings. And as the emperor's absence far exceeded expectation, this whole period provided me with an excellent opportunity for study, enabling me to
20 complete my major | treatise, *The Function of the Parts of the Body*, in seventeen books, and to add what remained to *The Doctrines of Hippocrates and Plato* <in ten>. <I wrote the second book of *The Function of the Parts* at the same period as these latter, having previously given the first to Boethus.> I was still search-ing for some of the anatomical studies which I had given to Boethus, <but failed to find any>. In the second book of *The Function of the Parts*, it is shown how I made the additional discovery of the muscles responsible for the motion of the joints of each finger after a long period in which I was ignorant of them—as were all my predecessors. In that treatise I also put off discussion of the motion of the upper eyelid, confining myself to demonstrating, once more, that the statements of certain persons were not true. Once I had persuaded both myself and others to whom I made the demonstration that I had discovered the truth of this too—along with a range of other matters which had been either misrep-resented or simply neglected by previous anatomists—at that point I wrote the *Anatomical Procedures*.

Meanwhile, however, *The Function of the Parts* had reached quite a wide readership; it became a focus of study for virtually every doctor who was involved with traditional medicine, as well as for philosophers of the Aristotelian
21 persuasion, for Aristotle himself | had written a treatise of a similar kind.[23] So, certain malicious individuals put about the city the slander that I was in the habit of describing things which were simply not visible in dissections, so as to gain a reputation for having made discoveries far beyond those of my predeces-sors; such matters, they said, could not have failed to be noticed by everyone before me. To these men my response was that of contemptuous amusement; but they excited the anger of my friends, who begged me to give a public dem-onstration, in one of the great auditoria, of the truth of the anatomical proposi-tions that I had written down. When I refused (for my disposition even then was to care nothing for public reputation), those slanderers attributed my adop-tion of this high-minded attitude to fear of refutation rather than to contempt for their stupidity; and every day they would go to the Temple of Peace—which even before the fire was the general meeting-place for all those interested in the pursuit of learning[24]—and mock me continually.

---

[23] The most explicit reference is probably to Aristotle's *Parts of Animals*; but the more funda-mental point is the convergence in intellectual project: both Aristotle and Galen in their biology are concerned to give an account which does justice to the *function*, understood in relation to its teleo-logical purpose, of every structural feature of an animal.

[24] In Greek, *logikai technai*, literally the arts related to reason, argumentation or logic: this would cover a wide range of intellectual, including scientific, subjects on which people would lecture and debate in this environment.

I was, then, compelled by my friends to give a public demonstration, wherein, over a period of several days, I proved that I had not been lying, and that there were many matters of which previous authorities had been ignorant; I and at   22 their behest I made written notes of what had been shown and argued; and these are entitled *Lycus' Areas of Ignorance in Anatomy*,[25] for the following reason.

When I came forward to demonstrate that I had not lied in my anatomical notes, I placed the works of all the anatomists in front of me and invited everyone present to choose whatever part he wished to be dissected. My claim was that I would show the extent of the divergence of the facts—which had been accurately described in my own works—from the accounts of my predecessors. And someone set me the topic of the chest. Now, as I was taking up the books of the most ancient of medical authorities, whom I intended as my starting-point, some of the very well-reputed doctors who were sitting in the front row suggested that I should not waste my time: Lycus of Macedon, who had been a disciple of Quintus, the greatest expert in anatomy, had written down all the discoveries made up to his own time, and so I should forget about the rest and subject his works alone to examination against mine. It was in accordance with this suggestion of theirs, then, that I proceeded in this way for all the topics that were set me on each day.

The reason that I feel compelled to mention all this is that the prospective I reader of my works should know at what age and for what reason each one was   23 written. Thus he will be in a position to distinguish works which give only partial accounts from those which are fully completed; and works written for the refutation of arrogant know-alls from works of instruction for pupils. I shall give further indications of these distinctions in what follows, as need arises. Let me now turn, however, to the list of my extant writings, beginning with the anatomical ones.

4 [3]. Works of anatomical science

First in this category is *Bones for Beginners*; after this, a number of other books written for beginners: one covering the anatomy of the veins and arteries, another that of the nerves, and a third which instructs the reader, in a summary but accurate account, of all that is said in *Anatomical Procedures* about muscles. The reader wishing to embark on *Anatomical Procedures* immediately after the anatomy of the bones may by-pass the works on vessels and nerves, and that on

---

[25] 'Notes' translates *hupomnēmata*. See *Freedom from Distress*, n. 17; and below n. 47. The work here referred to is not extant.

24 muscles too: for everything | concerning anatomy has been written down in the *Anatomical Procedures*. Its first book concerns the muscles and ligaments of the hands; the second, those of the legs; the third, the nerves and vessels in the limbs; the fourth, the muscles responsible for motion of the cheeks and lips, and the lower jaw, and also the head, neck and shoulder-blades; the fifth, the muscles of the chest, those in the area of the upper abdomen, the loin muscles and spinal muscles; the sixth concerns the organs of nutrition, namely the intestines, stomach, liver, spleen, kidneys, bladder and all other parts associated with them; the seventh and eighth cover the anatomy of the parts relevant to breathing, the seventh dealing with the parts in the heart, lungs and arteries, in both dead and living animals, while the eighth deals with those in the chest as a whole; the ninth covers the anatomy of the brain and spinal cord; the tenth, that of the eyes, tongue, the mouth of the stomach, and the parts connected with

25 them; the eleventh, that of the area of | the larynx[26] and what is known as the hyoid bone, and parts connected with them, as well as of the nerves attached to them; the twelfth, that of arteries and veins; the thirteenth, that of the nerves that come from the brain; the fourteenth, that of those that come from the spinal cord; the fifteenth, that of the parts concerned with generation.

These are the essential works of anatomical science; but in addition to the essential ones are a number of others which are also useful: a summary in four books of Marinus' twenty volumes of anatomy; and a summary of all of those of Lycus, in two. Let me list the main headings of each. The first volume of the summary of Marinus contains his first six books of anatomy; his first in these six gives an introduction to the science as a whole, before proceeding to skin, then hair, then nails, flesh and soft and hard fat; the second deals with glands, tunics and similar casings, <such as those around the heart, stomach, kidneys and liver>; with the peritoneum, the lining of the intestines, and the diaphragm; the third with those vessels whose existence is posited by theory, as well as the

26 dissection of veins and arteries, | and whether blood is naturally contained in the arteries; the fourth with the question of the activity, function and source of the arteries, and with the other questions which arise in relation to arteries; then with the ureters, with the uretic channel, the urachus,[27] the seminal vessels, the vessels, ducts and glands of bile; the vessels leading from the glands; the trachea; the vessels of the breasts, in which milk is secreted; with the liquids dispersed through the body and with which fluids are contained in which vessels; and with nutrition; the fifth book with the parts of the head, in particular the sutures of the skull; also with the sutures and natural junctions of the face, and all the bones of the head; with the perforations in both head and face;

---

[26] By 'mouth of stomach' is meant the oesophagus.
[27] By 'uretic channel' Galen refers to our urethra; the urachus is the remnant of a canal which drains the bladder in the foetus.

with the lower jaw and its perforations, and whether there is a natural join in it; with teeth, with the bone adjacent to the head of the trachea, and the parts which are contiguous with it and extend to the tonsils; the sixth with the spine, sacrum, hip-bone, ribs, | sternum, scapula and acromion; with the clavicle, with 27 the humerus, ulna and radius, the bones of the wrist and the fingers; with the thigh and the cartilaginous bones on either side of the knee;[28] and with the kneecap, the tibia and the bones of the foot.

The second of my sets of notes containing the summary of Marinus' anatomy covers the seventh, eighth, ninth and tenth of his volumes. The subjects of the seventh book are: the connection of the skull with the meninges and other membranes; the nerves of the whole of the face; the muscles of the temples, the masticatory muscles, the muscles leading from the sockets to the cheeks and lips; the muscles of the cheeks; then, the muscles within the lower jaw, as well as those around it (except for the masticatory muscles); the parts about the column-like outgrowths and those in the tongue; then the tongue and its muscles, and the muscles of the eye.

The subjects of the eighth book are: the mouth, lips, teeth, gums, | uvula and 28 pharynx; epiglottis, tonsils, *antiades*,[29] nose, nostrils, ears and neck; the muscles of the neck; the muscles around the ribs; those beneath the collarbone; and the nature of the neck. The subjects of the ninth are the muscles of the diaphragm, of the spine, of the intercostal region and upper abdomen; also those of the arm, scapula, forearm and hand; of the tenth hip-joint[30] and its muscles, the legs and their muscles, and the knee-joint.

The third of my summaries covers the eleventh to the fifteenth book of Marinus. In his eleventh book Marinus considered first of all the subject, 'Whether any fluid enters the lungs when one drinks, and whether during inhalation and exhalation any breath enters the stomach'; his second subject is the mouth of the stomach, followed by the trachea, lungs, heart, and membrane around the heart. In the twelfth book of his treatise Marinus considered the liver and the bile contained in it, the spleen, digestive cavity and mesentery; the thirteenth book begins with intestines, | proceeding to the kidneys, ureters, 29 bladder, urachus and urethra; then to the male member, the female genitals, the womb, the embryo and the testicles (which he calls 'twins'); and finally to the gland-like [parts].[31] In the fourteenth, he covers the anatomy of all veins above the liver; in the fifteenth, the vein which goes from the heart to the liver,[32] all

---

[28] Boudon-Millot suggests that the menisci are meant.
[29] Apparently a 'throat gland', distinguished by Marinus from the tonsils.
[30] This is conjectural; the MSS have a redundant further mention of 'forearm'.
[31] This term is apparently from Herophilus. Von Staden (1989, 167 and 212) argues that though it is possible that the prostate is meant, 'seminal vessels' is a better interpretation.
[32] As Boudon-Millot points out, the phrasing here reflects Marinus' view which, contrary to Galen's, has the heart, not the liver, as the source of the veins.

veins below the level of the diaphragm, and finally the arteries throughout the whole animal.

The fourth of my summaries covers the remaining five volumes of Marinus, from the sixteenth to the twentieth. The sixteenth contains questions and observations concerning the brain, such as whether there is a pulse-like motion in it, and whether we breathe into it; and then goes on to the spinal cord and meninges. The argument of the seventeenth concerns the commanding role of the brain; that of the eighteenth, voluntary activities and the distinctions between individual nerves, as well as between their different sources; that of the nineteenth, | the nerves which grow out from the brain; the sense of smell and the source of its organ of perception; and the nerves that go to the eyes, which Herophilus and Eudemus[33] call 'channels'; then[34] about the eyes themselves, and the nerves that reach them, by which they are moved; and after that, about the soft nerves, in which category he states to be also those that connect with the region of the palate; and after that, regarding the outgrowths to the ears, and the organ of perception relative to that; in the twentieth his discussion concerns the nerves that grow out from the base of the brain; the outgrowth of the spinal cord; and those from the brain and the spinal cord. As for the two books in which I epitomized the anatomical treatise of Lycus, the first contains nine of his books: the first, on the brain; the second, on the nerves from the brain and from the meninges; the third, on those from the spinal cord; the fourth, on those from the eyes; the fifth, on the head of the trachea; the sixth, after these, on the lungs in a dead animal, followed by the lungs in a living animal; the eighth, on the heart and the ninth on the diaphragm. The second part of the epitome of Lycus' anatomical books contains the epitome of ten books attributed to him, as follows: the first, on the liver; the second, in which he describes the anatomy of the omentum and the spleen; the third, on the kidney; the fourth, on the bladder and the genitals; the fifth, on the womb; the sixth, on the pregnant womb in a dead animal; the seventh, on the living embryo; the eighth, on the dead embryo; and after that, on the testicles; and then on the muscles.

These books contain what is necessary and useful within anatomical science; others have been written that relate to the same science, as an additional contribution. In this category are two books on *Disagreement in Anatomy*; one on *The Dissection of Cadavers*; and two more on *The Dissection of Living Bodies*; to this

---

[33] On the identity and dates of this Eudemus (often cited alongside Herophilus as a fellow-innovator in anatomy), see von Staden 1989, 62–3.

[34] The passage from here to p. 30 (see n. 40), covering the rest of this chapter, the whole of ch. 5 and the first lines of ch. 6, is attested only in the Vlatadon MS and in the Arabic version, and was missing from editions and translations of the text before that of Boudon-Millot.

class belongs also the book on *The Distinct Types of Uniform Part*.[35] And the *Anatomy of Hippocrates* and *of Erasistratus* have already been discussed. Four books were also added to these later, as an additional contribution, on *Lycus' Areas of Ignorance in Anatomy*; and some further works were written after later, too: two on *Points of Disagreement with Lycus in his Anatomical Writings*, and also regarding *The Function and Activity of the Parts of the Body*.[36]

These, then, are the books of anatomical science which give instruction on the parts of the body and the individual constitution of each. What follows on from these works is the discussion of the activities and function of each part, which is contained in the books listed below.

5. Which books contain the activities and functions of the parts made apparent in anatomy

There are three concerning *The Motion of the Chest and the Lungs*, as I said before, and another two on the *Causes of Breathing*; which are followed by four on *The Voice*; the two on *The Motion of the Muscles* belong within this branch of the science, too. For, in a sense, those of the activities which are known as the 'soul's' are covered in these works. As for the activities 'of nature', I have written three books with the title *Natural Capacities*, as well as on *Excretion of Urine, against the New Doctrine*. To this area of the science belong also the books: *The Function of the Pulse*; *The Function of Breathing*; *Whether Blood is Naturally Contained in the Arteries*; and *The Capacity of Purging Drugs*; and also what was [said][37] about the command centre of the soul and about the sources that maintain us, in *The Doctrines of Hippocrates and Plato*, in ten books. And following on from all those mentioned here are the seventeen books on *The Function of the Parts*.[38]

---

[35] The word *anatomē* may refer both to the practice of dissection and to anatomy as a study, and has been translated as either 'dissection' or 'anatomy' in different contexts, e.g. in these titles. The first and third of the works mentioned in this paragraph are lost; the second and third are preserved only in Arabic.

[36] This last work seems to be a further 'disagreement with Lycus' text; Boudon-Millot takes the last words as a repeated reference to *The Function of the Parts of the Human Body*, but it would be an oddly casual reference, and in any case the work is classified in the next section, rather than in the works of anatomy proper.

[37] There is a lacuna at this point in the Vlatadon MS, which may conceal something else.

[38] The works mentioned for the first time in this chapter are all extant, with the exception of that on urine, and of the tenth book of *The Doctrines of Hippocrates and Plato*. The conception of the 'command centre' (*hēgemonikon*), i.e. the source of voluntary motion and of the processing of perception, located in the brain, is central to Galen's psychology and physiology; see *The Doctrines of Hippocrates and Plato*, especially II.3, with n. 5. For the sense of the sources 'maintaining' (*dioikein*) the body, see *My Own Doctrines*, n. 14.

6. Necessary study preliminary to the method of healing

First in this area of the science is *The Elements according to Hippocrates*, in which it is shown that the hot, the cold, the wet and the dry are the elements common to all bodies which undergo generation and decay; or, if one uses the terms for their substances, they are earth, fire, air and water; and the elements of the human body[39]—as indeed of all blooded animals—are blood, phlegm and the two biles. Following on from *The Elements according to Hippocrates* are the three books on *Mixtures*, the third of which gives an account of mixtures in drugs. And one must join to these the eleven books on *The Capacity of Simple Drugs*. If a person wishes to read the first two books of *Mixtures*, and leave aside the treatment of the third book, as well as that of the *Simple Drugs*, and to read those later, that too is possible. After the first two books of *Mixtures* it is also admissible to read the following: *The Best Constitution of the Body*, *Good Condition* and *The Uneven Bad-Mixture*. After the reading of those mentioned so far come[40] *The Distinct Types of Disease* and *The Distinct Types of Symptom*. Following that on *The Distinct Types of Disease* is a single book teaching the causes of them; and following that on *The Distinct Types of Symptom* are three on *Causes of Symptoms*; following these, those on *Affected Places*. *The Opportune Moments in Diseases* also belongs to the category of those that precede the study[41] of therapy, as, too, are *The Distinct Types of Fever*, *Fulness*, *Unnatural Lumps*, and even *Antecedent Causes*, as well as *Containing Causes*; and *Tremor, Spasm, Convulsion and Rigor*, and the work entitled *The Art of Medicine*.[42]

7 [4]. Works of therapeutics

There is a fourteen-volume work on *The Therapeutic Method*, as well as two books on *The Therapeutic Method, to Glaucon*;[43] three ‖ on venesection, the first addressed to Erasistratus, the second to the followers of Erasistratus at Rome,

---

[39] I read *sōmatos*, ‘of the body’, for MSS *sōmata*, ‘bodies’, and earlier in the sentence *hapantōn*, ‘of all’ [bodies] for *apo tōn*, ‘from the’ [bodies], both of which emendations seem required by the sense.

[40] The passage available only in the Vlatadon MS and the Arabic version ends here.

[41] The word translated ‘study’, *pragmateia*, is also used to refer to a treatise on a subject, just as the word ‘method’ in the chapter title may have an abstract reference and a concrete one, here specifically to Galen’s *The Therapeutic Method*. The works of this chapter as a whole, then, can be understood either as necessary to read before the study of that method, or simply as before the reading of that actual book.

[42] All the works mentioned in this chapter are extant in Greek, except for *Antecedent Causes* and *Containing Causes*, which survive in Arabic and Latin.

[43] The former is Galen’s clinical *magnum opus*, the latter a shorter work which contains much of clinical interest and was used as part of an introductory course for students of medicine in late antiquity and early mediaeval times. All the works mentioned in this chapter are extant, except for

while the third is a therapeutic work composed in accordance with my own views on the subject. *Withering* is another in the category of therapeutics. There is also a very short work that I once gave to a friend, which then circulated very widely, and of which I now also have a copy, with the title: *Advice to an Epileptic Child.*

One might also place here the three-volume work on *The Capacities of Foodstuffs,* that on *The Thinning Diet* and that on *Good and Bad Humoral Fluid.* And no less part of the therapeutic œuvre are the volumes on *Erasistratus' Therapeutic Reasoning.* The work on Hippocrates' *Regimen in Acute Diseases* could be put in this category, or also in that of the commentaries on Hippocrates' works. These commentaries in fact contain a large number of observations relevant to therapeutics, as also to diagnostics and prognostics. | 32

8 [5]. The nature of the works of prognostic science[44]

First, there are three books on *Critical Days*; secondly, one should add the three on *Crises*; then the body of works on the pulse: four on *The Distinct Types of Pulse*; then the same number on *The Discernment of the Pulse*; the same number again on *Causes in the Pulse*; finally, four on *Prognosis by the Pulse*, which brings the total to sixteen. As well as these, one book was written on *The Function of the Pulse* and one on *The Pulse for Beginners.* In the context of this last work the question has been raised, why an account was not given of the pulse specific to those with fever; to which our answer was that that topic is too big a one for beginners, for it involves a long process of enquiry. This much I did say at the outset in that book, that there are two opinions among doctors, some claiming to be able to discern also the contraction of the arteries, others holding that it is indiscernible; and that we recommended that the beginner should first train himself on the basis of the easier doctrine, assuming it to be indiscernible.[45] Working within this framework, we retain the conviction that there is | no spe-   33 cific sign of fever in the pulse. But within the alternative framework, of which I have given an account in the large treatment of the subject in sixteen volumes,

Erasistratus' Therapeutic Reasoning; both a treatise and a commentary on Hippocrates' *Regimen in Acute Diseases* are extant (see further n. 55).

[44] Galen mentions here a range of works of particular importance for clinical practice (cf. his references to them in *Prognosis*, ch. 8 and ch. 13, pp. 60 and 64 below). The first two relate to the standard ancient medical view that diseases undergo a progression, the climax of which is known as the 'crisis', and that in the course of this progression there are particular moments at which medical intervention should be undertaken (or avoided). The central importance of the pulse in diagnosis and prognosis may be gathered from the other titles, which represent a major part of Galen's œuvre.

[45] Cf. *The Pulse for Beginners*, ch. 4, p. 355 below. Galen's view is that the contraction (*sustolē*) of the pulse can be detected, and used for diagnostic purposes, once one has sufficient experience and training, but that it is also legitimate, especially for beginners, to operate on the basis of its indiscernibility.

an account is given of this sign. Such enquiries are raised by those who have not learned with a teacher, but—according to the proverb—'navigate by books'. We stated right at the outset that the content of one's instruction is different in the case of beginners and in the case of those engaged in acquiring a thorough understanding of the whole subject.

I also wrote another short work giving a synopsis of the sixteen volumes. There are also eight volumes of commentary and criticism of Archigenes' major work on the pulse, separate from all these.[46] The three-volume work on *Difficulty in Breathing* may also be considered as belonging to this branch of the art.

9 [6]. Notes on Hippocrates[47]

As with my other works given to friends, so especially with the works of exegesis of Hippocratic writings, I had no expectation that they would reach a wider audience. To begin with, in fact, I wrote notes on those writings only as an exercise for myself[48]—as I did for each individual area of medical
34   science. Here, I prepared such notes for myself, | notes in which was transcribed all that Hippocrates had said of relevance to the art of medicine, [but] with the teaching made clear and fully elaborated. So, for example, I wrote specifically on *Critical Days* according to the opinions of Hippocrates, and also specifically on *Crises*, on *Difficulty in Breathing*, and on all the other subjects; and in the same way I produced *The Therapeutic Method*, in fourteen books,

---

[46] Archigenes was a doctor and medical author during the period of Trajan; his work on the pulse was probably a considerable influence on Galen's. The commentaries mentioned here are the only works in this chapter that have not survived; but Galen's extant works on the pulse contain a considerable amount of discussion of Archigenes' views, including some extracts from his work.

[47] On Galen's attitude to and use of Hippocrates, see the introduction, pp. xiv–xv, xviii–xix. 'Notes' here in the heading translates *hupomnēmata*, which has that original sense, although it came at some point to be the word regularly used for commentaries, and is sometimes used by Galen to refer to his treatises more generally. Except where further noted below, all the works on Hippocrates mentioned survive.

[48] Scholars have taken this phrase, on the basis of different emendations of the Greek text, to mean either 'I wrote notes on those writings not for distribution, but only as an exercise for myself' (Müller), 'I wrote notes on those writings as an exercise for myself' (Boudon-Millot, following the Arabic version, and followed here), or 'I never wrote notes . . . even as an exercise for myself (Singer 2019b, adopting a reading closest to that of the Greek MSS). No version is entirely unproblematic; the present one seems the least difficult, although the transition between talk of notes and talk of actual treatises (*Critical Days*, etc.) seems abrupt. On *any* account, however, it is clear that Galen claims that his major exegetical commentary activity was carried out in a later phase, whereas he had previously regarded his treatises as containing sufficient Hippocratic material in themselves. Cf. *The Order of My Own Books*, ch. 3, and for further discussion see Singer 2019b.

[containing] everything relevant to therapeutics, but also those things relating to his views.

As for word-by-word exegeses, these had already been written by many of my predecessors, and I knew their work pretty well. If I found what I considered errors in those writings, I thought it superfluous to refute them. This approach was manifest in whatever writings I gave people on request, at an earlier period, in which I seldom made remarks directed against such writers.[49]

In the first place, I did not even have those exegetical works with me in Rome, all those books in my possession having remained in Asia.[50] If, then, I remembered some particularly gross error on the part of one of them, such that anyone who believed it would suffer a severe setback in his medical practice, I would I draw attention to this; otherwise, I would confine myself to my own interpretation, without reference to the conflicting exegeses of others. The *Commentary on the Aphorisms* was written in this way, as were those on *Fractures* and on *Joints*; also those on the *Prognostic*, on *Regimen in Acute Diseases*, on *Wounds*, on *Injuries to the Head* and on book I of the *Epidemics*. 35

After I had composed the above works, I heard someone praising a false interpretation of one of the Aphorisms. From that point on, whenever I gave one of these works to anybody, it was composed with an eye to general distribution, not just to the specific level of attainment of the actual recipients.[51] In this category are: the commentaries on books II, III and VI of the *Epidemics*; then also those on *Humours*,[52] on *Nutrition*, on the *Prorrhetic*, on *The Nature of the Human Being* and on *In the Surgery*, as well as that on *Airs, Waters, Places*

---

[49] Though, as already suggested, Galen's account of the process by which he actually began to write (what became) the Hippocratic commentaries is somewhat obscure, what seems to be mentioned here is a process of writing up or dictating previously given lectures on a subject, at the request of an individual; one may compare the account of such a process in relation to Aristotle, in ch. 14 below.

[50] It seems unclear whether 'in the first place' (*tēn archēn*) should be taken temporally, or idiomatically, intensifying 'not even'. (Such an emphatic sense of the phrase is idiomatic in Greek, and indeed quite frequent in Galen.) If—as scholars have universally taken it—Galen is referring to an earlier phase of his commentary activity during which he did not have access to the works of previous commentators, and a later one during which he did, then he does not, as one would expect, specify in what follows the moment at which he is reunited with these works. Nor does such a distinction between earlier commentaries which make more detailed reference to other commentators, and later ones which make less such reference, seem to be borne out by the actual content of his commentaries.

[51] Again, previous scholarship has formed a misleading conclusion from these remarks, building on their basis a binary distinction between 'private' and 'public' commentaries. The claim Galen here makes, rather, is that he is in all cases writing such works *for individuals*, but that after a certain point he does so also 'with an eye to' their more general distribution—of which, however, he still claims not to be the instigator. A much more complex and nuanced account of the phases of his own Hippocratic compositions—but still insisting that all were written originally for friends or students—is given in Galen's commentary on *Epidemics* III; see again Singer 2019b.

[52] Although we possess a commentary on the *Humours* under Galen's name, it has been shown to be a Renaissance forgery.

(which I claim should be entitled rather *Habitations, Waters, Seasons and Lands*).[53]

The commentary on the *Aphorisms* is in seven volumes; that on *Fractures* in three; there are | four on *Joints*; three on the *Prognostic*; three on the genuine part of *Regimen in Acute Diseases* and two on the parts that were added to that text subsequently. I devoted one book of commentary each to *Wounds* and to *Injuries to the Head*; three to both the first and the third book of the *Epidemics*; six to the second book of *Epidemics* and eight to the sixth. On *Humours* I wrote three volumes, and the same number on the *Prorrhetic*, on *In the Surgery* and on *Airs, Waters, Places*; four on *Nutrition*, two on *The Nature of the Human Being*.

After the composition of this last commentary, I heard certain individuals attack that particular work as inauthentic; and so I wrote three more volumes, entitled *The Manifest Consistency of Hippocrates' Views Between 'The Nature of the Human Being' and His Other Writings*.[54] Also relevant to Hippocrates are: *Hippocrates on | Regimen in Acute Diseases*;[55] the *Glossary* of his terminology; the work addressed *To Lycus*, concerning the Aphorism which begins: 'Things growing have the most innate heat'; that *To Julianus*, the Methodist, on his criticisms of the Hippocratic *Aphorisms*. There is one other very short work which is also relevant to Hippocrates, in which I show definitively that *The Best Doctor is Also a Philosopher*. (The work appears also with the shorter title: *Galen's Hippocrates*.)

10 [7]. Works expressing differences with Erasistratus[56]

I have written three volumes of notes on book I of his *Fevers*; there are notes on the third book in the form of the first part of my treatise on Erasistratus' therapeutics. This treatise is entitled *Erasistratus' Therapeutic Reasoning*, and fills five volumes. There are also three volumes on *Erasistratus' Anatomy* and two on his venesection—one addressed to Erasistratus himself and the other to his followers at Rome. Also relevant | to Erasistratus is the work in which we investigate *Whether the Arteries Naturally Contain Blood*, as also that on *The Function of*

---

[53] This work is of particular importance to Galen for the support he finds in it for the humoral interpretation of individual bodily constitutions and environmental effects on them (see also *The Soul's Dependence on the Body*, ch. 8, pp. 446–9 below); Galen's commentary on it survives only in Arabic and in some Hebrew fragments. *The Nature of the Human Being*, in Galen's particular interpretation of it, is also central to his construction of Hippocrates; see further *The Elements according to Hippocrates*, esp. ch. 3.

[54] This work, mentioned also in *The Soul's Dependence on the Body*, does not survive.

[55] This work (distinct from the actual commentary on Hippocrates' work of this title, already mentioned) survives in an Arabic version, while the Greek work transmitted to us under that title is inauthentic. The *Glossary* and the remaining works mentioned in this paragraph are extant.

[56] Of the works mentioned in this chapter, those on venesection survive, as well as those that follow them.

Breathing, as well as the three volumes of *Natural Capacities*, which contain a critique of all that Erasistratus wrote on natural activities in his *General Discussions*.

11 [8]. Works relevant to Asclepiades

Eight volumes entitled *The Doctrines of Asclepiades*, and another short one with the title, *Asclepiades on the Substance of the Soul*.[57]

12 [9]. Works expressing differences with the Empiric doctors

Five volumes of notes on Theodas' *Introduction*; eleven on Menodotus' work *To Severus*; two on Serapion's work *Against the Sects*; *Outlines of Empiricism*; *Medical Experience*; three volumes on *Disagreement Amongst the Empirics*; *Against the Objections Raised to 'Disagreement Amongst the Empirics'*; three volumes on Theodas' *Summary*; an *Exhortation to Medicine*, related to Menodotus' work to Severus;[58] *Synopsis of the works of Heraclides* and seven volumes on *The Empirical Sect*.

13 [10]. Works expressing differences with the Methodists

Six volumes on *The Methodist Sect*; <two *Against Julianus' Objections to my Book on Sects*>; *Against Julianus' Criticisms of Hippocratic Aphorisms*.[59] | 39

14 [11]. Works useful for demonstrations

In disputes I had always observed how everyone makes the claim that he is engaged in performing demonstrations and seeks earnestly to refute his interlocutors. With this in mind I was eager to learn the science of demonstration, first of all things; and I desired the philosophers (who were reputed to be able to teach it) to put aside for the moment any other subject taught within the logical

[57] The works listed have not survived.
[58] The text relating to this title is uncertain; it is possible (as argued by Boudon 2002) that the work mentioned is that otherwise known to us as *An Exhortation to Study the Arts*, the lost second half of which, devoted explicitly to medicine, may have included material engaging directly with Menodotus. Apart from the first half of this work (if it is indeed the same), the *Outlines of Empiricism* (extant in a Latin translation) and *Medical Experience* (extant in Arabic), none of the works mentioned in this chapter survives.
[59] Only this last work, already mentioned above, has survived.

section of philosophy, if they could only ease the pang of my passion for demonstration. I wanted them to teach me the nature of that method which gives him who learns it the power to discern accurately whether a self-proclaimed 'demonstration' really is one, or whether, like some counterfeit coin, it appears similar to the genuine one while being in fact false; and enables him, also, in any field of enquiry, to use a particular way of proceeding in order to arrive at the discovery of the truth.

So I went to all the well-known Stoic and Peripatetic philosophers of the time; but while I learned many pieces of logical theory from them which, when I looked into them over a period of time subsequently, I found to be quite use-
40 less for the purpose of demonstration, I learned very few that they | had researched in any useful manner and which tended to lead to the goal in question. I found, additionally, that these pieces of logical theory were actually in conflict with each other, while some were even in conflict with our natural intuitions. Well, if I had had nothing but these teachers alone, I too would have succumbed to a Pyrrhonian despair of knowledge;[60] but I also had a grasp of the teachings of geometry, mathematics and arithmetic, in which subjects I had attained a very high level, having been educated in them from very early days by my father, who had himself had the science passed on to him from my grandfather and great-grandfather.

I had, however, observed the truths manifestly apparent in predictions of eclipses, as well as in the construction of sundials and water-clocks,[61] and in all sorts of other calculations made in the context of architecture; and so I thought that it would be better to employ the model of the geometrical demonstration. Indeed, I used to find that even the philosophers themselves, and those most versed in dialectic, although they would be in conflict not only with each other but even with themselves, nevertheless all bestowed equal praise on the geometrical proof. For this reason I realized yet more clearly that I must steer clear of the arguments of these people, and follow the pattern of the geometrical demonstration. (When I speak of philosophers in conflict with each other in
41 the | science of logic, by the way, I mean the Peripatetics, Stoics and Platonists; by 'in conflict with themselves' I refer to the differences *within* each sect; here the conflict among Peripatetics is comparatively small, while that within the Stoic and Platonist sects is very large.)

Now, to those who wish to train themselves in geometrical-style demonstrations, I suggest that they first get themselves educated in those, and then read

[60] Or 'perplexity', *aporia*: the term, common in philosophical Greek, refers to a logical or mental difficulty from which it seems impossible to extricate oneself; the Pyrrhonians or Sceptics, on the other hand, advanced arguments deliberately aimed at bringing about such a state (cf. *The Best Method of Instruction*).
[61] Further on these sundials and water-clocks, and their epistemological importance in Galen's view, see *Affections and Errors* II.5, pp. 488–90 below.

my work on *Demonstration*,[62] composed in fifteen volumes. I also wrote a large number of other works purely as a personal exercise; of these some were lost in the fire which consumed the Temple of Peace, others were given to friends and are now extant in many private collections, as is the case with my other works.

However, I also subsequently regained possession, via some third party, of those notes that had either been given by me to friends or stolen and distributed by members of my domestic staff. Among these are three volumes on Aristotle's *Interpretation*; four on the first of his books on syllogisms and the same number on the second. These texts are now l almost universally given the title *Prior Analytics*, while those on demonstration are given the title *Posterior Analytics*. But Aristotle himself refers to the former as his works 'on syllogism', and to the latter as 'on demonstration'. There are extant notes by me on the latter work too: six volumes on the first book, five on the second. 42

None of these sets of notes was written with a view to distribution; nor were the six volumes on Theophrastus' work on *Affirmation and Denial*; while that on Eudemus' work on *Language* was composed earlier at the request of friends. As for Aristotle's *The Ten Categories*, I had not at this stage either written any such work for myself, nor given one to others; and so when, at a later time, a student asked to have some notes of what he had heard on that work, regarding the solution of the questions posed in it, I wrote one, with the firm instruction that he should only show these notes to those who had already read the text with a teacher, or at least had some previous introduction from other works of commentary, such as those of l Adrastus and Aspasius.[63] 43

Even as a boy, when I was first sent by my father to study with someone who taught the logical theory of Chrysippus and the other famous Stoics, I wrote some notes for myself on Chrysippus' books of syllogistic; these were left behind in Pergamum along with a lot of other notes that I had made in my youth, but were handed out by a household servant to someone who asked for them, and later made public by those into whose possession they had passed.

Then there are a number of works composed after *Demonstration* which give a more expansive treatment of the matters covered concisely in that work: one volume on *What is Necessary for the Purposes of Demonstration*; one on *The Omission of Premisses in the Statement of Demonstrations*; one on *Premisses of Equal Weight*; one on *Demonstrations with 'Because'*; one on *The Number of Syllogisms*; two on *Example*; one on *Induction*; one on *The Probable*;[64] three on *Similarity*; one on *What is Meant by the Terminology of Genus and Species and*

---

[62] This major work of Galen's, to which he often refers, has survived only in fragments. None of the other works mentioned in this chapter has survived, with the exception of *The Best Method of Instruction, to Favorinus* (see below, pp. 117–22).

[63] Important commentators on Aristotle, and older contemporaries of Galen. See *Affections and Errors* I.8, p. 474 below, for Galen's own contact with a pupil of Aspasius.

[64] Or possibly on *Images* (following the MS reading, of which 'the probable' is an emendation).

44 *by Terms Used in Conjunction with Them in Ordinary Speech;* | one on *The Possible*; three volumes on *Words Used in More Than One Sense*; one on *The General and the Specific in the Arts*; one on *Arguments Which Undermine Themselves*; one on *Admissible Premises*; one on *Mixed Premises and Syllogisms*; one on *How to Distinguish the Enquiry of Practical Importance from the Verbal and Semantic*; one on *Clitomachus and the Solutions of his Demonstration*;[65] two on *The Shared Principle of Reason; The Best Method of Instruction, to Favorinus*; one *For Epictetus, against Favorinus*; <and another on *Teaching for Money;*> *The Function of Syllogisms*; two volumes on *The Function of Considerations Relative to Syllogisms*; one on *The Best Sect*; three on *Correctness of Terms; All Existents are Both One and Many*; one showing that *It is Impossible that One and the Same Thing Follows of Necessity from Opposed Propositions*; one on *Discovery by Demonstration*;[66] nine on *The Capacity and Science of Logic*; <one on *The Debate Concerning the Comprehension of Objects*>; dialogues with <a man who does not regard the science of the philosopher as a science>; a specific work regarding *The Common Conceptions*; one *Against Those Who*
45 *Interpret Words Maliciously*;[67] | three on *The Constitution of Arts*;[67] a one-volume *Summary of the Theory of Demonstration; Judgement Between Conflicts in Doctrines*; one showing that *The Quantity is Inseparable from the First Substance*; one on the *Demonstration per Impossibile*; one on *Things that Come to Be for a Purpose; The Enquiry Concerning Word and Meaning.*

15 [12].[68]

My opinions on questions of ethical philosophy have been stated in the following works: on *The Diagnosis of the Affections and Errors of Each Individual*, in two volumes; on *Character Traits*, in four volumes; *Against Favorinus on Socrates*;[69] one volume on *Freedom from Distress*; one on *The Goal according to Philosophy*; one on *The Relationship to his Hearers of One Making Public*

---

[65] Clitomachus (second century BC) was a Sceptical Academic, pupil and successor of Carneades; his 'demonstration' was presumably Sceptical in nature.

[66] Or on *The Demonstrative Sect*, but the Arabic text, offering 'discovery' in place of 'sect', seems clearly preferable. (The Arabic text gives the same substitution above, in the title *The Best Sect*, where, however, I have preferred the reading of the Greek manuscripts.)

[67] We possess one work by Galen *To Patrophilus, on the Constitution of the Art of Medicine*; but in *The Art of Medicine* he also mentions two other volumes that existed alongside this. With the exception of *The Best Method of Instruction*, and the arguable exception of this work, none of those listed in this chapter has survived.

[68] This chapter lacks a title in the manuscripts, although this could be supplied readily enough from the first sentence. Of the works mentioned, only the first (translated in this volume as *Affections and Errors of the Soul*), the second (but only in the form of an Arabic epitome, translated in Singer 2013) and the fourth (see above, pp. 3–15) survive.

[69] Scholars have variously interpreted this title as referring to a defence of Socrates against Favorinus or to a refutation of a work by Favorinus (for which there is some independent evidence) on 'Socrates on the art of love'.

Demonstrations; one on *People Who Read Surreptitiously*;[70] one on *To Make the Punishment Fit the Crime*; <one on *Laziness*;> one on *Consolation*; one on *The Discourse with Bacchides and Cyrus in the Villa of Menarchus*;[71] one on | *Interaction within Dialogues*; one *To Orators in the Forum*; one on *Pleasure and   46 Pain*; one on *What Follows from Each Chosen Aim in Life*; one on *Things Said in Public to the Adherents of Sects*; <on *The Epicureans*;> one on *Agreement*; two on *The Sense of Shame*; two on *Things Said in Public Against Flatterers*; a work on *Slander*, which also contains autobiographical material; seven *Temporal Accounts*[72] in one volume; <one on *Arguments Taken from Books*;> one on *Public Statements Made in the Reign of Pertinax*;[73] *To What Extent the Esteem and Opinion of the Public is to be Taken into Account*; *The Making of Wills.*

16 [13]. Works concerning the philosophy of Plato

One book on *The Platonist Sect*; notes on *The Medical Statements in the Timaeus*, in four volumes;[74] *To Those Whose Opinion on <Logical Theory> differs from that of Plato*, in three; on *Plato's Logical Theory*; eight volumes of summary of Plato's dialogues; one on *Analogical Procedures*[75] in the *Philebus*; three on *The Parts and Capacities of the Soul*; *The Capacities of the Soul Depend on the Mixtures of the Body*; *The Doctrines of Hippocrates and Plato*. | 47

17 [14]. Works concerning the philosophy of Aristotle

Three volumes of notes on *Interpretation*; four on the first book of the *Prior Analytics*, and four on the second; six on the first book of the *Posterior Analytics*, and five on the second; four on *The Ten Categories*; six on Theophrastus' *Affirmation and Denial*; three on the work on *The Number of Different Senses*; on *The First Mover is Itself Unmoved*; three on Eudemus' work on *Language*; one on *Demonstrations with 'Because'*; one on *Admissible Premises and Syllogisms*; one on *Mixed Premises and Syllogisms*; on *Linguistic Sophisms*.[76]

---

[70] The sense of this title is far from clear, but the most likely reference may be to the practice of 'passing works off as one's own', mentioned by Galen earlier in the text.

[71] The identity of these speakers (and even whether they appear in the correct form—'Marcus', or even 'the monarch' are other conjectured forms for the last name) is unknown.

[72] This title is again quite obscure.

[73] The emperor Pertinax reigned for the first three months of 193 after the death of Commodus.

[74] Apart from this work, which survives in fragmentary form, mainly through Arabic testimonia, only the last two books mentioned in this chapter survive.

[75] Or possibly 'transitions'; Galen presumably offered some account of the dialectical procedures in the dialogue

[76] This is the only surviving work amongst those listed in this chapter.

18 [15]. Works expressing differences
with the philosophy of the Stoics[77]

Three on *Logical Theory according to Chrysippus*; a three-volume *Commentary on Chrysippus' 'First Syllogistic'*, with one volume on his *Second Syllogistic*; seven on *The Power and Theory of Logic*; one volume demonstrating that *Analytical Geometry is Better than that of the Stoics*; two books on *The Function of Theoretical Considerations Relevant to Syllogisms.* |

19 [16]. Works concerning the philosophy of Epicurus

Two on *The Happy, Blessed Life according to Epicurus*; <one book on *Epicurus' Treatment of Dreaming*; one on *The Goal of Life according to Epicurus*;> *Epicurus' View of the Inflaming Pleasure*; one arguing that *The Causes that Produce Pleasure Are Inadequately Described by Epicurus*; on *The Hedonist Sect*; one discussing *Whether the Study of Natural Science is Useful for Ethical Philosophy*; on Metrodorus' nine volumes *To the Sophists*; a *Letter to Celsus the Epicurean*; a *Letter Relating to Pudentianus the Epicurean*.

20 [17]. Works of interest to both scholars and orators[78]

A forty-eight-book dictionary of words used by the Attic prose-writers;[79] three volumes on *Everyday Words in Eupolis*; five on *Everyday Words in Aristophanes*; two on *Everyday Words in Cratinus*; one of *Examples of Words Specific to the Writers of Comedy*; *Whether the Texts of Ancient Comedy are a Worthwhile Part of the Educational Curriculum*; six volumes *To Those who Criticize Linguistic Solecisms*; one on *False Atticisms*; *Clarity and Unclarity*; one volume on *Whether the Same Person can be a Critic and a Scholar*.

---

[77] None of the works in chs. 18–20 survives (although on the books on words from Attic prose and comedy mentioned at the beginning of ch. 20, see now *Freedom from Distress*, §20).

[78] 'Scholars' translates *grammatikoi*; see n. 4 above.

[79] This book, and the following ones on words from comedy, are described also in *Freedom from Distress* (23–8), where the former is said still to survive while the latter were lost in the fire. There is MS variation here on the number of books attributed to it, but the figure of forty-eight is consistent with both that work and *The Order of My Own Books*; on the question of length cf. *Freedom from Distress*, n. 16.

The Order of My Own Books

As with the previous text, considerable improvements were introduced through the discovery of the Vlatadon manuscript, including the restoration of a passage previously missing; see nn. 9 and 17 below.

Greek title: Περὶ τῆς τάξεως τῶν ἰδίων βιβλίων (*Peri tēs taxeōs tōn idiōn bibliōn*)
Kühn: XIX.49–61
Editions: Müller 1891; Boudon-Millot 2007 (with French translation)

1. You were quite right, Eugenianus, to suggest the need for some book which XIX.49 would explain the order of my writings; for they do not all have the same aim, function or scope. As you know, some were written at the request of friends, and are geared purely to their particular level; others were dictated for young beginners. In ǀ neither case was it my intention that they should be 50 handed on or preserved for posterity, since I had observed that even books written in previous ages are appreciated by a very small number of individuals. Doctors and philosophers form admirations for other doctors or philosophers without having learned their teachings, and without cultivating that demonstrative science which would enable them to sort false arguments from true ones. It is just that their father, or teacher, or friend—or some person who gained admiration in their city—happened to be an Empiric, or Dogmatic, or Methodist. So too with the different philosophical sects: there used to be a variety of reasons why one man became a Platonist, another a Peripatetic, or Stoic, or Epicurean; but now, just as there are chairs in each philosophical sect,[1] so too many people simply call themselves after the sect in which they were brought up—especially people who cannot think of any other basis for their life.

Convinced as I was that even if the Muses themselves were to write a book it would still not win more renown than the ǀ outpourings of complete imbeciles, 51 I never had any desire that any writing of mine be publicly circulated. Since, however, as you know, they were widely disseminated against my wishes, I became extremely hesitant to give any further written versions of my work to friends. For this reason I felt compelled to write a book on *The Best Sect*[2]—not the sort

---

[1] The term translated 'chairs' (*diadochai*) may also refer, more generally, to the 'succession' to headship that took place within each philosophical school; but it seems likely that Galen has in mind the establishment, by Marcus Aurelius, of official chairs in each of the four main schools, which further institutionalized their separate status.

[2] Although we possess a work of this title in the Galenic corpus, it is thought to be spurious.

of book that many doctors and philosophers had written previously, in which they praise their own sect by name, but one by which I indicated the actual way—the only way—in which the best sect should be constituted, in medicine or in any other specialized skill. In that work I stated and demonstrated the above proposition, that in order to become a reliable judge of sects one must first gain an understanding of demonstration. This requirement, however, is not sufficient on its own: it is also necessary to free oneself from the sort of affection which frequently causes the blind love or hatred of a sect; only one devoid of such affection, who is also willing to employ the scientific method so as to find 52   the truth for himself, or to judge the statements of others, | will be in a position to discover the best sect.

You will yourself be aware that the majority of doctors and philosophers, when it is proved against them that they do, indeed, have no training in the method of demonstration, proceed to adopt a quite opposite course. They either claim that there is actually no such thing as logical demonstration, or say that there is indeed such a thing, but that its nature is such as to be known by every- one, and therefore requires no process of learning or training. Against such an extreme of stupidity there can be no argument. And yet one of these individuals—they have an extraordinary confidence in their competence to pronounce on matters of which they are ignorant—will say, doubtless, that *I* am the arrogant one. Well, to escape such epithets, and to avoid having to return them to others, I had resolved to distribute none of my books. But those books which I had given to friends had become more widely disseminated; and it was because of them that I was compelled to write also on *The Best Sect* (the reason for its composition is stated in the work itself). One who wishes to read this material first of all will do well; if, further, he is persuaded by its arguments so 53   far as to wish to become an adept in demonstration, | before turning to the study and evaluation of all the sects, he has available to him my major treat- ment of the subject, *Demonstration*; and if he not only learns the methods set out there, but also schools himself in them, he will find out the truth in any subject of enquiry—if, that is, he is a lover of truth, not one to accept an opin- ion through some non-rational affection, like the supporters of different col- ours at the races.[3] Such a person, then, having recourse to the stated forms of argument, will find out the difference between what is truly known on the basis of them and what is falsely assumed.

2. This, then, is one starting-point in the reading of my writings; and it is for all those who are naturally intelligent and devoted to the truth. Even without this, however, someone who has put me, personally, to the test in respect of the entire conduct of my life and practice of my art; who realizes that the character of my

---

[3] The reference is to the extremely popular sport of chariot racing, in which the different teams were designated by the colours red, blue, white and green.

soul is such that all my actions are performed without enmity, competitiveness or non-rational love of any sect; who realizes, further, that the realities of the art in practice confirm the truth of my views ǀ —such a person will be able to derive 54 benefit from my writings even without the science of demonstration, but only inasmuch as he acquires correct opinion, not that accurate knowledge of the facts which is only available to those versed in demonstration. (Correct opinion was fairly characterized by the ancients as equal in value to knowledge in the practical context, but lacking the stable, secure nature of the latter.)[4]

This kind of person, then, will start by reading my works for beginners: that on sects (which is actually entitled *Sects for Beginners*); that on the pulse (similarly entitled); and thirdly, *Bones for Beginners*, which constitutes the first stage in my study of anatomy. One who wishes to undertake the whole of that study should begin with *Anatomical Procedures*: this work gives instruction in the parts of the body that are seen in dissection, in respect of their size, position, shaping, combination, colour and relationship with each other. One who ǀ has 55 been schooled in the observation of these parts in dissections will next learn their activities: those 'of nature', which have been treated in three volumes entitled *Natural Capacities*, and those which are known as 'the soul's', in several more. Preceding these is *The Dissection of Cadavers*, which is followed by two others on *The Dissection of Living Bodies*, and two more, on *Conflict in Anatomy*.[5] After these come the three books on *The Motion of the Chest and Lungs*; two on *Causes of Breathing*, and after those four books on *The Voice*. The books on *The Motion of the Muscles* belong to this field too[6] [...] and a demonstration was given concerning terminology.

The actual demonstration regarding the elements does not appear in full in that work [sc. *The Elements according to Hippocrates*], which confines itself rather to that part of it which was used by Hippocrates; to perfect one's understanding of the elements of the body one should turn to the relevant material in the thirteenth book on *Demonstration* and in the fifth and sixth books on *The Doctrines of Asclepiades*. Certain matters regarding the power of purgative drugs appear in ǀ *The Elements according to Hippocrates*, too, even though that 56 subject is treated monographically elsewhere. *The Elements according to*

---

[4] The distinction between 'knowledge' (*epistēmē*) and 'correct opinion' (*orthē doxa*) is Platonic in origin.

[5] See *My Own Books*, n. 35.

[6] For Galen's works on anatomy, see also *My Own Books*, chs. 2–5. Galen's presentation in the present text is confusing, as he moves from anatomy to capacities, then jumps back to mention four 'preceding' works of anatomy before proceeding to works which can be regarded as relating to capacities 'of soul'; compare *My Own Books*, ch. 5. There is also something missing in the MSS at this point; at the beginning of the next paragraph (as we have it), Galen is clearly already referring to *The Elements according to Hippocrates*. Before that, he doubtless mentioned a number of other works relevant to 'capacities' (again, cf. *My Own Books*, chs. 5–6). While Müller attempted an excessively confident reconstruction of the missing material, it seems overwhelmingly likely that, at least, both *The Doctrines of Hippocrates and Plato* and *The Function of the Parts* were mentioned here.

Hippocrates is followed by three volumes on *Mixtures*; and these by the major work on *The Capacity of Simple Drugs*; which in turn is followed by that on *The Composition of Drugs.*[7]

Now, the first books of *Mixtures* cover mixtures in animals, along with the specific indicators of each, while the third book contains a discussion of mixture in drugs. The correct order, then, is to read either the first two, or all three, books of *Mixtures*, followed by *The Best Constitution of Our Bodies, Good Condition* and *The Uneven Bad-Mixture*. These are three very short works dictated for friends at their request and later distributed by them—since, indeed, their function is contained in our treatise on *Health*,[8] where the different kinds of bodily constitution[9] have been described for all people; and it has been shown how each is to be preserved in health. After this comes another major work, on *The Therapeutic Method*. Now, all the above-mentioned works precede those two treatises; so, too, do the book on *The Distinct Types of Disease*, that on *The Distinct Types of Symptom* and yet a third, covering *Causes of Diseases*, as well as three more on *Causes of Symptoms*. So, all these precede *The Therapeutic Method*; and in addition to these also that on *Unnatural Lumps* and on *Fulness*, and the treatise on *The Distinct Types of Fever*. Now, these are necessary; but the same point applies here as in the case of the anatomical works, where I stated that some had been written as additional contributions. There are two specific works on therapeutics that were given to the philosopher Glaucon; another on *Venesection*; and in fact the work on *Antecedent Causes*, and that on *Containing Causes*, are both additional contributions. Certain other works are for the refutation of particular opinions, such as that on *Excretion of Urine, against the New Doctrine*. For when the false opinions have been refuted, the account of the true ones acquires a stronger foundation. Of this kind, too, is the work on *The Doctrines of Asclepiades*, and that on *The Methodist Sect*, as well as all that was written concerning the Empiricist method of the Empiric doctors. But as for those who come to my other treatises through first of all reading my treatise on *Demonstration*—for these people the first book of those entitled *The*

---

[7] *The Doctrines of Asclepiades* has not survived. The last two titles here refer respectively to the *magnum opus* on 'simples' and the work on 'compounds' or drug recipes, later divided into two treatises *The Composition of Drugs by Kind* and *The Composition of Drugs by Place*. The mention of this work on compounds here is puzzling in view both of its probable late date in Galen's output and of its absence from the supposedly later *My Own Books*, and is one of the features that suggests caution in assigning a clear date to either of the auto-bibliographical treatises.

[8] Galen's major treatise on lifestyle recommendations (diet, exercise, nurture, environment) for the maintenance of health. The work is intended for a non-specialist readership rather than for fellow doctors or medical students, as is perhaps emphasized by the word *pasin* ('for all people'), and thus in a sense stands outside the core curriculum of his works. Again (compare n. 7) the mention of the work, which may well be a late one, here and not in *My Own Books* seems odd, and may be due to a later updating.

[9] Directly after this word begins the passage attested only by the Vlatadon MS and by the Arabic tradition, but absent from the Ambrosianus manuscript and therefore from previous editions and translations of the work.

Constitution of the Arts[10] will be useful; and still more, another book following that one, entitled *Patrophilus, on the Constitution of the Art of Medicine.* *Thrasybulus* belongs to this category too—a work in which we consider the question, whether healthiness is a part of medicine or of athletic training.[11] But for all persons, whatever their starting-point in the study of the art of medicine, the book which we have entitled *The Art of Medicine* will be useful, since it contains the chief points of the art.

In addition to all the above-mentioned, there are other books belonging to the so-called 'semiotic' part of the art, which is divided into two branches: one involving diagnosis of the present state, the other involving prognosis of that which is going to obtain. The two overlap in many respects, and have a joint written exposition, sometimes also with the indication of what has been suffered in the past: addressed to this entire part of the art are the treatises we have written on *Critical Days* and on *Crises*, and, following on from and additional to these, that on *The Pulse*. This last itself has four parts: one, on *The Distinct Types of Pulse*; a second on *The Discernment*[12] *of the Pulse*; a third, entitled on *Causes in the Pulse*, and indeed a fourth, on *Prognosis by the Pulse*. [...][13] what we heard about the writers; when certain people had given a reading of a work of mine, he then sent it to be corrected; but at some point later my friend was away abroad, so that not only this work, but certain other similar writings, came to be quite widely circulated. For this reason it will be necessary for me to write another book, containing both an account and [...] of our own writings, and an indication of the chief points. For they are all consistent with each other, but they differ as to whether they are aimed at all those who are likely to read them, or written only for those who have received them directly from me.[14] It is, I suppose, natural also that the manner of expression will be better in those in the former class. And the manner of the demonstrations is useful in all; but that in those which I wrote meticulously follows the demonstrative methods precisely in all respects, while [it is different in the case of] works aimed at particular audiences, as it is with also in the case of some that came about on a particular occasion, with me dictating [..., or with some which] were given to

---

[10] See *My Own Books*, n. 67.

[11] By 'healthiness' (*to hugieinon*) is meant the art of health preservation through lifestyle recommendations—the subject matter dealt with much more fully in *Health*, as mentioned above. *Thrasybulus* is a dialectical and rhetorical work, aimed at proving the logical status of 'healthiness' as part of the medical art, and at attacking the claims of the rival expertise of athletic or sports trainers.

[12] *Diagnōsis* refers to a sensory and intellectual process of distinguishing or identifying different bodily phenomena, and categorizing them correctly, on the basis of the relevant criteria or signs, and is often better so translated than as 'diagnosis'.

[13] The beginning of this sentence is missing from the MSS.

[14] The Greek phrasing is confusing here, the literal translation being 'in those written by me for him' (*autōi*); but it seems that Galen must mean that his form of expression is clearer in those works for which he expects a wider readership.

servants.[15] Well, that is enough on these matters; I shall next proceed to speak about the notes written by us in interpretation of some of Hippocrates' writings.

3. Now, the most necessary points in his works relevant to the various functions of the art I have expounded in the above-mentioned treatises:[16] anatomical matters, in that which I dictated on *The Anatomy of Hippocrates*; similarly, on *Critical Days*, as also indeed on *Crises* and, in *The Elements according to Hippocrates*, the most essential points on the nature of the human being; and his statements on difficulty in breathing in my writings on *Difficulty in Breathing*. In the other treatises, similarly, there are the things that belong to each individual area; so that, after an acquaintance with my books, a person might be able to go directly to the books of Hippocrates—assuming that person to be both intelligent and educated in the fundamental studies—without recourse to those who have written commentaries on him; or, if not, at least with their help. It will be easy to carry out an evaluation[17] of the correctness or incorrectness of the interpretations for one who has first schooled himself in our treatises.

57 | For some of Hippocrates' works, you will find commentaries by me, too; and since these have already been written, I shall attempt to add the rest. Well, this may come to pass, if only I live. If I die before commenting on the most important treatises of Hippocrates, those who wish to know his opinions may consult my major works, as has been stated above, as well as those commentaries so far completed; and also, among previous Hippocratic commentators, the works of my teacher Pelops and, if by any chance they can get hold of them, those of Numisianus (very few have survived); in addition, the works of Sabinus and of Rufus of Ephesus. But Quintus and his pupils have not understood Hippocrates correctly, and therefore make many mistakes in interpretation; Lycus, meanwhile, actually criticizes Hippocrates, and accuses the man of errors without understanding his views. But the works of Lycus have become very widely known.[18]

Now, my teacher, Satyrus—I studied with him before moving on to Pelops—
58 did not offer the same interpretations of Hippocratic | texts as Lycus; and it is generally agreed that Satyrus preserves the doctrines of Quintus most accurately, without adding to or removing from them. Aeficianus, on the other hand,

---

[15] The sentence is lacunose, and it is impossible to recover the precise sense. The lacunae are shown by ellipses or by phrases in square brackets, which aim to provide the probable sense, at least in outline.

[16] Cf. *My Own Books*, ch. 9 with n. 48, for a similar account of the transition, or elision of categories, between medical treatises and commentaries on Hippocrates.

[17] After this word ends the lacuna in the Ambrosianus MS, and thus the section supplied on the basis of the Vlatadon and Arabic MSS alone.

[18] There may be a word missing here, in which case we should perhaps rather read 'clearly discredited' (or some other passive verb attached to 'clearly').

even gave them a somewhat Stoic slant. I had the two different experiences of, first, hearing Quintus' interpretations from Satyrus and then, sometime later, reading some of Lycus' works; and I convicted both of having misinterpreted Hippocrates' opinions. The followers of Sabinus and Rufus had a better understanding; but anyone with a preliminary schooling in my writings will have the capacity to evaluate their works too, and find out their correct statements as well as any blunders they may have made.

4. Enough, then, on Hippocratic commentaries. Let us turn to the remainder of my writings that belong to the study of logic. Among these, Eugenianus, the books on *Demonstration* should be sufficient for you, and for anyone whose only interest is medical; those who wish to spend their time on philosophy should read the other works also—unless of course the person in question is able to | do justice to both studies, that of medicine and that of philosophy. Such 59 a person, however, would have to be endowed with a sharp intellect, a good memory and a desire for hard work; and in addition to this he would have to have had the same good fortune as I did in the education I received from my father. My father brought me to a knowledge of mathematics, logic and language,[19] rearing me in the study of these subjects as well as the others necessary to the education of the young. In my fifteenth year he steered me towards the study of dialectic, with a view to my concentrating entirely on philosophy; in my seventeenth he was persuaded by clear dreams to have me train in medicine at the same time as philosophy. And yet even with this great good fortune, and the fact that I was able to learn whatever I was taught thoroughly and more quickly than anyone else, I would still have gained very little understanding if I had not devoted my whole life to the cultivation of medical and philosophical studies. Nor, indeed, is it any wonder that the great majority of people who do cultivate these studies do no good in either: they either lack the right natural endowments or the appropriate education— | or else they abandon these 60 disciplines and get sidetracked by political activity. Well, let that conclude this digression, which is in fact very much to the point.

My books of philosophical study, then, are to be read after the treatise on *Demonstration*; the nature and number of their arguments is given within each work, but will also be laid out clearly in the writing in which I will give a complete list of my books.

5. Now, you have also heard from me about my major work in which the terms used by Attic prose-writers have been collected and listed in alphabetical order. It will be well to repeat here the answer that I made you previously; for it is quite evident that others, too, are interested to know its purpose. I do not share

---

[19] *Grammatikē* refers to the field of study taught by a *grammatikos* (cf. *My Own Books*, n. 4), and included not just grammar but also linguistic and literary analysis.

the opinion of some of today's writers, who demand universal Atticism in language,[20] irrespective of whether a person is a doctor, a philosopher, a geometer, a musician, a lawyer, or indeed none of the above, but merely a gentleman of means, or for that matter just reasonably well-off. On the contrary, I consider
61 it wrong to | give blame or censure to those who commit solecisms. For solecism and barbarism of life are much worse than those of mere language. And I once wrote a treatise against those who censure the perpetrators of linguistic solecisms—so far am I from considering Atticism a part of correct education. It was because of the fact that many doctors and philosophers in their writings lay down new meanings for Greek terms, while actually criticizing the usage of others—this was why I undertook this work on vocabulary, too, making a selection from the Attic prose-writers which extends to forty-eight books.[21] I also made such a selection from the comic poets. The work is, as I have explained, written for the sake of the actual objects signified; at the same time, the reader automatically gains a knowledge of the Attic use of terms, though this is of no great value in itself. It was, however, on account of the those who use words badly that I composed another work, on their correct usage—a work, in fact, which would be best read first of all.

[20] Atticism was the linguistic or literary trend to keep (in vocabulary and grammar, and also in stylistic terms) to the usage of Attic Greek, that is the literary dialect of the major 'classical' prose authors of Athens, such as Plato, Xenophon and Demosthenes. This literary dialect formed the basis for the teaching of Greek in Roman imperial times, but there was a debate as to how closely or pedantically its classical features should be observed.

[21] Cf. Freedom from Distress, n. 16 and My Own Books, n. 79.

Prognosis (abridged)

This autobiographical and self-publicizing work provides us with a vivid account of some of Galen's most remarkable and well-known 'case histories' (in particular the diagnosis of a noble lady's lovesickness and of the emperor Marcus Aurelius' indigestion), and of the intensely competitive and conflictual nature of the practice of medicine in the Graeco-Roman world.

It also contains some of our best evidence for Galen's life, especially his early career at Rome, covering his first stay there (162–6), his return to Pergamum at the outbreak of the Plague, his return (169) and the stages—including dramatic successes and fierce medical rivalries—by which he was adopted both into the intellectual–cultural elite of Rome and into the imperial household, as court physician.

Greek title: Περὶ τοῦ προγινώσκειν (*Peri tou proginōskein*)
Kühn: XIV.599–672
Edition (with English translation): Nutton 1979

1. From the standpoint of the majority of doctors, Epigenes, it is impossible to XIV.599 predict what will happen to their patients in a given illness. Ever since the desire to *seem* has come to predominate over the desire to *be*, not only in medicine but in the other arts too, the finest things in those arts have been neglected, and what are cultivated are rather those things that will ǀ enhance one's popular 600 reputation: words and actions designed to give pleasure; flattery; constant fawning upon the rich and powerful in a city; the practice of accompanying such people about, of escorting them home, of acting as their dinner-time entertainer. Some go still further, relying on expensive clothes and rings, on the size of their entourage and on an array of silver utensils to persuade the uneducated of their superiority. They use all these means to delight or to impress persons who have no training in the true assessment of such matters, and thus gain great benefits—according to their own lights, that is. In my view, these are not genuine benefits, but appear so only in their false conception. Such, then, being their character, they have no hesitation in committing further outrages, in particular advertising their claim to teach arts within an extremely short space of time, and so acquiring large numbers of pupils who then increase their influence in the cities in which they live.

Our present-day life is vitiated by this sad fate of the arts in general; and the ǀ 601 forms this takes in the case of medicine are many. I should like to focus on one which has affected me especially. When a doctor who has learned the art systematically correctly predicts that a patient will suffer delirium, rigor, *kata-phora*, blood-flow, *parōtis*,[1] or an abscess in any other part of the body, or vomiting, sweating, digestive upset, collapse—or any other such thing—the phenomenon is perceived by the ordinary public as something weird and freak-ish, because of its unfamiliarity; and the person who makes such a prediction, so far from exciting their admiration, must be content not to be regarded as some kind of sorcerer. There are, it is true, some who do not reject the possibil-ity of such scientific knowledge; these immediately ask both the doctor who has made the prediction and the other doctors present whether any such know-ledge was discovered by their predecessors, or whether it is a discovery of this practitioner alone. At this point, it inevitably follows that the other doctors—either to cover up for their own failure to have learned it, or because they are genuinely unaware of the truth—claim that no previous doctor | wrote on such matters and that the one who has produced a prediction of this kind is a sor-cerer. It also follows that he himself does not dare, out of respect for the other doctors present, and fear of their hatred, to mention the work in this area by many previous writers, above all by Hippocrates, who leads us in all that is good. Nor, of course, does he dare state that he discovered the knowledge him-self: this would be not only to lie but also to provoke their hatred still further.

602

The person subjected from all sides to this impossible enquiry will naturally hesitate and deliberate. So, by his constant stalling, he will further increase the suspicion of sorcery; and in the end he will incur such enmity that he actually becomes the object of their plots—plots involving poison, or plots of the kind to which Quintus fell victim. Quintus was the best doctor of his time but was thrown out of the city because of an accusation that he was killing his patients.

[*Galen elaborates on the dangers experienced by one devoted to the true pursuit of the medical art, and the corruption of present-day culture.*]

605   2. During my first stay in Rome, completely unaware of all this, and suspecting nothing, I used to make manifest the prognoses of future states, and the rele-vant treatment, not just by words but by deeds, until the following events occurred—events indeed of which you are very well aware, since you were pre-sent from beginning to end during this illness of Eudemus the Peripatetic philosopher.[2]

[*Galen recounts how his own observations, including of Eudemus' pulse and urine, led him to suspect a quartan fever and thus predict precisely the time of its onset.*]

---

[1] For *kataphora*, a depressed or trance-like state, see *Affected Places*, n. 2; *parōtis* is a kind of abscess of the ear.

[2] As well as being an Aristotelian philosopher, Eudemus was an acquaintance of Galen's from his home city of Pergamum, who was well connected in Roman society and seems to have been instru-mental—as the following text suggests—in securing him access to its higher echelons.

A little later, | Eudemus received a visit from Sergius Paulus, who a short   611/612
time after this became Prefect of the City, and Flavius Boethus, who was himself
also already an ex-consul, and who was also, as Paulus was, a student of the
philosophy of Aristotle. He recounted to them everything that had happened in
relation to myself, saying that my prediction for that day, regarding the onset[3]
that was to come, still remained unfulfilled, and that he was paying close attention to the outcome. When this, too, occurred at the same hour as the previous
ones, Eudemus was full of admiration, and told all his visitors—which included
essentially all the most prominent men of Rome, in terms of both status and
education—of my predictions. It happened that Boethus, who had heard of my
high level of training in anatomical science, had already asked me to give a
demonstration on speech and breathing, and on the organs through which they
are performed. On recognizing my name, he told Paulus about this as well, and
said that after the present proof he would ask me to make some such demon-
stration to him too; for Paulus had expressed his desire to observe what can | be   613
seen through dissection. Barbarus, too, the uncle of the emperor Lucius, who
was at that time in charge of the region known as Mesopotamia, shared Paulus'
desire for such instruction; and so too, later, did Severus, a consul as well as a
student of the philosophy of Aristotle.

3. Well, you already know how those anatomical demonstrations turned out,
and will require only a short reminder of them, which I shall give presently. Let
me now go back to the case of Eudemus, who was suffering badly from three
quartan fevers in the middle of winter, and had been despaired of by his doctors. Now, both because I regarded him as my teacher, and also because I happened to be living nearby, I felt it my obligation to attend twice a day, if he
called for me. At this point I was ridiculed by Antigenes. Antigenes, who had
been a pupil of Quintus and an associate of Marinus, was looked upon as the
foremost doctor of the time and treated the most influential people. With what
motivation I do not know, but he now began to address my admirers mock-
ingly, saying that they would soon find out the true nature of the person that
they admired, when they saw Eudemus' body being carried out of the house.
| Those were the words he addressed to the general bystanders—in between   614
which he turned from time to time to the doctors, saying: 'Eudemus is in his
sixty-first year; he has three quartan fevers in the middle of winter; and Galen is
promising to heal him!'

---

[3] *Paroxusmos*: within the ancient understanding of fevers, this referred to the intensification, or
onset of strongly observed symptoms, that occurred periodically within the course of a fever. Fevers
were classified according to the length of this period, which was taken to be regular: the quartan
fevers mentioned below as afflicting Eudemus recurred every fourth day (counting inclusively),
tertian fevers every other day and ephemeral fevers every day.

Now I know, my dear Epigenes, that you continually told the world at large of my predictions, and my treatment, in this case; but this was the beginning of the envy that was felt towards me, as I provoked wonder both through the purity of my lifestyle and through my practice of the art. First, my prediction that the first of those quartan fevers to arise would cease that very day caused surprise; my correct foretelling of the dissolution of the second caused universal consternation; at the third, they began to pray the gods for my downfall. When, however, this too ceased at the time that I had predicted, I began to acquire a considerable reputation, both for my predictions and for my treatment.

615   Well, Antigenes might as well have been swallowed up by the earth, after his rash bad-mouthing of me; so too Martianus, who also I had a very great reputation amongst the young at that time, as indeed he had had for a considerable period, as the most expert anatomist: there were two anatomical writings of his which were very highly prized.[4] Martianus was also grieved by what Eudemus said, namely that I deserved not just universal praise but also admiration; and he began to spread the slander that my predictions arose not from medicine but from divination. When asked what kind of divination he meant, he stated, at different times, that it was from the flight of the birds, from animal sacrifice, from portents, or from astrology.

  What happened in the end with Eudemus was this. When the day came on which I had predicted his complete release from the third of the quartan fevers, Martianus came to Eudemus around the ninth hour,[5] stated that the onset which he was now experiencing was not just slightly, but very greatly, more vehement than that which had gone before, and departed with a radiant expression, clearly rejoicing in the failure of my prediction. Eudemus, meanwhile,

616   who was feeling for the first time a certain easing— I and at the same time a confidence that I would not be mistaken in my prediction—was awaiting the arrival of another doctor. In fact, not just one, but two, and even three, appeared, for all were keenly observing the outcome of the prediction, praying that I would fail at least in the prediction regarding the third quartan, as well as in its treatment; and Eudemus asked these, too, to declare what they thought was his situation. He received the same reply from them as he had from Martialius,

---

[4] Compare the account of this individual—a major anatomical authority of the time, and a follower of Erasistratus—in *My Own Books*, ch. 1, pp. 20–1 above. The manuscripts of the present work give the name in the form 'Martianos', those of that work in the form 'Martialios' (which would be the Greek transcription of the Latin name Martialis). It seems impossible to decide definitively between the two versions; I have followed Nutton (1979, 168–9) in preferring the former.

[5] i.e. in the middle of the afternoon. In Roman timekeeping, the whole period of daylight on each day is divided into twelve equal hours, which therefore vary in length seasonally. The completion of the ninth hour is thus half-way between noon (completion of the sixth hour) and sunset (twelfth hour).

and, noticing that they became equally radiant, realized that they, too, were rejoicing at what they took to be the failure of my prediction and treatment.

Now, it happened that I was later than usual, as I had been delayed by a visit, and he kept sending for me (I lived nearby, as I have said), wanting me to assess this easing that he had begun to feel. When I did arrive, he did not even wait for me to sit before extending his hand and instructing me to feel his pulse. I I smiled,   617 and said:

'You have nothing to expect but good things.'

'But tell me what precisely', he said.

'Is it not enough for you to hear that essential truth, and to rejoice at the future?'

'Indeed no', he said. 'I desire to hear every point from you in detail.'

'Well, then', I said, 'Listen. You will tonight be released from the entire disease state; and the dissolution of all resulting and future symptoms will follow.'

I stated, further, that the Nature which maintained[6] his body had indicated this to me through his pulse: this Nature had been awakened and was moving in such a way as to remove all the badness currently present in the humoral fluids of the body.

'But in what way do you mean that this has been indicated to you by this Nature? After all, Nature did not actually speak to you! Answer me that; for you know that I absolutely follow this kind of argument—far more so than any of these wretched doctors do.'

'Because it brought the motion of the arteries to a height greater than the lateral extension in either direction, and this typically happens when it is attempting to expel the source of distress from the body.'

At this Eudemus I responded: 618

'But there are many different channels of expulsion, which are separate in their nature: vomiting, evacuation of the bowels, perhaps also a large quantity of urine, copious sweating, blood-flow and the usual bleeding of haemorrhoids, all bring about intense evacuation. It must, then, be the proper function of your art to communicate the form of evacuation in question.'

I proceeded to mention the particular signs that precede blood-flow, and also those that precede sweating; and I added to my exposition also those that precede vomiting.

'We have, however', I continued, 'no particular, specific sign of intense, critical evacuation through the lower gut; it is, rather, the absence of all the others that leads one, by exclusion, to expect such an outcome in your case.'

---

[6] For the concept of the maintenance (*dioikēsis*), or internal regulation or control, of the body, understood especially as carried out through the three main 'sources', brain, heart and liver, and their respective networks in the body, see *The Art of Medicine*, n. 13 and *The Doctrines of Hippocrates and Plato*, passim.

'You have', said Eudemus, 'proceeded by inference to the discovery of the future event, in truly dialectical manner.'

This conversation had taken place in the evening; when you arrived the next morning, and were told of my prediction in outline, you found that the philosopher was no longer able keep to his usual, moderate manner of expressing himself, but cried to all of us friends as we entered that the Pythian Apollo had seen fit to prophesy to the sick through the | mouth of Galen, and after this to treat them, and to rid them of their sickness completely on the predicted day.

'In my own case, he foretold my recovery from this illness, which has just taken place—I am convinced that I am now completely well—a long time ago, and he was correct in both treatment and prediction. He has rid me of three quartan fevers to which I had fallen victim through a mistimed prescription of the theriac drug.[7] When the time *was* right for it, on the other hand, those doctors said nothing, and Galen administered it; and so he cured me, though he was mocked by them for his belief that he could cure an old man suffering from three quartans in winter.'

[*Galen encounters further hostility, a phenomenon he discusses with Eudemus, stating his own desire to return to his home city of Pergamum. He describes further successes in both treatment and anatomical demonstrations. The latter are admired by Flavius Boethus, as well as by Demetrius of Alexandria, a follower of Favorinus, and one Adrian (probably of Tyre, subsequently a famous orator), but they provoke the hostility of another philosopher, Alexander of Damascus (who is possibly to be identified with Alexander of Aphrodisias); the latter's sceptical provocation during an anatomical demonstration—'Should we in the first place concede to you the proposition that we should trust what is presented to us by the senses?'—causes Galen to storm off, regretting that he has wasted time with 'boorish Pyrrhonists'. The demonstrations also reach the attention of Severus, Paulus and Barbarus, 'and all the intellectuals of Rome', and are performed over several days in the presence of 'all those knowledgeable in medicine and philosophy'. Finally, he turns to an incident which recalls a famous story told of the doctor Erasistratus, who is supposed to have discovered a prince's love for his father's concubine (or, in some versions, his own step-mother), by observation of the pulse.*]

631   6. The woman whom I was called to examine was unable to sleep, and constantly moving the position of her body, throughout the night. I found, however, that she was free from fever. I therefore enquired about her recent experience of all those factors known to be relevant to insomnia, one by one. To these questions she gave little or no reply, as if to suggest that such enquiries were pointless; finally, she turned away, covered her whole body with the bed

---

[7] See *Freedom from Distress*, n. 4.

linen and her head with some little scarf and lay like a person wanting to sleep. As I left, I realized that there were two possible causes of her complaint. Either she was suffering from low spirits due to melancholy, or from some particular distress which she did not wish to communicate. I put off a more detailed investigation until the next day, | when, on my first arrival, I was told by the serving- 632 maid in attendance that it was impossible to see her at that time, and the same thing again at my second attempt.

I came a third time, and was told by the servant to leave, since the woman did not wish to be disturbed; I also found out that she had had a bath and taken her usual food after I left. On the following day I spoke to the servant alone, going over a range of subjects, and came to realize that the woman was very clearly suffering from some particular form of distress, the precise nature of which I then found out by chance. (This, I believe, was also what happened in the case of Erasistratus.)

Once I had understood that there was no ailment within the body, and that the woman was being disturbed by some kind of mental trouble, it happened that this fact was confirmed at the very moment when I was examining her. Someone arrived from the theatre and mentioned that he had seen Pylades perform. Both the look in her eye and the colour of her face changed, and when I observed this I put my hand on the woman's wrist, and found her pulse to have suddenly become irregular in a number of different ways. Such a phenomenon indicates that the soul has become disturbed; the same thing happens to people experiencing anxiety over some matter. | I therefore instructed one of my fol- 633 lowers to come the next day a little after my arrival for the examination of the woman, and to inform me that Morphus was dancing today. I found that her pulse was unchanged by this, and equally unchanged on the next day when I had someone inform me about a third dancer. Observing her very carefully throughout the fourth evening, and seeing, when it was announced that Pylades was dancing, that her pulse was disturbed in a number of different ways, I concluded that the woman was in love with Pylades; and this was definitely confirmed by careful observation over the subsequent days.

I also identified a similar pathology in the case of the slave house-manager of another rich man. This person was suffering distress at the prospect of having to produce the accounts, since he knew that a substantial sum of money was missing. He lost sleep as a result of the worry and was beginning to waste away from the distress. I ventured to tell his master that the old man had no bodily ailment, and also advised him to consider that he was afraid because his master was about to demand the accounts for which he was responsible, | and that he 634 was worried because of this, realizing that a large shortfall would be discovered. He agreed that this was a likely guess, and so I suggested, in the interest of achieving a definite diagnosis, to tell him that he was only demanding the money which he had in cash, as a precaution in case of his sudden death and the transfer of the household management to some other slave who was as yet untested; he was not demanding from him a statement of accounts. When the master said this, he realized that he would not be examined and so, within three days, was again free of distress and recovered his normal bodily condition.

What was it, then, that had eluded the doctors who had previously examined this woman and this household servant? Such matters may be discovered by inferences made on a general basis, even if one has little scientific understanding of medicine. The reason, I believe, is that they have no discernment of the ways in which the body is typically affected by the affections of the soul; nor, perhaps, do they even realize that the pulse is changed by challenges and fears which suddenly disturb the soul. It was through his understanding of this that Erasistratus | made his discovery—more easily, in that case, since the woman in question was in the same house as the patient, and was thus able to be seen more frequently by the young man, not just from time to time over a period of days, as was the case with Pylades. (Pylades was, indeed, not even present; the disturbance which he produced in the woman arose simply through the mention of his name.)

The notion of an 'erotic motion' of the pulse, then, is a great nonsense, put about by those who do not realize that there is no pulse actually indicative of love; rather, the pulse is altered, and departs from its normal evenness and rhythm, as a result of disturbance in the soul, whatever the cause of that disturbance.

7. Let me then add one more account before moving on to another subject. This was a case where Boethus was at first absolutely amazed but then, on hearing the explanation of the discovery, stated that he no longer found it surprising, but rather criticized the lack of education of those who were ignorant of the form of reasoning in question. One of his sons had fallen ill and then recovered; the illness had subsequently returned, before again ceasing; and after this the son was once more subject to attacks of fever. My response was that the boy was secretly eating food, for what was being given to him openly | was both appropriate in quality and of the right amount. Boethus set the boy's mother to watch over him, an office which she promised to perform assiduously; she sat with him all day, preventing visitors from entering, and slept in his room, which she took care to lock from the inside. After four days of this regime he became hot during the night. Boethus grabbed me and took me with him to the house to see the boy; we were accompanied also by some people who had met us in the street, yourself amongst them. I found that the boy had come out of the bedroom, with his mother, into a different room, which also contained a couch, on which the mother was sitting. A hammock had been attached, a little below the middle of this couch, on which she had laid the boy; and she was watching over

him so that no one might approach. There was one chair attached to the hammock at its other end, where the pillow was; and opposite it two low stools next to each other, by the top end of the bed. | Boethus had us sit down on these, 637 while he himself sat next to his wife, to whom he said:

'This is Galen. I have brought him hear so that you may tell him about your careful watch over the boy over the last few days, and how there has been no departure from the correct diet. He will observe whether the boy really had a fever in the night, or whether you were misled by your fear, telling me that he was hotter than normal and thinking that there was fever when the heat may have arisen for some other reason. He will then tell us clearly how the boy is doing and will instruct you in all matters concerning his diet.'

I then felt the boy's artery at the wrist, and declared both that he was free of fever and that I was about to be the object of further jibes from those who liked to refer to me as a prophet.

'Well', said Boethus, 'I too am in the habit of calling you a prophet, in front of those people, as you know, when you produce statements of the sort that your opponents in the art state are impossible to know on the basis of medical science.'

'And yet', I said, 'up till now I have shown you how such things are discovered through medical science and have even indicated some of the doctors | who 638 have written on these matters.'

So, all you who were present started telling me to deliver the prophecy. I asked you to allow me once more to feel the boy's pulse; and, after, doing this, I said:

'Boethus, you will be my witness that no one came out to meet me as I was on my way here, while you and I were in conversation together, and revealed to me the prophecy which is about to be uttered.'

He agreed that he would testify to that. Then, as you remember, I laughed as I told you all to pay attention and listen; the solemn utterance of the prophet, I said, was as follows:

'Young Cyrillus here has some food hidden in this room. So, whenever his mother goes off to her bath and locks the room, and then, for security, indicates this by pushing the key into the lock—I gather that this is what she does every time—her son takes out the food and eats it.'

On hearing this, Boethus immediately rushed over to the boy, grabbed him, moved him over to the couch, ordered the hammock to be stripped, and attempted to discover the hidden food at once. When all the blankets, as well as the undersheet, had been shaken out, he shook out the pillow too, | and even 639 picked up the chair, to see if anything could be found hidden underneath that. When this too revealed nothing, he returned the boy from the couch to the hammock, pulled all the covers off the couch, then finally ordered it to be covered again.

'Well', he said, with a laugh, 'what says the prophet now?'

Surprised as I was that he had found nothing in the places where he thought the food might be hidden, I picked up, and shook, the one thing that had remained unexamined, since no one had suspected that the object in question could be contained in it. This was a very small scarf belonging to his mother, which lay on the chair. As I shook it, a piece of bread that had been wrapped up within fell to the ground, and you all made a great noise, as did Boethus, laughing and praising this act of 'prophecy'. Boethus, laughing more than anyone, expressed his amazement that the pulse had the power not only to reveal the existence of hidden food but also to prophesy what was going to be done by a boy when his mother was in her bath. To this I replied:

'You are sharp, sir, indeed; but Galen did not arrive at this conclusion from 640 the indications of the pulse. Since, however, the door was locked carefully | for long periods of time, it is not difficult to infer that the boy was able to eat his food without fear of discovery. It is not the case that the pulse revealed to me either that there was something hidden or that that something was edible. I did, however, observe the disturbed state of the boy, and realized—as in the case of the woman in love and that of the terrified slave—that this disturbance arose from some affection of the soul, since indeed the boy was completely without fever.

'You may, then, ask on what grounds I was able to conclude that what was hidden was some sort of food. I will tell you that too. A boy who is preparing to argue a legal case, to wrestle, or to fight the *pankration*, or in general to engage in some competitive bodily or mental display—or one who is being accused of something—cannot succeed in holding in check the disturbance of his mind.'

When Boethus heard this, he swore by the gods, and expressed his astonishment that none of the doctors was aware of such well-known remedies. Quite evidently, he said, they have never displayed such achievements themselves, and of course they state that your achievements of this sort are based on anything but medicine. 'It seems', he said, 'not only that they are ignorant of the kind of pulse that is manifest in anxiety, but also that, even if one of them did by chance become aware of your reasoning in this area, he would not be able to perform a similar act of reasoning himself. For they are not intelligent by nature, nor have they schooled their rational faculties.'

Well, I said, they certainly are well schooled, and indeed sophisticated, in acts of malice.

641   8. I have you as my witness, Epigenes, to the truth of these accounts; and indeed I have many others who can verify all those things I achieved during my first stay at Rome. Moreover, you have yourself heard of them from the people treated by me.

There was one, though, which was genuinely so remarkable that doctors took to calling me a 'worker of wonders'—and not just 'teller of wonders', as I had been known before.

[*Galen proceeds to recount his amazing treatment of Boethus' wife, who suffered from the 'female flux', a condition involving fluid emissions from the uterus. Again departing from the opinions of the other doctors—as well as having to tend to her personally, in view of the useless interventions of her female attendants—he cures the condition by effecting a gradual evacuation through the skin, bladder and bowel, rather than through the womb.*]

When, at the end of the month, she again had a perfectly good complexion, 647 in no way different from that of her normal condition, and there was no sign of flux, he sent me four hundred gold pieces,[8] which increased the envy of those noble doctors in whose presence he had happened to praise me. Both he and Severus were prepared to inform the emperor Marcus Aurelius Antoninus, who was in Rome at that time, about me. (Lucius was at that time abroad because of the Parthian War that had flared up under Vologaeses.)[9]

9. Observing this inclination of theirs, and fearing that if they acted too 648 quickly, I should be prevented from returning to Asia, I asked them to refrain for a short time. I said that I would tell them the moment at which I would like this to happen. So, when I heard that the civil disorder [in Pergamum] had ceased, I immediately left Rome as if I were going to Campania, leaving one servant behind to look after the house. I gave him instructions to look out for a ship going to Asia, then, on the same day, get a salesman from the Subura to sell up the contents of the house and immediately embark on a ship to Sicily, and so return home. These instructions were carried out within a short space of time. I, meanwhile, hurried from Campania to Brundisium, where I was determined to cross on the first ship to sail, whether for Dyrrachium or for Greece, for I was afraid that I some very powerful man, or indeed the emperor himself, might 649 hear of my departure and, as with a runaway slave, send a soldier to order my return to Rome.

So, one day later, I sailed for Cassiope. My friends who looked for me in Rome asked the servant that I had left behind where I was and were told that I was staying in Campania. At first they were merely suspicious; but after some time passed, during which they saw neither me nor my man in Rome, they realized that I had indeed done what I said I was going to do in the first place. It was only then, and only with difficulty, that they were all convinced, in spite of their

---

[8] Equivalent to 40,000 sestertii, a vast sum; on the huge amounts earned by doctors in the imperial period, see Pliny, *Natural History* 29 and Nutton 1979, 179–80.
[9] This war ended in 165.

earlier disbelief, that I had genuinely intended to leave Rome, and that those claims of mine were true rather than false.

Lucius returned a short while later, but then another war, that against the Germans, broke out.[10] A discussion arose as to who were those persons who manifested the arts of medicine and philosophy in their deeds rather than merely in words, and a considerable number of those in the imperial entourage named me in this category. Since, then, they had already set out from the City 650 for the war, and had decided I to spend the winter at Aquileia, where they were preparing the army which they had assembled, they sent for me and commanded my presence. In the middle of the winter, however, Lucius was transported to the gods, and his brother accompanied the body back to Rome to perform the customary rites. After that he continued on his campaign path against the Germans, instructing me to join his retinue.

But the emperor was a fine and generous man, and, as you know, I succeeded in persuading him to leave me behind in Rome, partly on the basis of the expectation that he would, after all, return within a short time. My policy, for the whole period of his absence, as I was mindful of the habitual malice of the doctors and philosophers in the City, was to retreat to wherever his son Commodus was residing at any given time. Commodus' upbringing was in the hands of Peitholaus, who had instructions from the emperor himself to call upon me for the medical care of his son should he ever fall ill.

The emperor's prolonged absence on the German campaign was unexpected; and it was during this period that I wrote many treatises, both philosophical and medical, which I then gave to friends, at their request, after the emperor's return, in the expectation that they would remain in the hands of those indi-651 viduals.[11] I If I had realized that they would be distributed to unworthy persons, I would not have given them even to those friends. What I mean by that term is people of bad character, who read a text not in order to learn something but in order to find what they may criticize within it. It is these books, then, that contain the whole science of prognosis by the pulse and through the other prognostic signs. If, then, you wish to learn the scientific basis of the prognosis which I produced in the case of one of the sons of the Quintilii, Sextus, this will be clear and straightforward to you on the basis of a reading of the treatise on *Crises*, since you have from childhood schooled your reasoning faculty in geometry and dialectic. The majority of doctors, by contrast, have turned away from practical schooling and taken to the practice of villainy, training themselves in the art relevant to that; they are therefore unable to understand or train themselves in any of the matters written there.

[10] Galen is now referring to the year 168.
[11] Compare the account given of these events and of this period of Galen's literary production in *My Own Books*, ch. 3, pp. 23–4 above.

[*Galen describes his treatment of a young nobleman in the imperial entourage named Sextus,*[12] *and the way in which its understanding is related to his work on crises in diseases. Again Galen confounds expectations with his accurate prediction of the course of the disease.*]

This prediction, however, even if it appeared wonderful to the majority of doctors, in reality was not so; no more so the treatment, based on understanding of the present condition, of the young Commodus himself, during his visit to Rome. 657

11. What was genuinely remarkable was what happened in the case of the emperor himself at this time.[13] Both | he and those doctors in his entourage who had travelled with him on campaign believed that he was beginning to experience the onset of a fever, but all were misled, as was shown on the second and third days, both in the morning and at the eighth hour. On the previous day he had taken the bitter medicine composed of aloe at the first hour, followed by theriac, which he took as part of his daily routine, around the sixth hour.[14] He had then bathed around sunset, and taken a little nourishment. Throughout the night he experienced stomach cramps, as well as the voiding of his bowel, as a result of which he began to run a fever. The doctors in his entourage, on examining him first thing in the morning, ordered him to rest, then gave him some gruel to eat at the ninth hour. After this I was myself summoned to sleep in the Palace; and it was shortly after the lighting of the lamps that someone was sent to me from the emperor. 658

Now, since there were three doctors who had already seen him, both in the morning and around the eighth hour, and all had taken his pulse and diagnosed the beginning of an attack of fever, I stood still and said nothing; so that it was the emperor who looked at me and initiated the interrogation. | Why, he asked, had I, alone of the doctors, not made an investigation by touch? I replied that since the others had made two such investigations, and since, presumably, the specific nature of his pulse would be known to them by experience, as they had travelled with him on campaign, I would rather hope that they would be able to diagnose the state that had now arisen. His response to this was to instruct me to investigate by touch. It appeared to me that his pulse—considered in relation to the common measure of every age and nature—was far from that which indicates the beginning of an attack of fever. I therefore declared that this was 659

---

[12] Probably Sextus Quintilius Condianus; see Nutton 1979, 213–14.

[13] It seems most likely that the period referred to is that immediately after 176, following Marcus Aurelius' final return from campaign; alternatively, it is possible that Galen refers to the brief period, in 169, when the emperor and Galen were both in Rome; see Nutton 1979, 217–18.

[14] See n. 5 above: the first hour is an hour after dawn; the sixth midday; the eighth and ninth are in mid- to late afternoon. On theriac, see *Freedom from Distress*, n. 4.

not what was happening; rather, his stomach was being compacted by the food which he had taken, which had become phlegmatic before being voided, and was now making its presence clear.

At these words he gave what we may call a positive assessment of my diagnosis, repeating the following phrase three times:

'That is it. That is it—just as you have said. I feel that I am being weighed down by some cold sort of food.' And he asked what he should do. I responded on the basis of what I knew; and I said to him that had the patient been someone else, I would have given my usual prescription of wine sprinkled with pepper.

'In the case of monarchs such as yourself, however, it is proper for doctors to
660 employ only the safest of remedies; | it will thus be sufficient to make an external application to the region of the mouth of the digestive tract, using wool soaked thoroughly in warm nard ointment.'

He replied that whenever he had stomach trouble it was in fact his custom to use such an application, of warm nard ointment in purple wool; and he instructed Peitholaus to see to this and to dismiss me. After the application, in conjunction with the heating of his feet by masseurs with warm hands, he asked for Sabine wine, to which he added pepper before drinking it. After doing so, he said to Peitholaus: 'We have one doctor, a man of independent judgement.' He would constantly speak of me—as you yourself know—as 'first amongst doctors, but alone amongst philosophers'. For he had already had wide experience of those who were not only greedy for money, but also quarrelsome, obsessed with reputation, envious and malicious.

No other of my investigations, as I said, was more remarkable than this. The enquiry as to the specific sign of an attack of fever had already been made, before me, by all those doctors best trained in the pulse, including even
661 Archigenes, | some stating that it can be detected at the beginning of the arterial contraction, others that the contraction is in fact not discernible. I, however, was blessed with very great fortune; how else would one describe an extremely sensitive faculty of touch, able to discern minute distinctions in the pulse? And so I have personally had the experience of observing doctors be so badly mistaken that they sent patients who were actually beginning to experience an attack to the baths, or instructed them to be fed, and of being able to prevent this. I had thus thoroughly tested my own ability to diagnose the beginning of an onset; and it was on that basis that—rather rashly, perhaps, but nonetheless—I dared to go out on a limb and proffer to the emperor, after my first taking of his pulse, an account opposite to that which he himself had conjectured and which he had been told by the doctors.

12. What happened with Commodus, on the other hand, is generally said to be extraordinary, but in reality is very far from that.

[*Galen proceeds to relate his treatment of the boy Commodus, who has become feverish after a session in the gymnasium, and the reaction to it of a close relative of the emperor, Annia Faustina.*]

Faustina paused for a little, then took by the hand one of the Methodist doc-   663
tors who were in her entourage and led him forward. Jokingly, she remarked:

'You should know that Galen, here, combats you Methodists not with words but with deeds. He has frequently before now instructed bathing for people beginning a fever, and given them wine to drink; and he has allowed some to return to their usual activities on the first day, others on the third. You, mean-while, all instruct them always to fast for the first two days, | and to remain lying   664
down until the suspected hours have passed.[15] But now he has shown the reliability of his knowledge, when the son of the emperor, in his father's absence, had a violent fever on the first two days (as you yourselves heard yesterday), yet on the third day he did not wait for the eighth hour to pass, as you think right, but instructed bathing and nourishment. And even his guardian, Peitholaus, who is such a careful man in such matters that his care may seem to be timidity, was persuaded, by his previous experience of the man's skill, to allow washing and feeding before the suspected hour.'

Well, she uttered these words as she walked over to her carriage; and, taking my leave from her as she was about to get in, I said:

'You have made me a far greater object of hatred to the doctors than I was previously.'

Afterwards I recounted this all to Peitholaus, along with the fact that it was because of such doctors as these that I had just recently written three treatises, one on *The Distinct Types of Fever*, another on *Critical Days* and a third on *Crises*, in all of which I showed that the science by which one may predict what will happen to the sick has been written down by Hippocrates. | But these   665
people are so dull that they would not even be able to learn these things with the aid of my exposition of the texts....

13. The young man had had his illness for five days; and it seemed that an inter-vention involving venesection had been omitted, | although the ailment from its   666
outset demanded this on the second, the third or at the latest on the fourth day. Since, then, neither the season of the year nor the age of the patient—nor, indeed any weakness of vital capacity, nor the previous conduct of the illness—spoke against it, and all indications seemed to agree in pointing to venesection,

---

[15] A central tenet of the medical theory of the Methodist school of medicine—on Galen's doubt-less reductive account—was the indiscriminate prescription fasting until the third day (*diatritus*) for periodic fevers. The three days were counted inclusively, and ended at the same hour at which the first onset was observed (the 'suspected hour'). The total time of fasting was thus in principle forty-eight hours.

the doctors advised the vein to be cut, on the basis of very appropriate considerations. I had however observed that absolutely everything seen in this case coincided with Hippocrates' account of the signs of an imminent flow of blood. I therefore stated that they were correct to identify the importance of the removal of blood, but that Nature was arriving at this conclusion too, forcing the expulsion of the substance that was causing heaviness. This would, therefore, happen even if we did not intervene.

The doctors were surprised by these words; but at this point the patient rose from his bed as if wishing to jump up. Someone asked him why he had jumped up, since there was nothing to fear; and he said that he had seen a red snake 667   crawling out of | the roof and was afraid that it might fall and drop upon him, and that it was for this reason that he was leaving the place where he had been lying. The others thought that this was of no relevance to the likelihood of a blood-flow; but I, carrying out a thorough examination, especially of the right side of his nose, down to the cheek-bone, and observing a redness there, previously faint but just now much more evident, saw clearly that it was more probable than ever that the blood-flow would take place through the right nostril. I whispered to one of the patient's household servants to have under his cloak a vessel suitable to receive the blood; and then announced openly to all the doctors that if they would just wait a little while they would observe the man bleed through his right nostril. They laughed at this specific mention of the right nostril in my prediction, to which I replied that, on the contrary, either both predictions must be fulfilled or both be wrong; for the source of the forecast, in both cases, was science....

668   I encouraged the man concealing the vessel to pay close attention, so that as soon as he saw the blood flowing out from the nostril, he would hold the utensil in place underneath it. No sooner had I said this than the patient pulled out a blood-stained finger, and the man ran forward and put the vessel in place. At this point, as you know, there was an immense shout, and all the doctors fled. But you, on the other hand, questioned me; and I responded, revealing to you how I had learned the entire science of prognosis from the statements of Hippocrates; I added this, too, that I expected the blood-flow to be intense.

[*As predicted, Galen collects a large quantity of blood; he also succeeds in stopping the flow. The treatise concludes (ch. 14) with one more account of a successful prediction carried out on the basis of the pulse, and with a mention of the importance in this context of Galen's own specialist works on the pulse, especially* The Discernment of the Pulse; Causes in the Pulse; Prognosis by the Pulse.]

Anatomical Procedures (excerpts)

This is Galen's major work on both the practical techniques and the discoveries of anatomy, begun early in his career and revised and completed over a period of years.

Alongside its detailed account of anatomical structures, the work also gives invaluable information on the nature of anatomical research, teaching and practice in the Roman world, as well as on Galen's own anatomical education and approach to anatomy. It is these aspects, rather than Galen's anatomical knowledge more broadly, that are mainly illustrated by the brief extracts that follow.

We learn in particular about Galen's insistence on personal observation as opposed to reliance on books (even his own!), his focus on the use of apes (he typically dissected Barbary apes), given the impossibility of dissecting human cadavers in his time, but also his recommendation that human skeletons be observed—which was apparently still possible at Alexandria.

The text also presents us with Galen's account of the different values of different forms of anatomical knowledge, as well as a striking statement of Galen's—historically untenable—view that Hippocrates and his family and descendants (the 'Asclepiads') possessed a superior knowledge of anatomy.

Greek title: Περὶ ἀνατομικῶν ἐγχειρήσεων (*Peri anatomikōn encheirēseōn*)
Kühn: II.215–731
Edition: Garofalo 1991
Translation: Singer, C. 1956; Duckworth, Lyons and Towers 1962 (for later books, which are extant only in Arabic)

BOOK I

1. I had written an *Anatomical Procedures* earlier in my life, too, when I first II.215 came to Rome, shortly after the accession of our present emperor Marcus Aurelius Antoninus; but it became necessary to write a further such work, for two reasons. One is the history of that first work. It was written at the request of Flavius Boethus on the occasion of his departure from Rome for his home city of Ptolemais [in Syria]; he was a gentleman of consular rank who had conceived a fierce | passion for the study of anatomy, as much as any man who has ever 216 lived. I presented Boethus with a number of other works too at this time, but in particular with a two-volume *Anatomical Procedures*. He had asked me for such a work, as a reminder of the great many observations that he had made with me during a very short space of time, as he was afraid that he would forget them.

But he is now dead, and I have no copies of that work to give to my students, since those that I had at Rome have been lost.

The second reason is that a treatise written now will be greatly superior to that previous one, both because the exposition will be made at greater length, in several volumes, for the sake of clarity, and because it will be more accurate than the earlier work, since I have made many further anatomical observations in the intervening time.

When Boethus was still living in Rome, I wrote my works on the anatomy of
217   Hippocrates and | of Erasistratus, and those on the dissection of both living and dead animals, and also those on the causes of respiration and on the voice.[1] At the time of his departure I was writing a very large treatise on *The Function of the Parts*, which was later completed in seventeen books, and which I sent to Boethus while he was still alive. Much earlier, while still a youth, I had written three books on the motion of the chest and the lungs, for the benefit of a fellow student who was about to travel to his homeland for a long period: he wanted to be able to perform public demonstrations on these matters, but was not himself able to compose the appropriate text. When this person also died, these books came into the possession of a large number of people, although they were never intended for distribution. I had written them while I was still living in Smyrna, where I had moved because of Pelops, my second teacher after Satyrus, and I had at that time made no great new discovery of my own. Later I spent some time in Corinth because of Numisianus, who was also an eminent pupil of
218   Quintus, and I | went to Alexandria and several other places where I had heard that Numisianus was living, before returning to my home city, where I stayed for a fairly short time before moving to Rome. There I performed a large number of dissections, at which both Eudemus the Peripatetic and Alexander of Damascus, who now has the post of teacher of Peripatetic philosophy at Athens, were always present, and quite frequently also other prominent citizens, such as our present Prefect of Rome, Sergius Paulus, a man of absolutely the first rank in both the theory and the practice of philosophy. It was at that time, then, that I produced that previous *Anatomical Procedures* for Boethus, which were greatly inferior to the present work, not just in clarity, but also in accuracy.

So, then, let us turn our attention to the beginning of our account.

2. The bones in living beings are in their nature analogous to the poles of a tent,
219   or the walls of a house: the other parts are accommodated to them | and are
220   moved along with them ... | ... Since, then, the shape of the body is accommodated to the bones, and the nature of the other parts is such that they follow that outline, I recommend you first of all to gain a close familiarity with human bones; your observation of them should not be a casual one, nor based merely

---

[1] Compare *My Own Books*, ch. 1 with n. 9 and chs. 4 and 5 with n. 35.

on the reading of the books which some have written, with the title *Skeletons*, or simply *Bones*—even my own book with that title, which I believe to be superior to all those that preceded it, in accuracy, in concision of language and in clarity. No: your task and your endeavour should be not just to learn the form of each of the bones accurately from a book, but also to make direct and intensive observation of human bones.

This is very easy in Alexandria: the instruction given by the doctors there actually includes autopsy. You should try, for this reason if for no other, to make | the journey to Alexandria. If, however, you are unable to do so, it is still not   221 impossible to observe human bones directly. I myself have made such observations frequently, for example when a grave or a tomb has been broken open; there was even a case a few months ago when a river in spate destroyed a grave which had been hastily dug, the force of the water carrying the whole corpse— the flesh of which had already decayed, but the bones remained fully attached to each other—some 200 yards downstream. The course of the river passed some marshy, flat ground, on which the corpse was washed up; and it was accessible to view in just the same way as if a doctor had prepared it for the instruction of the young.

I also once observed the skeleton of a highway robber, lying on the mountainside a little way from the road. He had attacked a traveller who had however managed to kill him in the struggle, and of course none of the local inhabitants had any intention of burying him, their animosity being such that they actually took pleasure in seeing him eaten by scavenger birds. These indeed | ate the   222 flesh from the body within the space of two days, leaving the skeleton as though on purpose for the instruction of anyone who wished to observe it.

In your case, if you have not had the good fortune even to make observations in this way, you should then dissect an ape, and take careful note of every one of the bones, after removing the flesh. And you should choose those apes which are most similar to human beings, namely those which do not have long jaws nor large canines. You will find that such apes, which walk and run on two legs, are similar to human beings in the rest of their anatomy too...| ...So, amongst   223 apes, choose those which are most similar to humans, and thoroughly learn from these the nature of the bones, with reference to our own writings. You will quickly acclimatize yourself to their names, which will also be useful in the instruction on the anatomy of the other parts.

Thus, if you later encounter a human skeleton, you will readily understand and remember everything. If on the other hand you rely on reading alone, without a previous practice of observation of the bones of apes, you will neither understand the human skeleton accurately once | you see it, nor remember. For   224 the memory of perceptible things requires constant familiarity; it is for this reason, too, that we recognize those persons most quickly whom we have met most often, whereas we may pass by those whom we have only met once, or twice with a long interval in between, without experiencing either recognition or a recollection of having seen them before.

Thus the much vaunted 'anatomy by encounter', which is held in such high regard by some of our doctors, is not adequate to teach the nature of the things seen.[2] One must have first looked at each of the parts at great leisure, in order immediately to recognize what is seen on a subsequent occasion, and preferably have done so with human bodies themselves; if not, with animals similar to humans.

For example, when there was an outbreak of *anthrakes*[3] that occurred in many Asian cities, it happened that many people underwent the loss of their skin, or even of the flesh itself. I was living in my home city at that time, under the instruction of Satyrus, who had already been there for more than three
225 years, accompanying Cuspius Rufinus, the man who built | our temple of Zeus Asclepius; this was not long after the death of Satyrus' own teacher, Quintus. Those of us who had followed Satyrus' anatomical demonstrations were able to recognize any part thus laid bare, and to make a precise identification; we would ask the patient to make particular motions which we knew to be produced by this or that muscle, sometimes moving or displacing the muscles a little in order to observe a large artery, nerve or vein that lay next to it. But we found that everyone else seemed blind, completely ignorant of the parts exposed, so that inevitably one of two things happened: either they raised and moved aside many parts of the exposed muscles, annoying the patients with their pointless interference, or they did not even attempt such observation. When it came to telling the patient which was the muscle motion corresponding to the moving of a given part, a dumb animal would have understood it better. I realized from this that, for those who had previously undergone instruction, the observation
226 | of trauma was able to confirm what they had already learnt, whereas it was unable to teach anything to those who had no previous knowledge.

Let us return to the matter in hand. As I have already said, one must understand the nature of the bones, either through the body of a human being, if possible, or through those of apes, or even better through both. One should then move on to the anatomy of the muscles. For these two kinds of part underlie all others, as it were like foundations. After this you will be able to learn whatever you wish—whether arteries first, or veins, or nerves. Once you are familiar with the anatomy of these, there should follow an acquaintance with

---

[2] Galen means the Empirical school of doctors; 'encounter' translates *periptōsis*, and has the sense of one's first view of a phenomenon; see *Sects for Beginners*, ch. 2, with n. 5.

[3] A kind of eruption or boil on the skin associated with pestilential diseases, traditionally translated 'carbuncle' (the word also means coal or charcoal, and the Latin *carbunculus* is its translation, also bearing both senses).

the natures of the major organs. There will then come the knowledge of the digestive tract, of fat and of glands, all of which again should be examined individually in more detail....

3. ...Everything must be done very carefully by one trained in dissection, 231 including the actual removal of the skin; my predecessors remained ignorant of eight muscles, because they relied on others to remove the skin from the apes, as indeed I did in earlier days...ᴵ ...Many such matters have been overlooked 232 by anatomists throughout the whole body, because of their reluctance to perform the dissection with precision, preferring to make pronouncements based on what they find most plausible. It is no wonder, then, how great is their ignorance as regards the living animal. Given that they carelessly overlook matters which can be observed only through careful dissection of the cadaver, they would hardly be likely to engage in the practice of cutting the animal, and applying ligatures to parts of, while it is still alive, in order to learn which of the animal's activities are impaired by such cuts or ligatures.

Earlier on ᴵ I too used to have one of my assistants skin the apes, feeling a 233 natural reluctance to do so myself, and regarding the task as beneath me. One day, however, I observed, in the region of the armpit, a small piece of flesh, suspended from and connected in some way to the muscles there, and was unable to work out how to attach it to any of them. I then decided that I should skin another ape, properly. So I took one, which had been drowned in water. (This was my usual practice, to avoid compression of the parts in the neck.) I attempted to remove the skin, and only the skin, at the surface, without touching any of the parts beneath it. In this way there was found to be a fine, membraneous muscle, extended over the entirety of the flanks, and at its lower end extended beneath the whole of the skin in the region of the hollows of the ribs; and this muscle is continuous with the covering of the vertebrae of the lower back...ᴵ ...I became increasingly eager to remove the whole skin of the ani- 234 mal myself.

[*The book continues with the anatomy of muscles in general, then of the arms, hands and fingers, including detailed instructions on the actual procedures and tools to be used in the dissection.*]

BOOK II

1. I do not blame the ancients for *not* writing on anatomical procedures, any 280 more than I blame Marinus for doing so. For the former, it was unnecessary to write such notes for themselves or for others, since they were trained from childhood by their parents to dissect, as much as they were to read and write.

The ancients—not just doctors, but also philosophers—had a serious engagement with the practice of anatomy. There was thus no fear that people who had
281   learnt in this way would forget the ǀ manner of the procedures, any more than those who have practised the writing of letters from an early age would forget that. As time went on, however, it was decided to share the art not just with descendants, but with people outside the family—with people who were already adults, and were respected for their qualities. Once the childhood training was lost, however, it automatically followed that the learning deteriorated.

The power of such early training is, I believe, clearly indicated by all the ancients, who would use the word 'educated' not just for those who displayed an excellence in the arts, but also for all those who were well respected in their conduct of life as a whole. It was after the art had ceased to be kept within the family of the Asclepiads, and had then gradually deteriorated through a series of such transmissions, that written materials were needed to ensure its preservation.

282   ǀ In earlier times, there was no need either for works on anatomical procedures or for compositions of the sort first, as far as I know, produced by Diocles, and then by others of the earlier doctors, as well as by quite a few of the more
283   recent ones...ǀ ...For my part I have shared all that I have learnt from the beginning with those who have asked me for this information; my own wish would be for everyone to learn it, were that possible. And yet I already observe that some of those whom I have taught begrudge sharing their knowledge with others, so that if it happens that they die immediately after I do, the observations will be lost too.[4]

2. It is for this reason that I praise Marinus for having written down his *Anatomical Procedures*, and have myself been compelled to write another such work of my own, seeing his to be both deficient and lacking in clarity. And even more so since I believe that nearly all anatomists have failed to treat clearly of the most valuable part of their art. What could be more useful to a doctor for the treatment of war wounds, for the removal of arrows, for the cutting of bones, for dislocations, for fractures accompanied by ulceration, for the excision of fistulae, ulcers and abscesses, and for all other such things, than an accurate knowledge of all the parts of the arms and legs—and of all the parts

---

[4] The phenomenon of anatomical research or writing being preserved as secret knowledge and dying with its author is one that exercises Galen strongly, as shown by a later passage, in the part of the works surviving only in Arabic. There (XIV.1) Galen laments the fact that Quintus wrote no books that would communicate his considerable anatomical knowledge to others, and also tells of the fate of the highly valued writings of one of Quintus' best students, Numisianus. Desperate to have access to these works, Galen visited and cultivated his son Heraclianus in Alexandria, who guarded them jealously after his father's death. But in spite of repeated requests—and promises—Heraclianus never allowed Galen to see them, and was said to have had them burned before his own death.

nearer the surface | more than of those deeper within, the clavicle, forehead, 284
chest, flanks, upper abdominal region, neck and head. Doctors have to remove
arrows from these parts; they have to make incisions in the continuous parts of
the body; they have to excise matter or cause it to be ejected, in cases of putrid
wounds and abscesses, and in the surgical treatment of ulcers. In such cases,
one who does not know the location of an important nerve or muscle, or of a
large artery or vein, will sometimes cause death rather than healing for his
patient, and in other cases cause a permanent disability.

A knowledge of the muscles of the tongue, on the other hand, their number,
shape and characteristics, might be said to be valuable though superfluous, not
valuable in a primary sense, nor necessary. The reason that I say 'superfluous'
is that we are compelled to waste time on such matters for the sake of the
sophists, who are not content to keep the art concerning nature within the
bounds of what is actually useful, but constantly set us questions as to the reason
for which this or that | part came into existence, and why it is of this or that 285
nature or size. But a person of discernment in the art concerning nature is able
to understand matters sufficiently on the basis of one or two accurate dissections, in the course of which is revealed a great deal that is of direct value for
the art of medicine, but also, as an incidental benefit, the wisdom inherent
in nature.

I am in a particularly strong position to state that these latter findings of
anatomy are of no value for diagnosis, prognosis and cure, since I have escaped
the clutches of the sophists, who do not themselves deign to examine the argument, but turn to those who do make statements of it. The reason why such
sophists make the claim that they are exposing the uselessness of such observations is that they do not in fact understand them. It is because of these individuals, then, that I have offered a full account of what is surplus to requirements
alongside what is useful, to deny such sophists the possibility of using their
opponent's ignorance as a platform from which to build their counter-
arguments. I have demonstrated all this for their benefit in my treatise on *The
Function of the Parts*; but here too, equally, we shall state the anatomical pro-
cedures relevant to | all parts of the body.   286

As we do so, however, we shall distinguish between the different values of
different observations. The study of anatomy has one function for the natural
philosopher, who loves knowledge for its own sake; another, not for its own
sake but to enable one to show that nothing has been produced without purpose by Nature; another for one who wishes to be furnished by anatomy with
proofs relevant to the knowledge of some activity of Nature or of the soul; and
in addition to all these, another for one whose aim is the successful removal
of thorns or arrow-heads, the appropriate excision of a piece of bone, or the
correct surgical treatment of ulcers, fistulae or abscesses. These last matters are,

as I have pointed out, extremely necessary, and the best doctor must be trained in them particularly; but also, in the next phase, in the activities of the organs that lie within the body, and after that in their functions, insofar as these are of significance for the doctor for the diagnosis of disease—for some of these functions are of value to doctors rather than to philosophers, and in two ways, as

287   I have said: | either for the sake of the scientific study in its own right, or in order to show how the art of Nature acts appropriately within every part of the body.

[*In the remainder of the book, Galen polemicizes against previous anatomists, and then proceeds to the anatomy of the legs.*]

BOOK IV

[*In the course of a discussion of muscles of the back and shoulders, Galen digresses to consider the knowledge of his predecessors.*]

470   10. Those who wrote on the anatomy of the muscles previously were wrong about this [muscle extending to the shoulder-blade], as they were about many others. This is the case for example with Lycus, some of whose anatomical books are currently in circulation. I never actually met Lycus while he was alive, although I made contact with all the pupils of Quintus, being deterred neither by the length of a journey nor by the prospect of a sea voyage. But Lycus had no reputation in the Greek-speaking world during his lifetime; now that he is dead, certain of his books are the subject of considerable attention. I have no comment to make on his other books, which I have not encountered; but his works on anatomy, at least those which I have read so far, contain a large number of errors. Still, as I said before, it is not my present purpose to refute authors of previous generations, except where relevant, but only to write down the anatomical procedures themselves—a task also undertaken by Marinus, in a large book, which however is unclear in its language, and scientifically defective.

BOOK V

[*This following brief passage, coming in the context of his account of the muscles of the thorax, may serve as an example of Galen's detailed description of his practice with animal cadavers, as well as illuminating his relationship with his students or followers (hetairoi).*]

5. There is one muscle remaining, and it is by no means the least important,   503
known as the diaphragm.[5] Plato thought that this was merely a boundary
between two parts of the soul, the desiderative and the spirited. But it is more
than that; as has been shown in my work on *Causes of Breathing*, it is more
important than all those just mentioned for the activity of respiration. The ori-
gin of this muscle is of the same | form which I just described in the muscles in   504
the area of the ribs, namely that there are many fine ligaments which come out
from the bone, and which have simple flesh developed all around them. At the
very middle of the whole diaphragm is, as it were, a smaller circle within a
larger one, which is completely like a tendon in its nature, with none of that
flesh accumulated to it.

One may observe these features of the diaphragm by loosening the sternal
ribs from the upper parts, but it is not possible to understand its whole nature
clearly without first cutting away the eight muscles of the abdomen. Let us turn
to the dissection of these.

6. And I want to remind you of procedures which I perform constantly,
although I know that you in fact remember them. But this treatise is likely not
just to remain in the possession of my followers, but also to fall into the hands
of many others, some of whom will rush to malign them, though others will be
happy to select the best and learn from it. It is because of those people that |
I need to reiterate and state many times things well known to my followers—as   505
I am doing now.

[*Books V–XV continue with the anatomy of the rest of the body. The last part of the
work, from Book IX, chapter 6 to the end, is extant only in Arabic.*]

[5] Here 'diaphragm' translates *phrenes*, while 'boundary' in the next sentence translates *diaphragma*; but subsequently in the passage Galen himself uses the word *diaphragma* for diaphragm,
and in general the two words are interchangeable in his usage. (*Phrenes* is the older word, which in
earlier Greek writing often refers to the seat of a human being's mental or emotional experiences
rather than—or as well as—to this precise anatomical entity.)

An Exhortation to Study the Arts

This work belongs amongst those aimed at a wider audience, and is one in which Galen displays both his rhetorical skills and his literary knowledge to the full. He aims to establish both the practical and moral importance of arts (*technai*) and the status of medicine within the arts. The 'exhortation' (*protreptikos*) was an established genre, with the moralistic intent of converting or persuading people, for example towards the pursuit of virtue, or as in this case towards a particular study. The term *technē* (elsewhere also translated 'specialized skill') encompasses both the craft of the artisan and—with certain philosophical associations due to Plato and Aristotle—expertise of a more elevated or intellectually high-level kind.

The text is remarkable for the insights it gives us into the competitiveness of Roman intellectual life and its market-place of health, with its particularly aggressive attack on athletic training (a recurring theme in Galen's work), and also for the fact that it shows Galen as fully part of the literary culture of his time, disposing freely of quotations not just from medical and philosophical texts but also from a wide range of literary authors, as well as of a variety of other cultural and historical references.

Greek title: Προτρεπτικὸς λόγος ἐπὶ τὰς τέχνας[1] (*Protreptikos logos epi tas technas*)
Kühn: I.1–39
Edition: Barigazzi 1991 (with Italian translation); Boudon 2002 (with French translation)

I.1   1. It is not clear whether so-called 'dumb animals' are, in fact, entirely devoid of reason. Perhaps, though they are not endowed with that form of reason which achieves verbal expression, and which is known as 'external', they all nonetheless possess at least that form of reason within the soul which is called

2   'internal', although some to a more advanced degree than others.[2] | The crucial

---

[1] The title is in fact uncertain; it may have been, more specifically, an 'exhortation to the study of medicine', and may have been intended as a response to a work by an Empiric doctor, Menodotus, on the same subject (see *My Own Books*, ch. 12, with n. 58; and for full discussion see Boudon 2002, 35–42). If so, the extant text is the first part of a longer work which originally culminated with more specific material on medicine. In view of the uncertainty, however, and the fact that the extant text refers to 'arts' in general, I have here retained the traditional title.

[2] The terminology of 'external' (*prophorikos*) and internal (*endiathetos*) is thought to be Stoic in origin; in other sources for this distinction, however, it is—by contrast with the brief account here—the *internal* form of reason which is regarded as specific to humans. (The basic distinction itself between internal reason and that expressed in words can be traced to Aristotle, *Posterior Analytics*. I.10, 76b34ff.) Underlying the discussion is the fact that the Greek *logos* may be translated as both 'reason' and 'word'. The question of animals' possession of reason is an intriguing problem

difference between them and human beings, though, is seen in the great variety of arts which this latter animal performs, and from the fact that human beings alone have the capacity for knowledge, and can learn whichever art they wish. All other animals, with a very few exceptions, are practically without the capacity for Art; and these few acquire it by nature rather than by choice.

But it is not just that humans are practised in all their arts, mimicking the spider in weaving, moulding as does the bee, demonstrating considerable skill, too, in spite of being a land animal, in swimming. No: humans also follow the divine arts. They emulate Asclepius in the art of medicine; Apollo in this same art and in all the others which that god possesses—archery, music and prophecy—and each one of the Muses in her particular art. Humans are not ignorant of geometry, nor of astronomy; moreover they examine, as Pindar has it, 'the realm beneath the earth, the realm beyond the sky'.[3] | They have also by   3 conscientious labour acquired that greatest of divine goods: philosophy. So, even if other animals perhaps have some share in reason, it is the human being alone among them who is called 'rational' par excellence.

2. Is it not vile, then, to neglect the one part of us which we share with the gods, while squandering our energies on some other matter; to disregard the acquisition of Art, and give ourselves over to Fortune? The shabbiness of Fortune was the feature that the ancients wished to demonstrate when they portrayed her, not just as a woman—as if this were not a sufficient sign of inanity—but also holding a steering paddle in her hands, with a spherical support for her feet, and without eyes. All this was intended to indicate the unreliability of Fortune.[4]

On a ship that is fiercely tossed by a storm—buffeted by waves that threaten to sink her—you would be a fool to hand the rudder to a blind helmsman. But it seems to me that in life, too—where greater shipwrecks frequently befall a | house   4 than befall ships at sea—it is unintelligent, in such circumstances, to entrust oneself to a blind spirit, and one who is unstable into the bargain. She is so stupid and mindless that she frequently overlooks men of merit and enriches the worthless. But even these she does not enrich consistently: she frequently takes away again what she has given them. But this spirit is followed by a considerable crowd of uneducated men, though she is unable to remain in one place because

for Galen: on the one hand reason (in the sense which Galen proceeds to elaborate in this work) is the divine part of a human being's soul, that which clearly separates him from animals; in another sense, in Galen's psychological/physiological system, the rational part or 'command centre' of the soul, which controls motor function and processes sense perception, is clearly shared in very similar form at least by mammals. And indeed experiments on animals provide a major part of Galen's evidence for this theories in this area; see e.g. *The Doctrines of Hippocrates and Plato* I.6.

[3] Galen's citation of Pindar (the most famous of classical Greek lyric poets) seems to come via Plato's *Theaetetus* (173e).

[4] Galen is drawing on an established moralistic literary tradition in opposing Art (*Technē*) and Fortune (*Tuchē*), as well as referring to a specific pictorial tradition of representing Fortune in the way which he proceeds to describe (see Boudon 2002, 8–11 for more detail).

of the rolling of the base she stands on, which carries her this way and that, sometimes over cliffs and into the sea. And there all her followers go under together, while she alone emerges unscathed, mocking them as they lament and accuse her in vain.

3. Such, then, are the deeds of Fortune. Consider, by contrast, Hermes, and how differently the ancients I (both painters and sculptors) have adorned his picture: the lord of the Word and the practitioner of all Art. A fine young man he is, and his beauty is not a superficial, acquired beauty. It is natural, and the excellence of his soul immediately shines through it. He has radiant eyes, and a sharp gaze, and he stands on the firmest and most stable of all bases: the cube. Sometimes, in fact, the god himself is depicted in this shape. And you will see that his worshippers, too, are as radiant as the god who leads them, never blaming him (as Fortune's followers do her), never giving way nor retreating, but following and perpetually reaping the fruits of his providence.

4. Those who follow Fortune you will find to be idle and ignorant of the arts; they are borne up by hopes, they run with the spirit as she runs, some near her and some further away, and some even holding her hand. You will see amongst them, too, the famous Croesus, I the Lydian; and Polycrates of Samos;[5] and perhaps it will amaze you to see the River Pactolus flowing with gold from the former, the fish of the sea serving the latter. With them you will also see Cyrus and Priam and Dionysius; a little after this Polycrates crucified, and Croesus killed by Cyrus, and Cyrus himself by others; and you will also see Priam killed, too, and Dionysius in Corinth.[6] And if you consider the others, those who are rushing after the running spirit from further away, but failing to reach her, you will despise the whole band of them. Here are demagogues a-plenty, courtesans and prostitutes and betrayers of friends; and here are also murderers, grave-breakers and robbers; quite a few of them have not spared even the gods, but have robbed their altars.

5. The other band is a band of fine men: the practitioners of the arts. They do not run, nor do they shout, nor I fight each other. In their midst is the god, and about him they are all ranged in order, never leaving the place he has assigned them. Those nearest the god, forming a circle about him, are geometers, mathematicians, philosophers, doctors, astronomers and scholars.[7] After them

---

[5] The legendary power and wealth, and disastrous ends, of Croesus and Polycrates, as also of Cyrus, are recounted by Herodotus. (See also n. 17 below.)

[6] Priam was the legendary king of Troy, destroyed in the Trojan War; Dionysius was a tyrant of Syracuse who ended his life in poverty in Corinth after defeat by that city. It is possible that we should read 'imprisoned' instead of 'killed' after 'Priam'.

[7] Note that the term *astronomoi* may refer to students of astrology as well as astronomy, the two disciplines not being distinct in ancient categorization. On the term *grammatikos*, here translated

the second band: painters, sculptors, teachers, carpenters, architects[8] and stone-workers; and after them the third order: all the other arts. Each is drawn up in his individual place; but they all fix their gaze on the god as one, obedient to his instruction. You will find here, too, many who stand actually with the god—a sort of fourth rank, marked out from the others, unlike those who accompanied Fortune. For political reputation, noble family and wealth are not the criteria for this god. Rather, he honours those who lead a good life, excel in their arts and follow his injunctions, practising the art correctly; and these above all others ǀ he keeps about him always. The contemplation of this band 8 and of its character will, I fancy, conduce to emulation and, indeed, to adulation.

Socrates is among them, and Homer and Hippocrates, as well as Plato and his lovers—people we revere like gods, as they are the god's subjects and servants. The others too, though, without exception receive the god's attention. He not only cares for those about him; he goes to sea with the seafarers, and does not abandon the shipwrecks. Think of Aristippus' first reaction when in the course of a sea-voyage his ship was destroyed and he was washed up on the coast of Syracuse. It was a reaction of joy to see a geometrical diagram on the sand: he deduced that he had arrived among Greeks, and people of wisdom, not among barbarians. He then appeared in the Syracusan *gumnasion*[9] and uttered the following words:

> Who will receive the outcast Oedipus
> Upon this day, with gifts of any kind?[10]

As he stood there, people came up to him and, realizing who he was, ǀ immedi-   9 ately gave him all he needed. And when he was asked by some people who were about to set sail for Cyrene, his own homeland, if there were any order he wished to give to his family, he said: 'Tell them to acquire such possessions as would float with them in the case of a shipwreck.'

6. In similar situations mean-spirited men, obsessed with wealth, have frequently seized gold or silver to gird their bodies, and, in so doing, have lost not only these possessions but also their lives. Such people are guilty of inconsistency, for they are the first to prefer the skilled to the unskilled, even in the case of dumb animals. They prize horses trained for war, and dogs for hunting, more

---

'scholar', see *My Own Books*, n. 4; the related term *grammatistēs*, translated below as 'teacher', refers to the lower-level or elementary grammatical teacher.

[8] An *architektōn* was one responsible for the design and execution of building works, and could be equivalent, in modern terms, to a civil engineer as well as an architect (we note that this was, apparently, the profession of Galen's father); the term also has a broader connotation of master-craftsman or director of works.

[9] The *gumnasion* in a Greek city was a centre both of physical exercise and educational and intellectual pursuits.

[10] Sophocles, *Oedipus at Colonus* 3–4.

than any other kind; and they usually have their household slaves trained in some skill, often at considerable expense. Nonetheless they neglect their own education. But is it not disgraceful that the slave should be worth as much as 10,000 drachmas, while the master is not even worth one? One, did I say? No 10   one would | take such a fellow even as a gift.

Can it be, then, that their own persons are the *only* thing that these people neglect—such is their failure to learn a single skill from anyone? We have seen that these men give training to brute beasts, and despise slaves who are lazy or untrained; and they even take care that their land and other possessions achieve their full potential. But meanwhile they pay no attention to themselves: they are unaware even that they have a soul. They are, clearly, equivalent to the reject servants. One might reasonably say to such a man: 'Sir, your house, all your slaves, your horses, dogs, land and other possessions are in a fine state; but you yourself are sadly neglected.'

I am put in mind of two splendid observations, by Demosthenes and by Diogenes, the one referring to the uneducated rich as 'golden sheep', the other likening them to the figs that grow by on clifftops. The fruit of this tree is eaten not by men but by ravens and jackdaws; the wealth of the former individuals, 11   meanwhile, is of no use | to people of taste, but is enjoyed by flatterers—people who, once they have spent everything, will pass you in the street pretending not to recognize you. So perhaps even the comparison which someone once made of such men to wells was not an infelicitous one. When a well which once provided them with water dries up, people hitch up their clothes and urinate in it. And it is logical that those whose sole concern has been money should not only be deprived of that money, but at the same time also of everything that they have got by means of it. What else should they suffer, when they have attained no good of their own, but have always been borne up by other people's goods—or those of Lady Fortune?

7. In a similar case are those who set great store by their noble birth, and boast about it. They, too, are suffering from a dearth of goods which they can call their own, and so they hit on the notion of race. They fail to understand that this nobility on which they pride themselves is like the coinage of a particular 12   state, | which only has currency with the inhabitants of that state; to everyone else it is counterfeit.

—Did not your birth then raise you to the heights?
—Bad to have nothing; birth did not feed me.[11]

---

[11] Euripides, *Phoenissae* 404–5: the exchange is between the tragic Theban queen Jocasta, wife of Oedipus, and her son Polynices, who has lived as an impoverished exile, in which his noble birth was of no assistance.

The virtues of our fathers are, as Plato says, a fine treasure; but how much finer to be able to reply, with Sthenelus:

Greater by far than our fathers it is our boast to be.[12]

If noble birth has a function, it is surely just this: that it may produce the desire to emulate our ancestors' example. It will cause distress if we fall far short of their standards of virtue—not least to our forebears themselves, if they have some kind of consciousness. And the shame it will cause to us is greater in proportion to the distinction of the family. Ignorant people who come from an insignificant family derive a benefit from their birth: namely that most people will take no notice of their character. Those whose high, illustrious lineage allows them no such opportunity for obscurity I necessarily suffer all the more openly. Moreover,   13 a special disdain is reserved for those who fail to measure up to their breeding. If a fool makes reference to his illustrious lineage, his failing seems the less forgivable. For we do not judge or test ordinary men by the same yardstick as the highborn. The former are accepted even if they are quite mediocre, allowance being made for their poor birth; the latter will not gain admiration just for being much better than others, unless they also measure up to their forebears.

So, let anyone of good sense proceed to the practice of Art—that Art which will make you appear worthy of your family if it is a noble one; and, if not, will enable you to adorn it. Remember the great Themistocles of old,[13] who, when someone mocked him for his lowly birth, replied: 'But I shall begin a line. My family will begin with me; yours will end with you.' We see, too, that even the Scythian, Anacharsis, succeeded in being admired I for his wisdom, in spite of   14 his barbarian race. Anacharsis was once mocked as a barbarian and a Scythian. 'My fatherland', he said, 'disgraces me. But you disgrace your fatherland.' A very fine response to a worthless person who regarded country as the only source of honour. If you consider the facts, you will realize that citizens do not achieve renown by coming from such-and-such a city; in fact, the situation is exactly the opposite. It is good men—men who practise the arts—who cause their cities to be remembered. Whoever had heard of Stagira before Aristotle? Or of Soli, before Aratus and Chrysippus?[14] And indeed Athens herself has kept her fame living so long not through some virtue inherent in her soil but because of the people who were born there: a great number of outstanding men, who then shared their fame with their native land. You can best see the truth of this from a consideration of Hyperbolos and Cleon:[15] did they not gain more from

---

[12] Homer, *Iliad* IV.405.   [13] See further below, n. 36.

[14] Both Aratus, the author of an influential verse work on astronomy and meteorological phenomena, and Chrysippus, the major Stoic philosopher, were natives of Soli in Cilicia (modern-day southern Turkey) in the Hellenistic period.

[15] Political demagogues during the Peloponnesian War, in late fifth-century Athens.

15 Athens than they could have from anywhere else, ˡ in terms of the fame of their ill-deeds?

> Once their name was swine, the Boeotians

says Pindar. And again,

> If we escape the Boeotian swine![16]

hoping to destroy the whole nation's reputation for philistinism through his lyric poetry.

8. How praiseworthy, too, was that Athenian lawgiver who prevented anyone who had not taught him an art to be supported by his son.[17] For all Art must be studied precisely at the time when the body is at its peak of beauty. But it often happens that the young gain so much attention because of their good looks that they take no care of their souls. Then, when it is too late, they say:

> I wish this beauty that destroyed me so
> Had been destroyed.

16 ˡ At that point, too, Solon's saying comes to mind, that one should have a special regard for the end of one's life. Then they curse old age, as well they might, and value Euripides' words:

> It is not safe
> To have more beauty than the average.

It would be better to realize that a young man's prime is like the flower of spring, a short-lived pleasure, and to agree with the poetess of Lesbos:[18]

> The one is beautiful to eyes alone;
> The other, virtuous, has beauty too.

Solon, too, is persuasive when he says, in support of the same opinion, that one should prepare oneself for old age as for a hard winter ahead, fitting oneself out with shoes and clothes, with shelter, and with many other things besides. That is how a good helmsman would prepare, a long time ahead, for the bad weather. How wretched to have to say:

> The deed once done, he saw it.[19]

---

[16] The first quotation is available only as a fragment (no. 83), the second is from *Olympians* 6.90.

[17] The reference is to Solon, the legendary Athenian law reformer; the law in question is mentioned by Plutarch in his *Life of Solon* (22). The following reference to Solon's attitude to the end of life obliquely recalls his famous encounter with Croesus, and his caution to count no man happy until his end is known.

[18] The most famous female Greek poet, Sappho; the passage quoted is preserved as fragment 50.

[19] Homer, *Iliad* XX.198.

What use could a young man possibly be who was pretty but had no training? 17
Would he be any use in war? It might well be said to him:

> But you—go back to the soft delights of the bedroom![20]

or

> Home with you now and do your own work there![21]

And what about Nireus?

> He was the prettiest of all there at Troy,
> But feeble.[22]

That is the reason, it seems to me, that Homer mentions him only once, in the Catalogue of the Ships: to show that the prettiest men are useless if they have no other accomplishment.

Beauty is not even useful for the acquisition of money, as some wretches maintain. All free, respectable, reliable money-making comes about by Art: that which derives from bodily charm is disgusting, and universally despised. The young should follow the old | maxim: they should look at themselves in a mir- 18
ror and, if they are physically beautiful, take pains to make their soul so too, on the grounds that it would be absurd to have a bad soul in a fine body. If, though, the sight of the body is unpleasant, he should care for his soul all the more, so that he may say with Homer:

> That man then might be more feeble in body;
> But when God adorns his features with words, then
> All delight as they see him. Surely he speaks,
> Softly, with grace, and shines in the gathering of people.
> And as he goes through the town they think him a god.[23]

From all this it should be quite clear to all but the utterly stupid that neither distinction of family, nor wealth, nor beauty, gives grounds for a confidence which might allow one to despise the cultivation of Art.

The argument as it stands is sufficient. But it might be apposite to add, as a coda, a story about Diogenes. Diogenes was once dining with someone who lavished the greatest care on every aspect of his household— | with the sole excep- 19
tion that he neglected himself completely. It happened that Diogenes had cleared his throat, needing to spit. He looked all around him for a place to do so, then proceeded to spit, not at any of the surrounding objects, but directly at the master of the house. The man was incensed and asked him the reason for his action.

---

[20] Homer, *Iliad* V.429.   [21] Homer, *Iliad* VI.490.   [22] Homer, *Iliad* II.673, 675.
[23] Homer, *Odyssey* VIII.169–73.

Diogenes replied that he could see nothing else in the room that was equally neglected. The walls were all decorated with splendid pictures; the floor was constructed from valuable pieces of stone, which formed depictions of the gods; all the vessels were sparkling and clean; the couches and their covers were quite beautifully adorned; he alone was uncared-for. And it was the custom of all men to spit into the unworthiest place to hand. So, young man, do not allow it to happen that while everything else about you is quite splendid in appearance, you yourself are worthy to be spat at. Rarely do all these qualities co-exist in one

20   person: nobility, wealth | and beauty. If they do come together in one person, how terrible if he should be someone to be spat at, in spite of all he possesses.

9. Come then, my children, you have heard my words: dedicate yourselves at once to Art! And you must guard against those charlatans and mountebanks who make a big noise but teach 'arts' which are useless or wicked. You must understand that any practice whose end is not beneficial to life is not an art. In the case of other practices such as acrobatics—leaping, or tightrope-walking, or spinning in a circle without becoming dizzy, or feats such as those of Myrmecides of Athens or Callicrates of Sparta[24]—I am sure that I have already convinced you that none of these is an art. The only one that worries me is athletics. Athletics hold out the promise of strength, brings with it popular fame and is rewarded by our elders, at public expense, with daily financial payments similar

21   to those accorded to heroes. | There is a danger that it may deceive some young men into preferring it to an art. We had best investigate it, then; deception is always easy in any subject of which one has made no previous investigation.

The human race, my children, has something in common with the gods, and something in common with the brute beasts: with the former to the extent that it is possessed of reason, and with the latter to the extent that it is mortal. Better, then, to realize our kinship with the greater, and to procure a training by which we may attain the greatest of goods, if we apply it successfully—and, if unsuc-cessfully, at least we shall not suffer the shame of being worse than the most senseless of beasts. Now the athletic training of the body is, when it fails, the ugliest thing imaginable; its successful application, meanwhile, still makes us no better than dumb animals. Who is stronger than a lion or an elephant? Who faster than a hare? And surely everyone knows that, even as the gods are praised above all for artistic accomplishments, so too among men, the most excellent

22   are thought worthy of divine | honour, not for running well in a competition, or for throwing a discus or wrestling, but for the public benefits they may confer through the arts. Whether Asclepius and Dionysus were originally men or gods, the reason they deserve the greatest respect is the art of medicine, in the

---

[24] Galen here refers to a different kind of 'useless' performance: according to Pliny's *Natural History* (VII.85), Callicrates and Myrmecides produced minuscule statues.

former case, and, in the latter, the fact that he taught us the art of the grape. If you do not believe me, at least have some respect for the Pythian Apollo. It was this god who called Socrates the wisest of all mankind, and who addressed Lycurgus in these words:

> You come, Lycurgus, to my goodly home,
> Beloved of Zeus and all the gods on high.
> I doubt whether to call you man or god;
> But god, Lycurgus, do I rather choose.[25]

The same god, the Pythian Apollo, also displayed his considerable respect for Archilochus when he died. Archilochus' murderer tried to enter his temple, but was prevented by the words:

> O slayer of the Muses' friend, depart!

10. So tell me then, what are the noble forms of address associated with the 23 athlete? You cannot, because there is nothing to say; but perhaps you reject the evidence of that particular witness as unreliable. That is indeed the conclusion that seems to be indicated by your appeal to popular opinion, and your attempt to procure widespread adulation. And yet I am quite sure that if you were sick you would not turn to the masses for advice. You would turn to a very select few, namely those with the best medical training—just as, on board ship, you would trust one man, the pilot, rather than all your fellow travellers. The same applies in small matters. If you were building something, you would trust a carpenter; a cobbler, if you needed shoes. So how is it that in this matter of prime importance you allow yourself to be arbiter of the debate, and deny judgement to men wiser than you? (Never mind the necessity of consulting the gods.) Consider Euripides' opinion of athletes:

> Of every evil in this land of Greece,
> There is none worse than the athletic tribe.
> I First, they are ignorant of how to live,   24
> Unable, too—for how could such a man,
> The slave of jaw, the victim of his paunch,
> Attain a living to sustain his line?
> Yet ill prepared for chance or penury,
> Trained in bad habits from the first, such men
> Are lost and helpless when they suffer change.[26]

---

[25] Lycurgus was the semi-legendary founder of the Spartan constitution, and a byword for wisdom. The verses are quoted in Herodotus, *Histories* I.65.3.

[26] The quotation is a fragment from a lost play of Euripides, *Autolycus*.

He has something to say, too, about the uselessness of their individual practices. Listen to this:

> What wrestler, or what man of nimble foot,
> What discus-thrower, striker of the jaw,
> Is worthy of his city's laurel-prize?

Or consider, if you will, this even more detailed pronouncement:

> Will they then fight the enemy so armed
> With discus, or will running on the shields
> Scatter the nation's mortal enemies?
> | None with the iron close at hand raves so.

25

You may, perhaps, say that the testimony of Euripides and his ilk is not to be taken too seriously, and that we should rely rather on the philosophers for judgement. But they too are absolutely unanimous against this practice. Even the doctors—none of them has ever been in favour. You can listen to Hippocrates—who says 'The athletic state is not natural; better a healthy condition'[27]—or to any of the best doctors who followed him. Now, I did not want to rely on arguments from authority at all: that is the practice of a rhetorician rather than of a man who respects the truth. It is precisely because of the arguments of some who take refuge in the vacuities of popular opinion and reputation, and fail to investigate the practice in itself without reference to such external considerations, that I am none the less forced to provide witnesses here too, so that these people will realize that they can gain no advantage from that point of view either.

26   This might be a good moment to recount the story of Phryne. | This woman was at a drinking party once; and they started playing one of those games where everyone takes it in turn to give a command to their drinking-companions. Phryne had noticed that there were women present who had made themselves up with alkanet, white lead and orchil.[28] She ordered water to be brought; the women had to take some in their hands and dip their faces in it once; then immediately wipe them with a napkin. Phryne herself went first. The other women's faces were of course covered with slime, and they looked perfectly monstrous. But Phryne looked better than before: she alone had used no make-up, but relied on her natural beauty, without recourse to cosmetic tricks.

   Of true beauty, then, one can only make an accurate test when it is seen as it is, stripped clear of all extrinsic adornments. It is the same with athletics: you

---

[27] The quotation is from *Nutrition* (34), a work now considered to be a late addition to the Hippocratic corpus.

[28] Plant products used cosmetically on the face; a kind of rouge was extracted from orchil.

can only reasonably examine its worth by seeing whether it is of any benefit to the state as a whole or to the private individuals who practise it.

11. Of natural goods, some belong to the | soul, some to the body, and some   27 are external. There are no others that can be conceived apart from these three types.

Now, that athletes have never, even in a dream, enjoyed the benefits of the soul, is obvious to everyone. To begin with, they are unaware that they have a soul, so far are they from understanding its rational nature. Because they are always occupied in the business of amassing flesh and blood, their souls are as it were smothered in a heap of mire, unable to contemplate anything clearly, mindless as beasts without reason. There might be some dispute as to whether they possess some bodily good. Is it, then, the most precious of these, health, to which they lay claim? In fact, there exists no more dangerous bodily state, if Hippocrates is to be believed. He describes the 'peak of good condition' which these people pursue as 'dangerous'.[29] And again: 'Training for health, moderation in food, readiness in exertion'.[30] This is a very fine saying of Hippocrates, and universally respected. | But athletes do quite the opposite. They over-exert   28 themselves, over-fill themselves with food and completely ignore the great man's advice, just like drunken revellers. Hippocrates' prescription for the healthy life was: 'Labour, food, drink, sleep, sex—moderation in all'.[31] These people daily exceed the proper measure in exertions, and force themselves to eat; and they frequently carry on eating into the middle of the night. In fact, it might reasonably be said of them:

> Mortal warlords and gods were all sleeping soundly,
> Bound in the softness of dream-land all night long;
> But sleep came not to the *wretched souls of the athletes*.[32]

The pattern of their sleep itself is also immoderate. At the hour when ordinary men return from their labours and require food, athletes are just getting up from their sleep. Their life is thus like that of pigs—except that pigs do not over-exert nor | force-feed themselves. Athletes do both these things and in some   29 cases also have their backs lacerated by oleander branches.

The old master, Hippocrates, apart from the lines already quoted, also says this: 'Great and sudden changes are dangerous: filling or emptying, heating or cooling, or moving the body in any other way. For'—he adds—'all excess is inimical to Nature.'[33]

---

[29] Galen refers to *Aphorisms* 1.3.   [30] *Epidemics* VI.4.18.   [31] *Epidemics* VI.6.2.
[32] The verses are from Homer, *Iliad* XXIV.677–9, except that in the last line Galen has replaced a reference to Hermes with one to athletes.
[33] *Aphorisms* 2.51.

Athletes pay no heed to these words, nor to the others; they transgress all Hippocrates' excellent recommendations, and their every activity contravenes the dictates of health. I would say, in fact, that athletics is the cultivation not of health but of disease. And I think Hippocrates is of this opinion too, as shown by his statement: 'The athletic state is not natural; better a healthy condition.' By this he does not just mean that athletic practice has nothing to do with what is natural; he even uses the word 'state', refusing it the name of 'condition', which is always applied by the ancients to the truly healthy. A condition is a stable
30 state, | which is not readily altered; that of athletes is a peak, and is dangerous and liable to change. Further, it admits of no improvement precisely because it is a peak, and, since it cannot remain unchanged at the same level, it cannot but succumb to deterioration. Such is the state of the practising athlete's body; when he gives up, it is even worse. Some die after a short time; some live for a little longer; but even these do not reach old age. Or, if they do, they are as bad as Homer's Prayers:

Limping, all shrivelled up, deprived of sight[34]

at the end.

When walls have been shaken violently by siege-engines, they are easily swept away by any slight accident; they will not survive an earthquake, let alone some heavier attack. It is the same with the bodies of athletes: they have become weak and unsound because of the blows sustained in this regime, and are ready
31 | to succumb at the slightest provocation. Often hollow spaces have developed around their eyes, and, as their strength subsequently diminishes, these spaces fill with fluid. The teeth have been shaken up so much that when their power weakens a little, they tend to fall out; and those joints which have been twisted become too weak for the exigencies of life and are extremely susceptible to tearing and rupture. In terms of bodily health, then, it is clear that no other breed of men is as badly off as that of the athletes. One might, in fact, surmise that athletes had been well named—from the word *athlios*—or that this word for 'miserable' had derived from the word 'athlete'; or perhaps that both take their name from a common source, the term *athliotēs* ('misery').

12. We have been considering the greatest good of the body in health; let us turn to other bodily goods. As regards beauty, athletics is very far from contrib-
32 uting to it. | Indeed, men have frequently started off with very well-proportioned bodies, been taken by athletic trainers, stretched and rolled around in blood and flesh, and ended up in quite the opposite state. Some have had their faces quite distorted and disfigured, particularly the practitioners of all-in wrestling or of boxing.

---

[34] Homer, *Iliad* IX.503.

It is, however, when they get a limb completely broken off or mutilated, or lose an eye, that the full beauty of the sport appears in all its clarity. Such features scarcely constitute an adornment, even to someone in a state of good health; but once these athletes retire, their remaining organs of sense go too; and all their limbs, as I said, become distorted and cause all kinds of deformation.

13. Well, perhaps athletes lay no claim to health or beauty, but only to strength. For one thing is sure: they say that they are the strongest men in the world. Now just what kind of strength are they talking about, and what on earth is its point? Is it useful for agriculture? I should certainly ǀ like to see them digging or har- 33 vesting or doing anything of practical value on a farm. Is it useful for war? Call back Euripides, and listen again to his words of praise:

> Will they then fight the enemy so armed
> With discus?

For indeed:

> None with the iron close at hand raves so.

Does their strength then consist in a resistance to extremes of weather, enabling them—true followers of Heracles—to bare their bodies in winter and summer alike, to walk barefoot, to sleep in the open, to lie on the ground? Not at all: newborn babies are better than them at all these things. Where is it then that they can show off this strength? What is the source of their self-esteem? Surely not a capacity to beat shoemakers, carpenters or builders in the wrestling-school or on the track? It may be that they pride themselves on the ability to spend all day in the dust; but this ǀ they share with quails and partridges. And if 34 it is an accomplishment to be boasted of, so too, I suppose, is the ability to spend all day washing in muck.

But what about the famous Milo of Croton, who once did a lap of the stadium with a sacrificed bull on his shoulders? What an incredible act of stupidity that was! Not to realize that just a little earlier, while it was alive, the animal's body had been borne up by a soul which drove it with much less effort than Milo—and was able to run too. Of course, that soul counted for nothing in comparison with Milo's. But then Milo's death, too, bore witness to his stupidity. One day he saw a youth cutting a piece of wood along its length, by the insertion of wedges. He laughed at the fellow and pushed him aside, reckoning to split it with his bare hands. He expended all his energy on his first attempt, by which he pushed apart the two connected legs of the piece of wood. In the process the wedges fell away. Milo was unable to part the remainder of the log, in spite of a huge effort; in the end he gave up and, failing to get ǀ his hands out of 35 the way in time, had them crushed by the two parts coming together. First of all his hands were crushed; later they were the cause of Milo's own miserable end.[35] Much good his dead bull in the stadium did to prevent his suffering! Or perhaps you think that it was efforts such as that which Milo expended on the bull which saved Greece in the war against the barbarians? It could not rather have been Themistocles' good judgement, could it, first of all in interpreting the oracle correctly, and then in conducting an exemplary campaign?[36]

> A wise word will prevail against much force;
> The ill-directed masses do no good.[37]

It has been shown beyond all doubt that the athletes' training is of no use in any practical context; but it is possible to show too that even in their own field of endeavour they are worthless. Let me recount a story which was once turned 36 into an epic by a man of great talent.[38] | It goes like this.

If by Zeus' will it happened that there should be harmony and concord among the animals, with the result that the herald in Olympia could call on all kinds of animals, as well as men, to enter the stadium, not a single man would win a crown. For, he says,

> Best at long-distance racing is the horse;
> The hare will win the sprint quite easily;
> First in the double course is the gazelle;
> No mortal man would win a prize for running.
> O wretched race of men, who train for naught!

Nor would even a child of Heracles turn out stronger than an elephant or lion. Even a bull would win, I suppose—in the boxing. And the ass (he goes on to point out), if he so wishes, can use his foot as a weapon, and carry off the crown himself.

> In the vast chronicle the ass will be
> Set down: he once beat men in the all-in.
> The twenty-first Olympiad it was that saw
> His victory.

37 | This delightful tale demonstrates that athletic power is not one of the human accomplishments. And yet, if athletes do not hold the field over animals in strength, what good do they partake of?

---

[35] Milo of Croton (*c.* sixth century BC) was an Olympic athlete of legendary strength and apparently also a pupil of Pythagoras. The story of his death is that, trapped in the wood (usually specified as a tree trunk in a forest) in the manner described, he was eaten by wild beasts.

[36] The statesman Themistocles was renowned for his interpretation of an obscure Delphic oracle as an instruction to the Athenians to build a fleet, thus bringing them success at the Battle of Salamis (480 BC); the story is recounted by Herodotus, *Histories* VII.143.

[37] The lines are from Euripides' lost *Antiope*.   [38] The identity of the poet is not known.

14. You may say that bodily pleasure is a good; but they do not enjoy this either—not while they are training, certainly, nor afterwards. During their athletic activity they are in miserable pain, whether from their exercises or from the enforced eating. When they stop, most parts of their bodies give out. Again, you may say that they are respected for their money-making ability; in reality you will find that they are all in debt, both the practising athletes and the retired ones. One never comes across an athlete who is better off than the average estate manager of a wealthy individual. Besides, | making money by one's own   38
efforts is not in itself admirable; it is only admirable if one has true understanding of an art—the kind of art that will 'float with one in the case of a shipwreck'. This is not something which belongs to those who frequent the rich, nor to tax-farmers or merchants. Such people get more money from their activities than anyone; but, if they lose their money, they are also unable to perform these activities, since they require a certain minimum investment; without this they are unable to return to their former practices. And no one will lend them money without some pledge or security.

So, if what is required is a training that will lead to a secure livelihood which is at the same time honourable, the answer is a lifelong dedication to an art. Now, there is a basic distinction in kinds of art: there are the high arts, which are associated with reason, and there are the less respected arts, which are performed by bodily labour—the arts generally known as banausic or manual. Clearly the former kind is the more desirable accomplishment. The latter tends to give out | when   39
its practitioner reaches old age. The former includes rhetoric, music, geometry, mathematics, arithmetic, astronomy, grammar and jurisprudence. The arts of sculpture and drawing may also be included: though they are manual in their performance, they do not require the strength of a young man in his prime.

Unless, then, his soul is completely bestial, a young man should take up and cultivate one of these arts. And best of all would be the finest of them, which in my opinion is medicine. But this point will be demonstrated subsequently.[39]

---

[39] See n. 1 above. As cited by Boudon, the thirteenth-century Spanish Jewish philosopher Ibn Falaquera has preserved a few lines which apparently come from the missing sequel: in these, the argument for the superiority of medicine centres on the supreme importance of its aim, health.

II
SCIENTIFIC THEORY
AND METHODOLOGY

My Own Doctrines

In this work, thought by some to have been written towards the end of his life, Galen summarizes the essentials of his views and teachings in a range of philosophical and scientific areas; it functions in a sense as a companion piece to the works of 'auto-bibliography'. At the same time, it presents his views in some striking, in some cases even unique, formulations, especially in the context of his discussion of epistemology and the limits and purposes of human knowledge.

The full Greek text has only been available since the discovery of the Vlatadon 14 manuscript in Thessaloniki in 2005 (see the headnote to *Freedom from Distress*). Before that the work was available only in the form of some extracts in other Greek manuscripts, supplemented by a full Latin translation of a lost Arabic translation, as well as some quotations in Hebrew. Even after the discovery, the first new editions were based on inspection of a microfilm copy rather than access to the manuscript itself; only the last edition mentioned below had the benefit of the latter.[1]

Greek title: Περὶ τῶν ἑαυτῷ δοκούντων (*Peri tōn heautōi dokountōn*)
Kühn: not present
Editions: Nutton 1999 (based on a fragmentary Greek text and sources in Latin, Arabic and Hebrew); Boudon-Millot and Pietrobelli 2010 (the first edition based on the full Greek text; chapter and page numbers given here are those of this edition); Garofalo and Lami 2012; Polemis and Xenophontos 2023.

1. My present fate is, I believe, similar to that suffered many years ago by 172 Parthenius the poet.[2] The story has it that his poems had, during his own lifetime, come to be circulated very widely throughout the world; and that once, as he was walking through some city, he came upon two scholars[3] engaged in a dispute over a line of his poetry. One of them was giving an interpretation of the words which accorded with Parthenius' intention in composing them, the

---

[1] On scholarship on the manuscript since its discovery, see *Freedom from Distress*, n. 1. As mentioned there, the edition of Polemis and Xenophontos appeared after the present translation had been drafted and too late to be used systematically, though I have tried to take into account its main departures from previous editions.

[2] Parthenius of Nicaea, Greek poet of the first century BC, influential in bringing Hellenistic poetry to Rome. For the story and the reflections that follow, compare the preamble to *My Own Books*.

[3] The term is *grammatikos*, which refers both to a literary or linguistic specialist and to a teacher at a particular level (roughly, 'secondary' or 'middle', in modern Anglo-American terms) in a child's basic education, which focussed heavily on the literary classics; cf. *My Own Books*, n. 4.

other a completely opposite one. Parthenius himself attempted to show this second scholar that the line was meant in a different sense from that which he understood; but he absolutely refused to concede. 'And yet', said Parthenius, 'I actually
have it from Parthenius himself that the sense of this line is as I interpret it.'[4] When
even this failed to convince the man, he continued: 'Doubtless I will appear to be
suffering from some delusion, in claiming to be the author of these words; so I
will need to produce these servants of mine as witnesses. Then, perhaps, you
will believe that the Parthenius who wrote these words is, in fact, myself.'

Something similar seems to be happening to me now; and it comes about
because of the terrible fate that now afflicts both medicine and philosophy.
People who have had the instruction of neither scholar nor rhetor,[5] but who
rush straight to the specialized skills, misunderstand not just the writings of the
ancients, which are indeed often unclear, but even those written by me, which
are surely completely pellucid to anyone who has received a basic education.
The difference between my experience and Parthenius', however, is in the nature
of the witnesses. He had to resort to his slaves as witnesses of his true identity;
I, meanwhile, present my own writings as witnesses on my behalf, in relation to
those things about which I have declared secure knowledge, on the one hand, or
merely knowledge to the level of plausibility, on the other, as indeed there are
some things in relation to which I claim no secure knowledge at all, on the
grounds that I have no scientific understanding of them.[6]

2. I have decided to begin my account with these last, which include the following: whether the universe had a beginning or not, and whether or not there
is anything beyond it. And if I assert my ignorance of these points, then obviously I assert it also of the nature of the Craftsman of all that is in the universe:
whether he is incorporeal or possessed of a body; and still more so, what place
he inhabits. Do I, then, assert a complete ignorance regarding the gods, in the
173   manner of Protagoras,[7] or I do I rather, here too, state that I do not know the
nature of their *substance*, but that I do know that they exist, on the basis of their
effects?[8] For indeed, the constitution of animals is such an effect, as too are

---

[4] An alternative interpretation, suggested to me by David Leith, and arguably following the
grammar of the Greek manuscript as it stands more closely, would attribute this line to the scholar;
this would make the joke and point of the story slightly different. On balance I think that the present translation is to be preferred.

[5] The *rhētōr* or oratorical instructor provided the final stage of this literary-linguistic education.

[6] There is some doubt whether Galen is mentioning three different levels of epistemic certainty
here, or whether the final part of the sentence, from 'as indeed' glosses the second category, things
known only as plausible truths.

[7] Protagoras (fifth century BC) was famously credited with the statement: 'As regards the gods,
I am not able to know whether they exist, whether they do not exist, nor what is their nature' (as
quoted by Diogenes Laertius, *Lives of the Philosophers* IX.8.51).

[8] 'Substance' is *ousia*, also translatable as 'essence'; the term, with a Platonic and Aristotelian
heritage, refers to something's most fundamental nature, or definition; it may also however denote
something's physical substrate, what it is made of.

those things which they prefigure through portents, signs and dreams. Moreover, the god who is honoured by us in Pergamum has shown his power and providence in many contexts; in my own particular case, he once cured me.[9] I also have experience, at sea, not just of the providence of the Dioscuri but of their power too.[10] However, I do not believe that human beings are harmed in any way by ignorance of the *substance* of the gods. But I have determined to honour them, in accordance with ancient custom, just as Socrates encourages us to obey the instructions of the Pythian god.[11] This, then, is my position in relation to the gods.

3. My position in relation to human beings is as follows. I am convinced that we have a soul—as indeed is everybody, for I see that all people use the term 'soul' to refer to that which is responsible for voluntary movement and sensation through the instruments of perception. As to the identity of the substance of the soul, however, I confess my ignorance; and even more so, whether it is immortal or mortal. Indeed, when I wrote my notes on the doctrines of Hippocrates and Plato—which I did first of all purely for my own benefit, 'for the age of forgetfulness', as Plato has it,[12] though I later also shared them with friends, at their request—I nowhere made a declaration as to the mortal or immortal nature of the soul, nor as to whether it is incorporeal or has a body. I have, however, written down the demonstrations on the basis of which I am convinced that one source is in the brain, another in the heart and a third in the liver.[13] This was in the treatise in which I discussed *The Doctrines of Hippocrates and Plato*; I venture, too, to demonstrate that it is in the brain that arise our memories and intellective processes, those which involve the recognition of consistency and conflict and all other elements of logical theory engaged in by humans; and, more definitely still, that every part of the body has its impulsive, or voluntary (or whichever other term one may wish to use) motion directed

---

[9] The god meant is Asclepius; for his role in Galen's life see also *My Own Books*, ch. 3, with n. 22; see also *Health* I.6. The 'clear dreams' of his father in *The Order of My Own Books*, ch. 4, are probably also to be understood as involving Asclepius. The term translated 'providence', *pronoia*, has connotations both of foreknowledge (of the sort associated with divine beings) and care (of the sort that a doctor would provide); cf. *The Best Doctor is Also a Philosopher*, n. 1.

[10] The Dioscuri, twin sons of Apollo, were worshipped as protectors of ships and sailors. It has been suggested that this mention of their 'power' is a specific reference to the phenomenon of 'St Elmo's Fire', a kind of luminous electrical discharge sometimes observed on the rigging of ships during thunderstorms: the phenomenon was thought to be a manifestation of the Dioscuri, and a sign of deliverance.

[11] Socrates, while following traditional religious practice and (according to our most reliable sources) having strong religious commitments, constantly asserted his philosophical ignorance, especially on metaphysical matters. It is relevant too that it was the Pythian oracle—that of Apollo— which was responsible for the pronouncement, 'no one is wiser than Socrates'—the grounds for this pronouncement, according to Socrates, being that he alone was aware of his own ignorance.

[12] The quotation is from *Phaedrus* 276d.

[13] For this view, and the use of the terminology of 'source' (*archē*) in this context, see *The Doctrines of Hippocrates and Plato*, especially VII.3, pp. 274–5 below.

from the brain, as well as the discernment of all external perceptible objects, through the instruments of perception.

I also made a declaration that the heart was the source of the activity of the pulse, which takes place not just in it but also in all the arteries, and that the ferment, as it were, of the innate heat derives from this as from a furnace; the liver, 174 too, has some share in this heat, as do all plants, but | this is slight indeed, and at times requires the assistance of the heart; for there is such great heat in the blood (there) that it actually undergoes seething in episodes of rage.

I state that there is a source of motion in plants, too, and that they have capacities by which they are maintained; there are three books on these capacities,[14] where I show the existence of the capacity which is attractive of what is proper to them, as also of that which is expulsive of what is alien; then, of that which is transformative of nutrition and breath, and by which they assimilate these to themselves; and finally of that which is retentive of things proper to them; further, that nutrition, and also the growth of the embryo, are the task of the transformative capacity. I did not, however, at any point make a declaration on the capacity which shapes the embryo—whether it arises by nature from the same substance to which I have ascribed the four capacities (attractive, transformative, expulsive, retentive), or whether this capacity is something other and more powerful than these. This was discussed also in my work on *The Shaping of the Embryo*. Now, in discussion with Platonist philosophers, I refer to the substance which maintains plants as 'soul', whereas I use the term 'nature' in discussion with the Stoics—as, indeed, with people more widely: the capacities of this type of soul are referred to as 'natural' in the three books on *Natural Capacities*, a work whose argument in in this area is addressed both to all doctors and to humanity in general.

4. As regards the bodies in this world (I claim no secure knowledge of those in the heavens): I have shown, both that Hippocrates asserts that all arise from a mixture of fire, earth, water and air, and that this assertion was correct; moreover, that he himself refuted the opinions of those who take the elements of bodies to be unaffected and unchangeable in their qualities. My demonstrations of these matters appear not just in my work on *The Elements according to Hippocrates*, but also in three other books of commentary in which I give an explication of his work on *The Nature of the Human Being* along with certain other writings. I have also shown that Hippocrates maintains the same opinion in his other works.[15] Further, that the term 'hot' indicates (1) a completely hot

---

[14] Galen refers to his *Natural Capacities*, where he does indeed identify and distinguish these capacities, which are shared by plants and animals (albeit largely in the context of their role in the latter, and particularly in human beings). For the notion of maintenance or management (*dioikēsis*) of plants and animals by capacities (*dunameis*), see *The Art of Medicine*, n. 13 and *The Doctrines of Hippocrates and Plato*, passim.

[15] A lost work, referred to also in *My Own Books*, ch. 9.

body, unadulterated by opposite qualities, which we state to be one of the elements; (2) in another sense, that which is 'hot' through predominance of that quality; and (3) in yet another, different from both these, what Hippocrates customarily referred to as the 'connate hot', which has ǀ a specific balance in each   175 kind of animal.

I have offered demonstrations on this point in various works, especially in that addressed *To Lycus*, concerning his criticisms of Hippocrates' statement in the *Aphorisms*, 'things growing have the most innate hot'. Lycus' view was that Hippocrates had used the word 'most' in the sense of 'most vehement', not in that of the greatest extent of its own proper substance. The proper substance of the innate hot is semen and blood: our generation takes place through and from these. The correct understanding of the term 'most', which has also given rise to misinterpretation, was also demonstrated here: Hippocrates must be understood to have used the term in reference not to an intensification of the quality, but in relation to greater quantity.

It has been shown in our writings on *Mixtures*, which follow on from those on *The Elements according to Hippocrates*, that children are hotter than those in the prime of life in terms of the innate hot, while in terms of the acquired hot the latter are hotter than the former. Healthy people, similarly, have more innate hot than those suffering from fever; and the severity of the fever is in proportion to the inadequacy of the innate hot, for that which is acquired is unpleasant and biting, while the innate hot has no biting quality and causes no distress. Fevers arise through a distortion of the innate heat; I have shown that there are three primary kinds, which are called ephemeral, hectic and arising from putrefaction of fluids. This has been discussed in my writings on *The Distinct Types of Fever*.

5. In those on *Mixtures*, similarly, I showed that there are nine different types of mixture, four simple, four composite and finally one besides these which is the optimal and faultless one; that the simple bad-mixtures arise through the predominance of one of the elements, hot, cold, wet or dry, and the composite ones from the simultaneous domination of wet and cold, of hot and dry, of hot and wet, or of cold and dry. These, however, are not faultless, whereas the best mixture involves no predominance of one of the four elements, but represents a faultless mixture of them. In that work I also discussed at considerable length the wet, hot mixture, which many doctors and philosophers have claimed to be the best. ǀ This is not correct, if 'hot' and 'wet' are understood as   176 referring to a predominance of those qualities, which is indeed the sense stipulated by those same doctors and philosophers in their application of any of the terms 'hot', 'dry', 'cold' or 'wet' to a mixture. Since they use each of the quality terms in such cases to indicate an excess with regard to the state of good balance, here too we must, consistently, understand 'the hot, wet mixture' as that which involves a level of heat beyond the good balance, and an excess of wet

over dry. Yet, as I discussed there, some philosophers as well as doctors have stated that the best mixture is the wet, hot one, on the grounds that they observe that we have wetter and hotter bodies than dead animals or plants.

In a comparison between types of body, then, they have asserted that human beings in a natural state are wet and hot, and similarly that amongst the seasons spring is hot and wet, since it is wet by contrast with summer and hot by contrast with winter. If, however, you consider the mixture of spring in itself, you will there find a state of good balance in respect of both the oppositions. (By 'oppositions' I mean that of hot and cold and that of dry and wet.) Those states in which there is a predominance of hot over cold or of wet over dry must necessarily be bad ones. I showed, further, that Hippocrates gave an example of these in the second book of his *Epidemics*, where one particular spring season becomes distorted into such a state, as well as in the third, where this is the case for the entire year. In the second book of *Epidemics*, right at the beginning, he describes the state in which, he says: 'there was constant, violent rain in burning-hot weather'; and in the third, that in which 'the year was moist and rainy; there was an absence of wind throughout'.[16] In both states, he recounts the occurrence of plague-like illnesses. It thus seems clear that it is as a result of the homonymous usage of the terms that the dispute and disagreement in this area have arisen between myself and those who declare that the 'wet, hot' mixture is the best in animal bodies, and that, within the seasons, these are the qualities of spring.

A similar apparent disagreement arises in relation to old age, with some stating it to be wet and others dry. As regards the solid bodies themselves, it is correct to call them dry; as regards the residues, wet. For at this age there is a very large amount of phlegm, which is a cold, wet fluid. There thus appears to be a contradiction with the view of those who pay closer attention to the correct statements—as, again, in the case where we state that the nerves are tendentially wet in their mixture, while hot bodies have a greater potential for perception than cold ones. In such cases, one must therefore make the correct distinctions with regard to every statement, and understand correctly the sense in which it is meant.

177 |

6. We have shown—in accordance also with the opinion of the ancients—that the part in which the command centre of the soul is located is the primary [organ] of perception.[17] The capacity for perception, as well as that for voluntary motion, flows from that, through the nerves, to all parts of the body. (As has been already stated, it makes no difference whether one uses the term

---

[16] The quotations are from the Hippocratic *Epidemics*, II.1.1 and III.2, and are discussed by Galen further in *Mixtures* I.4.

[17] See *My Own Books*, n. 38, and *The Doctrines of Hippocrates and Plato* passim.

'voluntary' or 'impulsive'.) Further, that this capacity, on arriving at each part, renders it perceptive; and that the hotter parts more readily undergo the alteration due to this capacity, and thus become more able to perceive than the colder ones. The capacity that travels through the nerves, however, which function as it were as its vehicle, makes these, too, capable of sensation, but does not render them more so than the fleshy substance. You may realize this by laying bare a nerve in any animal you choose, and then pricking it with needles or stili; you will find that it makes more noise when the flesh or skin is pricked, since that causes it more pain. The majority of doctors, however, believe that the nerves are more capable of sensation than the flesh, because of the dangers attendant on the inflammation of the former, dangers which arise because these are offshoots of the primary sensory part. Thus, if you cut through the entire nerve, there is no attendant danger, as long as the source is not yet undergoing inflammation through sympathy; indeed, many doctors, fearing the dangers attendant on inflammation of the nerves, have on occasion cut through an entire pierced and inflamed nerve, without the patient becoming aware of this—which would be impossible if they had cut through some fleshy part.

During venesection, too, it sometimes happens that doctors accidentally sever a hair-like nerve which is extended | alongside the vein undergoing the 178 procedure. In such cases, the cut itself produces no greater pain than in patients not thus cut; it is only later, when numbness is experienced, that they realize that they have cut through a nerve. That the type of sensation of numbness that is consequent upon inflammation of the nerves is itself an indicator of faint pain, is quite obvious to all; and it is equally well known that such pain is consequent on the inflammation of the nerves.

It is quite frequent that patients who have suffered no significant pain during the inflammation of the nerves shortly afterwards manifest spasms. The presence of spasm indicates that the inflammation was a substantial one, while the moderate nature of the previous pain indicates that the pain attendant on inflammation of the nerves is not a powerful one.

Now, just as some have taken the nerves to be more capable of sensation than the fleshy parts, on the basis of the dangers attendant on inflammation of the nerves, thus attributing to these parts a greater share in sensation than they really have, Asclepiades has meanwhile gone to the other extreme, believing that they possess no sensation whatever. If one pays attention to the manifest evidence of the senses, one will find that the nerves are capable of sensation, but not in the same way as the fleshy parts. Yet we sometimes describe the nerves as 'more sensitive' on the grounds of the harm attendant [on such conditions].

7. Since I admit that I do not know the substance of the soul, nor whether it is mortal or immortal, and yet I see that it is consistent with both views that the soul is not capable of inhabiting all bodies, even if it is immortal, and indeed

even if it is incorporeal, I believe it reasonable to call the body which receives it—and which holds it so long as this body remains in an appropriate condition—'suited for sensation'; as, for example, the eye is suited for sight, the ear for hearing and the tongue for speech.

It is also reasonable to suppose that the generation of these is due to a particular mixture of the four elements; and if, indeed, it is the case that the soul has its generation at the same time as the shaping of the body, that this comes about through the mixture of the four elements, and that the generation of the soul and that of the sensory body are not two different things. For there is not, in that case, a substance of the soul considered in isolation; rather, it is what may be termed the form of the body (you should understand me here to mean 179 form ǀ in the sense of the opposition to matter, which we conceive of as being, in itself, without form).

I have shown, also, that this much is useful for the doctor to know, even if we are completely ignorant of the substance of the soul; for even if it is immortal and incorporeal, it is evident that it remains with the body for so long as it is able to perform the natural activities, so that we do not die so long as we preserve the body with its sensory mixture; and I have shown, further, in the first book of *Health*, that the mixture of the body is, necessarily, in a constant process of change towards the colder and drier, so that in old age it becomes completely dried out and cold, and when the dryness and coldness reach a certain point, the soul is no longer able to perform its proper functions, but these become withered even while we are still alive, in conjunction with the state of the body.

Thus, just as it is superfluous for a doctor to know whether the soul is immortal or not immortal, for the purpose of his cures, so it is, too, to know whether its substance is wholly incorporeal, as Plato supposed, or corporeal, as Chrysippus believes. The latter asserts that the soul is breath; but he does not specify clearly, as Erasistratus did, whether the soul breath is contained separately, within some empty space of the body, or whether it pervades all the solid bodies; nor whether it is divided into tiny parts, in accordance with Empedocles' view of our generation from the elements, or extended through every part of the solid bodies, so that none is without some share in it. The fact that he evidently says the same things throughout his work, but never clearly, has also been shown, in one book which I produced on the soul.[18] Nonetheless, as already stated, I am not able to venture a statement on the substance of the soul. But just as I call a certain body 'sensory', with the meaning given above, so too I refer to such a thing as 'psychic' breath.[19] And I have shown in a number of

---

[18] Or possibly, 'on his theory of the soul'. The textual self-reference here is somewhat unclear, but it seems most likely that Galen means one particular book of *The Doctrines of Hippocrates and Plato*.

[19] The words translated 'sensory' and 'psychic' could also be rendered 'suited to sensation' and 'suited to the soul', respectively.

places, especially the seventh book of *The Doctrines of Hippocrates and Plato*, that this breath is located in the ventricles of the brain, not in <its body>.

8. Now, many doctors are very ready to dispute any argument, as indeed are many philosophers, too; there are, for example, those who disbelieve the demonstrations of the truth that the sun is larger than the whole of the earth. You will find, on the other hand, that those who respect the truth do not have ⎸ disputation as their goal, and are not desirous to find an object for their attack; rather, when they hear someone making the claim that he will demonstrate a particular matter, these people are eager to hear the demonstrations. Then, subjecting them to assessment over a considerable period of time, they do one of two things: dispute the points which they reject, or refute those who are putting forward a counter-argument. What such people do not do is produce counter-arguments to propositions at all costs, even when these happen to be extraordinarily paradoxical.

It is for such people as these, then, that the present work has been written, with the intention of encouraging them to turn to the demonstrations which we have previously written regarding each of the doctrines mentioned; and to examine those demonstrations, rather than to attempt to assess their conclusions considered simply on their own.

So, for example, the knowledge that there are in us three sources, each of different kinds of motion, is immediately necessary, both for the discovery of the soul's virtues and in order to go about acquiring these virtues. The knowledge that one of these is located in the brain, one in the heart and one in the liver, on the other hand, is not necessary for these purposes. Plato indeed manifested this distinction by his own practice: while in the *Republic* he speaks of three forms of the soul without mention of the places in the body in which each resides, in the *Timaeus*, where he is giving an exposition of physical theory, he declares not just that our entire soul possesses three forms, but also that these have three separate locations—one in the brain, one in the liver, one in the heart.[20] Chrysippus and his followers, on the other hand, have written about the part of the body in which the command centre of the soul is located, but

180

---

[20] Galen is making a distinction between different purposes or values of different kinds of knowledge: the tripartite division of the soul is essential for ethical knowledge and therapeutics, while the anatomical locations of the three parts are not; the latter knowledge is, however, of importance in physiology or physical science. The distinction between the status of statements made by Plato in the *Republic* and in the *Timaeus* appears also in *The Doctrines of Hippocrates and Plato* (at IX.7, pp. 282–3; see also IX.9, pp. 285–6 below), there in the context of a somewhat different argument, about levels of epistemological certainty: Plato puts the argument of the *Republic*, which he takes to be certain, in the mouth of Socrates, and that of the *Timaeus*, which has a provisional or 'probable' status, in the mouth of Timaeus. That distinction is interesting in terms of Platonic hermeneutics, and also for the relationship between Plato's and Galen's views of epistemological certainty. Galen would regard the statements on the location of the three parts—which for Plato was merely part of a 'likely account'—as also firmly established (as indeed made explicit in *The Doctrines of Hippocrates and Plato* IX.9).

have not shown in what way this knowledge is useful for those engaged in social,[21] practical philosophy, any more than that of thunder, lightning, earthquakes, hail and snow, or of rainbows, parhelia, meteors or the halo that is frequently produced around the sun or the moon, which sometimes appears single, sometimes double or triple, or of all other meteorological science, as it is known. These things indeed constitute an appropriate subject of enquiry only for those engaged in the enquiry into theoretical philosophy; I demonstrated this very point, in fact, on a previous occasion, in a single volume which was addressed to a friend who was an Epicurean, and again in another addressed to a Stoic. I showed that the argument concerning the three sources is, however, useful for doctors; and some part of physical theory is also in a way necessary or useful for the understanding of the body.

181   9. I have also shown that the distinction between kinds of | alteration that take place in bodies is of value, although this is neglected by most. These are two in number: those which are accomplished through one or two of the active qualities—that is, hotness, coldness, wetness and dryness—and those, by contrast, which are accomplished through the whole specific nature of the active substance. It was shown, too, in my work on *The Capacities of Simple Drugs*, that some act through heating, cooling, moistening or drying alone, while others do so through a pair of these qualities—heating and moistening, or cooling and drying—but that there is a different class of drugs which act through the specific nature of their whole substance.[22] Purgatives, and those drugs known as 'destructive', which differ from those known simply as 'deadly'[23] in that the former are never of benefit to us, whereas deadly drugs may at times bring benefit, when taken in small quantities, and sometimes in a mixture with beneficial drugs. Amongst beneficial drugs, too, some act through one or two qualities, some through the specific nature of their whole substance, in a way similar to coction in the stomach or blood-production in the liver, and increase and nutrition. These capacities belong to every part of the animal; for each part maintains itself by virtue of the capacities known as 'natural'—which it has in common with the plants—functioning like a self-preserving animal by

---

[21] I so translate the adjective *politikos* (also in ch. 15 below). The word is derived from the noun *polis* and may be applied to a whole range of social activities or deliberations (and also to words; cf. *My Own Books*, ch. 20) connected with the life of the city, broadly conceived. Although 'political' would certainly be a possible alternative translation, it seems that Galen's focus here is on the practical and social concerns of everyday life, rather than on 'political philosophy' in any abstract sense. See the similar usage in *The Doctrines of Hippocrates and Plato* IX.7, p. 283 below.

[22] For this distinction between action by virtue of one or two qualities and 'whole substance' action, see *Mixtures* III.1 (with n. 16) and *Simple Drugs* I.3 (with n. 2), V.1, IX.2.1 and XI.24. The latter concept is discussed in detail by Singer 2020.

[23] Both *dēlētērios* ('destructive') and *thanasimos* ('deadly') might also be translated 'poisonous'; I have preserved the literal distinction that Galen makes between the two, although it may seem surprising to us.

attracting to itself what is proper to it, rejecting what is alien, and transforming, altering and assimilating to its own nature each of the things so attracted.

10. It was also shown that these parts require assistance in order to persist in their natural state: the liver both sends appropriate nourishment and augments the capacities if ever they weaken: this is as it were a furnace and source of the natural capacities, just as is, in plants, the part where the roots join the stem. As long as this retains its capacity, even if some individual root or branch becomes dried out, the plant survives. The capacity directed from the brain, on the other hand, is not similarly present in each of the parts; for the existence of this capacity consists not in a persistence, but in a process, | in the case both of 182 human bodies and of those animal ones which are not far from them in nature. The motion of the arteries, similarly, flows from the heart but does not remain in them, whereas those capacities known as natural are innate to, and persist constantly in, the substances of the parts. The persistence of the good-mixture of the substance, moreover, is significantly assisted by the pulse, as has been shown in my piece on *The Function of the Pulse*.

There is the possibility, if anyone is not paying careful attention, of a misunderstanding arising from my statement that we maintained by three sources: some may think that this refers not to the maintenance of the mature animal but to the shaping and generation of the animal in the womb. As previously stated, I declare my conviction that the animal, after birth, is maintained by three sources, but do not claim to know what capacity or substance it is that shapes the embryo.[24]

11. Those who think that it is the same as that which generates and shapes plants seem to me not to be aware of the artistry of the construction or our bodies; this I expounded in *The Function of the Parts*. However, I do not claim to know securely even which part is shaped first of all in the womb. In my youth I followed the view of certain men of distinction, that the heart was shaped first of all; but in later years I came to suspect this argument of being one that is plausible, but not, in fact, true. For this organ cannot be generated without blood, and blood is provided by the vessels in the womb, from which the embryo's generation takes place. It is evident, however, that this blood reaches the heart through a vein which is first implanted into the liver. If the arteries also functioned as conduits to the embryo's heart from its mother, either for breath alone or also for some amount of blood, this route would be longer than that via the veins. For the arteries leading from the womb to the heart pass through the chorion, go around the [embryo's] bladder and first proceed to a bone situated at the lower extremity of the spine, before then continuing in the

---

[24] For this statement of ignorance, as well as much of the argument that follows in the next chapter, see also *The Shaping of the Embryo*.

vertebrae of the lower back and the chest, and through the artery extended alongside them they bring to the left ventricle of the heart the substance pro-
183 vided from the womb—whether, as already mentioned, this is breath alone | or also an admixture of blood.

On this basis, then, it no longer seems logical or plausible that the heart should be generated before the chorion and the vessels which provide blood and breath in that place; and therefore also not plausible that it is shaped before the liver, since it is clearly observed that the vein which is generated from all those veins in the chorion reaches the liver before it reaches the heart. Still more incongruous seems to me the argument of those who believe that the parts in the womb are shaped by the heart; for surely it is reasonable to suppose that the power that shapes the heart itself, and indeed before it the arteries and the veins, proceeds to shape the remaining parts in the same way that it has these (and the liver along with them). Some take this power to be the semen which is ejaculated into the womb; others take it that the semen is, rather, the instrument, while that which shapes the embryo is something different, and more divine, without laying claim to any precise knowledge as to what that is.

12. As for the humoral fluids, as they are known, that is blood, phlegm, black bile and yellow bile, my views on these have been made clear both in my commentaries on Hippocrates' *The Nature of the Human Being* and in *The Elements according to Hippocrates*. Whereas Hippocrates states that these four fluids are produced in all bodies, even in a state of health, certain others claim that blood alone is the fluid proper to our nature, and that the others are not present in our natural state. Now, while the latter opinion may be plausible, that of Hippocrates is in fact far truer. The demonstration of this rests on a single doctrine, itself demonstrated previously, namely that each one of the purgative drugs draws to itself one of the fluids mentioned—phlegm, yellow bile and black bile respectively. Some also attract a small amount of the other two (either both of them or one). There are also those who would have it that the nature of the purgative does not simply draw to itself the relevant fluid contained in the body, but in the process of attraction actually alters all the fluids in the veins, transforming them into one type, namely that proper to itself. I discussed this not once or twice, but on many occasions; and later wrote a book on *The Capacity of Purgative Drugs*, in which it is shown that each of them has the nature to attract some particular fluid.

If their claim is that some small change takes place during the period of the attraction, I am happy to accept that; but it would evidently be an extremely small change, just as the time in question is an extremely short one. It has also been shown that, in the case of blooded animals, blood is only the fluid most
184 proper | to their nature, but that the generation of the others is also necessary,

although their function is limited; and that each of the bloodless animals, too, has its own proper fluid, equivalent to blood in our case. The fact that the fluids contained in the veins are each attracted by the respective type of purgative drug is made manifest by the fact that the administration of a hydragogic to one suffering from dropsy leads to the evacuation of a very large quantity of water, and that the volume of the body is reduced in accordance with the amount of this evacuation, and in the case of those suffering from jaundice, the jaundiced colour is cleansed away through the evacuation of yellow bile by a bile-drawing drug; if, on the other hand, one were to administer the hydragogic drug to one suffering from jaundice, and the bile-drawing drug to one suffering from dropsy, a very small quantity of the fluid appropriate to the drug would be drawn out, and that by force; and no benefit—and indeed probably harm— would result from the evacuation.

It has, moreover, been shown by Hippocrates in *The Nature of the Human Being* that not only blood, but also phlegm, yellow bile and black bile are produced from our food and drink. The question has, however, quite reasonably been raised, whether the generation of the three takes place as described in the preceding argument, or rather follows as a necessary consequence; and a plausible argument is advanced by those who say that blood alone is our proper fluid. Whatever the truth of this, however,—whether it is the only proper fluid or more proper than the others—it is in any case quite evident that one must, in a healthy daily regime, take care to remove the excesses of both biles, and of phlegm, avoiding the increase of these fluids that will arise from an excess of phlegmatic or bilious foods. Provided that we are agreed on this point, we will suffer no detriment to the practice of our art by adopting either point of view, that is, by regarding the four fluids as elemental, or by taking it that blood alone is produced by Nature according to her primary plan, and the other three fluids are necessary consequences of its generation. It is also quite evident that in cases of inflammation, induration or other problems of the spleen, which give rise to poor complexion, with a change towards a darker colour, there is again no detriment to our practice of the art even if we do not accept that melancholic fluid is being attracted by the spleen, but say rather that it is generated there. It is, however, absolutely clear that one must say one of these two things, as has also been stated (along with all other necessary enquiries regarding that fluid) in *Black Bile*.

There is, however, the very damaging practice of those who dispute the conclusions of a demonstration, without however refuting the actual arguments in question; and there are also those who cannot bother to read the argument—or who give it one, extremely hurried, reading— | but are not prepared to give it 185 consideration over a sustained period of time. It also happens quite frequently that people misunderstand the conclusions of the argument, if there is some homonymous usage, as is the case with the 'melancholic' fluid.

There are in fact two possible senses of this, not just the single one according to which it refers to 'black bile' itself. For the fluid generated in the liver, too, is not yet black bile, but is capable of turning into it, either if it persists in the veins for a long time or if some hot, dry bad-mixture takes hold of the animal; and this fluid is termed 'melancholic fluid', as too is black bile itself. The term 'melancholic' thus has two senses, the first, according to which it is the same as black bile (for this is also known as 'melancholic fluid'); the second, according to which it is a kind of sediment of the blood (rather like olive oil lees, or the dregs in wine). This too is referred to as 'melancholic fluid', since its nature is to produce black bile proper on the basis of a very slight provocation. It is on a similar basis that we refer to certain foods as 'phlegmatic' and certain others as 'melancholic'.

We demonstrated in *Natural Capacities* and also in *Capacities of Purgative Drugs* that it is through the same vessels that, on the one hand, nourishment is carried up from the digestive cavity to the whole of the body, and, conversely, melancholic or bitter-bilious or melancholic fluid is at times carried down from the body, as is, sometimes, blood itself; in response to this, some have rashly asserted that it is absolutely impossible for melancholic blood to be drawn through the vein which extends from the entrances of the liver to the spleen, for which it is to be the nourishment. Are we then to take it that it is possible for a purgative drug to perform this attraction upon a fluid, but not possible for each of the parts of the body undergoing nourishment? Or that there is but one fluid proper to each of them? Some say that this is blood; but they fail even to realize that there are a very large number of bloodless animals, each nourished by its own proper fluid, which is cold in comparison with blood, but which has its own proper, or connate, or innate—or whatever term one prefers—heat, just as does the liver and every other part of body.

13. And for this reason I state that the heart is as it were the furnace of the heat within animals, while I consider the kind of heat that exists in plants to be a different one. Our bodies, however, partake of this too, precisely as they partake of what is known as the 'natural' or 'nutritive'—which may be termed either a kind of 'nature', or, with Aristotle ǀ and Plato, a kind of soul. I hold, too, that the liver contains the same kind of source of natural heat as plants contain in what is termed their 'rooting', a source which is proper to their nature, while that which is conducted to the whole body from the heart is different from that in kind. This latter causes heating which is perceptible by our sense of touch, while the 'natural' kind is so small that it eludes perception, so that we in fact do not attribute the property of heat to plants, independently, at all, when making the comparison with animals and making the assessment on the basis of sense perception. We do not, then, either contradict those who make such an assertion or subscribe to this opinion—provided that the discussion is not being conducted in terms of full scientific accuracy.

It may even appear to some that there is a significant disagreement between this view and that of those who state that animals are hot and plants cold; but this is due to a failure to realize that there is a precise way of speaking, where we arrive at a completely scientific understanding, pursuing the subject under enquiry to the ultimate level of knowledge, and another, where statements are made about a matter in passing, while the focus of the enquiry is a different one; and that in this latter case the immediate sensation of heat or cold is sufficient.

Indeed, Plato himself regularly refers to animals as endowed with soul, but states that stones, herbs, wood and plants in general belong amongst the non-souled bodies; when, however, in the *Timaeus*, expounding his views on natural philosophy for the very small audience which is able to follow scientific arguments, he states that the soul of the universe is extended throughout it, one should not consider that this is a discrepancy, or that the man is making contradictory statements—any more than is Aristotle or Theophrastus, who wrote certain works for the wider public, but lectures for their own students. When a doctrine which belongs in the category of those which are completely inaccessible to our perception, one which requires a great deal of argument for its demonstration, is stated prematurely, it will have a discordant effect on the audience. One should not, then, make assertions on such points before one has gone through the painstaking process to the conclusion of the entire argument; nor, in other contexts, assert that the soul of the universe permeates stones, shells, sand, and indeed dead bodies undergoing cremation or putrefaction. If Plato had made such a straightforward statement in front of a large audience, he would have had an unfavourable reception from all those present. Now, I have shown in a different work what considerations brought him to adopt this opinion, without myself declaring either my agreement or my disagreement with it. Indeed, Plato himself does not make declarations, in this sense, in relation to natural philosophy, claiming rather that this may advance only as far as what is plausible and likely. Now, I hold it true that plants have within them a source of motion, and that they have ⎮ perception of what is proper and what is foreign to   187 them; but I avoid making hasty pronouncements on such matters, even more than Plato did himself.

If, however, I am asked in what way animals are superior to plants, my response is that they have perception and voluntary motion; and as for the capacities which I mentioned previously, those of attraction, expulsion, retention and alteration, I refer to these as 'natural' capacities, not capacities 'of soul',[25] since I can discern no harm either to the art of medicine or to ethical

---

[25] The distinction in Greek is between the adjectives *phusikos*, related to *phusis* (nature) and *psuchikos*, related to *psuchē* (soul); another possible translation would use the terms 'physical' and 'psychical'; cf. a few lines below, 'natural or physical' (also translating the adjective *phusikos*).

philosophy arising from such a usage. When, however, it becomes necessary for me to speak of Plato's view on the natural or physical part of ethical philosophy, I approve his opinion and declare my agreement with it in some respects, while in others I am prepared to proceed as far as the plausible; and on yet other matters I am completely at a loss, having no inclination one way or the other as to which is the more plausible of the positions under dispute.

14.[26] For example, that we *have* a soul, I regard as a matter securely known—as do all people, on the basis of the manifest observation of actions performed [by it] through the body: walking, running, even wrestling, carrying out a variety of sensory functions. We realize that there are certain causes of these actions, on the basis of a certain postulate of natural philosophy which commands universal consent, namely that nothing happens without a cause; since, however, we do not understand the identity of the cause of these actions, we attribute to it a name derived from its *capability* of bringing about the effects that it does, that is, we speak of the 'effective *capacity*' of each of these events. In the same way, it is standard to speak of scammony as possessing a purgative *capacity*, and of the medlar as having a stopping *capacity*, in relation to the stomach.[27]

Those who exert themselves upon natural philosophy have persuaded themselves of various different propositions: some, that certain non-bodily capacities inhabit the perceptible substances, others, that those substances themselves act, each one by virtue of its own specific nature, which itself has arisen from the mixture of the four elements, or from a particular composition of the primary bodies—which some state to be atoms, some 'unjointeds', some the 'partless'.[28] And as regards our soul itself, too: there are those who believe it to be some non-bodily substance, I while others believe it to be breath, and others deny that it has any independent existence of its own, saying rather that the specificity of the substance of the body is stated to have the capacities for those things which it by nature does; that is, that those [capacities] are not particular substances with their own particular nature, but rather that the active substance

188

---

[26] At this point the Vlatadon manuscript has the indented phrase: 'Galen on the substance of the natural capacities'; the remainder of the Greek text from this point on circulated under that title as a separate treatise, which was also translated into Latin. Some modern editors have omitted the phrase from the text, others have emended 'natural' (*phusikos*) to 'of the soul' (*psuchikos*) in light of the argument that follows. It seems better to regard the words as an editorial gloss or subtitle which came to define a section of the text rather than as belonging to the text itself.

[27] Cf. the similar discussion of the concept of capacity in *The Soul's Dependence on the Body*, ch. 2, pp. 433–4 below.

[28] Galen here refers to a number of doctrines concerning the fundamental constituents of the universe, in particular those of various Atomists and of the followers of Asclepiades of Bithynia, with his theory of the 'partless bulks' (*anarmoi onkoi*). One Greek manuscript adds 'and some uniform [parts]' (*homoiomerē*), a possible reference to the view attributed to Anaxagoras that the most basic elements were a kind of uniform ('homoiomerous') part. Compare *The Elements according to Hippocrates*, n. 5 and n. 10.

should be said to have capacities in a particular respect in relation to those things that come about through it and by it.[29]

The position which I have myself adopted in relation to this is, one might say, a middle one. On other doctrines I have made a straightforward assertion, either of my knowledge of the truth or of my complete lack of such knowledge, depending on the case; but with respect to those which I just outlined, I proceed as far as the plausible: my position is that though it would be desirable to have such knowledge of them as to be able to make these assertions, as in the case of the others, I am not persuaded—as others are—that I have secure knowledge of matters about which I have not received a secure demonstration.

I should like, then, to speak also about all those matters the knowledge of which is not necessary either for health of the body or for the ethical virtues of the soul, but which would, if they were securely known, be an adornment to those things accomplished by medicine and by ethical philosophy. (This latter discipline, meanwhile, I claim to be both useful and possible for all who wish to cultivate; and indeed I have written two short books on the subject.) Now, however, I shall continue the argument as promised, beginning with the following point.

15. It is, I claim, securely known that everything within our bodies comes into being from the four elements—and, furthermore, that this takes place through their total mixture, and not, as Empedocles believed, through their division into tiny particles. Whether, on the other hand, the *substances* of the bodies penetrate each other, or their *qualities* only, I claim to be an unnecessary question to decide, and I make no assertion on it. I believe, however, that it is more plausible that the mixtures arise through the qualities. As for the soul, I make no claim to secure knowledge as to whether it is an immortal substance which becomes mixed with bodily substances and thus governs animals, or indeed whether there is no substance of the soul, considered in itself. This, however, is quite apparent to me: that, even if the soul enters the body [from outside], it becomes enslaved to the physical nature of the body, which, as already stated, arises from particular mixtures of the four elements. Accordingly, I do not believe that anyone will suffer any setback, in respect of the art of medicine, through ignorance on the subject of empsychosis and metempsychosis (as they are known).

I The body which is to receive the soul must be suitable for it, and if the for-   189 mer suffers any great alteration in regard to its mixture, the latter will immediately depart. Such an alteration would be the extreme cooling which the body undergoes through loss of blood or through the consumption of cooling

---

[29] Both argument and manuscript tradition here are somewhat difficult; but the proposition is essentially the same one made about capacities in *The Soul's Dependence on the Body*, ch. 2, pp. 433–4 below.

drugs, or when the ambient air is extremely cold, on the one hand, or the immoderate heating that takes place in cases of fever, inhalation of flame or consumption of heating drugs, on the other. Nor is it only in such cases of alteration of the mixture of the body that we observe the soul to become separated from it, but also when it is completely deprived of breath; this too leads to an alteration in the body. It seems to me a matter of certain knowledge that so long as the natural good-mixture of the body is preserved, it is impossible for the soul to be separated from it. And for this reason the knowledge of the identity of the soul's substance is not necessary either for the curing of disease or for the preservation of health, or, indeed, for the purposes of ethical, practical or social philosophy (one may use any of these terms, distinguishing this kind of philosophy from the theoretical; and I have discussed this further in other writings).

Once the distinction of natural capacities has been made, in terms of both kind and number, a further enquiry will arise as to *how* we are to say that they attract to them what is proper and expel what is alien. Such action would appear to be impossible without the ability first to *identify* what is proper and what is alien, before then bringing about the attraction of the proper and the expulsion of the alien; and such identification would seem to be a function that belongs to a perceptive capacity.

It is for this reason that a misunderstanding arises, even though Plato stated clearly that it is a different kind of perceptive capacity that exists in plants, as some who read this phrase may take it that there is some capacity within plants which *recognizes* what is proper and what is alien.[30] They have a capacity which extends only to the distinguishing of those two kinds—whether that capacity arises through pleasure and pain or through some similar and analogous phenomena that take place in them; the vegetative soul is not capable of identifying things through any other form of perceptual activity. For they have no ability to distinguish visual, auditory, olfactory, gustatory or tactile qualities, but merely between those things which have the capacity to nourish them and those which do not. They accumulate those things which do have this capacity, attracting them to themselves, retaining them, subjecting them to coction and transform-
190   ing them into the substances proper to those to be nourished, | and do not accumulate those which do not have this capacity. It thus seems to me that Plato is correct to describe plants as possessing perception, namely that of what is proper and what is alien; and that in this respect—as well as in respect of the

---

[30] The language seems a little odd, since the word used to denote the capacity denied to plants (that 'which recognizes', *gnōristikē*) is closely related to that used to denote the capacity which they are indeed said to possess (that of 'distinguishing', *diagnōsis*). The fundamental point, however, seems clear, namely that the sense in which the faculty of perception can be attributed to plants is a narrowly circumscribed one.

fact that they are not devoid of a form of self-movement—they may legitimately be called animals.[31]

Since, however, this knowledge, too, is unnecessary for the purposes of medicine and ethical philosophy, I confine myself to a statement—proceeding only to the level of the plausible, on the basis of logical consequence—of agreement with Plato, in his view that plants too are animals and participate in sensation. This claim of his refers to that form of sensation which identifies what is proper and what is alien, a form which, if one considers the matter carefully, belongs within the class [that relates to the identification] of what is pleasant and what is not pleasant. For one cannot state any other basis upon which it is possible for plants to attract, and to assimilate to themselves, what is proper, other than enjoyment and pleasure arising within them. Nonetheless, as stated, it is sufficient for medical purposes to understand this alone: that they do attract what is proper—that is to say, that by which they are by nature nourished—and repel what is alien. Moreover, the precise knowledge of such matters is even less valuable from the point of view of ethical philosophy; which is why Plato himself does not discuss it.

[31] The term *zōia* may also be translated 'living beings', and there is a dual use in Greek biological texts (especially for example in Aristotle), whereby it sometimes indeed includes plants in its reference; here, however, Galen seems to be insisting precisely on a stronger claim on the relationship between the two.

The Best Doctor is Also a Philosopher

In this short text Galen rhetorically exalts the status of medicine as an art, and the model supposedly represented by Hippocrates in both ethics and scientific method. The best doctor is a philosopher, the argument suggests, precisely to the extent and in the senses that Hippocrates was one.

Greek title: Ὅτι ὁ ἄριστος ἰατρὸς καὶ φιλόσοφος (*Hoti ho aristos iatros kai philosophos*)
Kühn: I.53–63
Edition: Boudon-Millot 2007

I.53 1. There is a malaise very frequently encountered in athletes: in spite of a desire to become Olympic champions, they take no regular exercise which might lead to the realization of that desire. A similar problem obtains in the case of doctors. Doctors will pay lip service to Hippocrates, to be sure, and look up to him as to a man without peer; but when it comes to taking the necessary steps to reach the same rank themselves—well, they do quite the opposite.

The opinion of Hippocrates was that astronomy, and therefore clearly the study which is prior to astronomy, too, that is geometry, are of central relevance to the study of medicine; these people are not only personally ignorant of both disciplines— | they actually censure others who are not equally ignorant. Furthermore, Hippocrates set great store by accurate knowledge of the body, as the starting-point for the whole science of medicine; these doctors' zeal for this study is such that they do not know the substance, conformation, shaping, size, or relationship to its neighbours, of each part of the body—nor even its position. Hippocrates also pointed out that an inability to distinguish diseases by species and genus leads to the failure of the doctor in his therapeutic aims; his attempt was to encourage us to train ourselves in logical theory. But the present generation of doctors, so far from enjoying a training in logical theory, in fact blame those who do have this training for wasting their energies on useless pursuits. Again, Hippocrates says that one should employ great foresight[1] in the

---

[1] *Pronoia*: the word includes the connotation of 'care', in the medical sense, and foreknowledge or forethought (including that exercised by divine powers: see *Affections and Errors* I.4, with n. 11); it is also related to the noun *prognōsis* and related verb *proginōskein*, which Galen here invokes in a paraphrase of the famous opening lines of the Hippocratic *Prognostic*—a highly influential text, on which Galen wrote a voluminous commentary. These lines were considered in some ways programmatic of the whole methodology and status of the doctor. Here the inclusion of past and present

construction of a prognosis of the present, past and future state of the patient. Today's doctors are so perfectly studied in this branch of the art that if someone predicts a blood-flow or a sweat | they denounce him as a sorcerer or diviner.[2] 55 Such fellows are hardly likely to tolerate one who is able to predict other matters beyond these; nor are they likely to establish a diet based on the expected peak of the disease—in spite of the fact that Hippocrates himself advocated such diets.

What remains, then, for them to admire in the man? Certainly not his skill in exposition. Such skill is, indeed, another of Hippocrates' qualities; but it is one so lacking in these authors that they may sometimes be observed making two mistakes in one word—something which is quite difficult even to imagine.

2. So I decided to try and find the reason why this universal admiration for the man is not backed up by a reading of his texts. Or, if someone actually does read them, he does not understand them; or, if by great good fortune he does both, he baulks at actually training himself in the theory with the intention of learning it securely and incorporating it in his practice. In my experience, all accomplishments may follow if one is well endowed with will and ability; if either | of these is lacking, it is quite impossible for the goal to be attained. We 56 can readily observe athletes failing to reach their goals, either through the natural deficiencies of their bodies or through a neglect of training. But if someone has a physique that equips him for victory, and undertakes the appropriate training as he should, what can possibly prevent him from running off with a whole series of crowns? So, are today's doctors deficient on both counts? Do they lack both potential and sufficient eagerness in their preparation for the art? Or do they have one but lack the other?

That no one should be born with sufficient mental powers to learn an art which is so beneficial to mankind seems absurd, since the world is essentially the same as it was in previous times: the seasons have not changed order, nor has the sun's course altered, nor has any one of the stars—either a fixed star or a planet—undergone any change. It must be because of the bad upbringing current in our times, and because of the | higher value accorded to wealth as 57 opposed to virtue, that we no longer get anyone of the quality of Pheidias amongst our sculptors, of Apelles[3] amongst our painters, or of Hippocrates

within the remit of 'prognosis' may seem puzzling; but the sense of 'prognosis' includes that of knowing or understanding something of the condition *before being informed of it by the patient*; and precisely this was thought to be an essential component of the doctor's art.

   [2] One may compare the vivid account of his own experience given by Galen in *Prognosis*.

   [3] Pheidias was the fifth-century-BC sculptor most famed for his supervision of the Parthenon sculptures, and for his colossal chryselephantine statues of Pallas Athene (in the Parthenon) and of Zeus at Olympia, the latter considered one of the wonders of the ancient world; Apelles (a contemporary of Alexander the Great) was the most famous of ancient painters. By Hellenistic and late antique times they had acquired an emblematic status, their names synonymous with 'the best' in their respective fields. Compare the attitude to Homer and Sappho indicated in *The Soul's Dependence on the Body*, ch. 2, p. 434 below.

amongst our doctors. And yet the fact that we were born later than the ancients, and have inherited from them arts which they developed to such a high degree, should have been a considerable advantage. So, for example, it should be easy to learn thoroughly in a very few years what Hippocrates discovered over a very long period of time; and then to devote the rest of one's life to the discovery of what remains. But it is impossible for someone who puts wealth before virtue, and studies the art for the sake of personal gain rather than public benefit, to make the goal of the art his own; people with those aims in view will succeed in enriching themselves long before we attain the goal of this art. It is impossible to pursue financial gain at the same time as training oneself in so great an art; someone who is really enthusiastic about one of these aims will inevitably despise the other.

Can it, then, be said of any of our contemporaries that his desire for financial
58   gain is limited to ‖ what will provide for his simple bodily needs? Is there any-one who has the ability not only to make a verbal formulation, but also to give an actual example, of this: the limitation of wealth to Nature's requirements for the prevention of hunger, thirst or cold?

3. If such a person does exist, he will scorn Artaxerxes and Perdiccas.[4] He would never come into the sight of the former; as for the latter, he would heal him of the disease he suffers, regarding him as a man in need of the Hippocratic art. He would not, however, think it right to spend all his time with Perdiccas, but would treat the poor people of Kranon and Thasos and the other small towns. He will leave Polybus and [Hippocrates'] other disciples to the citizens of Cos, and will himself travel through the whole of Greece; for he must take notes on the natures of different places.[5] So as to test from his own experience what he has learnt from reading, he will at all costs have to make a personal inspection of different cities: those turned towards the south or the north, and
59   those turned towards the rising or the ‖ setting sun.[6] He must visit cities that are located in valleys as well as those on heights, and cities that use seawater as well as those that use spring- or rain-water, or water from lakes and rivers. Nor should he neglect to consider whether they use excessively cold or hot waters, or waters with natron in them, waters with astringent qualities, or any other such waters. He should look at a city on the banks of a large river, one on a lakeside, one on a hill, one by the sea—and consider everything else about which Hippocrates taught.

---

[4] Artaxerxes was the name of two kings of Persia in the late fifth century; Perdiccas was a general of Alexander the Great, and after his death regent of the Macedonian empire.

[5] Polybus was Hippocrates' son-in-law and disciple, thought by many to have written several of the 'Hippocratic' works, including *The Nature of the Human Being*. The place names are also chosen for their Hippocratic significance: Hippocrates was from Cos, and Kranon and Thasos feature in the Hippocratic *Epidemics*.

[6] There is a verbal echo here of the Hippocratic *Airs, Waters, Places*, a crucial text for Galen.

So, the person who wishes to attain to such a character will, necessarily, not only despise money, but also be extremely hardworking. And one cannot be hardworking if one is continually drinking or eating or indulging in sex: if, to put it briefly, one is a slave to genitals and belly. The real doctor has been found to be a lover of self-restraint and a follower of truth. Furthermore, he must train himself in logical method, to know how many diseases ǀ there are, by species   60 and by genus, and how one may discover some indication of the treatment in each case. This same method also provides the foundations for knowledge of the body's very nature, which is to be understood on three levels. First, the level of the primary elements, which are in a state of total mixture with each other; secondly, the level of the perceptible, which is also called the 'uniform'; thirdly, that which derives from the organic parts.[7]

The function and activity of each of these parts for the living being are also taught by the logical method; and these must be learned, not uncritically, but with the support of demonstration. What grounds then are left for any doctor who wishes to be trained in the art in a way worthy of Hippocrates not to be a philosopher? He must be schooled in logical theory in order to discover the nature of the body, the differences between diseases and the indications as to treatment; he must despise money and cultivate self-restraint in order to continue assiduously in this training. He must, therefore, possess all the parts of philosophy: the logical, ǀ the physical and the ethical.[8] In that case there will be   61 no danger of his performing any evil action, since he cultivates self-restraint and despises money: all evil actions that men undertake are done either at the prompting of greed or under the seductive spell of pleasure. And so he is bound to be in possession of the other virtues too, for they all go together. It is impossible to gain one without acquiring all the others as an automatic consequence; they are connected as if by one string.[9]

If, then, philosophy is necessary to doctors with regard both to preliminary learning and to subsequent training, obviously one who would be a doctor must definitely also be a philosopher. That doctors need philosophy in order to employ their art in the right way seems to me to require no demonstration, when it has so frequently been observed that those who are interested in financial gain are druggists, not doctors, and use the art for the opposite of its natural purpose.

4. I hope that no one is going to quibble over words, and come out with some piece of disputatious ǀ nonsense, such as that 'the doctor should of course be a   62

---

[7] For the three-level theory of bodily composition see also *The Best Constitution* and *The Art of Medicine*; on element theory and the notion of 'total mixture' see *The Elements according to Hippocrates*, ch. 3, with n. 10.

[8] The division of philosophy into these three branches was probably standard by Galen's time, although it is particularly associated with Stoicism.

[9] The doctrine of the unity of virtues is originally a Socratic–Platonic one, though there may again be Stoic echoes in the present formulation.

person with the qualities of self-control and self-restraint, above monetary matters, and a just man, and yet not a philosopher'; or that 'he should know the
nature of the body, the activities of the organs, the function of the parts, the
differences between diseases and the indications as to treatment, and yet not be
trained in logical theory'. This would be to agree on the factual issue, but shame-
lessly concoct a disagreement on the basis of semantics. We do not have time
for this sort of thing. You would do better to return to your senses, and not
indulge in a pointless quarrel over sounds, like a jackdaw or raven, but interest
yourself in the actual truth of the matter. You cannot surely claim that, though a
weaver or shoemaker could never achieve competence without teaching and
practice, people may suddenly display the accomplishments of morality, self-
restraint, logical ability, or skill in relation to the natural world, without having
had recourse to teachers, or without having trained himself. One prepared to
make such brazen claims on these matters is a person indulging in a verbal, not
a factual, dispute.

We must, then, practise philosophy, if we are true followers of Hippocrates.
And, if we practise philosophy, there is nothing to prevent us, not only from
reaching a similar attainment, but even from becoming better than him. For it
is open to us to learn everything which he gave us a good account of, and then
to find out the rest for ourselves.

The Best Method of Instruction

This short treatise attacks the views of Favorinus of Arles, a successful orator in the generation before Galen and a proponent of Academic Scepticism, a movement which espoused sceptical philosophy within the Platonist tradition. It is one of three polemical works addressed to this author (see *My Own Books*, chs. 14 and 15), who, although none of his philosophical works survive, was clearly for Galen a central representative of the sceptical threat which he strongly feels the need to counter. Through the polemic, the work gives a succinct account of the fundamentals of Galen's own epistemology.

Greek title: Περὶ ἀρίστης διδασκαλίας (*Peri aristēs didaskalias*)
Kühn: I.40–52
Edition: Barigazzi 1991 (with Italian translation)

1. Favorinus states that 'the argumentation for both sides' is the best method of   I.40
instruction: this is the terminology used by the Academics for that form of instruction in which they approve of arguments placed in opposition to each other. Now, the earlier Academics take it that this argumentation ends in 'suspension'[1]—the name they apply to what one might call 'indeterminacy', that is, the abstention from definitions or secure assertions about anything. A more recent group, of which Favorinus is by no means the only example, sometimes advances this 'suspension' to such a degree that they do not agree even that the sun is 'graspable',[2] but on other occasions | advance the possibility of knowledge   41
to such a degree that they allow it to their pupils without these having first been taught a scientific evaluative principle;[3] for this is undoubtedly what Favorinus says in his work on the Academic disposition, entitled *Plutarch*; and he says the same too in his *To Epictetus*, which has Onesimus, the slave of Plutarch, in discussion with Epictetus.

---

[1] *Epochē*: standard Sceptic term for that withholding of belief which is the desired outcome of the argumentative process.

[2] *Katalēpton*: in Stoic epistemology, this term and its cognates refer to a kind of impression which is so strong as to guarantee its own veracity. The sense could thus also be rendered as e.g. 'certain', 'perceived or known with certainty'. I have preferred a translation which renders both the more literal connotations of the word (similar, in fact, to the etymological sense of the Latin-based equivalent 'comprehend') and its peculiarity as a technical term in school philosophy.

[3] 'Evaluative principle' translates *kritērion*; 'criterion' partially captures the sense, but what is meant is also an internal mental capacity, not just an objective standard.

Indeed, in the book written after these, the *Alcibiades*, he also praises the other Academics, who approve each of the arguments opposed to each other, but allow their pupils to choose which are truer. In this latter work, however, he says that it appears plausible to him that nothing is graspable, while in the *Plutarch* he seems to concede that there is such a thing as the securely knowable. (It is better to use this terminology for the 'graspable', and to depart from Stoic usage.)

Indeed, I must say that it always used to amaze me that Favorinus, who customarily changes every term into its Attic equivalent, still continually uses the
42 words 'graspable', 'grasping', 'grasping impression', as well as their negative forms, | the 'non-grasping impression', or indeed, as a noun, 'the non-grasping'; so that he has even written three books, one to Adrian, another to Druso and a third to Aristarchus, all entitled *The Grasping Impression*—in all of which, to be sure, he nobly strives and contends to show that it does not exist.

2. But I do not believe that 'the graspable' means anything other than the <securely> knowable, nor 'to grasp' something anything other than to know it securely; and similarly with the sense of 'grasping' and 'the grasping impression'.

For since we think that we see, hear, or in general, perceive some things as in dreams and in states of *mania*, while in other cases we do not just think that we see them or perceive them but in fact do so in truth, the latter cases are thought by all except Academics and Pyrrhonists to reach the level of secure knowledge, and the impressions that the soul has in dreams or in states of delirium to be all
43 false. Now, if | they themselves concede that this is so, let them erase those books of theirs in which they write that the mentally sound individual is no more trustworthy, in terms of knowledge of reality, than the one suffering from *mania*, nor the healthy than the sick, nor one who is awake than one asleep. If, on the other hand, nothing is knowable by those persons any more than by those who are in the opposite state, the evaluative principles of truth have, then, become confused, and neither the Academic teacher himself nor his pupil will be able to evaluate the arguments made on either side of an opposition.

Moreover, we shall not have any need of such teachers in the first place, since in that case we are able ourselves to read the writings of the adherents of the sects, and to know them no less than the Academics do; and if there is anything unclear in them, it will be safer to refer that to the Stoics, in the case of Chrysippus, and to the Peripatetics, in the case of Aristotle and Theophrastus. And so on with the others, too; so that there would be nothing left for the Academics to teach us, according to Favorinus' argument.

Amongst the older generation [of Academics] this was indeed the instruc-
44 tion: that there is no evaluative principle provided by nature to human beings, | by reference to which one may accurately identify each thing; and therefore they thought it right, too, that one should make no assertion on any matter, but should suspend judgement about everything. If, however, they will concede to

us that perception is sufficient for 'natural evaluative principles', we shall then have no further need of the argument on both sides, but of something different; and we shall turn rather to the practitioners of specialized skills, who offer their pupils straightaway, for example, the skill of calculation (which is known by the masses as 'counting'), and in this process whoever supervises a person being trained pays attention to the mistakes he makes, and corrects only these.

In the same way the trainer, too, corrects the errors of those who exercise in the wrestling-school, and the scholar, the rhetor[4] and the musician teach in this manner, not undermining nor swaying their pupils' trust in the natural evaluative principles, but supervising them in their training, until they manifest error-free performance of the individual activities. They will not employ [...] and so introduce 'suspension', as would be the practice of those who persuade people to distrust the manifest perceptions and to scorn things | securely known.   45

Indeed, Carneades does not concede that one should believe even this most manifest of all things, that amounts equal to the same amount are also equal to each other. We actually still now possess the arguments by which he attempts to destroy these and so many other propositions which appear manifest to you and are believed by you, because these arguments are treasured and stored in writings by the disciples. These 'solutions' have not, however, been repeated either by them or by any subsequent Academic. Well, he did successfully demonstrate this, I suppose, if nothing else: that all these arguments are sophisms, and that you, the pupils, should seek the solution of the sophisms. That is a miserable activity, to be sure, but at least less so than that carried out by those who wrote down these arguments, but have not shown us their true nature.

3. If Favorinus were present, I would gladly ask him whether he intends me to be persuaded by all these arguments, or to investigate whether they are true or false. For if he | conceded that I should investigate them, I would then addition-   46
ally of course ask him whether it is available to all human beings by nature to distinguish true and false arguments, or whether there is a method for the recognition of each. If the former, how is it that we do not all agree with each other, nor make the same assertions about the same matters? If, on the other hand, there is some method, I would have earnestly entreated him that I might first of all learn it, and then undertake all kinds of exercise, with his guidance, using many different examples, just in the same way as those do who learn athletic skills, cobbling, house-building, ship-building, speech-making, reading or writing—or, in quite general terms, the performance of any specialized skill whatever.

Now, if any of the Academics has written what kind of thing is a demonstration, and what kind a sophism, how one should distinguish the one from the other and how one should train oneself in that, then it is reasonable for Favorinus to entrust the evaluation of the arguments advanced on either side to

---

[4] See *My Own Books*, n. 4 on scholars and rhetors.

his pupils—except that it is otiose for the Academic to teach each of the subjects mentioned, if indeed we each have our own [internal] teachers of our doctrines.

47   If, however, none of them has either written | about the difference between them, nor given schooling in this, his practice is similar to that of a carpenter who instructs his pupil to measure, to weigh, to extend a line, or to draw a circle, without giving him a measuring-rod, scales, a ruler or a compass. Perhaps he will say that there is no such thing, in the realm of philosophy and of doctrines. Cease, then, your claim to know anything; cease to make declarations; do not retreat from the suspension of judgement that was introduced by the earlier Academics; and do not pride yourself on performing the task of a scholar who has learnt thoroughly the statements of your predecessors, since you will obviously realize that there is nothing in this that is sound. For such a procedure is not a mode of instruction, but rather idle chatter and nonsense.

Since, then, no hope remains of the discovery of what is true—for one who has no evaluative principle of what is true and false has no hope of gaining knowledge of that—you ought to have directed this teaching, that we have no inborn evaluative principle, only to the sophists, so as to then have the audacity to say: 'A person may, perhaps, allow us, who state that perception and intellection are manifest evaluative principles of the truth, to wallow in logical

48   lucubrations, | provided it is understood that this person is feasting on vain hopes.' But those who have removed all hope, as he has, are gibbering in vain. And so it is quite evident that Favorinus is loath to overturn everything and to state that he knows of the existence of no [evaluative principle] (precisely that principle denied by the Academics and Pyrrhonists before him); but that he rather claims to allow the evaluation to his pupils; whereas his predecessors did not even allow it to themselves.

4. The procedure conceived by Favorinus, then, of instructing students in any subject, is not only not the best of all; it is not in fact a procedure of instruction at all. That much, I suppose, has by now been clearly shown. As for those procedures conceived by the rest of them—well, these are at least procedures of instruction; whether they are best, we should investigate systematically, starting from the same considerations again. To us it appears manifest that there is something securely knowable,[5] even if the sophists do all they can to make it untrustworthy, saying that there is no such thing as a natural evaluative principle: for the compass draws the circle, the ruler determines lengths, as the scales do weights. It is human beings themselves who have

49   fashioned these, | taking their natural instruments[6] and evaluative principles

---

[5] These last six words correspond to a conjectural insertion in the text, which seems required by the sense.

[6] *Organa*: the word corresponds to 'organs' in the body as well as to 'instruments'.

as their starting-point. We have no evaluative principle either more valuable or more noble than these. If, indeed, one must proceed from these—for, again, our intellect tells us that while it is possible for us to trust or to distrust the natural evaluative principle, it is not possible to evaluate this evaluative principle on the basis of anything else, for how could that by which everything else is evaluated itself be evaluated by something else?—are you willing to trust your eyes when they see quite clearly, and your tongue when it tastes that this is an apple, but this a fig? If you are not so willing, I will submit to whatever you wish to do to me; but if you are keen to have a discussion, [I am ready to talk to you if you do trust them], but to shun you as one who is an unnatural state if you do not.

Let us first posit the case that you do not trust them; then you may hope to learn nothing from me; I have just finished making this point. Let us assume that you do trust them; then, you may hope to learn from me to make evaluations, but I [evaluate] what is perceptible by things manifestly apparent to the senses, and the intellective realm by things that are manifest to the intellect. But since all the specialized skills fashion instruments | and specialized evaluative 50 principles by which they both themselves construct and also evaluate what has been constructed by others, I too will teach you, in general terms, the instruments and evaluative principles, with which you will both fashion true arguments and evaluate those which arise from other people. The general principle is this: if something appears in itself manifest to the senses or to the intellect, this does not need enquiry. Something which is not so requires knowledge based on something else.

Now, my claim is that I will teach you certain things which are analogous to the instruments of the specialized skills, on the basis of which you will find out the object under enquiry, and certain things analogous to the evaluative principles, on the basis of which you will evaluate what seems to have been found out. Once you have learnt these, I shall school you, by use of many examples, to find out and evaluate the object of enquiry both swiftly and accurately, so that you will not need either any book or any other instruction for the finding-out of what is true; and, naturally, you will also readily discern those who are saying something other than what you find out. Just as one who recognizes the single nature of the correct road does not need any further | instruction in order to 51 dismiss the ones that lead astray, so too the person who learns the correct path of demonstration immediately also discerns, by virtue of this, the paths that lead astray.

5. Favorinus seems to me to do something similar to one who states that [Dion] is blind, but that he can evaluate which of us is dirtier and which cleaner, not realizing that one who is to make that evaluation must first be endowed with the faculty of sight. Of course, it makes no difference from the

point of view of the evaluation whether one actually has no faculty of vision, or whether one has it, but does not trust it. In the same way, what we evaluate with our minds—for example, that those things which are equal to the same thing are also equal to each other—one would not allow to human beings who do not have a trustworthy mind, any more than one would to asses who have no mind at all. Again, it makes no difference for the purposes of the teaching of the evaluation of matters, exactly what the nature of this person is—whether he does not have an evaluative principle or whether he does not trust it.

And so it is ridiculous of Favorinus to allow the evaluation to his pupils without conceding trustworthiness to the evaluative principles; for if nothing is 52 manifest to the mind | or trustworthy on its basis, the evaluation of all things is destroyed. But if the mind within our souls is just like the eyes within our body—that is, they are not equally sharp in every person—then it is possible that, just as one whose sight is sharper may lead one who sees less clearly to vision, in the same way in matters of the intellect too, one who is less sharp may be led to the sight of a matter of intellect by one who is quicker to see it clearly. And this person (as Plato states, and as I, too, am persuaded) is the teacher. I have written further on these matters in my treatise on *Demonstration*, where it is shown that the instruction of the intellect is, manifestly, of this kind. I also wrote how best one may, starting from the elements and principles in each case, demonstrate everything which is capable of demonstration—not, like our extraordinary friend Favorinus, writing one whole book in which he shows that not even the sun is 'graspable', and then elsewhere speaking to us as if we had forgotten this, and both conceding that there is something securely knowable and allowing this to his pupils.

Sects for Beginners

This introductory work on medical methodology or epistemology is important as a summary of the positions of the main rival medical sects of Galen's time, and his relationship to these. Galen mentions it as a work that should occupy a prominent place early on in the medical curriculum; and it was so used also in medical education at various subsequent periods.

Greek title: Περὶ αἱρέσεων τοῖς εἰσαγομένοις (*Peri haireseōn tois eisagomenois*)
Kühn: I.64–105
Edition: Helmreich 1893

1. The aim of the art of medicine is health, and its goal is the acquisition of I.64 health. It is necessary for doctors to know by what means one may bring about health when it is not present, or preserve it when it is. Those things which bring about health when it did not exist are called 'cures' and 'remedies', while those which preserve existent health are called 'regimes for health'. The traditional account says that medicine is the knowledge of things healthy and diseased;[1] those that preserve existent health, or restore health when it has been destroyed, are referred to as healthy, I and the opposite of these as diseased: the doctor 65 needs a knowledge of both in order to choose certain things and avoid others.

The source of this knowledge, however, is not equally well agreed by all, some stating that experience alone is sufficient for the art, others that reasoning appears to play a considerable role. Those who proceed on the basis of experience alone take their name from that term and are called Empirics, and similarly those who proceed on the basis of reasoning are called Rationalists; and these are the two fundamental sects in medicine, the one using testing to arrive at the discovery of cures, the other using indication.[2] The names 'Empiric' and 'Rationalist' have been accorded to these sects; but the former is frequently known as 'observation-' or 'memory-based', the latter as 'dogmatic' or 'analogistic'.[3] The

---

[1] Compare the lengthy account, using this basic distinction, in *The Art of Medicine*. (The term *nosōdes*, there translated 'morbid', is essentially synonymous with *noseros*, 'diseased'.)
[2] The Greek terms here translated, which help explain the etymological connections mentioned, are: *empeiria* ('experience'); *empeirikos* ('Empiric'); *logos* ('reasoning'); *logikos* ('Rationalist'); *peira* ('testing', related to *empeiria*, and in some cases also translated 'trial' or 'experience'). The term *endeixis* ('indication') refers to inference from observation or evidence to a hypothesized cause or physical reality, or from known facts about the patient, the history and the environment to the appropriate intervention.
[3] The process understood by 'analogism' is explained below, ch. 5. As suggested here, the terms 'Dogmatic' and 'Rationalist' are used interchangeably in this medical epistemological context.

practitioners, too, as well as the sects, are given names derived from these terms: 'Empiric', 'observational' and 'memorialist of the phenomena', for those who choose experience, and 'Dogmatic' and 'analogistic' for those who attach themselves to reason.

66   2. The Empirics state that the art is constituted in the following manner.[4] They have observed many ailments befalling human beings. Some of these arise spontaneously, in both diseased and healthy individuals, such as nosebleed, sweat, diarrhoea, or other similar things which bring with them either harm or benefit but do not have a perceptible effective cause. Others have an evident cause, but arise not from our own decisions but from some chance event, such as a flow of blood resulting from a fall, a blow or some other wound, or the drinking of cold water or wine in disease to satisfy one's desire; each of these, too, has either a beneficial or a harmful effect. They call the former class of beneficial or harmful things 'natural', the latter 'chance'; but they refer to the first sight of each of them as an 'encounter',[5] using that term because one encountered the thing without the involvement of his or her will. This, then, is the 'encounter-based' part of Empiricism; then there is the 'improvisatory',
67   where the person deliberately | puts something to the test, either at the behest of a dream or through some other conjecture. There is, however, a third part of Empiricism, namely the 'imitative': this is where any one of the beneficial or harmful factors—whether 'natural', 'chance' or 'improvised'—is again tested for the same ailments; and this last is the main element in the constitution of their art.

They imitate something which has previously been beneficial, and do so not twice or thrice but very many times; then, finding that it for the most part has the same effect in the same ailments, they call this kind of memory a 'theorem', and at this point regard it as a reliable part of the art. And when many such theorems have been 'assembled', the whole 'assemblage' is medicine and the person who assembles it a doctor. Such an assemblage is also called by them 'autopsy', being the memory of what has been seen frequently and identically. This very thing they also refer to as 'Empiricism', while the communication of it they call 'history';[6] for the same thing is autopsy for the person who observes it and history for the one learning of the observation.

---

[4] Galen frequently uses the terminology of the 'constitution' (*sustasis*) of an art, and even wrote a work entitled *The Constitution of the Art of Medicine* (the word is sometimes also translated 'composition'). What is meant is the way that an art acquires its overall structure and rationale on the basis of its constituent elements.

[5] Galen is here listing a series of words which had a technical sense within the Empirical school; 'encounter' translates *periptōsis*, on which see also *Anatomical Procedures* I.2.

[6] The term *historia* in Greek had the general senses of 'enquiry', 'observation' and 'narrative'. In the present usage, especially associated with the Empirics, it comes to have a sense close to the modern medical one of a 'case history'.

Since, further, they | at some point came upon diseases which had not been   68
previously seen, or diseases which were known, but in places where there was
no supply of those cures which had been observed by trial, they produced as an
instrument for discovery of remedies the 'transition from the similar'. By the
use of this they frequently transfer the same medicine from one ailment to
another, or from one bodily location to another, and also make the transition
from a previously known medicine to a similar one. An example of the first
kind of transition would be that from *erysipelas* to *herpēs*; of the second, from
arm to thigh; of the third—in a case of, say, diarrhoea—from quince to medlar.
But all such transition is a pathway towards discovery; there is no discovery,
yet, before testing; but whenever the expected result is brought to the test, what
is evidenced by this test is considered no less reliable than if it had been
observed very many times and identically. This particular kind of test, then,
which follows from the transition from the similar, they call 'skilled', since one
who is to make discoveries in this way must become skilled | in the art; all the   69
other tests, on the other hand, which the art needs for its constitution, but
which precede experience, can be performed by any non-expert. Such, then, is
the pathway, via trial, towards the goal of the art.

3. The pathway via reasoning, on the other hand, exhorts us to learn the nature
of the body which it attempts to cure, and the capacities of all the causes which
the body encounters on a daily basis and which make it either healthier or more
diseased than before. Further, the Rationalists also claim that the doctor must
be an expert in airs, waters, places, actions, food, drink and customary practices,
so that he may discover the cause of all diseases and the capacities of the cures,
and be able to compare them and reason that, for such-and-such a type of
cause, the introduction of a remedy with such-and-such a capacity will by
nature produce such-and-such a result. Without a thorough and varied schooling in all these matters, they claim, he will not be able to provide cures.

The following | brief example will enable you to grasp the whole point. Say   70
that some part of the body is in pain, hard, rigid and enlarged. In this case,
[according to the Rationalists,] the doctor must first discover the cause of the
fact that a larger amount of moisture than normal has flowed to that part, raised
it and stretched it so that it is in pain; next, if that flow is still taking place, he
must stop it; if and when the flow has ceased, he must then evacuate the part.
How, then, are you to prevent the flow, on the one hand, and evacuate the moisture, on the other? You will stop the flow by cooling and constricting the part,
and you will evacuate the accumulated fluid by warming and loosening. Thus,
the indication of what is beneficial comes to them from the actual state; but
their claim is that this is not sufficient on its own, but that there is another indication from the capacity of the person diseased, another from his or her age,
another from the specific nature of the patient; and, similarly, that a specific

indication of what is beneficial arises from the season, the year, the nature of the place, the actions and the customary practices. This too may be more clearly understood by way of example. Say that someone is suffering from an acute

71 fever, | is reluctant to move and feels that his body is heavy; say, too, that he has more bodily mass than previously and more red in his colouring, and that his veins are also enlarged. It should be evident to all that such a person is suffering from an excess build-up of hot blood. What, then, is the cure? Evacuation, of course; for this is opposite to build-up, and opposites cure opposites. How, then, shall we evacuate it, and to what extent? This we cannot know from the cause alone: we have additionally to consider capacity, age, season, place and all the other factors just mentioned. If the person is strong in capacity, in the prime in terms of age, if the season is spring and the place well balanced in mixture, then it will be perfectly appropriate to cut a vein and evacuate as much blood as the cause demands. If, however, the person is feeble in capacity, or either very young or very old, or if the place has a freezing climate, like Scythia, or a sun-baked one, like Ethiopia, and if the season is either very hot or very cold, then it

72 would be highly inadvisable to cut a vein. | The Rationalist would also tell you to consider customary practices and actions, as well as the nature of the body, on the grounds that there arises from all these a specific indication of what is beneficial.

4. But the source of 'indication of the beneficial' for the Dogmatics is the same as that of 'observation' for the Empirics. For the assemblage of symptoms just mentioned in the case of the person with fever—which the latter customarily call a 'syndrome'—enjoins the Dogmatic doctor to evacuation and the Empiric to recollection of his observation. Having seen evacuation be beneficial to people in this state on many occasions, he hopes that he will provide benefit by using it on this occasion too. He knows, furthermore, on the basis of frequent observation, that people in their prime can endure a substantial evacuation without suffering distress. So too with the point about spring as opposed to summer, the well-balanced mixture of the place, and whether the patient has any customary practice of evacuation, such as haemorrhoids or nosebleeds: the Dogmatic would take these, too, as grounds for a large evacuation, using as his starting-point the nature of the thing, while the Empiric would have as his

73 starting-point the fact that he had made such observations. In short, | both Dogmatic and Empiric adopt the same cures for the same ailments, but have a dispute as to the manner of their discovery. On the basis of the same observed symptoms in the body, the Dogmatic has an indication of the cause, from which he discovers the treatment, while the Empiric has a recollection of things observed very frequently and identically.

In cases, however, where the Dogmatic has no observed symptom providing an indication of the cause, he does not hesitate to enquire about what is known as the 'antecedent' cause—for example, whether what bit the patient was a mad dog, a viper, or something else of this sort. For the wound appears no different in these cases, throughout the course of the ailment, or certainly to begin with. In the case of a mad dog, the wound appears similar to that caused by some other creature, throughout; in the case of a viper, it appears similar in the first days, but later, when the patient's state is already very poor, certain additional ailments arise in the body, which are fatal in tendency. Indeed, all such symptoms arising from the | venomous animals (as they are known) are utterly fatal 74 unless they are treated well right from the start. What, then, is the right treatment? It is, of course, the evacuation of the venom that entered the body at the moment of the bite. One must not, then, attempt to make such a wound scar over, or close it up, but on the contrary make many incisions, albeit extremely small ones, and also, for the same reason, employ drugs which are hot and acrid and capable of drawing out and drying the venom. The Empirics apply the same drugs, too, but are led to their discovery not by the nature of the thing, but remembering what was apparent to them in the course of the testing. So, just as they learnt the treatment by experience in the case of age, season, place and each of the other things mentioned, so too in the case of the antecedent causes. If, then, they agreed with each other that both pathways of discovery were truth-giving, there would be no need of further arguments.

5. Since, however, the Dogmatics accuse experience[7] of being either 75 incoherent,[8] incomplete, or lacking in the quality of an art, while Empirics, conversely, accuse Reasoning of being plausible but untrue, there thus arises a twofold argument on both sides, and a very long one, too, as each by turns engages in accusation and defence. On the one hand one has the statements of Asclepiades against experience, indicating that he thought that nothing could be observed many times and identically, and proposing therefore that it was completely incoherent and insufficient for the discovery of anything at all. On the other, we have those of Erasistratus, who concedes that simple remedies, for simple cases, are discovered by experience—for example purslane for tooth sensitivity—but not composite ones for composite cases. His proposition, then, is that it is not impossible for experience to find out anything at all, but that it is not sufficient for everything. There is also the position of those who accept that such things are discovered by experience, but who find fault with its long, limitless nature, and with what they themselves[9] refer to as its unmethodical

---

[7] One might also translate *empeiria* here and in what follows as 'Empiricism': what is meant is experience as understood by the Empirics, and with the specific claims they make for it.

[8] The Greek term is *asustatos*, a negative adjective related to the 'constitution' of an art (see n. 4 above); so, the claim is that the art as defined by the Empirics lacks the formal or epistemological level of 'constitution' required for an art.

[9] It seems not quite clear whether 'themselves' refers to the critics or the Empirics; but the use of the Greek word *autoi* seems odd unless the Empirics are meant. In that case, the Empirics openly

76   character, | and who therefore introduce reasoning, on the grounds that experience is not in fact incoherent or without basis, but lacking in the quality of an art.

Against these verbal attacks the Empiricist defend themselves, attempting to show that experience is both coherent and sufficient and that it has the quality of an art; they themselves also mount a multi-faceted attack on analogism, so that it is then necessary for the Dogmatics to defend themselves against each kind of accusation. The Empirics lock swords with the Dogmatics on the latters' claim to know the nature of the body, the origins of all diseases and the capacities of cures, on the grounds that they proceed no further than the plausible and the likely, and have no secure knowledge. Sometimes, on the other hand, they accept that they do have knowledge, but attempt to show its uselessness; or, conceding that point, again accuse it of being superfluous.

Such, then, in general terms, is the dispute between the Empirics and the Dogmatics. But the specific points, on each side, are many. On the question of
77   the | enquiry into the discovery of non-evident facts, for example, the latter support anatomy, indication and dialectical theory, taking these to be tools in the quest for the non-evident. The Empirics, meanwhile, neither accept that anatomy discovers anything nor, if it did, that this would be necessary for the art; moreover they altogether deny the existence of indication, as well as the notion that one thing can be known on the basis of another. Their claim is that everything requires to be known on the basis of itself, and that there is no such thing as a sign of something which is in its nature non-evident; nor do they admit that any art requires dialectic. They also advance an argument against the presuppositions of dialectic, and against definitions, and deny that demonstration exists in the first place. They have something to say both about the faulty modes of demonstration which the Dogmatics habitually use and also about the process of analogism itself, and the impossibility of its finding out what it claims to; nor, so the claim goes, does it contribute either to the constitution of any other art or to the progress of human life.

78   The process of epilogism, on the other hand, which | they state to be a reasoning about what is apparent, is useful for the discovery of 'immediate non-evidents': this is the term which they themselves use for things which belong within the category of the perceptible but have not yet become apparent; it is useful, too, for the refutation of those who venture to say something against what is apparent. Moreover, it is useful in showing what is being overlooked within the category of the apparent, without at any point departing from things

---

admit that their form of medicine lacks *methodos*, whereas it is the view of their critics that this lack—which corresponds to a lack of reasoning—is precisely what needs to be remedied to make it a true art (*technē*).

evident, but always concerning itself with those. Analogism, however, they say, does not do this: it starts from the apparent, but proceeds to the permanently non-evident and for that reason is multifarious; for, from the same things apparent, it arrives, at different times, at various non-evidents. Here they point to the fact that there is a kind of disagreement which admits of no criterion to decide it, saying that this is a sign of non-graspability; for they themselves use the term 'grasping' for true and reliable knowledge, and 'non-graspability' for the opposite of that. It is, they say, this non-graspability that is the cause of the disagreement, and, conversely, disagreement is a sign of non-graspability. | They   79 state that disagreement on non-evident matters admits of no criterion to decide it, whereas this is not true of disagreement on things apparent. For in the latter case each thing which has become apparent bears witness of what it is like on the side of those who tell the truth, and refutes those who lie. The Empirics and the Dogmatics conduct countless such disputes while—at least in the case of those who have been trained properly within either sect—producing the same treatment for the same ailments.

6. Let us turn then to those known as the 'Methodists'. (This is the name that they have given themselves—as though the Dogmatics of previous times would not also state claim to undertake the art methodically.) Now, in this case it is clear that the dispute with the traditional sects is not just a verbal one; on the contrary: they transform much in the actual practice of the art, denying the usefulness for indication of treatment not only of affected place but also of cause, age, season, place, or consideration of the capacity, nature or condition of the person diseased. They dismiss customary practices, too, stating that that indication of what is beneficial which arises from the ailments alone is sufficient for them; furthermore, they posit these as common and universal rather than divided into types. | Indeed, they use the term 'commonalities' for precisely these   80 features which they say pervade all the particulars; and they attempt to show that there are two commonalities (as well as a third, 'mixed one'), either of the diseases in relation to daily regime, or, as some claim, of all diseases absolutely.

The names that they have given to these are 'constriction' and 'flow'; and they state that every disease is either constrictive or fluid or a complex of the two. If the body's natural evacuations are restrained, they call this constrictive, whereas if they are too active they call that fluid; and when they are both restrained and too active, they say that a complexity arises, as in the case of an eye which is simultaneously inflamed and suffering from flux. For inflammation is a constrictive ailment, but since in this case it arose not alone but together with a flux in the same place, this makes the ailment as a whole a complex one. And the beneficial thing indicated is loosening, in the case of constrictive affections, and stoppage, in the case of fluid ones. So, for example, in the case of inflammation of the knee, they claim that one should use loosening, whereas one should

81 restrain and stop the digestive cavity | or eye when it is flowing; and in complex cases one should work against the more urgent factor: for they state that one should oppose that which is causing trouble and bringing danger, which is to say that which is stronger, rather than the other.

Why, then, do these people not call themselves Dogmatics, since they prescribe remedies on the basis of indications? The reason they give is: 'The Dogmatics enquire into the non-evident, whereas we concern ourselves with what is apparent.' Indeed, they define their whole sect in this way, as the 'knowledge of apparent commonalities'; and, so that the definition may not seem to be shared with all the other arts (for they hold that they, too, are forms of knowledge of apparent commonalities), they make the addition: 'consequent upon the goal of medicine'. Some prefer the phrase 'in agreement with' to 'consequent upon'; most, however, add both phrases, stating that 'the Method is knowledge of apparent commonalities which are in agreement with and consequent upon the aim of medicine'. Some, including Thessalus, add the phrase

82 'and necessary to health'. In these respects, then, | they propose that they should neither be called Dogmatic, for they have no need of the non-evident, as these do, nor Empiric, even though they are concerned especially with the apparent, for they are distinguished from the latter by the use of indication.

They say, further, that they disagree with the Empirics on the actual mode of involvement with the apparent; for the Empirics reject the non-evident as unknowable, whereas they reject it as not useful; and the Empirics take 'observation' on the basis of what is apparent, whereas they take 'indication'. These, then, are the ways in which they say that they differ from each of the others, and especially in their exclusion of seasons, places, ages and all such matters—things which are manifestly useless, in their view, although held in very high esteem by previous doctors.

This they claim as the greatest good of the Methodist sect, and it is for this that they pride themselves and seek admiration, criticizing the one who said that life was short but the art long. Quite to the contrary, they say: the art is

83 short, but life is long. | If we remove all those elements that have been falsely supposed to benefit the art, and pay attention only to the commonalities, then, they claim, the medical art is neither long nor difficult, but extremely easy, clear and possible to learn in its entirety within six months. In this way not only are those diseases related to daily regime reduced to a narrow compass, but so too those involving surgery and drugs. In these too they seek to find out certain commonalities and posit a small number of remedies—so much so that one would think that, so far from requiring the six months of their famous slogan, the entire art could actually be mastered much more quickly than that. If, then, their claims are not false ones, one should be grateful to them for the concision of their instruction; if they are, one should take them to task for its inadequacy.

7. Let me now state how, in my view, one may rightly decide whether they are blind to what is useful or whether they alone correctly avoid what is super-fluous. Such an investigation seems undoubtedly important; nor does the dis-pute appear to be a merely verbal one, | as do the those of the Dogmatics and 84 Empirics who quarrel over the first discovery of remedies, while agreeing with each other on their use. Rather, the practice of the art must either be greatly harmed, or greatly improved, by the Methodist sect. There are two modes of judgement on matters of fact: one through reasoning alone, the other through things manifestly apparent. The first, through reasoning alone, involves a longer argument than is appropriate for beginners, and therefore this is not the place for it; but the second, through what is apparent, is common to all human beings. Why, then, should we not address this first, since it is both clear to beginners and approved by the Methodists themselves? Certainly, they are always singing the praises of the apparent, and nothing but the apparent; they accord it a place of honour in every case, saying that the non-evident is wholly useless. Well, let us consider first the antecedent causes, taking the apparent as the yardstick for our judgement.

Let the Methodist come forward and make his speech first.

'Why, o Dogmatics and Empirics, do you | waste so much time talking about 85 cooling and heating, drunkenness and failure of coction, filling and emptiness, fatigue and idleness, qualities of food and modifications of customary practice? Are you going to pass over the actual states within the body, and cure *those* things—things which are not even present in the first place? Those things are no longer there; it is that which has arisen in the body as a result of them that remains and needs to be cured. This, after all, is the ailment. One must there-fore consider what sort of a thing this ailment is. If it is constrictive, one should loosen it, and if flowing, one should stop it, irrespective of the cause from which either of these has arisen. What benefit, indeed, does the cause retain, when what is fluid never requires loosening, nor what is constrictive stopping? No benefit at all, as the fact itself shows.'

A similar argument will be advanced by the Methodists also in relation to the non-evident 'containing' causes, as they are known. They claim that these too are superfluous, since the ailment indicates its proper treatment even without knowledge of the cause from which it arose. With the same type of argument, too, | they will move on to seasons, places and ages, expressing their amaze- 86 ment, here too, at the doctors of previous ages, in their failure to understand such a manifest fact. For inflammation, they say, since it is a constrictive ail-ment, will surely not require loosening remedies if it occurs in summer but some others in winter; it will require the same remedies in both cases. Nor will it require loosening remedies in childhood but stopping ones in older age; nor loosening ones in Egypt but restraining ones in Athens. So too in the opposite case to inflammation: a fluid ailment will never require loosening remedies, but always stopping ones—whether in winter, in spring, in summer or in autumn, and whether the sufferer is a child, one in the prime or an old man, and, for that matter, whether in Thrace, Scythia or Ionia. They claim, then, that no such consideration is useful in any respect, and that this whole discussion is a massive waste of time.

87 'Why, further, should one consider the parts of the body? Are these, too, not valueless for the indication of treatment? Or would anyone dare | to say that an inflammation should be loosened in a part consisting of nerve, but stopped in one consisting of artery or vein? Indeed, would anyone dare to say, in quite general terms, that anything constrictive that arises in any part of the body should not be loosened, or that anything fluid should not be stopped? Since, then, the nature of the part does not in any way alter the mode of treatment, and the discovery of the medicines depends on the kind of ailment, then consideration of the part will, obviously, be pointless.'

Such, then, is the Methodist, to summarize his views in outline.

8. Let the Empiric step forward next. His argument will be roughly as follows.

'I know nothing beyond what is apparent, and make no claim to any greater knowledge than that of what I have frequently observed. Now, if you reject what is apparent—and I feel that I have heard some sophist in the past speaking along those lines—then it is time for us to move on to those who do not reject it; and in that case you will win a "Cadmean" victory.[10] If, however, as I heard

88 you say at the beginning, you state the non-evident to be entirely useless, | and concede that you follow manifest appearances, perhaps I may show you what you are overlooking, by reminding you of what is apparent.

'Two persons were bitten by a mad dog, and went to the usual doctors, requiring a cure. In each case the wound was small: the skin had not been completely separated. The first doctor provided treatment addressed to the wound alone, without paying attention to any other considerations, and rendered the part healthy within a few days. The other, since he knew that the dog was mad, so far from attempting to make the wound scar over, on the contrary made the wound larger and larger, using strong, acrid drugs for a considerable period of time, and simultaneously compelled the person to drink drugs which he claimed were a remedy for madness. And the following was the outcome in each case: the one who drank the drugs was saved and returned to health, while the other, believing that there was nothing wrong with him, suddenly started to fear water, experienced spasms, and died. Does it then appear to you pointless

---

[10] A 'Cadmean' victory is one of the type more often known now as 'Pyrrhic', i.e. providing no benefit to the victor.

to enquire into the antecedent cause in these cases? Did that person die for any other reason I than the inadequacy of the doctor, who failed either to make any enquiry about the cause or to adopt the treatment that had been observed in the case of that cause? It certainly seems clear to me that there is no other reason. 89

'Since I follow what is apparent, I cannot pass by any such cause; nor, similarly, can I ignore or reject the age of the patient; for here too what is apparent compels me to the confident view that the same ailments do not always indicate the same treatment; rather, the differences are sometimes so great at different ages that they do not just affect the level, but also the whole kind, of medicine given. I have frequently seen doctors, including yourselves, administer venesection to sufferers from pleuritis who are strong and in their prime, but even you never dared to perform evacuation through the veins on a person in extreme old age or on a very small child; nor, indeed, has anyone ever done so.

'And what of Hippocrates, when he says, "During the time of the Dog, and before it, drugs are troublesome," or again, "In summer one should apply drugs rather to the upper parts, in winter I to the lower"? Do you think that he is telling the truth or not? It seems to me that either reply will cause you problems. If you say that he is lying, you will be rejecting the apparent, which you were claiming to accept; for the truth is, quite apparently, as Hippocrates states it. If, on the other hand, you say that he is telling the truth, then you are paying attention to the seasons, which you declared to be useless. But I think that you have never even travelled far from your own region, nor made any trial of the differences between places; otherwise you would know that those in the northern regions do not withstand substantial evacuations of blood, nor, indeed, those in Egypt and the south in general, while those midway between those areas frequently derive a manifest benefit from venesection. 90

'Your failure to consider the parts of the body, too, seems to me quite extraordinary, as well as terribly incongruous: it stands in contradiction, not just of what is true but also of your own actions. Does an inflammation, for heavens' sake, require the same treatment wherever it occurs—in I the leg, in the ear, in the mouth or in the eye? Why, then, have I frequently observed you opening inflammations of the leg with a knife and applying oil to them, but never doing this to the eye? Why do you cure eyes which are suffering inflammation with constrictive drugs, but do not apply the same to the legs? Why do you not cure inflamed ears with the remedies used for the eyes, and vice versa? The drug used for inflammation of the ears is quite different from that used for inflammation of the eyes. Vinegar with rose oil is a good remedy for inflammation in the ears; I do not think that anyone would venture to pour that mixture over inflamed eyes. Indeed, if someone actually did embark upon such a venture, he would undoubtedly be liable to a significant punishment. In the case of inflammation of the uvula, the fruit of Egyptian thorn is a good remedy, as is crushed 91 alum. Will this then also be the case for inflammation of the eyes, or would that not rather cause extreme harm?

92   'And all this has been said on the basis of my conceding to | you the initial assumption that one should loosen inflammation when it occurs in the legs or hands, but not when it occurs in the eyes, uvula or ears. When, however, I remind you that even inflammation in the legs and hands should not in every case be loosened, surely at this point the only sensible course for you is to acknowledge the extent of your error. Here too the argument will rely on recollection of the apparent. For in cases of inflammation arising in any part spontaneously, without the patient having previously suffered any injury, and where the state known as plethoric is present, there is no need to loosen the part before evacuation of the whole body. Such an intervention would increase the existing inflammation rather than diminishing it. This is why we administer constrictive and cooling medicines to the part on such occasions; when we then come to evacuate the whole body, the inflamed part is able to withstand the loosening agents. If I do not persuade you with this argument, then, as I said at the outset of the discussion, the moment has come for me to move on to those

93   who do pay attention to what is evidently apparent.' |

9. That, then, is the speech of the Empiric. Let the Dogmatic now come forward; his speech will be along the following lines.

'What has already been said might be sufficient to persuade a person of sense that neither age, nor season, nor place, nor, indeed, antecedent causes, nor the particular part of the body, should be considered irrelevant. If, however, the Empiric has not yet persuaded you, with his reminders of what is evidently apparent, and you require some further argument, let me then add the following one. In the process I shall demonstrate that the underlying assumption of your sect is unsound.

'I hear you talking of "knowledge of the evident commonalities"; but, however often I ask you in what this commonality consists and how we are to recognize it, I still remain unable to understand the answer. The reason? You agree with each other in purely verbal terms, but you differ when it comes to the actuality. Some of you define what is constrictive or fluid on the basis of the degree of the excretions' departure from the norm, calling the ailment "constriction" when these are held in and "flux" when there is excessive excretion. Others (and quite a considerable number) state that the ailments consist in the bodily states them-

94   selves, | and severely criticize those who pay attention to the excretions.

'Let me then show what appears to be the blunder of each of these groups. The argument will first address those who assess ailments on the basis of normal excretions. It is extraordinary to me that they have never seen the beneficial evacuation of larger than normal quantities of sweat, urine, vomit or faeces, in the course of a disease; and most bizarre of all that they have never observed a nosebleed as a critical event.[11] In the latter case, it is not just the quantity that is abnormal: this kind of excretion is abnormal in kind, whereas sweat, urine and excretions through stomach and vomiting are not abnormal in kind, though they may be immoderate in amount—so much so, indeed, that I have seen some individuals sweat so much that they soak their pillows, and others evacuating more than thirty cups through their digestive tract. In none of these cases did I intervene to stop the evacuation, because it was the source of distress that was being evacuated. Yet if one were using the normal level of excretion as the yardstick in all cases, ∣ such symptoms should have been prevented.   95

'I thus find the proponents of the alternative view, that the states within the bodies themselves are the commonalities, in some ways more plausible; but how on earth, in that case, is this compatible with their claim that these commonalities are evidently apparent? For if the "flux" is not actually that which flows from the digestive cavity, but the state of the bodies as a result of which it flows—a state which cannot possibly be apparent to any of the senses—how then can the commonalities still be apparent? The state of flux may, after all, be located within a limb, in the small intestine, the jejunum, the stomach, the mesentery, or in many other internal regions, none of which, nor any ailment of which, can be grasped by perception. How, then, can they still maintain that the commonalities are evidently apparent—unless one were to use such terminology to refer to something's being recognized by signs? But if that is their meaning, then I do not know what their point of difference would be with the doctors of old. And how then do they claim to teach the art thoroughly within six months? For they would require a very substantial method in order to recognize those things which escape perception; moreover, a ∣ good practitioner of 96 this will have need of anatomy to teach him the nature of each internal part, as well as a considerable body of theory of nature, so that he may examine the task and function of each. Without the discovery of these, it is impossible to identify the ailment of any of the parts in the interior of the body. Need one add that there will also be a great need of dialectic, to provide clear knowledge of what follows from what, and so not to be led astray at any point by sophisms, whether these are uttered by others or arise from our own reasoning or from someone else's? (For it does sometimes happen that we deceive ourselves in this way.)

'I should also like to ask them—if they *have* learned to have a dialectical discussion—what kind of thing is a fluxion? It does not seem to me sufficient to state merely, as some of them do, that it is a certain abnormal state. For until we are told which state it is, we will have no better idea whether it is a loosening, a softness, or a porousness; and it is impossible to get a clear answer from them

---

[11] 'Critical' is understood in the technical sense as taking place at, or leading to, the 'crisis' of a disease; cf. *Prognosis*, ch. 13 for Galen's account of this very phenomenon.

on this question. They say whatever occurs to them: first that it is one of those, then another, and quite frequently even ǀ that it is all of them at once, as if there were no difference; and if someone tries to explain to them the way in which these things differ from each other, and how each of them requires a specific treatment, not only do they not stop to listen; they actually criticize the ancients for having made such pointless distinctions.

'That is the wretched level of these people when it comes to the search for the truth. They cannot even bear to hear the propositions that what is tensed is opposite to what is loosened, the hard to the soft, the dense to the porous, and, beyond this, that it is one thing for the natural excretions to be restrained and another for them to flow; and that all these distinctions were made by Hippocrates. They make rash declaration on all these matters, and state, immediately and without examination, that inflammation (which they call a dry, rigid, painful, hot swelling) is a constrictive ailment. They also have another category of 'complex' inflammations, such as those in the eyes which are accompanied by watering, and those in the tonsils, the uvula, the roof of the mouth and the gums. ǀ Then, they postulate that there are channels, some of which have become narrow and some dilated, and give this as the basis for either kind of ailment. Some even go so far as to state that both flux and constriction arise in the same channel, something which it is not easy even to conceive. Such is the extent of their audacity. There are, however, some few amongst them who can bear to listen to and investigate all these points at greater length, and who eventually, with great difficulty, reconsider and move towards a truer position. For these people, and for all who wish to learn with some precision about the primary and generic ailments, we have written a separate work. It will nonetheless be appropriate to address some brief remarks to them here too, insofar as these remarks may be of use to beginners. I would hope that some of those others may benefit from them too, as would be possible if they could abandon their competitiveness and examine the argument itself, independently.

'The argument goes like this. Inflammation, as even they themselves call it, is an abnormal, painful, rigid, hard and hot swelling; it does not by its own nature make the part either more porous ǀ or denser than normal, nor harder, but rather makes it full of superfluous fluid, and for that reason tensed. Yet it is not the case that everything that is tensed becomes denser or harder than normal. You can understand this from the case of leather skins or straps, or wicker, if you attempt to stretch them as tight as possible.

'So, too, the cure for filling is evacuation: for this is the opposite to filling. And it follows from a part's being evacuated that it becomes more loosened. Tension necessarily follows from filling, just as loosening does from emptying, whereas becoming denser or more porous does not necessarily follow, no more than flux or retention. For the fact that a part is porous does not automatically and necessarily mean that there will be flow from it: what is contained within it might be dense and small in quantity. Nor does it automatically follow that in the case of a dense part there will be retention; for something that is fine in its consistency and large in quantity will flow out, even through dense channels. It would therefore have been better for these people too to read the books of the ancients and learn how many different ways there are in which something which has been constricted in a part may again be excreted. For this may happen through the part that contains it becoming porous, | through the substance   100 itself being thinned, growing larger in quantity, being moved more vehemently, being drawn towards something external to it, or pushed or as it were sucked back by something internal. One who ignores all this and considers there to be only one cause of evacuation, namely making the channels porous, would appear not even to be acquainted with everyday observations.

'For example, we observe quite clearly in the case of a piece of wool or a sponge, or other such porous objects, that if they contain a small amount of water they constrict it and do not let it through, but that if there is more they let it out. How is it, then, that these people have not noticed that the same applies to eyes, too, to the nostrils and the mouth, and to other such porous parts— namely, that sometimes something flows out because of the build-up of moisture contained in them, not because of the porous nature of the channels? Moreover, we have often seen earthen pots that are so porous that water flows through them; but if you pour honey into them, it does not flow through, for the substance of honey is denser than the channels of the pot. Nor would it have been out of place to observe that a substance frequently flows through because of the fineness of its consistency, even if the | body containing it is not by nature   101 perforated; and it should not be difficult, for one closely familiar with artificial mechanisms, to conceive that Nature, which maintains the animal, uses a very vehement impulse to evacuate all that is superfluous, as it were squeezing and pushing it out; indeed, crises of diseases for the most part take place in this sort of way.

'I pass over the other causes of evacuation, as also those of retention. (The latter, being the opposite of the former, are equal to them in number.) The present discussion is not the place for such a lecture; but I return again to a proposition which I think they might at some point understand, namely that it is possible sometimes for an eye to water because the fluid has become either large in quantity or fine in consistency, or because it is pushed out through this part by Nature, although the bodies themselves undergo no alteration from the normal state. In such cases one should, obviously, densify the fine liquid, evacuate the large quantity, and accept the impulse of Nature, provided that it takes place at the right time; one should not concern oneself at all with the actual bodies of the eyes, since these were not the cause of the flux. The | belief that   102 there is a certain inflammation which is a constrictive ailment and another which is complex seems to me to make no sense at all. Those who hold this have, to begin with, forgotten their own argument that one's criterion of the "fluid" should not be evacuation, nor one's criterion of the "constrictive" retention, but that one must rather look to the actual bodily states. When, then, these are similar in every respect, and the present inflammation shows no apparent difference from the previous one except in that one has an outflow whereas this one does not, is it not terribly illogical to consider one complex and the other constricted?

'How, moreover, did the following line of reasoning, which is the most obvious of all, not occur to them: that this kind of inflammation, in which something flows away to the outside, has never been seen to arise in a hand, a foot, on the forearm or upper arm, on the upper or lower leg, or on any other part of the body, but that this only exists in the mouth, the eyes and the nose? Is it that 103 Zeus gave strict instructions to all the complex commonalities, that | none of them must ever go to any other part of the body, but must attack only the eyes, the nose and the mouth? After all, inflammation is capable of taking hold of any part which by nature is such as to receive the causes of its generation. It is because some of these parts are porous in their nature and some dense that in some the liquid flows out and in some it is retained. If you fill a wineskin or some other such container with a wet substance, nothing flows out; but if you fill a sponge, or some such porous thing, immediately all the excess water flows out. It should not have been difficult for them, by considering how much more constraining the rest of the skin is than that in the regions of the eyes, the nostrils and the mouth, to assign the cause to the nature of the part, and to forget about complexity and such lengthy verbiage.

'The truth of this is shown by inflammations arising in conjunction with ulceration in other parts of the body. In these cases, too, the finer substance flows out, as it does in eyes, nose and mouth. But so long as the skin remains unaffected and provides a complete covering, this, and not the type of the 104 inflammation, is the cause of nothing flowing out. | Imagine, again, that you drench a sponge or some wool in honey or wet pitch in a fairly small quantity: nothing will flow out because of the density of the wet substance; or if you do the same with water or some such fine substance, but in extremely small quantity, then too none of it will flow out because of the small quantity of the wet substance. It is for the same reason, surely, that matter does not flow out of the eyes all the time—either because of the density of the moisture or because it is not in excess; and this, indeed, is the case with people in their normal state. It is thus possible for the same type of inflammation, differing in nothing except the density of the substance in flux, to produce an inflammation of the eyes without watering; this is called "constrictive", and thought to differ from the "complex" kind, by those brilliant Methodists—forgetting their own arguments, as they turn everything upside down, and suggest that the constitutions of the ailments are bodily, rather than consisting in the types of wet substance. How, therefore, when the same state exists in the body, differing in nothing other than whether the nature of the wet substances is fine or dense, so that in one case something flows out and in the other it is retained, ⎮ do you take it that there are different   105 commonalities?

'This "complex" category of yours is also unintelligible. At some point in the future, perhaps, you will become aware of all your other individual errors, too, not just in the context of daily regime but also in those of surgery and pharmacy, if this has not been sufficient to persuade you. Now, however, since this is enough for beginners, I shall end the present argument here.'

The Art of Medicine

This text, apparently written late in Galen's career, came to have a huge significance in the history of medicine. It was used as one of the central texts in a medical curriculum as early as the sixth century and, taken as a summary of his most important medical doctrines, was the most frequently copied, translated, commentated and taught work of the author in mediaeval and early modern times, both in the Islamic-Arabic tradition and in the west. Through a Latinization of the Greek title, it became widely known as the *Tegni*, and was also sometimes referred to as the *Ars parva* or 'Small Art', by contrast with Galen's other *Ars*, the fourteen-volume magnum opus *Methodus medendi* (*The Therapeutic Method*).

It also became a crucial, and introductory, part of the *Articella*, a collection of medical texts and synopses that functioned as a medical textbook in late mediaeval western medical instruction, for example at Paris, Bologna or Montpellier, before a wider range of Galenic texts started to become available through new waves of translation.

The use of *The Art of Medicine* as a Galenic 'summary' is understandable, as a function both of the range of topics it covers and in particular of the focus on the relationship of sign to bodily condition (i.e. practical diagnosis). The work systematically discusses: the definition of medicine, health and disease; the health and ill-health of a full range of bodily locations; the notion of humoral or elemental balance itself (in a way closely connected to the discussion of *Mixtures*); and the key notion of different levels of composition.

The text is also notable for a number of discussion and formulations which are distinctive or even unique within Galen's corpus, in particular: the account of 'method' or teaching in medicine in the preface (which provoked much discussion in mediaeval and early modern times); the discussion of health and its causes, including the concept of the 'neither' or neutral; the discussion of signs, including an extended account of the supposed relationship between external features of the body and the constitution or psychological make-up; an account of the chief 'sources' or organs of the body which includes the reproductive organs alongside the usual trio of brain, heart and liver.

Some of the above features, especially the last mentioned, have been perceived as so unusual within Galen's work that the text's authenticity was even called into question; but the prevailing view is now in favour of authenticity, seeing these discussions rather as distinctive developments by Galen at a moment late in his career. Even one who doubted that the work was composed by Galen must still admit that it undoubtedly contains, in concentrated form (in some cases, in more interesting form than elsewhere) much Galenic material; and there can hardly be a work of greater influence in medical education.

Finally, the treatise also contains a bibliography—similar to but much more condensed than those of *My Own Books* and *The Order of My Own Books*—designed to give the reader guidance with regard to the most important of Galen's other writings.

Greek title: Τέχνη ἰατρική (*Technē iatrikē*)
Kühn: I.305–412
Edition: Boudon 2002 (with French translation)

Preface

There are three types of instruction in all, each with its place in the order. First is that which derives from the notion of an end, and is performed by *analysis*. Second is that from the *synthesis* of the findings of the *analysis*; third is that from the *dialysis* of a definition; and it is this on which we are now engaged. This type of *dialysis* may be referred to not only as '*dialysis* of a definition', but also, according to various people's usage, unfolding, *analysis*, division, simplification or explanation.[1]

Now, some of the followers of Herophilus have attempted to produce an instruction of this kind, as has Heraclides the Erythraean. Instruction by *synthesis*, too, has been attempted by ⏐ these same Herophileans, and also by some of the 306 followers of Erasistratus, and by Athenaeus of Attalia. But no one before us has written a course of instruction beginning from the notion of an end, from which notion all arts are constituted methodically. We have expounded such instruction elsewhere; here we shall produce one based on the definition. For while this falls short, in both status and method, of that by *analysis*, we shall find, equally, that it excels it in terms of both the overview of the whole and the memorization of individual points. Everything that arises from the *dialysis* of a definition is easy to remember, because the best definition contains within it the principal points of the entire art. Such a definition is called by some 'essential', in contradistinction to those definitions referred to as 'notional': the latter derive from features incidental to the object under definition, the former from its very essence.[2]

---

[1] *Synthesis* means literally 'putting-together', *dialysis* 'untying' or 'loosening'. The terms *synthesis* and *analysis*, and argument in this first paragraph more broadly, have been the subject of debate from the earliest times (for details see Boudon 2002, 164–76). *Didaskalia*, the term here translated 'instruction', was rendered in Latin as *doctrina*; and the distinction between *analysis* and *synthesis* was interpreted by mediaeval Aristotelians as mapping on to one between types of logical *demonstration* ('quare' and 'quia'), with the 'notion of an end' also understood in Aristotelian logical or metaphysical terms; but it seems more relevant to focus on Galen's practical and didactic aims. The third procedure—that adopted in the treatise—is simply that which takes the definition as a given, rather than as something subject to enquiry, and uses the explication of this definition as the means of practical instruction. The other pair of procedures, *analysis* and *synthesis* (about which Galen admittedly gives very little detail, but which involve respectively abstract definitional reasoning about the 'end', here health, and the placing of a variety of phenomena in their correct place in relation to that defined end) are those by which one establishes or 'constitutes' medicine, or indeed any art, according to a fuller, more epistemologically sound, method—as Galen here claims to have done in other of his works. Further on *analysis* and *synthesis* see *Affections and Errors of the Soul* II.5, pp. 488–9 below.

[2] For this usage of 'essence' in relation to a definition, see *The Doctrines of Hippocrates and Plato* II.3, with n. 6. 'Essence' translates *ousia*; see also *My Own Doctrines*, n. 8.

The elaboration of the whole of medical theory, part by part, has been con-
307   signed to the page in many other of our treatises, and these may be ∣ consulted
for the purpose of the three forms of instruction. Now, however, let us embark
on the definitional one, adding this caveat, that only the chief points—as it
were, the conclusions of the precise demonstrations—will be mentioned here.

1. Medicine is the knowledge of things healthy, morbid and neutral. It makes
no difference if one uses the term 'diseased' instead of 'morbid'. The term 'knowledge' is to be understood in its common, not its technical, sense.

'Healthy', 'morbid' and 'neutral'—each of these is applied in three different
contexts, that of body, that of cause and that of sign.³ Greek usage applies the
adjective 'healthy' to the body which is the recipient of health, to the cause
which is productive and preservative of health, and to the sign which is indicative of health. In the same way, 'morbid' is used for recipient bodies, productive
and preservative causes, and indicative signs. And so also for 'neutral'. Medicine
308   is in a primary sense the knowledge of 'healthy' ∣ causes, and because of them,
also of the others: it is secondarily the knowledge of morbid causes, and thirdly
of causes which are 'neutral'. Next after this, it is the knowledge of bodies—
again, first of the healthy, then of the morbid and finally of the neutral. And the
same applies to signs. In practice, however, the discernment⁴ of bodies, on
the basis of signs, is of course carried out first; after this comes the discovery of
the causes in each case.

But since the terms 'productive', 'indicative' and 'recipient' are each of them
applied in two ways, without qualification or with reference to the present,
it should be understood that medicine is the knowledge of both. The term
'without qualification' also has two senses, that of 'always' and that of 'for the
most part'; and medicine is the knowledge of both these, too. The 'neutral', as
cause, sign and body, both without qualification and with reference to the present, has three senses in each case. The first is that of having no part in either of
the opposites; the second that of participating in both; the third that of partici-
309   pating sometimes in one, sometimes in the other. ∣ The second of these admits
of yet another distinction: it may participate in both equally, or in one more
than the other.

There is a further linguistic ambiguity, which we should also resolve, applying to the definition as a whole. For when one says that medicine is the knowledge of things healthy, morbid and neutral, this may mean the knowledge of *all*
individual things which are either healthy, morbid or neutral; the knowledge of

---

³ This three-part definition involving the notion of the neutral or 'neither' apparently derives
from Herophilus. The tripartite distinction of bodies, causes and signs, meanwhile, is paralleled by
the distinction of symptoms, states and causes at *Health* IV.2.

⁴ The word is *diagnōsis*, also in some cases translated 'diagnosis'; in Galen's linguistic usage however *diagnōsis* is usually 'of' bodies or states of the body, not of diseases.

some things which are healthy, morbid or neutral; or the knowledge of *what kind of* things are healthy, morbid or neutral. But the knowledge of all would be boundless and impossible; the knowledge of some would be deficient and unscientific. The knowledge of what kind of things fall into each category is both scientific and sufficient for all the individual parts of the art, and this, we state, is what is contained in the definition of medicine. Let us, then, begin first with bodies, and consider of what kind are the healthy, the morbid and those which are neutral. We shall then give an exposition of signs and of causes.

2. A body is healthy without qualification when it has from birth a good-mixture in its simple, primary parts, | and a good balance in the organs which   310
are composed of these. A body is healthy with reference to the present when it enjoys this healthy state for the time being. Such a body will also be (for the duration of its healthy state) of good-mixture and balance; but it will not be possessed of the best type of mixture and balance, rather of that proper to itself. Of bodies which are healthy without qualification, the 'always' healthy is the one with the best mixture and balance, while the 'for the most part' healthy is that which falls short of the best constitution by only a little.

A body is morbid without qualification when it has from birth either a bad-mixture in the uniform parts, or a bad balance in the organic ones, or both. A body is morbid in the present when it is suffering from a disease at the time when this term is used of it. Clearly such a body too—for the duration of its morbid state—will have either bad-mixture in the uniform parts or bad balance in the organic, or both. The 'always morbid' is that body which from birth is either of a very poor mixture in all its simple, primary parts, or in some of them, or in the most important; or, equally, of extremely poor balance in the organic parts—here, again, | either in all, in some or in the most important.   311
A body is morbid for the most part when it is in a less bad state than this last one, but still not situated in the mean position.

Now, the neutral body has three subdivisions, that whereby it participates in neither of the extreme states, that whereby it participates in both and that whereby it participates sometimes in one, sometimes in the other. According to the first usage, then, the neutral body will be that which is at the precise mid-point between the most healthy and the most morbid. And this one is further subdivided into that which is so without qualification—having such a constitution from birth—and that which is so in the present—being temporarily situated in this middle position between most healthy and most morbid. And again, 'without qualification' may mean 'always', when it remains such through-out all stages of life, or 'for the most part', where some changes are involved. According to the second usage, a 'neutral' body will be one which has from birth some share in both the opposing states, either in one part, or in two differ-ent ones. It will happen in one part if that part | is well-mixed with respect to   312 *one* of the oppositions of active qualities, or even if it is well-mixed in both respects, but has some flaw in the shaping, size, number, or position, of the parts; it may, conversely, be perfect in all these respects (or in some of them), but wanting in respect of mixture.

This simultaneous sharing of opposites may occur in different parts, too; and it may take place with respect to all the opposed pairs of qualities. And a body which is 'always' of this sort will remain the same throughout all times of life, while that which is so 'for the most part' will undergo certain small changes. There is a body which is 'neutral' in the present, in the second sense, too, either with respect to one part, in that some of its characteristics are healthy and some diseased, or with respect to different parts. In the third sense, a 'neutral' body will be one which is by turns healthy and diseased, as for example it sometimes happens that a healthy child becomes a diseased youth, or vice versa. This type of 'neutral' cannot strictly speaking occur at one time; but it may do so on a broader definition: we should be aware that 'the present' has two senses.

The various senses of healthy, morbid and neutral in the context of body, and the characteristics of each, have now been adequately distinguished.

3. Next in sequence comes the consideration of signs. Here, too, we have the healthy—those which discern present health, which foretell[5] future health, or which recall past health—and the morbid—those which discern present, foretell future, or recall past disease. And similarly the 'neutral', which discern, foretell or recall 'neutral' states, as well as those which indicate nothing at all about states, or do not indicate a healthy state more than a diseased one; those indicative of a state which is healthy in some respects but diseased in others; and those which sometimes indicate a healthy and sometimes a morbid one. And these apply to the three time-frames in just the same way as the healthy and morbid. (In the terminology of some of the ancient doctors, all these kinds of signs come under the heading 'foreseeing',[6] even if they are indicative of states present or past.) The discerning and foretelling signs are of great practical use, those which recall less so.

4. In the case of bodies, the healthy were divided into those which are so without qualification and those which are so in the present (which are also called 'in health'); and those which are so without qualification further into those which are so always and those so for the most part. The former of these were those with the best possible constitution, the latter those which were not far short of

---

[5] The Greek words translated 'discern' and 'predict' are *diagnōstikos* and *prognōstikos*; see n. 4 above and n. 6 below.

[6] Or 'prognostic'. One may compare the beginning of Hippocrates' *Prognostic* (in conjunction with Galen's commentary on it), where it is stated that the doctor should 'foresee and foretell…what is present, what has happened before, and what is going to happen' (1.2): on this usage see *The Best Doctor is Also a Philosopher*, n. 1.

them. Now, the discernment of these must proceed from characteristics that belong to these bodies by virtue of their actual essence, and from the activities and symptoms that pertain to them as a necessary consequence of this; the latter are also known as 'specific attributes'.[7]

What proceeds from the essence itself of the best-constituted bodies is the balance of the uniform parts ⏐ in respect of heat, cold, dryness and moisture; and the balance of the organic parts in respect of quantity and magnitude of their component elements, and also in shaping and position of each of its parts and of the organ as a whole. Proceeding from characteristics which are necessary consequences of these uniform parts are: with respect to the sense of touch, a balance between hardness and softness; with respect to the sense of sight, a good complexion and balance between smoothness and roughness;[8] in the context of activities, the perfect performance of them, which is also called 'excellence'. What proceeds from the necessary consequences of these organic parts consists in the balance and beauty of the organs of the body as a whole, and also in the excellence of their activities.

Such are the signs by which one discerns the best constitution of the body. As for those which fall short of them while still remaining within the bounds of the healthy, these have either some small fault in the mixture of the uniform parts, or some equally small fault in the balance of the organic parts—either in all of them, or in some of them, or some in each category. The classes of fault correspond to ⏐ the types of excellence: mixture in the uniform parts; number, shaping, size and position in the organic. But common to both is the quality of unity, which is also known as 'continuity'.

The bad state of a morbid body, too, falls into these same classes, in accordance with each of the meanings of the term 'morbid'. The line of demarcation between the two is provided by the perceptible impairment of the activity. Bodies which fall short of the optimum constitution by only a little are also, in the strictest sense, impaired; but such impairment is not yet perceptible. The distinctive feature is the degree of impairment, in terms of both performance of the activity and ability to withstand the causes of disease. Bodies that are morbid without qualification are distinguished both by the readiness with which they succumb to such causes and by a significant deterioration of the excellence of their activities.

Midway between the two come the 'neutral'—both those precisely so and those so called with a certain latitude. This latitude, or spectrum, of health as a whole can be divided into three parts, ⏐ each of which itself involves a considerable spectrum. The first would be that of healthy bodies, the second that of the

315

316

317

---

[7] For 'specific attributes' see *The Doctrines of Hippocrates and Plato* VI.3, with n. 44; and for the distinction between what belongs to something in its essence and what follows a necessary consequence, compare *Mixtures*, n. 13 and *The Function of the Parts* XI.13, with n. 11.

[8] Or simply 'hairiness'.

'neutral', the third that of morbid bodies. Next in sequence are bodies that are actually ill, which are marked off by perceptible impairments in their activities. Now, bodies in pain, and bodies whose motions are faulty, or have been completely destroyed, are clearly defined. But those whose activities are only somewhat lacking in intensity,[9] although these too are easily distinguished when the departure from the norm is a very large one, are less so when it is smaller. In relation to this class of impairment, then, arises the state which participates in neither of the opposites; and this too, as we have said, is called 'neutral'. All these matters are decided by the senses, not on the basis of the actual nature of the facts; otherwise there would be a danger of our falling into the doctrine of 'perpetual pathology'.[10]

Now, the signs of bodies which are currently 'in health', but are in fact healthy, morbid or neutral,[11] will differ by virtue of the extent of the distance: we posit 318 two opposed extremes, that of the best constitution and that of a | disease that has just appeared, and we consider to which of these the body in question is nearer. That which is nearer to the best constitution is healthy, and that which is further from that and nearer to the actually diseased is morbid. The one which appears between the two, equidistant from each, is the one we should call 'neutral'.

The indicators of the best state of the body have been enumerated. The classes of the inferior ones are innumerable, since they may be divided according to degree. Having established this tripartite distinction, then, let us begin with the signs of the body that is morbid 'without qualification'; for the other two kinds of latitude will be evident from these. A generic account has already been given in the work on *The Best Constitution of our Bodies*; we shall now be more specific. Let us first distinguish the parts.

5.[12] There are four different kinds of part in all: some are sources; others grow out from these; yet others are neither sources of maintenance of others, nor are 319 themselves maintained by others, | but possess innately the capacities that maintain them. Some, finally, are maintained by both innate and external capacities.[13]

---

[9] The Greek word is *tonos*, which may refer both to tension in the physical sense, e.g. of muscles, and to the intensity or energy with which activities are performed.

[10] The insistence on actual distress to the subject as the criterion of ill health, and also on the need to avoid this absurd theoretical position, whereby (almost) all bodies are defined as ill, appears also at *Health* I.5, where there is also further discussion of the notion of the latitude or spectrum of health.

[11] There is some MS uncertainty here, regarding the inclusion of the word 'healthy' and/or the word 'morbid'; but it does seem from the argument immediately following that (in spite of the apparent paradox of a body 'in health' being ultimately defined as morbid) Galen intends all three possibilities to be available in this case.

[12] N.b. I follow Boudon's relocation (on the basis of the Arabic tradition and the sense of the argument) of the beginning of ch. 5 to this paragraph, rather than the preceding one; a similar change applies to the positioning of the ch. 18 heading below.

[13] The notions of source (*archē*) and maintenance (*dioikēsis*) are central to Galen's physiology (see *My Own Doctrines*, n. 14 and *The Doctrines of Hippocrates and Plato* passim). The major

The sources are: brain, heart, liver and testicles.[14] Growing out from them, and subservient to them, are: for the brain, nerves and the spinal cord; for the heart, arteries; for the liver, veins; for the genitals, the spermatic ducts. Parts which maintain themselves are: cartilage, bone, ligament, membrane, gland, fat and simple flesh. All the other parts which have in common with these the feature of being self-maintained also require arteries, veins and nerves. Hair and nails are not maintained, but only generated. So much for the different kinds of part.

6. Next let us consider the signs of the mixture of each. We shall start with the brain. There are five innate kinds of indicator:[15] first, the state of the head as a whole; secondly, the excellence or badness of the sensory activities; thirdly, the excellence or badness of the motor activities; fourthly, of the commanding activities; | fifthly, of the natural activities.

Another type in addition to all these is alteration arising from external influences. The state of the brain as a whole is gathered from its size and shape and from the nature of the hair. A small head is the specific sign of a poor constitution of the brain. A large head, however, is not necessarily a sign of a good constitution: if it has become so as a result of the vigour of the capacity located there, which has crafted this abundance of matter for its use, it is a good sign; but if as a result merely of the quantity of matter, it is not good. The two may be distinguished by the shape of the head and by the parts growing from it. The shape should be well proportioned; this is always a good sign. The parts growing from it: it should be strong-necked and in the best state in relation to the other bones; its nerve-like parts should all have good growth and good tension.

The proper shape of the head is just like that of a precisely spherical piece of wax, depressed slightly on each side. It will thus follow that the front and back parts will be more curved than is the case with a sphere, | and the sides straighter. If the extent of the protrusion at the occiput is diminished in someone, examine also the nerves and the neck, as well as the other bones. If these are normal, then the defect has come about through a lack of matter, not a weakness of capacity. If they are inferior, then the source is weak. Usually these deficiencies of the occiput are attended by weakness of the above-mentioned parts; cases where it is not so are in fact quite rare. And examine the head which

320

321

organs—usually just the first three, without mention of the genitals—are regarded as control centres which maintain, and direct the function of, other parts of the body through the three networks or nerves, arteries and veins. (*Dioikēsis* could also be translated 'management', 'control' or 'regulation'.)

[14] *Orcheis*: the term may also be used to refer to ovaries, but it does seem from what follows both that Galen has the male of the species exclusively in mind and that he is considering the *orcheis* as an observable external part of the body from which inferences may be made about the nature and behaviour of the individual.

[15] Or possibly: 'five kinds of indicator in all.'

is pointed at the occiput with the same criteria which apply when the whole head is large. Here too, if the cerebellum has a well-proportioned shape, it is usually a good sign.

This part is called by some doctors the 'hindbrain', which accurately describes its position, the limit of which is defined by the lambdoid suture; and it is the source of the spinal cord, and through it of all the motor nerves throughout the animal. This hinder part in itself is connected with very few sensory nerves, but a very large number of the motor ones; similarly the other part, situated in front, 322 ⎸is connected with a great number of sensory but few motor nerves. A good state in either of these, then, will lead to strength in the parts growing out from them.

The same distinctions apply in the parts to the front of the head, at the face. One should examine whether this is small or large; the shape; and the relevant senses—sight, taste and smell. The parts that grow from a source, and the source, are reciprocal indicators of each other's excellence or badness. In the case of the commanding activities, however, their excellence or badness is an indicator of the source alone and in itself. What I mean by commanding activities is those which arise from the source alone. Quick-wittedness is an indicator of a fine substance in the brain, while slowness of intellect is an indicator of a dense one; aptitude to learn is an indicator of a substance which takes impressions easily; and memory of a stable one. Similarly, inability to learn indicates a substance which takes impressions with difficulty; and forgetfulness one which is fluid. Changeability of opinion indicates a hot one, while stability indicates a cold one.

323   ⎸I believe then that of those types of indicator that we initially undertook to discuss, two still remain: that of the natural activities and that of external influences. These are both covered by one argument. If the brain is well balanced in respect of the four qualities, it will be at the mean in terms of all the factors already mentioned; and also at the mean with respect to the residues (those evacuated by palate, ears, nostrils or eyes); and will be very little harmed by any external influence—things which heat, cool, dry or moisten. Such people have reddish hair as infants, fairish hair as children and genuinely fair hair as adults; it is halfway between straight and really curly; they are not prone to hair loss. These and subsequent indicators are to be understood as referring to well-balanced habitations; the remarks on hair as referring not just to places, but to 324 the mixture of the humoral fluids, which is related ⎸to the mixture of humoral fluids in the brain. If it is hotter than the mean, but well balanced in respect of the other opposition, then if the excess of heat is considerable all the above indicators will be very marked; if the excess is small, hardly noticeable. This point should be taken to apply equally to all the parts, regarding the indicators that we shall mention for all the mixtures.

7. The signs, then, of heat in the brain, apart from those already mentioned, are that all the parts about the head are red and hot; the veins in the eyes are visible;

after birth the hair grows quickly on the head. Where the brain is much hotter than the point of good-mixture, they become black, strong and curly; in cases of a small excess, they are first fairish, later turning black; as the person grows older there is hair loss, more so the hotter it is. In such people the residues evacuated by palate and nostrils, eyes and ears, are small and well 'cooked', so long as they are enjoying perfect health. I But when the head is filled—and this 325 happens in these cases continually, especially where care is not taken over diet—these residues become larger in quantity, but still fairly well 'cooked'. The cause of this filling and heaviness of the head is the consumption of heating foods and drinks, and smells, and indeed all external influences, including the ambient air. And still more so if these are not only hot but also wet. People with this kind of mixture are content with little sleep, and quite light sleep at that.

The indicators of a brain that is colder than it should be are: greater evacuation of residues, by those proper channels; the hair straight and red, not liable to fall, growing a long time after birth, being at first fine and insubstantial. Such persons are easily harmed by cold influences, and at the same time that they undergo such harm they succumb to catarrh and mucus. It may be observed, too, that the parts about the head are not hot to the touch, nor red, and the veins in the eyes are invisible; and the subjects are rather prone to sleep.

I The indicators of a dry brain are a lack of residues in those channels, and 326 sensory acuteness; such people are prone to insomnia, and have very strong hair, which grows very quickly at birth, curly rather than straight; and they become bald early.

The wetter brain has straight[16] hair, which is not liable to baldness at all; its sensations are hazy; there is a build-up of residues; sleep is long and deep.

So much for the simple bad-mixtures.

8. First of the compound bad-mixtures is the hot and dry. In this case the person is lacking in residues, endowed with acute sensation, extremely insomniac, and prone to early baldness. The first growth of the hair is very fast and vigorous; it is black and curly; the head is hot to the touch, and red up to the time of full growth.

Where heat is combined with wetness, then if each of these qualities is only slightly in excess, there is a good complexion; heat; the veins in the eyes are large; the I residues considerable and moderately 'cooked'; the hair straight and 327 fairish, not prone to baldness; but the head is liable to being filled and made heavy by heating substances. And even more so if such people become moistened, since they then acquire a large quantity of residues, too. If they reach a very high level of wetness and heat, the head will be morbid, full of residues, and easily harmed by moistening or heating influences. The south wind is the

---

[16] Or perhaps 'delicate'.

constant enemy in such cases. They are best off in north winds. They find difficulty in staying awake for long periods; but when they try to sleep they are sluggish but at the same time insomniac, and prone to vivid dreams. Their vision is hazy, and their sensation imprecise. If the brain is much hotter than the norm, but only a little wetter, the indicators of the hot mixture will predominate, but with a faint trace of those of wetness; conversely, if it is much wetter, but only a little hotter, the indicators of wetness will be manifest and pronounced, and those of heat faint. (A similar argument applies to all the

328   compound bad-mixtures.)

The mixtures of the brain which are at once cold and dry render the head cold and devoid of colour—as far as their own effects are concerned; for the distinction which was made at the outset should always be borne in mind: we should consider to what extent the parts within it are altered by the mixture of the humoral fluids. To begin with, people with such mixtures are lacking in veins in the eyes, and liable to harm from cold influences; so that their state of health is an uneven one: they are sometimes extremely light in the head, and lacking in residues; sometimes apt to succumb to catarrh and mucus and small influences. Their sensation is in youth acute and perfect in every respect; as they grow older this quickly deteriorates; in brief they are quick to grow old in all matters concerning the head. For this reason they also go grey early. At birth their hair comes with difficulty, is lacking in vigour, and red; in the fulness of time, if cold comes to predominate more than dryness, they do not go bald. But

329   conversely, if it happens that dryness comes to predominate greatly over the wetness, and the cold slightly over heat, such people will go bald.

The wet and cold mixtures of the brain make people sluggish and somnolent; of poor sensation; full of residues; their heads easily cooled and easily filled; susceptible to catarrh and mucus. But such people do not go bald.

Such are the signs of the mixtures of the brain; on the basis of these you will by extension know how to discern those for each of the organs of sensation.

9. It will suffice to give an account of the eyes. All those which are clearly hot to the touch, which move readily and often, and which have thick veins, are hot. The cold are those opposite to these; the wet, those which are both soft and full of moisture; the dry, those which are both rough and hard.

All are easily harmed by influences of the same kind as their own mixture, and improved by the opposite sort, when these are applied in moderation. (This

330   point should be borne in mind in the context of every discernment of mixture, in every part of the body.) Large eyes, in association with good proportion and excellence of the activity, indicate the large quantity of the well-balanced substance from which they have been formed. When not associated with these features, they show that that substance is large in quantity but not well-mixed. Small eyes in association with good proportion and excellence of the activity indicate the substance to be small in quantity but well-mixed; in association

with poor proportion and poor activity they signal that this substance is not only small but also bad.

The distinctions with regard to colour are as follows. Bright[17] eyes, shining with a moisture which is both small in amount and clear, become so by the abundance of bright light; and black eyes in the opposite manner. Eyes of shades between these come about through causes intermediate in nature. Now an eye can be bright because of the size, the brightness or forward position of the glassy substance, or the small quantity and clearness of the fine, watery moisture in the pupil. The co-existence of all these factors produces the brightest eye of all; if | some of them are present but not others, this brings about different   331 degrees of brightness. Black eyes come about through the small quantity of the glassy substance, or its sunken position, or because it is not genuinely bright and light-like; or because the fine moisture is greater in quantity, or not clear. Either some or all of these may be the causes. And degrees of blackness come about in the manner already outlined.

If the fine moisture is on the watery side, and greater in quantity, this renders the eye moister. If, on the other hand, it is on the dense side, or less in quantity, this renders the eye drier. As for the glassy substance, if this is harder, it makes the eye drier; if softer, moister; so, too, if this substance is excessively fine, this too makes it drier, and if deficiently so, the opposite.

10. Let us turn now to the mixtures of the heart, first reminding the reader that when we speak of greater heat, cold, dryness or moisture of a part, these terms are relative to that part itself, not to some other object. Thus, even if a | heart is   332 comparatively cold by nature, its mixture will still be much hotter than that of the hottest brain. Of the signs of heat (relative to the proper balance of a heart) some are inseparable and specific to the heart, such as the volume of breath, the speed and frequency of the pulse, courage and fearlessness in action; a very high degree of heat is reached, we see quick temper and crazy rashness. Such people have a hairy chest, especially in the region of the sternum and the upper abdomen. Usually with a hot heart the whole body will be hot, too, unless the liver counteracts this effect powerfully. But we shall come to the indicators for the whole body shortly.

Thickness of the chest is also an indicator of heat, unless, again, the brain provides a powerful counterbalance. For the size of the spinal cord is on the whole in proportion to the brain, and the size of the vertebrae corresponds to that of the spinal cord; thus, the whole spine, too, is on the same scale. And the

---

[17] The term is *glaukos*, which, in common with a number of other Greek colour terms, is notoriously difficult to translate. Traditional translations include 'blue', 'green' and 'grey'; but research has suggested—as indeed seems confirmed by the present passage—that such terms to some extent correspond more closely to different *intensities* of light, rather than different *hues*. I have therefore preferred the translation 'bright' to any of the above possibilities, in this context. But it seems that eyes that are (in our terms) either blue or green are probably be covered by the word.

333   chest is connected to that part of it which is in the upper region of the ⎢ back, in the same way as a ship is connected to its keel, so that of necessity its length will be equal to that of the upper back. As for its width, if the connection comes about in proportion to the thickness of the vertebrae, it will accord with them; but if from birth the heat of the heart predominates, inflating and widening throughout, the width will accord with the heat of this part. For this reason, too, a small head combined with a broad chest is the clearest indicator of heat in the heart; while a big head combined with a small chest is a very specific indicator of a cold heart. If the head is in proportion with it, then you must judge the heart by the other signs, for you will gather nothing from size of the chest.

In the case of a cold heart, the pulse is smaller than the norm, but not necessarily slower or less frequent. Breathing will be proportionate to the pulse, provided that the smallness of the chest is in proportion to the coldness of the heart; if the chest is larger than accords with the degree of coldness, the breathing will be not only smaller, but also slower and less frequent. Such people are

334   timid by nature, ⎢ lacking in courage, sluggish and hesitant; their chests are smooth, without hair. In the case of its smallness, the same distinctions apply as above; and similarly regarding the heat of the body as a whole.

Dryness in the heart makes the pulse harder, and the spirit not readily aroused, but fierce and difficult to placate. For the most part the body as a whole, too, will be drier, unless the parts about the liver counteract this. Signs of a moist heart are: a soft pulse, a spirit readily moved to anger but also easily placated, and the whole body moist, unless the parts about the liver counteract this.

11. The bad-mixtures of the heart arising from combinations of the fundamental qualities, meanwhile, are as follows. With a hot and dry heart, the pulse is hard and large, fast and frequent; and breathing is of large volume, fast and frequent; and much faster and more frequent in cases where the chest has not grown in proportion to the heart. These people are the hairiest of all in the

335   region of sternum ⎢ and upper abdomen. They are easily roused and quick to action, spirited, tyrannical in character; for they are quick-tempered and difficult to placate. As regards the mixture of their bodies as a whole, and also the broadness of the chest, one must apply the same kind of distinctions as above.

Those with a predominance of both moisture and heat are less hairy than those just mentioned, but no less easily roused to action. Their spirit is not wild, merely quick to anger. Their pulse is soft, large, quick and frequent. In cases where the chest is in proportion to the heart, breathing follows the same pattern as the pulse. If it is smaller, breathing is faster and more frequent than the previous case by the same degree that the chest is smaller. If the deviation in mixture is a large one, especially in cases of deviation towards the moist, there arise, in addition to the phenomena mentioned, diseases of putrefaction, as the humoral

fluids become corrupted and putrefy; and exhalation is | greater and faster than   336
inhalation; and in the pulse the contraction is fast.

With a moist, cold heart the pulse is soft, and the character timid, fearful and
hesitant. Such people are also devoid of hair around the sternum, and the least
prone to nursing resentment, being also slow to anger. In respect of the chest
and the body as a whole, the same distinctions apply as above.

A cold and dry heart renders the pulse hard and small, and breathing—in
cases where the chest is small, in line with the coldness—well proportioned. If
the chest is larger, breathing will be infrequent and slow. Such people are the
least irascible of all; but if they are in some way constrained to anger, they retain
the resentment. Their chests are the least hairy of all. The previous distinctions
apply regarding smallness of the chest and also coldness of the whole body.

But the following reminder should be given, which holds for all these statements equally. Whatever has been said on the subject of moral characteristics,
here or in any other discussion of discernment of the mixture, does not | apply   337
to those character traits—good or bad—which come about through philosophy,
but to those which are innate.[18]

12. The indicators of a hot liver are: broadness of the veins; excess of yellow bile
and, in the prime of life, also of black bile; warmth of the blood, and by virtue of
this also of the body as a whole, unless the characteristics of the heart counteract this; hairiness of the areas of upper abdomen and stomach. The indicators of
a cold liver are: narrowness of the veins; excess of phlegm; coldness of blood,
and a cold condition of the body as a whole, unless it is somewhat warmed by
the heart; upper abdomen and stomach free of hair. A dry liver: the blood is
dense, dry and small in quantity; the veins hard; the condition of the body as a
whole dry. A wet liver: a large volume of moist blood; the veins soft; and the
whole body so too, unless this is counteracted by the heart.

The indicators of a hot and dry liver: the upper abdomen extremely hairy;
the blood dense and also dry; a very large quantity of yellow bile and, in the
prime, of black bile too; | broadness and hardness of the veins. And the whole   338
body will be similar. Now, the warmth proceeding from the heart may override
the cold proceeding from the liver, as also its cold may override the warmth.
But dryness of the liver cannot be changed to its opposite by a moist heart.
Moisture of the liver stands between these two: it has a greater capacity to be
overridden by dryness from the heart than, in the case of its dryness, by moisture of the heart; but a lesser capacity to be overridden than warmth, and still
less than cold—that is the most easily overridden of all the qualities arising in

---

[18] It is noteworthy that Galen here allows a distinct domain for educational and philosophical
development and control of one's character traits or emotions—a domain explored more fully in the
ethical works *Affections and Errors* and *Freedom from Distress*.

the liver. It is, then, obvious that if the mixtures of both these sources coincide, the entire body will be disposed according to them. (The indicators of this will be mentioned shortly.)

The liver which is simultaneously moist and hot renders the area of the upper abdomen less hairy than does the hot and dry liver; the blood is extremely plentiful; the veins large; the condition moist and hot, unless counteracted by 339 the heart. If there is an abnormal excess of both these qualities, I the subject is vulnerable to diseases of putrefaction and bad humoral fluid; and especially so if it is the moisture that predominates rather than the heat. If, conversely, there is a great excess of heat but very little of moisture, such people are least prone to bad humoral fluid.

A cold and moist liver has a hairless upper abdomen; it produces phlegmatic blood, and narrowness of veins; and the whole body of the same nature, unless converted to an opposite state by the heart. A cold, dry liver renders the body short of blood, with narrow veins, and cold, and the upper abdomen bare— unless, again, the heart overrides this.

13. Of mixtures of the testicles, the hot is the most erotic, while also being prone to the production of males, and fertile; it leads to early growth of hair in the region of the genitals, extending also to neighbouring areas. The cold is opposite in effect. The moist mixture produces a large quantity of wet sperm, while the dry produces a small quantity, reasonably dense.

340 The hot I and dry mixture is productive of the densest and most fertile sperm, and from the beginning urges the animal most quickly towards congress. Such persons also grow hair most quickly in the genitals and all surrounding areas— above, up to the region of the navel, and below, down to the middle of the thighs. Though this mixture is highly prone to the sexual urge, it is also very quickly sated, and, if forced, liable to harm.

If the heat is combined with moisture, the subject is less hairy, but has a greater quantity of sperm. He does not, however, have greater desire than the other type, but can undergo more encounters with impunity. If, indeed, both moisture and heat are present to a considerable degree, the subject cannot safely abstain from congress.

If the mixture of the testicles is moist and cold, the surrounding parts will be free of hair, and the subject will be late in embarking on sexual activity. He will not be prone to the sexual urge; and his sperm will be watery, thin, of poor fertility and liable to produce females. The cold and dry mixture is in other respects 341 similar to this I one, but the sperm is denser, and extremely small in quantity.

14. The conditions of the body as a whole have been mentioned already, to the extent that they accord with heart and liver. Whichever part is more strongly endowed with one of the fundamental qualities (which are also known as 'active'), will impose that quality over the rest. But the phrase 'condition of the

whole body' is used with particular reference to those parts which the observer encounters first. Such are, for example, the muscles, which surround all the bones, and are composed of both flesh pure and simple and the fibres around which they grow. The substance specific to muscles is both of these. And the vessels which come to them are like waterpipes, which do not supply their substance, but only serve for their maintenance.

Let us then mention the indicators of mixture of the muscles, in the context of a habitation which enjoys good-mixture. For those with bad-mixture affect the skin, imprinting it with their own nature and thus destroying certain of the indicators. Thus, if in a region with good-mixture, in | summer, one exposes 342 oneself naked to the sun, this will affect all those indicators which regard colour, and the relationship of soft and hard. But if both the region and the lifestyle of the subject are good in their mixture—so that he does not bake himself naked in the sun for a large part of every day, nor (as some do) perpetually seek the shade in the manner of young maids—then the indicators of mixture will be accurate.

Now, since our argument is to consider this, let us turn our precise attention to the matter. The indicators of a well-balanced mixture with respect to the whole condition of the animal are: complexion a harmony of red and white; hair fair and generally quite curly; and a good balance of flesh in terms of quantity and quality. Such a body is precisely at the mid-point between all excesses, which are, indeed, considered and defined by reference to it. A thick body, for example, is called 'thick' in relation to this one, and similarly one which is thin, or fleshy, lacking in flesh, fat, hard, soft, hairy or | bare. None of these terms 343 refers to the well-balanced state, like that of the Canon of Polyclitus, which represents the perfection of every type of good balance, appears neither soft nor hard to the touch, nor hot nor cold; and, on inspection, neither hairy nor bare, thick nor thin—nor endowed with any other imbalance.

15. Bodies which are warmer than the correct balance, but not moister or drier in their fleshy parts, which are those with which the present argument is concerned, appear warmer to the touch to the same degree that they are warmer in mixture. They will also be hairier to that same extent, with less fat, very red in complexion and black-haired. Signs of a cold mixture are: lack of hair, fat, coldness to the touch; and their complexion, as well as their hair, will be reddish. If the cooling is great, the body will be a sort of blue-grey colour; some doctors refer to such cases as 'leaden-skinned'. The drier mixture is thinner and harder than the | well balanced, to the same degree that it is drier, but in other respects 344 similar. The moist mixture is similar, too, except that it is better endowed with flesh and softer.

16. Bad-mixtures arising from combinations of the primary qualities give rise to a composite form of indicators. That which is hot and dry will be hairy,

hot, hard, lacking in fat, thin and black-haired. If the heat predominates, it will also be black-skinned. A hot, moist mixture is smooth and fleshy, and hotter than the best mixture to the same degree as the increase in both these qualities. But when the increase is very great, there is vulnerability to the diseases of putrefaction, and poor humoral fluid may readily arise. If the increase in moisture is small, while the increase in heat is very great, such subjects will be only slightly softer and fleshier than the norm, but considerably hairier; and they will also be considerably hotter to the touch. Their hair will be black, and
345   their flesh lacking in fat. If the increase in heat is small, and that in [|] moisture very great, the flesh will be soft, of great quantity, of a complexion which is a combination of red and white; and they will be slightly hotter than usual to the touch. We may sum up the composite mixtures by saying that the indicators of the dominant quality will always dominate.

The cold, moist mixture, when both these qualities are only slightly increased, is hairless, white, soft, dense and fatty. If the increase is greater, the changes will be in proportion with such increase in these qualities; furthermore, the complexion and hair will be red, or blue-grey when the increase in both qualities is extreme. With an unequal increase in the qualities, there will be a dominance of the specific signs of that which undergoes the greater increase. If cold and dryness are both equally increased, the nature of the body will be hard, thin, hairless and cold to the touch. In these cases, in spite of their being thin, the fat is dispersed through the flesh. The nature of the hair and complexion is in accord with the degree of cold. When a hot, dry mixture changes, at an age beyond the
346   prime, into a dry, [|] cold one, the condition will be thin and hard; also melancholic; and because of this the hair will be both black and thick. If one of these qualities is greatly dominant, while the other deviates only slightly from the norm, the indicators of the dominant one will dominate, while those of the other will be faint.

The following indicator is of quite general validity, in all the matters discussed so far and still to be discussed: if a body is easily cooled, this indicates either cold or porousness of the flesh; if it is cooled with difficulty, this indicates heat or density; if it is damaged by drying influences, and becomes rough, dry and hard to move, this indicates dryness; and if it is weighed down by moistening influences, moisture.

One should also examine whether the muscles are all of a similar mixture, or whether some are different, bearing in mind the size of the bone beneath them in each case. Sometimes a part appears to be thin although that quality is not in fact present in the muscle, the illusion deriving from the narrowness of the bone. So also it may not infrequently appear thick, not because of the broadness
347   [|] of the bones but because of the quantity of flesh; the fluctuations in amount of flesh, and in its hardness or softness, render this part either dry or moist. Small quantity and hardness make it dry; large quantity and softness, moist. So, too,

the places between the uniform parts, by containing more or less moisture in them, or by being denser or finer, make the part either moist or dry: moist, when the moisture is fine and large in quantity; dry, when it is dense and small in quantity. For though the solid parts of the body—the genuinely solid, primary parts, that is—can in no way be made moist, it is sufficient if they are prevented from drying out quickly; and the spaces between them may be filled with moisture, of one sort or another; this in fact is the proper nourishment of the uniform parts: that which is brought to them by placement alongside, rather than conveyed through vessels.

A common argument applies also to all the parts mentioned and will be repeated in ┃ our instruction on the causes of health and disease. But let us now   348 turn to the next topic.

17. Indicators for the stomach: if it is dry, the subject becomes thirsty quickly, but is sated with little drink, and weighed down by larger quantities, and has 'waves'; the excess comes to the surface of the stomach; such a person takes pleasure in dry foods. With a moist stomach the subject will have no thirst, but will have an ability to take larger quantities of water with impunity, and will take pleasure in moist foods. A hot stomach has a better digestion than appetite, and is particularly good at digesting those foods which are by nature hard and difficult to transform. Easily transformed foods tend to be destroyed in such a stomach. It takes pleasure in hot foods and drinks, but is not harmed by a moderate intake of cold ones. A cold stomach has good appetite, but poor digestion, especially of foods which are difficult to transform and cold. Such foods tend to be made acidic in a cold stomach; and so it is also prone to acidic belching. ┃ It enjoys cold foods, but is easily harmed by excessive use of them.   349 Similarly, it cannot endure prolonged contact with cold influences from outside; the same applies to the hot stomach, in the case of cold external influences.

Bad-mixtures of the stomach due to disease, however, differ from the innate ones in the following respect, that they desire opposites, not similars, as do the latter. Composite bad-mixtures of the stomach will be recognized by their combination of the simple ones.

The above statements must be studied carefully, and distinguished from those that follow. For it is not the digestive cavity alone that causes thirst or lack of thirst, and appetite for cold and hot drinks, but the organs of the chest, too—the heart and lungs. But those whose thirst is due to the heat of these organs inhale more deeply, and produce long exhalations; and they feel the burning in their chest, not, as those whose thirst is due to the stomach, in the upper abdomen. Nor do such cases gain relief immediately on drinking; a cold drink, however, assuages their thirst better than ┃ a very hot one. They are also cooled by the inhalation of   350 cold air, which brings no relief to the thirsty because of their stomachs. Conversely, those in an opposite state are discernibly pained by the inhalation of cold air.

That, in fact, is the best indicator of cold in the lung. And just as they experience a clear sensation of pain and cooling on inhaling cold air, such subjects also find the hot pleasurable. They feel the need to clear their throats and cough, expectorating phlegmatic residues.

18. Dryness of the lung involves an absence of residues, cleanness of phlegm and clearness of voice; conversely, wetness leads to an unclear, hoarse type of voice; and if the subject tries to produce louder, or higher-pitched, utterances, residues get in the way. It is not that the heat itself is the cause of the volume of the voice, nor the cold of its quietness; rather, loudness is a consequence of the broadness of the windpipe, and of the vehemence of the exhalation, and softness of the opposite. Loudness and softness thus do not constitute a constant, or primary feature, but an incidental one, and ones which are a consequence only of the innate | mixture, not of acquired ones. Since the organs have acquired their particular nature by virtue of the mixture, and since a particular type of voice comes about as a consequence of that nature, one may make inferences about the innate mixture on the basis of the voice. So, also, a smooth voice is a consequence of softness of the trachea, and a rough voice, of its roughness. Now, smoothness of the trachea is a consequence of a well-balanced mixture, and roughness a consequence of a dry one: roughness is an uneven state which comes about in a hard body, through imbalance. The trachea is rendered hard by dryness of the uniform parts of it, and uneven by a lack of dispersion of moisture through these parts. Similarly, a naturally high-pitched voice is indissociable from narrowness of the pharynx, as also a deep voice from its the broadness of that part. And narrowness is the result of innate cold, broadness of innate heat.

351

The various pathological states of the voice follow the same basic distinctions as apply in the natural ones, and function, here too, as indicators of their efficient causes. (We have covered all these matters sufficiently in our treatise on *The Voice*.)

352

The other internal parts of the animal have | only faint indicators regarding their mixture. One should nevertheless attempt their discernment, by observation both of the influences that do them benefit or damage, and of the actions of the natural capacities. In the third book of *Causes of Symptoms* it was stated which mixture precedes[19] the excellence or deficiency of every capacity. And the indicators of the mixtures have already been mentioned.

19. The situation regarding defects in size, shaping, number or position, meanwhile, is the following. These are easy to discern when they are

[19] 'Precedes' may be taken here as meaning 'functions as the preceding cause of'; for Galen's technical notion of preceding causes, see *Affected Places* III.7 with n. 6.

immediately present to our perceptions; when they are not thus present, they are either difficult to discern or actually indiscernible.

The size and shape of the head, for example, and with it of the brain, are evident, and these have been discussed above. The same is true of the chest; so too it is easy to make out the characteristics of shoulder-blades, shoulders, upper arms, forearms, hands; or of hip, thigh, calf or feet, whether there is a defect in the shaping in one of these parts, or in the size, | , number, or composition of   353 the parts that constitute it. Malfunctions of the activity of any of these parts are also evident. But not all internal features can be ascertained. Now I have, it is true, seen a stomach that was so small and round, and in such a forward position in the upper abdomen, that its shape was clear in outline both to the eye and to the touch. And I once saw a bladder which was so protruberant and small, that if the subject delayed in the passing of urine, a clearly demarcated lump would appear. But none of the other internal parts has ever been manifestly discernible to me in this way.

One must, however, attempt the discernment of their excellences and defects, if not by secure knowledge, at least by a form of skilled conjecture. Take the case of the liver. I have frequently observed that people with a large number of narrow veins, and a lack of colour in the body as a whole, if they take food even slightly to excess, especially flatulent, dense, viscous food, | get a sensation as of   354 a weight inserted or suspended deep within their right upper abdomen, in some cases accompanied by a painful tension. It thus seems likely that their livers are small, with narrow passages.

Another case I have observed is that of a man, phlegmatic in his whole constitution, who nevertheless would vomit yellow bile daily. I realized the necessity of examining his excretions too; and they contained very little bile. From this I inferred that the passage which carries bilious fluid was sending a sizeable portion of that substance into the pylorus of the stomach—a phenomenon we observe in a number of animals. It is therefore obvious that, in the parts not evident to sense-perception, a knowledge of anatomical facts, and the discovery of activities and functions, are of great value for our discernment. Those who wish to discern the kinds of bodily defect outlined just now must first train themselves in anatomy, and in the discovery of activities and functions. We have written specifically about all these matters in other works, which | will be   355 enumerated right at the end of this book, so that those who are eager to learn may know in which particular treatises to continue their study. But enough, now, on these matters.

20. States of bodies which are morbid with reference to the present, that is bodies which are in a state of disease, may also be discerned, insofar as they present to our senses changes from the normal state, for example changes in size, colour, shape, number, position, hardness and softness, or heat and cold. But

the states of non-observable morbid bodies are to be discerned too, by means of—in summary—impairments of the activities; excretions; pains; or unnatural lumps. These phenomena may occur in some combination or all together.

Let us consider here the individual parts.

Morbid states of the brain may be discerned through the various types of derangement; through impairment of the activities of sensation, impression-formation or voluntary motion, through the excretions by palate, nostrils or ears; or through different types of pains within the brain itself.

Morbid states of the heart are to be discerned from the various types of dif-
356 ficulty in breathing, and by palpitations; | also from the pulse in the heart and arteries; from quickness of temper or depression of the spirit; fevers; chills; differences in colour; and pains in the heart. Morbid states of the liver, from deficiency or excess of the humoral fluids, deviation of these into unnatural states, lack of colour, and also from changes within the process of distribution, nutrition or the evacuation of waste substances; further, from heaviness within the liver itself, as well as lumps, and pains not just in the liver but occurring elsewhere by sympathy, involving certain kinds of difficulty in respiration, and coughing.

Morbid states of the stomach, similarly, can be diagnosed by defects in diges-tion of and appetite for moist and dry food offered, or in the evacuation of res-idues; and also by retching, belching, nausea, vomiting, and by the nature of the vomit. For morbid states of the chest, the indicators are: difficulty in respiration, coughing, pains in the chest, the varieties in the substance coughed up. For dis-eases of the windpipe, indicators are: difficulty in breathing; coughing; pain in
357 that place; the substance | spat out; vocal impairments. And in the same way with the remaining parts, the discernment will be made from these phenomena: lumps, pain, impairment of activity and the nature of the substances excreted.

Unnatural lumps are to be divided into: inflammations, erysipelas, indur-ations and oedemas. A pain affecting a particular part indicates either a dissol-ution of continuity there or a sudden alteration.[20] Continuity is dissolved by cutting, erosion, compression or tension. The substance is altered by heat, cold, dryness or moisture. Activity is impaired in three different ways: it is either weak, faulty or completely non-existent. Substances excreted may be divided into: parts of the affected area, residues, and matter contained within the part in its natural state; and each will provide its own specific indications. This topic has been explored further in my work on *Affected Places*; no previous writer had treated that subject-matter methodically or completely, as is the case
358 with all those enquiries which the ancients embarked on | but did not finish.

---

[20] By 'dissolution of continuity' is meant simply a tear or physical division in a part of the body, especially in the flesh, e.g. as in the case of a wound.

The indicators of diseased bodies should be learnt from that treatise. The indicators of those which are about to suffer disease and of those which are about to return to health, on the other hand, can be gathered from the present method.

21. Those of bodies about to be ill are intermediate in form between those which occur in the states of health and disease. In healthy people all indicators are normal; in people suffering disease, they are abnormal, to the extent to which the person is diseased. Midway between these are the signs indicative of an incipient state of disease: some belong to the class of the 'normal', but altered in quantity, quality or time; others belong to the class of the 'abnormal', but are lesser signs than in the cases of disease proper. And therefore these states, too, of bodies that we have shown to be on the verge of disease, belong to the class of the 'neutral', as do the signs which indicate them. For these signs are primarily indicative of health, but secondarily of disease. And the same signs, considered relationally, are both 'neutral' and I morbid: those which indicate an already 359 existing state are 'neutral', while those which prefigure a future one are morbid. By the same token, too, those signs which announce release from a disease may be referred to as healthy, in that they prefigure a future state of health; but also as diseased, in that they indicate a present state of disease; and so it is obvious that, being indicative of both states, such signs should be called 'neutral' according to one sense of that term. Nor should it surprise us that the same signs acquire all three appellations, healthy, diseased and neutral, in different relational contexts. In another sense, we refer to all signs relating to recovery from disease as 'neutral', as also to those relating to old age.

So all these types of sign fall within a number of different conceptual categories and arguments. Those signs relating to perfect health, on the other hand, come only within the conceptual category of 'healthy'; equally, in cases of disease, those which are not indicative of a future state of health belong in the conceptual category of 'morbid' alone. I We shall return to these in due course. First 360 let us consider the signs predictive of incipient disease. There is a twofold division here; let us turn first to those which deviate from the normal state not in their actual forms but in amount, quality or time. Examples are people whose appetites are larger than normal, or smaller, or not at the usual time, or not for the usual foods, or whose residues become smaller, or larger, moister or harder. Similarly, there is the lack of moist residues, or their excess beyond what is normal, or changes in their colour or composition, or in the time of evacuation; also insomnia or increase in sleep, or sleeping at unusual times. There may also be an unusual desire for more or less drink than normal, or for hot or cold drink. Or also: an immoderate desire for sex; desire for it at inappropriate times; sweating more or less than normal; reluctance to move, or heaviness when movement is attempted; great dissipation; suppression of menstrual flow, or its

361   evacuation in greater or smaller quantity; and the same with haemorrhoids. ❘
Change in the amount of pleasure taken in food or drink is another indicator of
incipient disease. So, too, is an abnormal obtuseness of the intellectual faculties,
unaccustomed forgetfulness, or sleep more than normally filled with dreams.
Also, the faculties of hearing, smell and sight affected by obtuseness or obscurity.

In brief, there is increase, decrease or alteration in time, amount or quality of
all those things which were previously normal. The bulk of the body, too,
becomes smaller or greater, redder or whiter, more blue-grey, as it were, or
blacker; there is increase or decrease from the natural amount of belching,
sneezing and flatulence; and changes in the amount, quality and times of the
evacuations by which the brain is cleansed: those by nostrils, palate and ears.
All these belong in the class of the normal.

Biting sensations in the stomach, the stomach mouth, or some part of the
362   gut, meanwhile, or ❘ moderate pain during defaecation, vomiting or urination,
or some other form of moderate pain, belong in the class of the abnormal; but
those suffering from these complaints are not considered to be yet in an actual
state of disease. The same applies to heaviness or pain in the head, provided that
these have not reached the point of impairing the usual performance of one's
activities. That is the demarcator of disease in such states. Therefore the same
state will be regarded as either actually diseased or neutral, according to context. Each of the above will be a disease or a 'neutral' state, depending whether
the capacity is strong enough to bear it with ease, or is quickly overcome by it.
Thus, if we turn to the capacities of sensation, the distinctions here are not of
degree; here; rather, this whole class of impairments is abnormal. These too are
signs of disease, so long as they are small, and not yet sufficient to detract from
the performance of customary activities.

Such impairments, in the case of taste, would be: the perception of saltiness,
bitterness or some other quality in all the substances that are eaten or drunk;
363   also ❘ when the saliva acquires one of these qualities even without anything
being taken. In the case of smell: experiencing a particular kind of smell when
none is actually present, or experiencing a variety of different smells as the
same. It is quite common that the sense of smell is lost altogether, or that there
is the sensation of a foul smell even though there is no foul-smelling substance
to give rise to it. In the case of hearing, the hallucination of sounds and noises is
abnormal; in the case of sight, things which appear to float in front of the eyes;
these may be black and murky, blue, red or yellow, round or oblong, narrow or
wide. In the case of touch: when some unusual sensation, be it of density,
weight, tension or of a wound-like state, is manifested in the whole condition of
the body; or equally, when a feeling of tension, compression, biting or heaviness
arises in any individual part of the body. Such sensations, provided they are
minor and not lasting, indicate a state which is neutral, but prefigure disease.

22. Signs arising in bodies which are already in a state of disease are divided   364
into those which indicate health and those which indicate death. The former
are healthy signs, the latter belong to the class of the morbid, and within that, to
the specific type known as fatal.

To summarize: these signs are drawn from the excellence or otherwise of the
bodily activities, and individually from the individual activities. The different
classes of the latter have already been enumerated: first, that of the sources; secondly, that of the parts which grow out from these; thirdly, that of those which
are responsible for their own maintenance but are connected by some kind of
outgrowth to the sources. The fourth class previously mentioned is in itself not
of use for prediction; but may be so in an incidental sense, and in fact predictions are made on the basis of these parts, as also on the basis of the residues.
They are made on the basis of the former by virtue of a sympathy in their
nature, on the basis of the latter because there are signs of digestion or non-
digestion present in them, as a result of which it is not possible that there be no
indication present at any given time. Either there will be an indication of the
subjugation of matter by nature, or of | the subjugation of nature by matter, or of   365
the subjugation of neither by the other. In the first of these cases the signs will
be called healthy; in the second, morbid; in the last, neutral. Signs that food has
been definitely digested are healthy; that it has definitely not, morbid; signs
which give no definite indication one way or the other are neutral. Also in this
last category are those signs which for some time indicate the one state, and for
some time the other, as is the case with fingers turning black. Symptoms that
indicate a crisis are also of this nature.

All these have been discussed in my work on *Crises*; and all those which
involve individual bodily activities have been discussed in *Causes of Symptoms*.
These books must be consulted for all the individual subject matter in each
case; here, in the interest of avoiding excessive length, I shall end the discussion
of signs, and shall turn rather to that of causes.

23. Of causes, too, some are healthy, some morbid, some 'neutral'. Let us first
consider the healthy. These are further divided into the preservative and the | 366
productive of health; the former are prior to the latter both in chronological
terms and in terms of importance, and we shall turn our attention first to that.

Now, since there are not just one, but many kinds of healthy bodies—as distinguished above—each will have its own cause of preservation, since, indeed,
every cause is a cause in relation to something. We should, then, begin once
more from the best constitution of the body, and consider which are the causes
of health in relation to that. And the discovery of these is suggested by the
nature of the object itself. For if the body were immune from affection and not
subject to alteration, the best constitution would endure permanently, and there
would be no need of an art to watch over it. Since, however, it is subject to

alteration, decay and change, and does not preserve the state which it had from
the outset, it requires assistance, to precisely the extent of that alteration. There
are therefore as many varieties of assistance as modalities of alteration.
'Assistance' in this context means 'preservative causes': as has already been
made quite evident by the above, these causes belong to the class of the restora-
tive. Since the restorations in question are very small ones, which are carried
367 out before I the damage reaches any considerable size, they are referred to by
doctors not as 'prophylactic against incipient illness', but 'preservative of the
existing constitution'.

The causes of alteration in the body are divided into the 'necessary' and the
'not necessary'. By 'necessary' I mean those which it is impossible for a body not
to encounter; by 'not necessary', all others. Constant contact with the ambient
air is necessary, as are eating and drinking, waking and sleeping; contact with
swords and wild beasts is not. The art concerned with the body is thus performed by means of the former, not of the latter. And if we make a classification
of all the necessary factors which alter the body, to each of these will correspond a specific class of healthy cause. One such class is contact with the ambient air; another is motion and rest of the body as a whole or of its individual
parts. A third is sleep and waking; a fourth, substances taken; a fifth, substances
evacuated or retained; a sixth, the affections of the soul.[21]

368 I The body cannot but be in some state or other with regard to all these. By the
effects of the ambient air it will either be heated, cooled, dried or moistened, or
will undergo some combination of these, or even an alteration in its whole substance. It will also be heated, dried, cooled or moistened, or will undergo some
combination of these, through the effects of motion or rest, if either becomes
immoderate. So, too, it must be affected in some way by sleep and waking; and
in the same way as a result of substances taken, evacuated or retained; and by
the affections of the soul. All these cause alteration in the body, whether directly
or through the action of other, intermediate, causes and, if such alteration continues and is of great extent, loss of health. Each of them has been considered
specifically in my *Health*.

Now, all these classes of healthy causes which we are now discussing are
materials: the correct employment renders them causative of preservation
and healthy, while errors with regard to their proper balance renders them
morbid. From which it is obvious that there is no separate set of things,
369 beyond these, which are materials of health I as distinct from materials of ill

---

[21] The mention in this context of the affections of the soul (*pathē psuchēs*) makes a connection
between the medical diagnostic project and the ethical discourse of *Affections and Errors of the
Soul*: these ethical, or emotional, states for Galen had distinctly discernible physical consequences.
The passage is also of interest for its 'classic' statement of the six necessary factors, later developed
and formalized in mediaeval Galenism as the well-known 'six non-naturals'. See also *The Pulse for
Beginners*, ch. 9 with n. 7.

health; rather, it is the same substances which, according to context, are either healthy or morbid. When, for example, the body is in need of motion, exercise is healthy and rest morbid; when it is in need of a break, rest is healthy and exercise morbid. The same sort of argument applies to food, drink, and all the others. Each is healthy when the right sort is given in the right quantity to a body which is in need of it; when given to a body which does not need it, or given in the wrong measure, it is morbid. Quantity and quality of what is offered are the two variables to be borne in mind generally in matters of the healthy and morbid. The addition of a third variable, time,[22] is not correct, since this is included in those already mentioned. If a body needs such-and-such a substance, then clearly that substance is to be offered at the time when it is needed. The importance of time derives from the fact that mortal bodies are constantly subject to flux and change, so that they require different kinds of treatment on different occasions. | 'Time' is thus not a third class with respect to those already   370 discussed, although for teaching purposes we often treat it as a third, for the reason given.

24. Now the consideration of these variables applies equally in the case of the healthy causes previously listed and in the case of the class which we are considering now; let us return, then, to these healthy causes.

When the constitution of the body is optimal, and the ambient air of a good-mixture, then a perfect balance of all those elements mentioned above—rest and motion, sleep and waking, substances taken and evacuated—will be suitable. When it is not of a good-mixture, the balance of these elements should be modified in accordance with that departure from good-mixture. The points to be borne in mind are: that the ambient air should be such as neither to cause shivering from the cold nor sweating from the heat; that exercise should be discontinued as soon as the body begins to suffer from the exertion; that food should be properly digested, and excretions preserve a good balance in both quantity and quality. In such persons appetite will be well attuned to digestion, | so that they   371 will need no supervisor measuring out the amount of each of the substances taken. The best natures only desire as much as they are able to digest well. The amount of sleep, too, is naturally regulated in cases of optimal constitution: such people will finish sleeping when their bodies no longer require sleep. And if their lifestyle follows this pattern, then the expulsion of residues—through the stomach, the urine and the body as a whole—will be free from problems.

The former sort of excretions are rendered healthy by a balanced diet, transpiration from the whole body by the employment of exercise. Of course one must also avoid all immoderate affections of the soul: anger, distress, rage, fear, envy and worry; for these too cause alteration and move the body

---

[22] *Kairos*: also sometimes translated 'occasion' or 'opportune moment'.

away from its natural constitution.[23] As for sex, it was Epicurus' view that no indulgence in it is ever healthy; the truth is that it should be engaged in at sufficient intervals of time that there is no sensation of dissipation consequent on the act, but that one rather gains the impression of becoming lighter and in better breath. The correct time for sexual activity is when the body is in a pre-
372 cisely medial state | with respect to all external influences: neither over-filled nor empty, neither excessively heated nor cooled, dried nor moistened. And if there is any error in these respects it must be a small one; and it is better to err on the side of a hot state rather than a cold one, of full rather than empty, and of wet rather than dry, when performing the sexual act.

The quality of each of the factors mentioned must also be chosen; in the case of the best constitution, exercise will be such that each part of the body moves in proportion, none being worked either too hard or not hard enough. Food and drink will be of the best-mixed varieties, these being most appropriate to the natures which enjoy best mixture. And the same goes for all the other factors.

25. In cases where the body has departed only a little from the optimal constitution, the preservative causes, too, will be modified to an equally small extent. There is, however, a wide range of such types of body, and each must be considered individually. Now, that which causes alteration to the mixture of the
373 uniform parts, | but not to the balance of the organic parts, is divided into two kinds of healthy cause: that which preserves the mixture and that which moves it towards the best.

The former type of cause will differ from that applicable in the case of the optimal constitution to exactly the same degree that the mixture of the body as a whole differs from that state. Hotter bodies require hotter regimes, colder bodies require colder ones, and so too with drier and wetter bodies. And in composite cases: hotter, drier bodies require hotter, drier regimes, and so too with each of the remaining three pairings. The materials of these causes will be employed correctly by one who has a proper understanding of their innate capacities—for example, that motion, emptiness, sleeplessness, evacuation and all the soul's affections dry the body, while their opposites moisten it. Similarly in the case of practices which dry or moisten, or food or drink with these
374 effects; in short, with respect to everything which is | in the body, one who knows the different materials and their capacities will employ healthy causes, applying like to like when the desire is to preserve the mixture of the body which already exists.

---

[23] There is some variation in the precise list of affections in the manuscript tradition; the Arabic and Latin transmission adds 'joy', while only a few Greek manuscripts give 'worry'; however, joy is not usually mentioned by Galen in such lists of emotional states with physical consequences, while worry regularly is.

When, on the other hand, he wishes to alter and improve it, then we come to a different type of healthy cause, opposite in effect to those just mentioned, differing from the well-mixed, medial ones which we stated to be appropriate for the best natures to exactly the same degree in the other direction. A hot, dry mixture, for example, will not achieve a perfect state of mixture under the influence of a hot, dry regime, but under the influence of one which is colder and wetter to the same degree that that mixture is too hot and too dry. This type of cause is corrective of the innate bad-mixtures, while the former is preservative. For the doctor, each of them has its proper place. The corrective is to be employed at great leisure, in the context of a gradual process of amelioration; for natures cannot endure great alterations all at once. I When necessity dictates   375
a lack of leisure, the preservative must be employed.

Why, then, is this type of cause also defined as 'preservative'? It might appear to be rather 'alterative', 'healing', or 'corrective' of the innate errors in the body. But the term is used by reference to the class of health as a whole, not to the specific differences within it; so that whatever preserves someone in a state of health is called 'preservative', whether it also has the effect of improving the entire mixture of the body, or that of preserving that which existed originally. Causes which make it worse, meanwhile, are 'morbid'. Now, where the bad-mixture is distributed evenly throughout the body, the treatment of all the parts will be the same; where it is not so distributed, it will not. The stomach, for example, might be colder than it should, but the head hotter: each will need its own remedy. Of the other parts, similarly, one might be too moist, too dry, too hot or too cold; and each of these will require its own regime for this bad-mixture. We would not exercise I all parts of the body to the same extent in such   376
a patient, nor moisten or dry them all to the same extent—and so on with the other factors. We have given a fuller account of these matters in our *Health*.

26. In the case of the organic parts, too, healthy causes are distinguished from each other by reference to the deviation from the best constitution. The healthy causes in respect of defects of shaping are different from those with respect to size, or again number, or position. Defects of shaping, in fact, are more numerous: it is not just the shape of the part, but also any hollow, opening, channel, or roughness or smoothness, that it naturally possesses, that may deviate from the proper state of balance. If it undergoes such aberration for a short period, it will still be referred to as a healthy body; if for a long period, as a morbid body; and if it reaches the point where the activity is impaired, we then say that it was actually diseased.

Quantitative excess or deficiency leads to the same distinctions. There may also be a numerical lack or superabundance, I in one or more of the uniform   377
parts. In this class, too, belong any sorts of substance arising in us which are contrary to our nature. There remains the class of position of each of the simple

parts; here too there are four distinct types in all. First, we have the best; secondly, that which is only a little way from the best, and which still gives us a healthy body; thirdly, the morbid, where the deviation is greater; fourthly, when it is greatest of all, the actually diseased.

Parts with some defect in their shape—limbs, for example, which are distorted, bent or bandy—may, provided they are treated in early childhood while they are still soft, be returned to the natural state by shaping and binding. Once they are allowed to grow and harden, this is no longer possible. Defects in the hollowness of a body, too, may be rectified while the body is still growing, but not once growth is completed. Hollows are reduced in size by binding and rest, and increased by activity of the parts and retention of breath. Defects in the 378 channels or | openings in a body are treated in a similar manner: those which are larger than they should be are reduced by rest and an appropriate binding. They are augmented by natural motion and moderate massage, as well as all other factors which cause the attraction of greater quantities of blood.

As for the remaining parts, those which are generated from blood are possible to restore; those generated from sperm almost impossible—though it is sometimes possible to create others which fulfil an equivalent function.[24] (Of all these parts Nature is the true artificer, the doctor merely her servant.) When there is a numerical excess, a healthy cause will be removal; but one must first investigate whether or not that is possible; if it becomes clear that it is impossible, then one should attempt the transfer of the part to some other place. The same applies in the case of defects in position.

Of course, it is quite frequently the case that one part has two or three defects. An example would be the patient whose stomach was both small and round, and pressing into the diaphragm: in this case there were defects in size, shaping 379 and position. Furthermore, the mixture of the stomach was | too cold. To restore the natural state was not feasible; what one was able to do was lessen his distress. Since a full stomach would occasion shortness of breath, he was given smaller, but nourishing, food, three times a day. Another patient, who was suffering very frequent blockages of the liver because of the narrowness of the vessels, found a healthy cause in the thinning diet.

27. There remains one class which applies equally to uniform and to organic parts, and this is the dissolution of continuity. Some will deny that this can ever be present in flawless states of health, on the grounds that it is always an ailment. But this is to ignore the fact that a similar problem would arise with regard to all the classes. If we do not take discernible impairment of function as

---

[24] The distinction seems related to that made between form and matter in Galen's account of reproduction and embryology: blood constitutes the matter from which the embryo is made; sperm or seed (though it also provides some of the matter) contains the form or active cause of the embryo's development.

our criterion for distinguishing illness from health, but rather consider the exact qualitative condition in each case, we shall have to adopt the doctrine of 'perpetual pathology', since there is no one whose activities are all in an optimal state. This, however, is a more theoretical sort of enquiry, and should be treated separately.

28. We proceed to consider the healthy causes in relation to those who are uni- 380
versally agreed to be ill. Let us begin with bad-mixture. The first distinction to be made (which is omitted by nearly all doctors) is that different things are healthy causes in the case of a bad-mixture which is already there, one which is in the process of coming about and one which is about to happen. In the last case, the relevant causes will be found both in the prophylactic branch and in the healthful branch of the art; in the first case, in the healing branch only; in the middle case, in the branches of prophylactic and healing. For a disease which has come about and is already present must be healed; while one which has not yet come about, but threatens to emerge from the present state of the body, must be prevented; and one which is coming to be, to the extent that it has already happened, must be healed, to the extent that it is in the future, prevented. And this prevention will be accomplished by the removal of that state in which it would naturally come about; and such a state is called a 'pre-ceding cause'.

І Disease which has already come about will be treated by the dissolution of 381
the condition by which the normal activity is primarily impaired—which is, in fact, what we call the cause of the disease. The one primary and general aim of a cure is this: the opposite of that which is to be removed. All causes which are productive of health belong to this class, while in the case of individual parts we are concerned with what is opposite in each case. For a hot state, a cold cause will be the opposite; a hot one for a cold one, and so on. If everything that is contrary to nature[25] is ill-balanced, and everything that is in accord with nature well-balanced, then it is necessary that the ill balance be restored to a good bal-ance by something which is equally ill-balanced in the opposite direction. With the terms 'heating', 'cold' and so on we are of course referring to capacities, not impressions. By capacity I mean what genuinely and truly has the property attributed to it, by impression what is imagined to have that property on the basis of superficial perceptions, but in fact does not. How these are to be recog-nized is discussed in my treatise on *The Capacities of Simple Drugs*. І The discov- 382
ery of healthful causes in the context of already existent disease must employ that method which distinguishes impressions from capacities. Their discovery in the case of a disease which is in the process of inception must employ this same method, but additionally that which finds out the causes of diseases. Say,

---

[25] *Para phusin*: the same phrase is also translated above as 'abnormal'.

for example, that a fever arises from some putrefied humoral fluids. In such cases alteration and evacuation are indicated; the former will halt the putrefaction without touching the underlying substance, the latter will remove the entire substance from the body. The type of alteration used in this case is coction; so once one has discovered which causes may bring this about, one automatically has the knowledge of healthful causes of this type. The evacuations in question are performed by venesection, enemas, urine, or transpiration through the skin, as well as by the repulsion and transfer of fluids to elsewhere. In this class belong also the provocation of menses, the opening of haemorrhoids and |

383 cleansing by nostrils and palate. Here too, once we discover the materials by the application of which—in whatever particular quality, quantity, time and manner—evacuation is effected, we will have found the healthful causes relevant to this branch of the art. The discovery of all of them is indeed laid out in *The Therapeutic Method*.

With the other three bad-mixtures, equally, we have the same single aim, namely to cast out the effective cause in each case, and so then to come at the disease caused by it. In this way we shall discover the healthful causes. In cases of composite bad-mixture, the combination of the simple elements will point us towards the prescription for health; here too we will require remedies proportioned to the extent of the bad-mixture. If, for example, a body deviates from the norm by being, in numerical terms, ten times hotter and seven times drier, then the healthful cause in such states must be ten times colder and seven drier.

384 And if such a drug is to be applied to the actual part affected, | its degree of coldness and moisture must be determined by the indicators in each case. If, for example, the affected part lies deep, one must attempt to engineer it that the healthful drug does not lose its power on the way. Say it is to be hotter than the norm; then it must not be only as much hotter as the ailment requires; the amount of cooling it will undergo because of the position must also be taken into account. Say it is to be colder; one must also consider the kind of stuff it is made of. For a very dense substance will not penetrate to a great depth; in fact, it will have a quite opposite effect, densifying the surface. If it is a fine substance, it may penetrate to a greater depth. In the cases of moistening and drying substances, too, their density or thinness has to be considered.

So the position of the affected part provides an indication as to the healthful cause, in the way just described. An indication is provided by both shaping and position in cases where the visible outlets are perforated in such a way as to

385 communicate with another part, or where such outlets are not there at all. | For we will divert those outlets that lead to the most important parts, and stimulate those which lead to the less important.

It is evident, then, that the cure of the effective causes of bad-mixture is through evacuation, while the cure of bad-mixture itself is merely alteration.

29. With dissolution of unity, the aim of treatment—unification—is impossible to achieve in the case of the organic parts. It is not always impossible, however, in the case of the uniform. In some cases, such as the flesh-like parts, the cure is an agglutination, which may equally be referred to as 'growing together'. Where the wound is large this must be preceded by a drawing together of the parts which have been sundered—a process which belongs to the class of shaping. In order for the effect to be a lasting one, we use binding, which brings the parts together, *anktēres*,[26] and stitches. But it is Nature that closes the wound up and restores the original unity. Our task is: first of all, as stated, to bring together the parts that have been divided; secondly, once brought together, to keep them in this state; thirdly, to take care that nothing enters between the two sides of the wound; | fourthly, to preserve the health of the actual substance of the part.   386

The first two of these activities have already been described. The third involves the process of drawing the parts together, at which point one must be careful not to allow anything to fall in from outside; often a bit of hair, or oil, or some other moist substance comes between the two parts that are to be closed up, preventing their unification. This third task is also performed subsequently, in the act of draining a wound, a process which consists in the making of additional incisions, the making of compensatory incisions, and in the production of an appropriate shape. And health of the substance of the part is preserved by moderate drying agents.

So much for the cure of dissolution of unity in a flesh-like part when this occurs on its own. If, however, it is combined with another illness, the number of approaches indicated will be greater; these will be discussed in due course, in the context of composite or complex illnesses (which may also be referred to in a number of other ways). For the present let us turn to the remaining types of dissolution of unity.

30. In the case of bone, the dissolution of unity is a fracture. This is incurable 387
in terms of the first aim; but there is a kind of cure which may be effected in terms of the second. For our first aim, that of 'growing together', cannot be performed because of the hardness of this kind of part. The second is possible, by means of the binding effect of a callus which forms around the fracture. Now the generation of callus, to the extent that it is due to matter and the operation of Nature, is the same as that of any other part; but by virtue of its closeness to bone in form, it takes its origin from the stuff that nourishes bone. In the case of soft bones of the sort found in children a successful 'growing together' may even be possible.

It is quite rare for this kind of injury to be sustained without some kind of complication. Generally the surrounding muscles, as well as other adjacent

---

[26] An instrument for closing up wounds.

parts, are damaged when a bone is broken; and therefore the aim of treatment is twofold—that of the bones and that of other bodies adjacent to them. These matters will be dealt with in our discussion of the complex states of fleshy parts. For now let us confine ourselves to fractures.

The cure of fractures consists in the formation of a callus; and for this to be
388   achieved, | through the function of the nutritive substance specific to the bones, a residue must form the natural basis for the generation of the callus, this residue being well balanced in terms of both quality and quantity. Therefore a regime is required which will cause the blood which flows to the bones to acquire the quality and the quantity suited to the formation of the callus. And since this blood flows through the fissures of the broken bone, one must examine it with regard to amount and quality, and on that basis decide whether to make the regime drier or wetter. (This subject has been more fully discussed in *The Therapeutic Method*.)

31. Lesions of nerves or tendons will readily give rise to convulsions, because of the extreme nature of the sensation in these cases and because of the connection between this part and the source. This is especially so when there is not transpiration to the outside, because the injury of the skin has been covered over. This must be opened, and dried by some substance of a sufficiently fine composition to be able to penetrate right down to the injured nerve. This sub-
389   ject too has been fully discussed in *The Therapeutic Method*. | So much for healthy causes in simple states of this class.

32. As for composite ones, the first factor which causes a complication of the wound is hollowness. This is commonly regarded not as a different state, but as a distinct type of wound; in reality this is not just a distinct type, but a completely different class of illness, in which there is actual loss of physical substance. The manner of cure of this twofold type of ailment must involve a twofold aim: on the one hand, the reunification of the continuity which has been dissolved; on the other, the regeneration of lost substance.

The aims of generation were stated earlier; now, it is evident from the nature of the phenomena that one must first cure this latter state, before then attempting unification. If, then, the empty space is refilled, and the wound achieves evenness in its substance, it follows that the other aim is removed from view: the two sides of the wound cannot be brought together when there is newly generated flesh standing between them. Our cure must therefore have some other
390   aim, which is found in the normal state that should obtain in the case of | this part. Its normal state is to be covered by skin. We should therefore attempt to produce skin, or failing that, some substance similar to skin. We must, in short, produce flesh which is skin-like in nature—which will be the case if it is dried and made callous. What are required, then, are drugs which will have the effect of drying and contracting (without causing a biting sensation), for the purpose

of scarring over. In the same way, if any dirt appears in the wound, the aim is to cleanse it, and the healthy drug will be a cleansing one. The materials used for these are stated in my works on drugs. If, furthermore, there is any inflammation, compression, induration or swelling in the wound, this must be treated first, by the methods already mentioned. Again, if there is some fluxion in the wound, one must employ the remedies for that; or if there is some bad-mixture in the wounded area, one must first have recourse to the remedies for bad-mixture. We have said sufficient on this subject.

33. Let us turn now to the class of shaping, which itself is divided into many distinct types. And ⏐ we shall begin with the clearest of these, which is that   391 related to the change of shape.

In bodies which are still growing, most parts are able to be rectified in shape; in bodies which have completed their growth this is not possible. The aim of treatment will then be, as far as possible, to move in the opposite direction from the distortion. If a fracture has been badly set, so that the shape of one of the limbs has been distorted, and the callus is already hard, one must leave it be; if it is still at an earlier stage, one should break it again and set it properly before the hard callus forms.

Blockages, too, belong to this type of illness, and have a variety of causes. They may come about as a result of viscous, dense humoral fluids; here too the aim will be the single one of producing the effect opposite to that of the ailment: the healthy causes will be cleansing, cutting drugs. Another cause may be a hard piece of faeces stuck in the intestine, in which case the first job is to counteract this hardness with wet, smooth enemas, then to evacuate with acrid ones. Another cause is a stone in the bladder, the immediate cure for which is transferral; the complete cure is surgical removal.

The treatment of abnormal ⏐ moisture contained in a part consists in its com-   392 plete evacuation, as in the case of suppurations. An immoderate state of fulness is treated by immoderate evacuation, as for example of the blood in the veins. Any pus or blood in the stomach, intestines, trachea or lungs, similarly, requires complete evacuation. An excessive intake of food or drink—provided that it is recent—should also be corrected by evacuation.

Substances contained in the lungs or chest are evacuated by coughing, which is assisted by thinning drugs; substances contained in the liver, veins, arteries, kidneys, either by urination or through the stomach. Evacuation by urine takes place under the influence of powerful thinning drugs; evacuation by the stomach under that of drugs with the effects of attracting and opening. What is in the upper part of the stomach is evacuated by vomiting, while what is in the lower part is evacuated by defaecation. Substances under the skin are treated by surgery, by burning, or by drugs with a burning effect. The same applies to some cases of substances contained in a natural cavity, for example in the chest.

In short, the aim, in the case of whatever falls within the class of the abnormal, must be removal; or, where this is impossible, transferral elsewhere. Whatever is not in this class, but is abnormal only by virtue of its degree, must be evacuated. The discovery of the appropriate cures is derived partly from consideration of the actual state of the patient, but mainly from the parts affected. Parts which have acquired an abnormal roughness should have their normal smoothness reintroduced: in the case of bones this will mean a filing operation, in the case of the trachea or tongue the application of non-biting, viscous fluids to smooth them out. Parts which have acquired an abnormal smoothness must have their normal roughness reintroduced, by drugs with a marked cleansing effect and by a brief astringent process.

34. Where any form of blockage or narrowness follows as a result of another illness, the latter must be treated first. It was demonstrated in *The Distinct Types of Disease* that the above conditions frequently follow from inflammations, indurations, oedemas, or excessive dryness, as well as from poor states of the actual body in which they are contained; l and also from certain lumps in the bodies in the surrounding area.

394

If, additionally, there is some combination of more than one of the above, the indications of this will be complex. Let it suffice for our argument to mention one example; all these matters are dealt with in greater detail in my therapeutic works. Let us assume that an excess of blood flows into some part or other, causing distension of the vessels in that part—and not only the large vessels but even those which are so small as to have been previously invisible, but which are evident now because of the quantity of blood in them. (They are also sometimes clearly seen in the eyes, because of the whiteness of the membrane.) And it is reasonable to suppose that there are still smaller vessels which are similarly filled and distended, but which are too small to be seen. Now, in such cases, there is a danger that some excess fluid may flow out from the vessels into the empty spaces between them, or indeed that a small amount will be discharged externally.

The cure of this kind of ailment has evacuation as its aim—or, to be more precise, the removal of voided substance. Since the ailment consists in the unnatural filling of the part in question, the requirement is l to evacuate the excess, either by forcing it to return in the direction from which it came, or through the affected part itself. The means by which it may return are by being pushed, by being pulled or attracted, by being conveyed, or by some combination of these processes. The means by which it may be evacuated through the part itself are: either in large, visible amounts or by being broken down into vapours. Now, if the body in question is as a whole fairly plethoric,[27] then one

395

---

[27] i.e. filled with excess residues in need of evacuation.

should not evacuate through the affected part. For if we bring about a notice-able evacuation by means of scratches and cuts, which at the same time cause pain, we will cause the part to draw more matter towards it; and if we attempt to disperse the substance by the use of heating agents, the effect of the heat will be to attract more matter into the part than will be dispersed. And if we wish to send the substance back where it came from, this will not be possible in the case of a full body.

We must have these two points in mind when we attempt to evacuate the body as a whole. We must then proceed to draw the substance that is flowing into the affected part away to a different region. In doing this, the substance should be expelled from the part, before the attempt is made at dispersion. For evacuation will be easier to effect if it is through larger passages; and we shall succeed in driving the substance out of the ˡ affected part by the use of astrin- 396 gent and cooling agents. The substances evacuated will, additionally, attract to themselves that which is being driven out. (This point was also shown in our *Natural Capacities*.) The vessels, furthermore, having been toned up by these astringents, will contribute their conveyance.

Now, the best case is that in which all the substance is caused to return in this manner. If, however, some matter remains in the part, this must be inferred to be viscous, or dense, and so to have become indissolubly lodged; even if it does not possess those qualities, in fact, it may still flow out into the surrounding spaces.[28] It is at this point, then, that we should turn to evacuation through the affected part itself, by applications to the surface above that part which have the capacity to drive out inflowing substance. And if you have reason to infer that anything has remained in those spaces, you should make particular use for the evacuation of scarification and at the same time of drugs with dispersing prop-erties. But all dispersing drugs are hot in their effects, and what is excessively hot also has a biting effect; therefore a high degree of heat is to be avoided, especially when the affected part is on the surface. ˡ For if in addition to the 397 original problem there is also a biting sensation, the pain will be considerable, and all pain has an exacerbating effect on fluxions. Drugs which are moderately hot will not be painful in these cases, and especially not if they are also moist. Such drugs will be sufficient to disperse what is at the surface, even if the dis-persing effect is not very strong. But if the surface is completely unaffected, and the part in need of evacuation is at some depth, the heat of the dispersing agent must be intensified and increased; for the danger is that it will lose its power before reaching that depth. And there will not be any distress caused when the drug makes contact with the surface, since this is not the affected part. So both circumstances conduce to the use of drugs of considerable heat and

---

[28] Or, according to the Arabic and Latin tradition, 'into the uniform parts'.

acridity—the fact that the parts at the surface can tolerate them, and the fact that those within are in need of them.

Now, the above indication was taken from the position of the affected part. We should next consider whether anything relevant to treatment has been omitted through this consideration; and in fact there seems to be a matter of considerable importance. Of the affected parts themselves, those which contain

398   the excess | fluid, some are spare, porous and soft in their natures, some dense, compacted and hard. The former are easily evacuated; the evacuation of the latter requires quite acrid drugs, which must also be very fine in their substance. If the part is at a considerable depth, these qualities must be even stronger. Here, then, is a further indication, that based on the substance of the part affected.

Another is that derived from shaping and position together. Take, for example, a case in which the liver is suffering from the state which we have been considering; and there is fluid lodged in the narrow extremities of the vessels—fluid which is either viscous, dense, or of considerable quantity. Should we not first employ thinning foods and drinks to render this dense, viscous quality finer? And should we not then proceed to evacuate the offending matter, not only through the narrow, invisible passages (as in the case of other parts) but also through the wide ones? For the veins in the liver are quite wide, as well as being very numerous; and those in the convex parts terminate in the vena cava, those in the concave parts in the portal vein. It should therefore be easy to evacuate the lodged matter, in whichever of these veins it happens to be.

399 | Liquid lodged in the veins in the concave parts can be drawn into the stomach by attracting and opening agents, while that lodged in the veins leading to the vena cava can be expelled into the urine via the vena cava.

A further indication in addition to the above is that which is derived from the liver in its capacity as source of the veins. For since it is in the nature of this organ not only to maintain itself, like most parts of the animal, but also to transmit a capacity into the veins, there is a risk that in loosening its tension with slackening baths and poultices we will not only render it devoid of the necessary tension for the performance of its own activity, but also have a similar effect on all the veins. When treating the liver we must therefore add a small amount of some astringent drug. Since, however, it is at a considerable depth, there is a danger that this astringent property will be lost, unless it is helped on its way by some other fine substance, such as that of aromatic herbs. It is even better if the astringent drug is itself also aromatic; for its intrinsic possession of

400   these two capacities will | render the effect stronger.

Now, imagine that the unnatural fluxion into the part has been evacuated, and that the humoral fluids have been returned to their normal balance. We must at this point consider whether the mixture itself may have been altered in some way by the quality of the fluid. If, for example, the fluid was phlegmatic, it may have had a cooling effect, if bilious, a heating effect. We must cure this bad-mixture too if we are to restore the body to perfect health; and this is achieved by the introduction of the opposite quality (as was discussed in the context of the treatment of bad-mixtures); if any part has been heated, for example, we introduce a cooling effect equal to that heating. Here again, therefore, it is essential to have knowledge of the body's normal good-mixture. How other-wise will we know to what degree it is colder or hotter than its normal state, or when to stop cooling it, if we do not actually know its normal degree of heat? So too if we are heating a body which has become too cold: unless we know what its normal degree of coldness is, we shall not be able either to identify the drug with the correct heating effect, or to be sure when to stop heating.

35. We have said enough on this subject, too; and it is time to turn to those   401 which are in an abnormal state as regards number. There is a twofold division here. If some part is lacking, the aim is to bring this into being; this is of course to be done in subservience to Nature, in the manner described a little earlier. When there is some part in excess, this must be removed, either by the knife, by fire or by a caustic drug. Now, it is possible for nearly all these parts to be cured, but not for all of them to be regenerated (as was demonstrated in my work on *Semen*). Some, however, though not themselves capable of regeneration, may be replaced by a substitute. For example, a bone may be completely removed and replaced with a substance different from bone and flesh. The substance that arises in this place is like a sort of callous flesh, or flesh-like callus; it is more like flesh to begin with, but becomes increasingly callous as time proceeds.

Wherever a part which has been destroyed cannot be replaced by substance either the same in type or similar, our third option is to find some cosmetic solution, as I in the case of mutilations. This whole class obviously has some-   402 thing in common with that of magnitude. In matters regarding the normal state it is adjacent to that class; the only difference arises with regard to the abnormal state. Here one's first aim will be to remove a part, where that is possible; where it is not, one's aim will then be to transfer one to another place, as in the case of cataracts. Where the excess or deficiency is not in a whole part, but in a part of that part, one must attempt the recuperation or regeneration of the deficient parts, and the removal or diminution of the excessive. There is thus no separate aim in these cases, nor any type of medication of a distinct class.

Let us turn then to the remaining class of causes of health: those which rect-ify wrong position within a body, such as dislocated bones, or intestines in the scrotum. The former problem arises from violent tension or pressure, the latter from a dilatation or rupture of the membrane that surrounds it. Thus, the cure in the first case is to exert a compensatory strain and to push it back in the opposite direction; in the second case, to I make the membrane impermeable.   403 The methods for finding out the treatment in individual cases are laid out in my treatise on therapeutics.

36. It remains to mention those causes which we put off in the previous part of the work. These are known as the 'prophylactic'; and within this too there are three classes. First is that relevant to a person in a state of perfect health; second, to one in imperfect health; and third, to a person in a state of disease. The first class—which, as we have said, is itself twofold—belongs to the discourse of health; the second, to that of prophylaxis, and the third to that of healing.

Now, this class as a whole consists mainly in consideration of the humoral fluids: these must be neither viscous, nor dense, nor watery, nor excessive in amount, nor too hot or cold; nor biting, nor liable to putrefaction, nor destructive.[29] For when such humoral fluids increase, they become the causes of disease. The causes of such increase are in some cases the same as those which produced these humoral fluids in the first place, sometimes the sympa-
404 thetic alteration that the fluids perform Ⅰ on those throughout the body. Here, too, the cure involves two aims: alteration and evacuation. Alteration may be brought about by the coction of the humoral fluids by the body itself, or by the capacities of certain drugs, such as those which treat the venom from animals known as venomous, and those which transform the 'destructive' drugs. Evacuation takes place by means of drugs with a strong heating effect, and by purgatives, enemas, sweats and vomiting.

These are the means of evacuation, in general terms; but specific kinds of evacuation are prescribed on the basis of the particular places in which the excess is collected. This is clarified in *Health*, in the third and fourth books, and especially in our account of kinds of fatigue and of other states related to fatigue. Thus, excesses collected in the first veins[30] are more easily voided through the stomach; those around the liver, through urine; those which affect the condition as a whole, through sweating; those in the head, through palate, through
405 nostrils, or through both; those in the open spaces of the chest, Ⅰ through the pharynx, by coughing; those in the kidneys or bladder, through urine. For all parts, repulsion is indicated, towards the parts furthest way, and transfer, towards the near ones.

So, everything that heals such states is referred to as a healthy cause, just as whatever increases them as a morbid cause, and what does not hurt or help as 'neutral'. Some may deny the application of the term 'cause' to these altogether— the majority of the sophists, for example, people who have no interest in discovering the actual distinctions in matters, but prefer to waste their time on

---

[29] An alternative translation for the term (*dēlētērios*) would be 'poisonous'; but Galen distinguishes more specifically, amongst drugs, between the 'destructive' and the 'deadly'. See further below in this paragraph, and compare *My Own Doctrines*, ch. 9, with n. 23 and *Simple Drugs* V.1, p. 416 below.

[30] Galen regards the liver as the source of the veins, and thus by 'first veins' means those which connect the liver to the intestines; cf. the distinction between different kinds of vein in relation to different parts of the liver (and different forms of evacuation) made in ch. 34 above.

terminology. I have addressed myself to these more fully elsewhere. So much, then, for the prophylactic part of the art.

37. That part which relates to recovery from illness, and also to old age, is known as the 'recuperative' or 'convalescent'. This nature of the relevant state, and the particular causes by which it is returned to the normal state, I have been   406
shown very comprehensively in my writings on *The Therapeutic Method*; here let us recapitulate the main points. The state is as follows. The blood is good, but small in quantity; so too the breaths known as vital and psychic. The solid parts themselves are dry, and therefore their capacities weak, and in consequence of this weakness the whole body is cold. The healthy causes—those which will correct such a state—may be summed up in general terms as those which bring about quick and safe nourishment. Specifically, these consist in well-balanced motions, food, drink and sleep. The motions break down into passive exercise,[31] perambulation, massages and baths; and, if the subjects' improvement while performing these is great, they may also engage to a small degree in their regular tasks. The food should to begin with be moist, easily digestible, not cold; they should then gradually proceed to take the more nourishing foods. Suitable drink is wine, of a balance suited to the person's age, and of a clear, translucent type: white or very light in colour; moderately sweet-smelling, and neither completely watery in taste I nor manifesting any one very marked quality—   407
neither sweetness, bitterness, sourness nor acridity.

As I have just remarked, much more has been said on this in *The Therapeutic Method*. Our present task is not to go through every individual point, but merely to call to mind the principal points, of which I have given a full account in other works. I shall now list those works, setting down their number and their subject matter; and with that I shall conclude the present treatise.

I mentioned earlier that there is one other book in which I discuss *The Constitution of the Art of Medicine*. This is preceded by the previous two, on *The Constitution of Arts*.[32] But these works, along with this present one, stand apart from the systematic treatises. The latter have the following order. There is one book on *The Elements according to Hippocrates*; and following on from that, three on *Mixtures*. Of these, two concern mixtures in animals, while the third concerns mixtures in drug. Thus, the treatise on *The Capacities of Simple Drugs* cannot be properly understood without a I careful reading of the third book of   408
Mixtures. I also wrote another small book, which follows on from the first two of *Mixtures*, namely *The Uneven Bad-Mixture*; and similarly two other small ones, on *The Best Constitution of the Body* and on *Good Condition*. There is

---

[31] The term refers specifically to motions in which the subject is carried, especially in a litter or horse-drawn carriage.

[32] Only the last of these three, with the fuller title *To Patrophilus on the Constitution of the Art of Medicine*, has survived.

another treatise, in three volumes, on *Natural Capacities*; this may be read either next in order after the two books of *Mixtures* or after *The Elements*. After this, there are a number of treatises in which we have examined the activities of the soul. But since the findings of anatomy are of considerable importance for the demonstrations employed there, one should first train oneself in those works. Of these, the most useful is *Anatomical Procedures*. There are, however, many others in addition to this: two books on *Disagreement in Anatomy*, one on *The Dissection of Dead Bodies*; and, following on from these, two on *The Dissection of Living Bodies*. Certain other works cover individual subjects and were written for beginners, such as that on the dissection of bones; on the dis-

409   section of muscles, nerves, | arteries and veins,[33] and some other similar ones. Among these, too, belongs the treatise *Whether Blood is Naturally Contained in the Arteries*.

Then we have those which demonstrate the activities of the parts: two books on *The Motion of the Muscles*, three on *The Motion of the Chest and the Lungs*, following which are the *Causes of Breathing* and the work on *The Voice*. Matters concerning the leading-part of the brain, and in general all other questions regarding natural and psychic capacities, have been made clear in a many-volume treatise entitled *The Doctrines of Hippocrates and Plato*. The work specifically devoted to *Semen*, as also that on *The Anatomy of Hippocrates*, also belong to this type of enquiry. *The Function of the Parts* follows, in turn, after all these.

For diagnosis of diseases, *Affected Places* and the work on the pulse are useful; in the latter we also give instruction on prognosis. But before the work on

410   the pulse come two books, on *The Function of Breathing* | and on *The Function of the Pulse*. The work on the pulse is itself divided into four parts: first, on *Distinct Types of Pulse*, secondly, on *The Discernment of the Pulse*, thirdly, on *Causes in the Pulse*; and fourthly, on *Prognosis by the Pulse*. In this class too is the work written on *The Pulse for Beginners*. I intend, also, to write one more book as a kind of summary of them all, which will be entitled either *The Art of the Pulse* or *The Synopsis*. In this field, my work of commentary and criticism on Archigenes' *Pulse* is also of use. On prognosis, the most useful treatise of all is that on *Crises*; but preceding that is *Critical Days*. But *Difficulty in Breathing* is of value, too, both for diagnosis of the present state and for prognosis of the future good and ill that will befall the patient.

All these are useful to read, and with them a handful of single-volume works,

411   too, such as that on *Antecedent Causes*, | on *Medical Experience*, and on *The Thinning Diet*; and also on *Venesection, to Erasistratus*, and on *Unnatural Lumps*. Similarly, the work on *Fulness*, and a number of similar ones.

---

[33] Exactly how many different titles are meant here, and the precise form of the titles, are not entirely clear; cf. *My Own Books*, ch. 4 [3].

Most necessary of all for the method of healing is the work on *The Distinct Types of Disease*, and that on *Symptoms in Diseases*, and a third in addition to these, in which we consider the *Causes of Diseases*; then three more, in which we discuss the *Causes of Symptoms*. There are also the books on *The Capacities of Simple Drugs*, mentioned above, as well as those on *The Composition of Drugs*; these are followed by those specifically devoted to the subject of *The Therapeutic Method*, as well as those concerned with *Health*. That one should also—before all these—train oneself by means of the treatise on *Demonstration*, if one is to embark upon the art in a rational manner, I showed in the work on *The Best Method of Instruction*.

It is not necessary now to go through all the other treatises and sets of notes that we have written; | we shall produce a comprehensive list on another occa- 412 sion—a work of one or perhaps two books, which will be entitled: Galen, *My Own Books*.

III

HUMAN BODIES

Composition, Physiology, Embryology

The Elements according to Hippocrates (excerpts)

This is Galen's fundamental work on the elements and on the physical composition of human beings and animals, and indeed all things in the natural world. He refers to it frequently elsewhere as providing the demonstrations, and laying the foundations, of his physical theory as assumed in other works. This 'demonstration' is expressed in complex terms; a large part of it is an argument against the coherence of ancient Atomism.

If, Galen argues, we take the fundamental elements to be 'unaffected' (*apathē*), that is, not liable to alteration of any kind, and also themselves not sentient, then such elements cannot explain the phenomena of change in the natural world, and in particular the phenomena of pain and sensation. According to the Atomists, at least on Galen's interpretation, all atoms are themselves indistinguishable ('one in form') and unchanging in their properties; they give rise to different discernible properties in the observable world, and to pain and sensation, merely through the different combinations and configurations of bodies which are themselves all of one kind, and immune to change.

Against this, Galen argues that unless the elements *themselves* undergo alteration, there can be no 'new' properties in the observable world other than those that belong to those fundamental particles themselves. The unchanging, unaffected atoms of Epicurus and Democritus can give rise to no discernible properties that are not properties of the atoms themselves; thus, since they are not themselves capable of sensation, they cannot give rise to sensation or pain.

On Galen's opposing view, there are four elements (earth, air, fire and water), or at an even more fundamental level of analysis, four basic qualities (the hot, the cold, the dry and the wet). It is the varying combinations of these, and the interactions between them, that explain both the different natures of, e.g., animals and plants, and the changes that they give rise to and undergo. Crucial to his view is the notion of 'mixture' (or 'blending': *krasis*), a process which involves alteration of the underlying substances, not merely different combinations or configurations of them.

The exposition of this view leads to another central feature of this work, and indeed of Galen's project: the exegesis of Hippocrates. Galen takes himself to be following, in his own theoretical views, the 'Hippocratic' *The Nature of the Human Being*—a text which does not clearly support the four-element theory (earth, air, fire, water) at all, and moreover focuses on four *fluids* (or 'humours', *chumoi*: blood, phlegm, yellow bile and black bile) as constituents of human bodies, rather than on four fundamental qualities. For Galen, conversely, while the four fluids or humours do have an important role in his understanding of health and disease, they are—with the exception of blood—essentially bodily residues produced in the digestive process, rather than the actual constituents of the healthy body. (See ch. 10 with n. 20 below.)

The work manifests some tension, then, in the reconciling of the 'Hippocratic' view with Galen's own, and in particular in the exegetical challenge of presenting *The Nature of the Human Being* as concordant with Galenic element theory—a theory which seems much more closely indebted to Aristotle's. In the process, it provides a vivid insight into the nature of ancient debates in this area, both through Galen's painstaking use of philological argument to support his interpretation and in the glimpse it gives of an alternative—apparently a less theoretically dogmatic—view, that of the followers of Athenaeus, with which Galen belligerently engages.[1]

Greek title: Περὶ τῶν καθ' Ἱπποκράτην στοιχείων (*Peri tōn kath' Hippokratēn stoicheiōn*)
Kühn: I.413–508
Edition: De Lacy 1996 (with English translation)

I.413   1. Since an element is the smallest part of that of which it is an element, and what is smallest in terms of sense perception and in reality are not the same thing—after all, there are many things that elude our perception on account of their smallness—it is quite evident that sense perception cannot be the judge[2] of what are by nature and in reality the elements of each object. So, for example, if you decided to crush rust, cadmia, litharge or copper ore finely, then mix them together thoroughly to form a powder, and leave it to sense perception to make the discernment, all these different items will appear to you to be one

414   thing. Indeed, | if you were to combine together many more than these four, they would still appear to you to be one, although in fact they are not. It is for this reason, then, that Hippocrates, when considering the elements of the human being, rejects those which are simplest and primary in relation to sense perception, seeking out those which are so in reality and by nature.

Moreover, the usefulness of the latter for cures is no less than that of those which are primary in sense perception, as has been shown in other works. One may concede that these [primary] perceptibles *appear* to be elements, but not that they actually are. For what is in reality the element is not the part which is apparently simplest, and primary, but that which is so in nature. If we were to say that what appears to be the smallest and primary part in each case actually was the natural element, then what was an element would be a different thing for Lynkeus,[3] for an eagle, or for any other exceptionally sharp-sighted human

415   being or non-rational animal, and for the rest of us. | So, if we intend to gain

---

[1] It is at least arguable that the position of Athenaeus, his argument against which he reports in ch. 6, represents a more accurate representation of Hippocratic 'element theory' (or its absence) than does Galen's.

[2] *Kritērion*: see *The Best Method of Instruction*, n. 3.

[3] According to legend, a companion of Jason's in the quest for the Golden Fleece, who was able to see even below the earth.

precise knowledge of the nature of the human being, or of any other thing which exists, let us then not pursue the enquiry in this way but rather enquire which are primary and simplest by nature, and not liable to any further dissolution.

2. What, then, is the method of discovery of these? It is surely none other than that introduced by Hippocrates. One should distinguish, first, whether the element is one in form, or whether there are many elements, various and dissimilar from each other; secondly, if they are indeed many, various and dissimilar, how many there are, what they are, and what are their characteristics and the nature of their relationship with each other. Now, Hippocrates shows that the first element, from which both our bodies and those of all other living beings have come about, is not a single thing; he does this in the following words (I shall set down his actual statement, and then give an exegesis of it):

> I say that if human beings were one, they would never feel pain; for there would exist nothing by which they could be caused to feel pain, if they were one.[4]

Here it appears to me that he gives a perfect statement, while nonetheless using the briefest possible form of words, | of the essential point of his demonstration   416 that there cannot be just one single element, in both form and capacity. To say that what exists is numerically single would obviously be an utter absurdity, and very definitely the statement of one with no concern for evident facts. One might, however, say that all things are one in their form and capacity; this, indeed, is what the followers of Epicurus and Democritus say in relation to atoms. Those who posit as elements 'minima', 'unjointeds' or the 'partless' also belong to this band.[5] Hippocrates produces a single counter-argument to all such people, demonstrating that there is not just one single element, in terms of its form and capacity—and not even mentioning, on the grounds that they are completely out of their minds, those who state that what exists is single numerically.

Let us then see whether he reasoned correctly, and appropriately countered those who take as their fundamental assumption that there is a single element in nature—whether | these persons wish to give that element the appellation   417 'atom', 'unjointed', 'minimum', or 'partless'. We shall not need to consider their particular points of difference, if we refute what is shared in common by all the sects. For it is the common postulate of them all that the primary element is

---

[4] *The Nature of the Human Being* 2.
[5] The technical concept of the 'unjointed' (*anarmes*) or 'unjointed bulk' (*anarmēs onkos*) was that of Asclepiades of Bithynia, while the theory of the 'partless' (*ameres*), which could also be described as a theory of minima, was associated with Diodorus Cronus. Galen lumps together all these theories, including with them those of the various Atomists, claiming that they support the same essential doctrine. Compare *My Own Doctrines*, n. 28.

without quality, having no inherent whiteness, blackness, or any other colour; nor sweetness, bitterness, heat or coldness—nor, indeed, any other quality.

'For colour is by convention, sweet is by convention, bitter is by convention; but in truth there are atoms and void', says Democritus, who holds that all perceptible qualities, as perceived by us, arise from the coming-together of atoms, whereas in nature itself nothing is white, black, yellow, red, bitter or sweet. This is what he means by the phrase 'by convention', namely that these qualities exist only conventionally and in relation to us, not in the actual nature of the things....

418   All the atoms are small bodies, without qualities, while the void is a place in which they are carried upwards and downwards for all eternity,[6] becoming in various ways entwined with each other, hitting and bouncing off each other, separating from and combining with each other in the course of such encounters, and thus producing not only all other compounds but our bodies themselves, as well as their experiences and perceptions. But their postulate is that the primary bodies remain themselves unaffected.[7] Some, like Epicurus, hold

419 that they are unbreakable because of their hardness; others, | like the followers of <Diodorus and>[8] Leucippus, that they are indivisible because of their smallness; but in any case that they are not capable of being altered in any respect in those processes of alteration that all human beings are convinced, on the basis of sense perception, take place. They cannot, for example, be heated nor cooled, nor dried nor moistened, still less blackened or whitened; nor can they admit of any qualitative change at all.

It is, then, reasonable for Hippocrates to state as a counter-argument to them that human beings would never feel pain if this were their nature. For what feels pain must, necessarily, have these two characteristics: it must be both liable to alteration and capable of sensation. If it were never to admit of any alteration, it would preserve forever the state which it had at the outset; but that which feels pain does not thus preserve its state. If, however, it did indeed change its state, like stones or wood when they are heated, cooled or split apart, but there were

420 no sensation present in it by nature, | it would not perceive the condition arising in relation to it—any more than a stone does. Now, the elements posited by these people lack both these characteristics, since no atom is by nature either liable to alteration or capable of sensation. If, then, we consisted of some kind of

---

[6] There is some doubt about the inclusion of the words 'upwards and', which are omitted by some of the manuscripts. The view that the atoms move downwards only, and do so for all eternity, would be an authentic reflection of Epicurus' view.

[7] It is worth noting that the word for 'unaffected', *apathē*, which could also be translated 'immune from change', is cognate with that for 'experience' (*pathēma*) in the previous sentence. An experience, *pathos* or *pathēma* (also sometimes translated 'affection', 'ailment', 'suffering') is conceived as a process of being affected by something else.

[8] These words appear in the extant Arabic version of the text; compare n. 5 above.

atoms, or of any other such single-form nature, we would not suffer pain; but we do suffer pain; it is therefore evident that we do not consist of some simple or single-form substance.

This is the chief point of the argument. It is immediately evident to all who have been schooled in logical theory, and basically establishes our demonstrandum. Since, however, those who introduce such elements not only are *not* schooled in reasoning but are also argumentative in other respects—they consider any sort of change for the better to be an evil!—one must attempt to expound the general argument with the help of individual examples.

So, if someone pierces an animal's skin with an extremely fine needle, that animal will undoubtedly feel pain. Yet the needle must be in contact with either one or two atoms—or indeed more. Let us assume first that it is in contact with one atom. Now, | each of these atoms is itself incapable or being pierced, and 421 incapable of sensation. The animal will not, then, be affected[9] in any way by the needle; nor, if it were affected, will it perceive that affection. For if the feeling of pain arises from two things, namely from that which is capable of being affected being so affected, and from the perception of this affection, and atoms have no part in either of these, then the animal will not feel pain when the needle is in contact with one atom.

Let us then suppose that it touches not one but two atoms. But what was just now stated in relation to one atom will now apply equally to both of them....

It would be quite remarkable if, in a case where none of the parts either were 422 affected or experienced sensation [of it], the whole became capable of perception and affection.

There are two instruments for the discovery of such propositions, experience and reason; and by neither of them will it ever be found that something composed of non-perceptive and unaffected things is capable of perception and affection....

If you concede that [atoms] are unaffected but are perceptive, they will not 424 feel pain, because they will not undergo an affection; and if they do undergo an affection but are non-perceptive, they will not suffer pain because they do not perceive the affection. For that which is to feel pain must both undergo affection and perceive that affection.

What is capable of perception, then, cannot consist of elements that are both unaffected and non-perceptive, nor of ones which are both unaffected | and 425 perceptive; for in this latter case too it will not feel pain, since is does not undergo an affection: it would be capable of perception but would not actually ever perceive, just as our bodies, which manifestly are capable of perception, nonetheless do not perceive anything before they are affected in some way. The

---

[9] The verb is *paschein*, cognate with *pathos* and *apathē*; see n. 7 above. In the present context one could also translate 'suffer'.

opinion of those who introduce 'homoiomeries',[10] too, is clearly confounded by this argument; for if certain of their elements are capable of perception, and yet completely unaffected, how will the perceptive element perceive anything, when it is perpetually outside the realm of affectedness?

It remains, then, that the perceptive body must consist of things which are both perceptive and affected or of ones which are affected but are not perceptive. Which of these two is the case, we shall consider later; but it has been clearly shown that the perceptive body could never come about from elements which are both non-perceptive and unaffected nor from ones which are perceptive but unaffected. | But common to both these [rejected] views is the notion of 'from what is unaffected'; so, then, the element cannot be one in form, since it is not unaffected. The demonstration that what is one is unaffected is a short one: a single element does not have either anything into which it can change or anything by whose agency it can be affected. For what changes must change into something else, and what is affected must be affected by the agency of something else. How, then, will it be preserved as one? Hippocrates, then, was right to reason that there must be more than one element, if anything that exists is to feel pain. 'For', he said, 'there would not exist anything by which [human beings] could be caused to feel pain, if they were one.' Undoubtedly, then, the number of the elements is greater than one.

3. How large that total is, however, not yet evident; and this should be our next enquiry. But we should first give an account of the remaining two views, which I mentioned a little earlier: those which share the proposition that any body by nature capable of feeling pain must consist of primary elements which undergo alteration.

426 (margin)

427 | For we find that there are in all four distinct types of view. First, there is that of non-perceptive and unaffected elements; secondly that of perceptive but unaffected elements. These two share the notion of 'unaffected', which we showed to be impossible, so rejecting both opinions. There remain two: one basing the composition of the perceptive body on primary elements which are both perceptive and affected, the other basing it on ones which are non-perceptive but do undergo affection. These both share the notion of 'affected'. Let us then see whether one of these views, too, is impossible, or whether both are equally possible, and in that case which one is not only possible but actually true.

You will find, then, if you consider the matter, that both are possible. For if you wish to test the actual parts | and investigate them by the use of reason, all

428 (margin)

---

[10] The reference is probably to Anaxagoras, to whom was attributed the cosmological or biological theory of a kind of uniform or 'homoiomerous' animal parts, which in some way exist as indivisible elements of the larger entities.

those belonging to bodies capable of perception are themselves both capable of perception and liable to affection, as we said a little earlier with regard to flesh. But if you investigate the primary elements, it is possible that these underlying elements are non-perceptive, but are of such a nature as to act upon and be acted upon by each other in a variety of ways, and that the perceptive body comes about at some point as a result of these many individual alterations. Any composition from a plurality will not, if those components remain permanently as they are, acquire a single new form from outside, unless this was present in the components. If, however, those components may be altered and changed in various ways, then the composite object may acquire some property which is different in kind and was not a property of the primary elements....

Now, those who favour the view that a certain composite body may become 430 perceptive as a result of fire, water, air and earth changing and being mixed and altered in their totality,[11] are stating possibilities, | while those who favour the 431 view that the latter remain as they are and are only combined together with each other in the same way that one might combine wheat, barley, chickpeas and beans in a pile, are attempting the impossible. It makes no difference at all whether one states that fire, water, air or earth come together to produce a perceptive body or—as people in the past did—that atoms do so. It is impossible, so long as the elements remain unaffected, that a single perceptive body be produced from the coming-together of many non-perceptive ones. For it has been shown that nothing of a different kind may accrue to the components; and perception is indeed something of a completely different kind from shape, weight and hardness—the properties of atoms—and, equally, from those things which are the properties of fire, earth, air and water. Even when considered in relation to colour, flavour, aroma and, in short, all other properties of bodies, perception is different in kind, so that a body capable of perception cannot come about either from atoms or from fire, earth, water and air, if these remain | unchanged 432 and just as they are in their own nature. It is necessarily the case that a body which is to perceive is composed either from primary elements which are perceptive or from ones which are not perceptive, but are of a nature to change and undergo alteration.

---

[11] The phrase 'in their totality', more literally 'through the whole' (*di' holōn*, or *hola di' holōn*) is taken from Stoic technical language, where it refers to the specific notion of bodies interpenetrating each other. Elsewhere Galen presents this 'total mixture' as one of the possible theoretical options, but remains agnostic about whether bodies do undergo 'total mixture' with each other in this sense, or whether what become intermixed are the *qualities* of the bodies rather than their *substances*; see e.g. *The Therapeutic Method* I.2, where Galen contrasts the Aristotelian position (qualities alone undergo such mixture) with the Stoic one, and regards this as an issue that he does not have to decide.

These considerations, then, show that the number of elements is definitely greater than one, and that they are capable of suffering; whether it is from primary elements which are capable of perception or not, is not yet shown....

438   Let us enquire no longer, then, into what was stated by him [Hippocrates] in the beginning of the work, nor give an interpretation of it which goes beyond our statements here, since by now we have a clear understanding of the man's overall view. When, then, he says:

> One who habitually listens to people speaking on the nature of the human being in terms that go beyond those relevant to medicine—the present discussion is not for him. For I say that human beings are not, absolutely, air, nor fire, nor water, nor earth—nor anything else which is not evidently ENEON in the human being.[12]

When he says this, we are not to read that ENEON as one word [= *being present*], without an aspiration, as do many of the Hippocratic commentators, but rather add an aspiration and separate it into two words [HEN EON = *being one thing*]. So, it is as if he had said:

> For I say that human beings are not, absolutely, air, nor fire, nor water—nor any-
439 thing else which is not *evident as being | one single substance* in the human being.[13]

For the first part of his work is entirely about the proposition that the element is not one, as has been demonstrated both by what I said a little earlier and, equally, by what he adds, at the very beginning, just after the statement quoted above:

> For they state that what exists is one, and that this is the one and the all; but they do not agree with each other on names. One says that this one and all is air, another that it is fire, another water, another earth.[14]

And again, just after this:

> Amongst doctors, some say that the human being is blood alone, some that it is bile, some others that it is phlegm.[15]

Then, after that, in commencing his refutation of these people, he begins by writing that statement of which I gave the exegesis first, which stands against both natural philosophers and doctors, then specifically counters the doctors in this passage:

---

[12] *The Nature of the Human Being* 1.
[13] According to the interpretation which Galen rejects—and which at least arguably gives a much more natural reading of the Hippocratic text—we would translate: '...nor anything else which is not evidently present in the human being.'
[14] *The Nature of the Human Being* 1.   [15] *The Nature of the Human Being* 2.

As for myself, I would urge one who states that the human being is blood alone,
| and nothing else, to show that that human being does not change form, nor   440
become varied in characteristics, but show some season of the year or time of
life in which blood alone appears to be the one thing [*or*, appears to be present]
in the human being.[16] . . .

4. And it is rather a cause of amazement that those who say such things were   442
held in high repute in human society than of difficulty in finding their refutation... for those who said that there was one element did not employ any plausible arguments, nor ones which were difficult to dispel; rather their absurdity is
ready to hand and extremely easy to detect. For those who say that water is the
element, because this when densified and as it were compressed becomes earth,
and when rarefied and as it were dispersed, air, and when further rarefied and
dispersed, fire, state for this reason | that this is the element; those who say that   443
it is air also state that it becomes fire when rarefied and water if its thickened;
those who say that it is earth, claiming that water arises from its moderate dis-
persal and air from its further rarefaction, and that if it suffers this to an extreme
degree, it turns to fire, reason on these grounds that earth is the element; and
similarly with the proponents of fire, who claim that it comes together and is
densified to become air, undergoes this to a greater extent and is more vehemently compressed to become water, and when most completely densified
forms earth—these too reason that this is the element.

The absurdity of these arguments, though, is right there in front of you. All
these have spoken of the change of the elements into each other; and yet they
do not believe that this is what they are showing. They think that they are showing what each of them believes to be *the element*. Yet it is not the same thing to
speak of the change into each other of air and fire | and water and earth as to   444
speak of the elements. It is not by virtue of their changing into each other that
each of these things is an element, but by virtue of its being primary and simplest. Now, Plato too spoke of their change into each other, in the *Timaeus*, supporting the view that there is a single, common matter which underlies them
all. He, however, used the change of the primary bodies into each other as one
who knows how to make a demonstration in an appropriate manner; but
Thales, Anaximenes, Anaximander and Heraclitus attempted to demonstrate,
on the basis of their change into each other, that whichever one each had posited was the element.

What these people seem to me to be vaguely gesturing towards is the common matter which underlies all the elements; they see that this is single, and
therefore assume that the element is single as well. Then, when they should
have said, if anything, that that which underlies all—air, water, fire and

---

[16] *The Nature of the Human Being* 2.

earth—in common is the element, they bypassed this and declared some one of the four as the element, all of them using the same judgement in respect of the | demonstration, but choosing different elements. This indeed is what Hippocrates ridicules, at the very start of the work....

445

Thus, they all use one justification for different hypotheses. But, first of all, they do not draw the appropriate conclusion: it would have been appropriate to say, on that basis, that the substrate and substance which *underlies* the primary bodies is one. Then, they do not realize this very point, that they are all attempting to give one and the same demonstration of four different hypotheses....

451   5. ...It appears indeed that Aristotle and Hippocrates have laid out their arguments in exactly the same way, but that their commentators have not followed them. Hippocrates' statement that his discussion is not suited to those who habitually listen to people speaking on the subject of the nature of the human being 'in terms that go beyond those relevant to medicine' is not motivated by a rejection of those who posit fire, air, water and earth as elements, but—from beginning to end—by criticism of those who state this of *one* of those four. | It would be terribly illogical if all four were to be rejected on the grounds

452   that no single one of them appears in unadulterated form in the body; by the same reasoning, surely, one would then reject the proposition that the *tetrapharmakon*, as it is known, is composed of wax, resin, pitch and tallow, since no one of these appears in it whole and complete.[17] Actually, one does not need to refer to such cases, where things are mixed in their totality. Even dry drugs, those composed of cadmia, antimony and smelted copper, when these have been reduced to a fine powder, retain nothing in adulterated form, and it is impossible to get hold of even a most minute part of them in which one of the substances mentioned may be observed unmixed and uncombined.

Nor, certainly, should one reject the proposition that the bodies of animals consist of a mixture of the four elements, on the grounds that here too none of

453   these is unadulterated or complete; | nor should one for this reason concede that the cosmos consists of the four, but take animals out of the realm of what comes into being from these, as though they had arrived from somewhere else and had not come about within the cosmos. Or are you asking me to show you earth in unadulterated and uncombined form in the bodies of animals, when you cannot yourself point to such a thing even in the cosmos? Whatever part of this you take will unavoidably also have some degree of heat, of moisture and of airy substance, whereas that uncombined earth which we conceive also as the element, is to the extreme degree thick, heavy, dry and cold. Rather, just as,

---

[17] The *tetrapharmakon* (or *tetrapharmakos*) was a mixture of the four products mentioned, used as an external application for wounds or inflammations of the skin. The word came to be better known through its metaphorical use by the Epicureans to refer to a fourfold set of precepts designed to summarize the school's doctrines and dispel distress.

within the cosmos, you will point out to me a stone as an example of an earthy body, so in the realm of animals I will point out to you the class of bone, and also that of cartilage, and of hair. To the same class belongs also the shell, as it is known,[18] in shelled animals, which is completely dried out and compacted, so as to be equivalent in form to earth.

And so, if you look for earth amongst the animals, you will be able to observe it in the same form as it is in the | cosmos. You will not easily find it alone,   454 uncombined and complete—any more will you find water pure and unmixed with all the others, or fire, or air. All have been adulterated and mixed up with things of a different kind, partaking in each other to a larger or smaller degree. Even in this combination, however, the form of the dominant [element] is apparent to a person of intelligence. Do not, then, seek something uncombined in animal bodies either; rather, let it suffice for you, when you see that some-thing is cold, dry and thick, to be reminded of earth, and when you see some-thing rarefied, wet and fluid, to arrive at the concept of water. Great heat in an animal body, meanwhile, should remind you of fire; and the nature of breath, without which no animal can be put together, should remind you particularly of air. So do not ask me for earth *as such* in the body of an animal, nor for any other of the elements | in unmixed form—or else show me, first, the wax in the   455 *tetrapharmakon.*

It would amaze me if you did not think that wheat, barley, acorns, figs and all the other kinds of pulse and fruit had come about from earth and water, when you see clearly that they have their origin there. Do they, then, not partake of air or fire at all, for the origin of their substance? Yet if you submerge earth in water, all you will have is mud; but each of the pulses and fruits is not this same mud, because it has partaken of fire and air, mixed with each other in totality. Is it, perhaps, that you concede that acorns and figs have come about from the elements of the cosmos, and before them the plants themselves—since you observe that a small seed of each is thrown onto the ground, this seed being not even a ten-thousandth part of the fully grown plant—and yet, in spite of seeing how all other substance comes about from the elements of the cosmos, you have a doubt about animals, as if they, too, had not been nurtured by the same source? Sheep | feed on grass, pigs on grass and acorns, goats on these things   456 and also on new shoots of trees; and from these their blood is generated, their body nourished, and the embryos are put together and grow....

[Galen continues his argument against those who deny the existence of the under-lying elements in the sense he has outlined, with particular reference to a debate in which he engaged with a follower of Athenaeus of Attalia. He accuses his interlocu-

---

[18] In its primary meaning *ostrakon* in Greek refers to an earthenware vessel, the shells of testa-ceans or molluscs (*ostrakoderma*) acquiring that name by extension.

tor of confusion, as expressed in a statement that elements are 'clearly visible and need no proof'.]

461   I did not know whether he was applying 'hot', 'cold', 'wet', 'dry' and any other such terms to some underlying object.

'*White*', I said, 'may refer both to the colour itself, as when we say that one colour is white, another black, another red, another yellow, another pale yellow, and also to the bodies that receive these colours, as when we say that a swan or milk is white, or that a crow or an Ethiopian is black. So, with the term *hot*, I sometimes hear people using it with reference to a body, for example fire, and sometimes with reference to the quality alone. I do not understand, then', I said, 'when you say *hot*, what you wish to indicate: the quality or the body which receives it.' To this he replied, very readily, that he did not mean the quality 462 alone, | agreeing that the whole body should be termed *hot* too.

Next, I asked the further question:

'Do you refer to that body which is at the peak of hot as an element, or will a body which is moderately hot also be an element?'

I also put the same question regarding cold, dry and wet.

'What difference does this make to you?' he said, already in a state of unease, and not as ready with his answers as before.

'There is a great difference', I said, 'as to whether one takes as one's supposition an infinite number of elements or a finite one. If you suppose that something moderately hot, cold, dry or wet is an element, the number will be infinite; if that something at the peak is an element, then it will be finite. For in this latter case there will be one [extreme] in each category, so that there will be a finite total of four elements.'

'Well, then', he said, 'you may conceive of it this way, as four.'

'It is evident, then', I said, 'that they are at the peak of their qualities, and that they are simple and primary.'

463   'But why', said he, 'are you insisting on this | at such length?'

'So that I may have a precise conception of what is meant.'

'All right, then', he said, 'that is what I mean, and you may conceive it so.'

'How is it', I replied again, 'that you are asking me to conceive of the element which is at a peak of hot or cold?'

By now he was becoming irritated and quite ill-at-ease. He said:

'Where the hot is dominant, I call that a hot body; and similarly with wet, dry and cold. It is that in which each of those preponderates or dominates.'

'Well', I said, 'there is nothing to prevent you calling them so. After all, bread may also be called hot, and so may a dish of lentils or barley porridge, or a bath; but I don't think that you are suggesting that I conceive of each of these things as an element. Rather, that would apply only to what is at a peak of hotness;

similarly with what is at a peak of coldness, dryness and wetness. For the element must be simple and uncombined, not composite or in combination.'

'So use that conception, then', he said. 'I would not say that barley porridge or a dish of lentils was an element.'

'But', I said, 'if I am to conceive of I the body at a peak of hotness as the elem-   464
ent, my conception is immediately of fire and nothing else.'

'Very well, then', he said. 'Let that be your conception of fire.'

'Are you, then', I said, 'willing for me to have water as my conception of the peak of wetness?'

Very reluctantly, he conceded this point too.

'We have, then', I said, 'found ourselves back with fire, air, water and earth, from which we originally departed.'

'That', he said, 'is because you mix up the argument in this way', and, turning to his other pupils, he continued: 'This man, who has been brought up in dialectic and afflicted with the itch that that gives one',—this was the term he actually used—'turns everything upside down, and twists it round and about, confusing us with his sophisms, in order to display his expertise in logic. So, then, he comes here and tells us to conceive of *hot* as ambiguous—applying first to a quality (in a similar way to the colour white), secondly to the body which receives that quality to the extreme degree, and thirdly to a body which has that quality dominant in it, such as a bath. But we have not learned to solve sophisms', he said. 'Let him resolve it himself, since he was the one who created it.'

[*The argument continues on Athenaeus' confusion of perceptible with primary elements, and his refusal to accept fire, earth, air and water as the latter.*]

To concede that the element must be at an extreme of wet, but at the same   469
time to claim that one thinks it something other than water, is perfectly stupid—unless, perhaps, you claim that the qualities themselves are alone the elements, and not the bodies that receive them. Thus, moisture will be the element, rather than water, and heat rather than fire. But if so...he will be clearly exposed as failing to apprehend the difference between an element and a principle.[19] All the philosophers whom Athenaeus is keen to follow agree that extreme heat is simpler than fire, and that fire is produced when it enters into matter; it is equally well agreed, furthermore, that the principle of the fire's origin is [the combination of] that matter which is itself without quality but underlies all the elements and I extreme heat entering into that matter; that while this matter   470
exists constantly throughout eternity, ungenerated and undecaying, what comes to be and passes away is its quality; and that an element must be of the same

---

[19] *Stoicheion* and *archē* in Greek.

class as that of which it is the element. This is the point of distinction between a principle and an element, namely that principles are not necessarily of the same class as the things of which they are principles, while elements definitely are of the same class as the things of which they are elements. For a simple quality is an element of a composite quality, and a simple body an element of a non-simple body. Now, if the terms 'hot', 'cold', 'dry' and 'wet' are used in three senses—as quality, as uncombined body or as body [formed from] combination—then it is evident that neither the quality nor the mixed, combined body is the element. The remaining possibility, then, is that the unmixed, uncombined body, which is simple in terms of its qualities, is the element. So, then, you come back to fire, air, water and earth—the primary [bodies] in which exist heat, cold, dryness and wetness....

473 7. ...All bodies subject to coming-to-be and decay undergo two types of change: the alteration of their substance, and at the same time its flowing-away. It is altered by being cooled, heated, dried and moistened—these qualities are the only ones which change the substance totally throughout, as will be stated a

474 little later— ǀ while it flows away in the observable processes of expulsion, and also in one which is not evident, called transpiration. In order to be preserved, therefore, the body requires a twofold restoration, on the one hand correcting those qualities which are in excess, on the other replenishing the actual stuff lost. Now, that which removes the imbalance is, of course, the quality opposite to that which is in excess, while that which replenishes the lack is not a quality, but should be as similar as possible to the substance which was previously evacuated; for it is to replace that for the animal. This is in fact what nourishment is in a body; it comes about from some substance similar to that previously evacuated, and so, indeed we call that substance nourishment. When, however, we wish to alter the underlying matter in quality alone, we term the means by which we accomplish this not nourishment but drugs. Since, however, we cannot find even one quality existing without substance, we are compelled to administer qualities together with substances to the bodies in need. When what

475 they need is the extreme of a quality, ǀ we administer the element itself: fire, water, earth or air; but when a moderate quality is needed, we administer some combination of these; for example, if we wish the body to be warmed, we choose a drug in which the portion of fire is greater than that of its opposite, and if we wish to cool, the reverse. Sometimes, when we have decided to do both at once—to alter and to nourish—we seek a substance which provides the function of both food and drug....

[*There is further discussion of Hippocrates' correct views on the primary elements, and on the relationship of these elements with the 'proximate' ones discernible in the human body, namely the four fluids, blood, phlegm, yellow bile and black bile. There is then some consideration of other views.*]

10. Let us then turn to the second discourse. Hippocrates, after demonstrating   492
that the hot, the cold, the dry and the wet are the elements common to all existent things, proceeds to another kind of element—not primary or common,
this time, but specific to blooded animals. For blood, phlegm, yellow bile and
black bile are the elements of generation of all blooded animals, not just of
human beings. The parts specific to human beings are the smallest, | which are   493
termed *uniform*—these too, however, are shared with some of the blooded animals, such as horses, oxen, dogs and any others of this sort: all these also have
arteries, veins, nerves, ligaments, membranes and flesh, though they are not in
every respect completely similar to human one; moreover, there are some which
are different in kind, such as hooves, horns, spurs, beaks and scales. As, then,
the hot, the cold, the dry and the wet are common elements of all, in exactly the
same way, in turn, the parts which are primary from the point of view of perception are those which are specific to each animal; these are discussed in my
Anatomical Procedures. Between the former and the latter are, in our case, the
four fluids,[20] and in the case of each of the other animals, whatever is the 'proximate' matter of its generation (this is the customary term employed for that
matter from which something primarily arises, without any intermediate
change).

11. Now, it is immediately obvious to all that all the parts of blooded ani-   494
mals have been generated from the blood of the mother; since, however, this
blood partakes both of phlegm and of the two biles, it is understandable that
there has been a point of disagreement here, with some stating that our generation is from blood alone, others that it is from the four fluids. The demonstration of the truth is not equally possible here as in the case of the primary
elements: each argument in fact contains a certain plausibility. I shall try,
though, to show the grounds which moved Hippocrates to consider the truer
account to be that which has the four fluids as the material of human generation; and I shall begin with this: both flesh and nerve are uniform, flesh is
blooded, hot and soft, while nerve has the opposite qualities: lacking in blood,
hard and cold. It is not, however, the case that the former is completely soft and
hot, nor that nerve is completely hard and cold; but blood is softer and hotter
than flesh, | while bone is harder and drier than nerve. So, too, with all the   495

---

[20] While this remark seems to posit the four fluids (or humours, *chumoi*) as an intermediate
stage, or level of bodily composition, between the elements and uniform parts, and such an account
is sometimes given of Galen's views in this area, this analysis is somewhat problematic. Galen in
general regards the fluids rather as residues or by-products of digestion—with the exception of
blood, which is clearly taken to be the chief building block in the generation or composition of
human bodies. The clearest sense in which the other three fluids are intermediate between elements
and uniform parts, or form the basis of the composition of the latter, seems to be (as indeed is
implied in what follows) that blood, from which the uniform parts definitely *are* composed, never
appears simply as pure blood, but itself always has some admixture of the other three fluids. See
also *My Own Doctrines*, ch. 12.

other parts: one is colder, one hotter, one softer, one harder. Is it, then, that they all came into being from the same substance, or rather that Nature, being a good craftsman, when first generating and shaping the embryo from the blood that comes from the mother into the womb, drew from it what is thicker for the purpose of solidification of the harder bodies, and what is wetter for that of the softer bodies—and similarly what is hotter for the hotter bodies and what is colder for the colder? This seems to me to be by far the more natural way: it is from its own proper matter that the embryo has been shaped, right from the very beginning, and that all the parts subsequently continue to gain their nourishment and growth. For blood appears to be a single thing, as indeed does milk. But reason teaches us that it in fact neither blood nor milk is single....

[*The argument continues in the remaining chapters, 12–14, with further detail of the nature and actions of the fluids in the human body, again with positive references to Hippocrates' views as expressed in* The Nature of the Human Being, *and with negative references to the views of Asclepiades.*]

Mixtures (excerpts)

Following on from *The Elements according to Hippocrates*, this major work presents Galen's main statement of his theory of the physical composition of, and differences between, human bodies, and of the medical significance of this theory. Human bodies—like all other bodies in the universe—come about through a particular 'mixture' (or 'blending', *krasis*) of the four fundamental elements or qualities. So too do the different characteristics or states of different human bodies, both those which they have from birth or as a result of environment and early nurture, and those which are acquired (either temporarily or chronically) during their lives as a result of diet, lifestyle factors and the aging process. Where there is an imbalance or 'bad-mixture' (*duskrasia*) this is a pathological state, which may give rise to further specific diseases.

The Galenic theory of mixtures developed in mediaeval times into the hugely influential theory of 'temperaments' (*temperamentum* being a Latin translation of *krasis*). It should be noted, however, that the understanding of different temperaments as character dispositions—sanguine, choleric, phlegmatic, melancholic—is a later development, and not part of Galen's view. For Galen, excesses of phlegm, black bile and the other fluids (or humours, *chumoi*) are indeed relevant to disease, and sometimes related to emotional states; and such excesses may be present in chronic form in a human being. But there is no such categorization of human beings into distinct physiological or character types on the basis of their humours.

Two other ways may be noted in which Galen's theory of *krasis* differs, both from the 'Hippocratic' theory and on that which came to be widespread in Europe and beyond. First, and as we saw also in *The Elements according to Hippocrates*, Galen's foundational 'Hippocratic' text, *The Nature of the Human Being*, presents the four fluids or humours (*chumoi*: blood, yellow bile, black bile, phlegm) as the components of the human body, while for Galen it is the four basic *qualities* (hot, cold, wet and dry) that are fundamental. These are the ultimate explainers of the discernible qualities of bodies in the cosmos and of physical change. The fluids, by contrast, though of importance in relation to health and disease and though in a close causal relationship with the four basic qualities, are conceived (with the exception of blood) essentially as residues or by-products of the digestive process. Here, as discussed also in the prefatory remarks to *The Elements according to Hippocrates*, Galen's view seems fundamentally Aristotelian rather than 'Hippocratic'.

Secondly, in the 'Hippocratic' view there is a clear correspondence between the four fluids and the four qualities, on the one hand, and the four seasons, on the other: each fluid represents a predominance of two qualities over the other two, and each such predominance or imbalance has a corresponding time of year (and also a stage of life). The correspondences can be neatly presented in a circular diagram, of the sort which is frequently seen in illustrations of mediaeval manuscripts. Yet Galen devotes considerable space to an attack on precisely this neat correspondence view: the association of 'hot and wet', and so of a predominance of blood, with spring, he argues, rests on a confusion.[1] Spring is not 'hot and wet' in the sense that it has an excess or predominance of those qualities; rather, it is the only truly well-balanced season.

As well as its presentation of Galen's physical and medical theories, the text also offers some fascinating but frustratingly cursory discussions of fundamental questions of causation in the natural world, whereby Galen presents the 'bottom-up' four-quality theory of physical explanation alongside—or arguably as in conflict with—a 'higher-level' account in terms of divine craftsmanship or design. These passages are again indebted to the Aristotelian discussions, especially in the biological works; they also show Galen wrestling with a problem that in some ways runs through his work.[2]

Greek title: Περὶ κράσεων (*Peri kraseōn*)
Kühn: I.509–694
Edition: Helmreich 1904
Translation: Singer 1997a; Singer and van der Eijk 2018

BOOK I

I.509   1. Animal bodies are a mixture of hot, cold, wet and dry; and these qualities are not mixed equally in each case. This was adequately demonstrated in ancient times, by the best philosophers and doctors. There is also a work of mine covering the apparent facts of the case—the one in which I investigate *The Elements according to Hippocrates.*

In this work I shall deal with the subject that follows on from that, namely, the discovery of the number and nature of the different kinds of mixture, and 510   the classification of these into classes and types.[3] | Let me begin with a discussion of terminology. When we say that bodies are a mixture of hot, cold, dry and wet, we understand by this the extreme case of each of those qualities, in other words the actual elements: air, fire, water and earth. When we describe an animal or plant as hot, cold, dry or wet, on the other hand, we do not understand these qualities in that same sense. No animal is hot in the absolute sense, like fire, nor wet in the absolute sense, like water. Nor does it have an extreme

---

[1] It is worth remarking that it seems fairly clear that the people he polemicizes against on this point reflect that Hippocratic picture more accurately than he does, in spite of his protestations that he is the authentic representative of Hippocrates. (For a similar point see *The Elements according to Hippocrates,* n. 1.)

[2] See I.9 and II.6 below, and for discussion of Galen's engagement with this philosophical issue, Singer 1997b and Singer and van der Eijk 2018.

[3] 'Class' translates *genos* and 'type' *eidos.* The traditional translations are 'genus' and 'species', but the two terms are more fluid in Galen's application than those equivalents would suggest. Both refer to some kind of division or classification according to kind, the former to a broader and the latter to a narrower one, but the distinction between them is not always clear-cut. For example *genos* is often used (including in this text, below) in cases where we would say 'species'.

degree of either wet or dry. Such epithets derive rather from the predominance of any one of these qualities in the mixture. We say that a body is wet, when its share of wetness is larger, and dry when its share of dryness is larger; and similarly in the cases of hot and cold. So much then for the terminology.

[*In chapter 2, Galen surveys the views of predecessors in this area, most of whom identify four types of mixture (hot–wet, hot–dry, cold–wet and cold–dry), though some conflate the effect of the hot with that of the dry, and the effect of the cold with that of the wet.*]

3. Such are the positions of the most distinguished of our predecessors, both 518 doctors and philosophers. Let me now proceed to outline the points on which I depart from them. I First of all, they have completely left out of their account 519 the well-balanced[4] mixture, which is actually superior to all those above mentioned, in both excellence and potential. They have simply disregarded its existence, in spite of the fact that it is impossible even to make any statement about the others without reference to it. The very concept of a predominance of heat, in the case of a hot mixture, or of cold, in the case of a cold one, is intellectually impossible without the prior assumption of a well-balanced mixture. Nor can the healthy regime be discovered otherwise than by reference to this well-balanced state of nature; for the aim is to cool any body which is hotter than it should be, to heat any which is colder, and similarly to dry any which is wetter and moisten any which is drier. In each case the attempt is, of course, to remedy an excess by the introduction of what is missing, in order to bring about a state which may be described as well-balanced or medial.

And so I should like them to state, before all other mixtures, which one it is that they have always as their goal, and by reference to which they attempt to remedy poor states of mixture. Yet such people, far from mentioning this goal at the outset, I omit it entirely. But, they may say, it has not been omitted: the con- 520 cept is contained within that of the hot and wet mixture. How, then, do you arrive at the figure of four rather than five mixtures, if you are making reference to the best one? There are only two possible explanations: either one of the poor mixtures must have been omitted, or the well-balanced one. It is in fact perfectly clear to me from their recommendations that they are omitting the latter....

Let us grant that the well-balanced is the same as the hot, wet mixture—which accords with their opinion. But then they have omitted the bad-mixture which is opposite in nature to the cold, dry one—that in which there is a predominance of heat and moisture. Well, they say, that is the one we are talking about. But how is it that heat can both predominate and not predominate, I and 521 that cold can be both dominated and not dominated?

---

[4] Literally, 'well-mixed' (*eukratos*).

[*Galen proceeds to take issue with the views of followers of Athenaeus of Attalia, that a 'hot, wet' state is never associated with disease.*]

524   4. ...The opinion that spring is hot and wet, and simultaneously also well-balanced, is a manifest confusion. Spring is neither wet to the same degree as winter, nor hot to the same degree as summer, and thus possesses neither quality in a disproportionate sense. And yet each of the above terms—as these people themselves agree—is indicative of disproportion. Their mistake is in fact twofold, consisting both in the desire at all costs to find in the seasons the fourth pairing of mixtures, and secondly in the assumption that spring is hotter than winter and wetter than summer. It is not necessary to identify a fourth pairing of mixtures in the seasons, if such an identification does not accord with the evidence; and the comparison with the seasons on either side of it does not reveal spring as 'hot and wet' any more than 'cold and dry'. If the terms 'hot' and 'wet' refer to an excess of those qualities, their statement is not correct. Spring is well-balanced in all respects.

[*The argument is further elaborated, with supporting reference to the Hippocratic dictum 'Spring is the most healthy and least fatal' (Aphorisms 3.9)*]

529   My own view is that 'hot and wet', so far from being the characteristics of spring, or of good-mixture in general, in fact constitute the worst possible state of the ambient air; a state which does not occur naturally within the seasons at

530   all, but sometimes comes about in conjunction with states of disease or ⎮ plague.

[*The chapter continues with supporting references to passages from Hippocrates's* Epidemics *which describe the occurrence of certain pathological conditions (e.g. pustules and putrefaction of the skin) in hot, wet climatic conditions. In chapters 5–7 Galen points to the different applications of such terms as 'hot', and the confusions that arise from the failure to distinguish them. He specifies three distinct senses in which such terms are used: the absolute sense (applicable only to the elements or fundamental qualities); that by reference to the medial item in a class or species; and that indicating comparison with some other object. In chapter 6 he also clarifies the inextricable relationship between the concept of the 'best mixture' within a particular species and the optimal functioning of that species. On these points see further Book II, chapter 1.*]

554   8. ...There are the pure, unadulterated qualities: heat, coldness, dryness and moisture. Clearly the bodies that have received those qualities will be hot, cold, dry or wet in the full, precise sense. Now, you should conceive of these bodies ⎮

555   as the elements of all things that are subject to growth and decay, and of the other bodies—those of animals, plants and all inanimate things, such as bronze, iron, stone and wood—as having some intermediate status between these primary elements.

[Imbalances arise through the domination of either one or two of these qualities.]

As has been observed previously, these latter four types of bad-mixture [i.e. 556 those in which two qualities predominate] are recognized by the majority of doctors and philosophers. The four other bad-mixtures, which come about from one half of each of the above, have for some reason been overlooked, as has the first mixture of all—the best. Yet it appears to me abundantly obvious from what has been said above that it is quite possible for the hot to predominate while there is no greater tendency, within the other opposition, to either moisture or dryness. Even if the above statements were not sufficient, however, it is perfectly easy to make this deduction, once it is agreed that 'wet and hot' and 'dry and hot' are two different mixtures. For if a hot mixture is not necessarily dry, but may equally be wet, then it is obvious that it may I also be midway 557 between the two; for a medial mixture is closer to a dry one than is a wet one.

By the same token there exists a distinct item called a cold mixture, in which the cold is the dominant element; and it does not follow that this mixture must be either wet or dry. It may equally well be midway between the two: the same argument applies as in the previous case. (That is: if the cold state is not necessarily wet, but may equally be dry, it is obvious that it may also be midway between the two, since the medial state is closer to the wet than is the dry.) And in the same way that we have shown the existence of these two bad-mixtures within the one opposition—one which is hot only, one which is cold—there will be two more corresponding to these within the other opposition—one which is dry only, one which is wet—in both of which there will be a state of balance between hot and cold. Here again we will employ the same argument: if it is not necessary that a dry mixture be automatically hot, but possible, equally, for it to be cold, then it cannot be impossible for it to be neither hot nor cold, but rather well-balanced with respect to this opposition, though dry I in the terms of the 558 other. And a wet mixture, finally, need not necessarily be either hot or cold, but may be in the medial state between the two terms of this opposition.

But if a certain kind of bad-mixture in terms of the opposition of dry and wet is not a necessary consequence of a certain kind of imbalance in the opposition of hot and cold, nor vice versa, then there is the possibility that a state well-balanced between heat and coldness may be either dry or wet, and that a state well-balanced between these latter qualities may be either hot or cold. And so we have four more bad-mixtures in addition to those which our medical and philosophical predecessors have bequeathed us; and these four have a position halfway between the well-balanced state and those states which are ill-balanced in virtue of both oppositions. For the perfectly well-balanced mixture has an excess in neither of the oppositions, while that which is opposite to it has a poor state in both of them. But midway between these is that which is well-balanced in one opposition, but ill-balanced in the other; this type is half well-balanced

559   and I half ill-balanced, and may thus appropriately be termed medial between the fully well-balanced and the fully ill-balanced.

If the above is a correct account—and it is—then we may confidently assert that there are nine different kinds of mixture in all: one well-balanced, the other eight not well-balanced; and that of these eight there are four which are simple (wet, dry, cold or hot) and another four which are composite (wet and hot, dry and hot, cold and wet, cold and dry).

9. In each of these mixtures there are great differences of degree, both within the mixtures considered in absolute terms and within existence as a whole and within any individual class. One who wishes to gain expertise in the identification of mixtures should begin his training with the well-balanced, medial types within each class. Using this as a reference point he will easily discover what is I
560   excessive or deficient in each case.

We should, then, first consider the mixtures which are well-balanced and ill-balanced in absolute terms, those which we said were to be judged in the context of all that exists in the generated world, not just in the context of animals and plants. Here again a linguistic distinction must be made, in that there is a difference between the mixture which is hot actually and that which is hot potentially.[5] By 'potentially' we refer to a quality which is not yet present in the object of which it is predicated, but which may very readily come to be present by virtue of a natural tendency that that object has for this to happen. First, then, let us consider those things which are actually hot, cold, dry and wet, first in the context of existence as a whole, then in that of plants and animals. In this way the project before us will be perfectly completed.

Now, since the medial within any class—but most obviously within that of all existent things—consists in a mixing together of the extremes, our conception and identification of it must also come about from the same starting-point.
561   Conceptually the matter is very simple. We begin with the hottest I of all perceptible things, fire, say, or violently boiling water, and imagine a line drawn from that down to the coldest we know, ice, say, or snow; and we mark this line exactly in the middle. This will give us the point of good proportion conceptually—that which is equidistant from each of the extremes. We may also create it physically, by mixing equal amounts of ice and boiling water. For that which is made from a mixture of both these will be equidistant from the two extremes of burning and of that which causes death by cooling. It is thus a simple matter, by getting hold of this mixture, to have an example of the medial state of all existence with regard to the opposition of hot and cold. One may then remember this, and use it as a standard[6] against which to measure everything else.

---

⁵ 'Actually' translates *energeiai* (more literally, 'in [its] activity'), 'potentially' *dunamei* (more literally, 'in [its] capacity').

⁶ For *kanōn*, 'standard', see n. 9 below.

A similar procedure will produce a body halfway in the opposition between dry and wet. A quantity of dry earth, ash, or some such completely dried-out substance may be placed in an equal amount of water. Here again, it is a simple matter to learn the characteristics of this object by sight and by touch, | to con- 562 sign them to the memory and to use the object as the standard or criterion for identification of substances with deficiency or excess within this opposition. Of course, the object under examination should be in a medium state of heat. For if an object which is midway between wet and dry is at an extreme of either heat or cold, this will sometimes create the illusion that it is either wetter or dryer than the norm. In cases of excessive heating, the resulting melting or flow will produce the impression of a wetter body; excessive cooling may lead to solidifi-cation or freezing, and lack of motion, causing the body to appear hard to the touch; and this in turn will create a false impression of dryness. If, however, a body which is equally wet and dry is also in a medial state between heat and cooling, such a body will not appear hard or soft to the touch.

A total mixture of one with the other—of hot, cold, dry and wet, that is—is not humanly possible to achieve.[7] When one mixes earth with moisture, | this 563 creates the illusion of a total mixture of the two substances; but what takes place in reality is a placing alongside each other of very small parts, not a total mix-ture. The total mixture of the two, on the other hand, is a task for God or for Nature, and even more so in the case of a total mixture of the hot with cold. But setting substances alongside each other in such a way that each of the individual substances in the mixture becomes imperceptible is an accomplishment which is not unique to Nature or God, but may be performed by us too. It is not diffi-cult by this kind of combining to create a sort of mud which is midway between wet and dry and also between hot and cold; and such a body will appear to you well-balanced in terms of heat, as well as halfway between hardness and softness.

Human skin is an object of this sort, being exactly midway between all the extremes—hot, cold, hard and soft. And this is especially true of the skin of the hands. For this part was designed to be the instrument of assessment of all per-ceptible objects; it was crafted by Nature as the organ | of touch suited to the 564 most intelligent of all animals. It therefore had to be equidistant from all extremes, whether of hot, cold, dry or wet. Moreover, it was created from this equal balance not just by a process of combining, but by total mixture, some-thing which none of us may ever bring about, since it is the work of Nature.

Now, those parts which are harder than skin, such as bones, gristle, horns, hair, nails, ligaments, hooves and spurs, have more dryness in them; while those which are softer, such as blood, phlegm, hard and soft fat, marrow, brain and the spinal cord, have a greater proportion of moisture than dryness. And the degree by

---

[7] For the language and conception of 'total mixture', see *The Elements according to Hippocrates*, n. 11.

which the driest of all parts in the human body exceeds the skin in hardness is the same as that by which the skin in turn exceeds the wettest part. The extraordinary value of this information lies in the fact that man is the best balanced, 565 not only of animals, but in fact of all bodies quite generally, | and that, furthermore, the skin on the inside of the hand is, properly speaking, immune from all the excesses.

So let us again concentrate our attention on this point, and investigate the question, within the human race, which individual has the best mixture of all? Such a person must be placed in the middle with respect to the whole of existence, let alone with respect to animals in general, and to human beings. He may be regarded as a kind of standard or yardstick by comparison with which all others will be called hot, cold, dry or wet. For such a case we require the co-existence of a number of indicators. The person in question must be clearly in the medial state with respect to the whole of existence, but especially so with respect to humans and animals. Now the indicators which apply in the context of all existent things general have been mentioned above. Those applicable to animal species, on the other hand, are assessed in relation to the perfection of the activity appropriate in each case.

In the case of a human being, for example, it is appropriate to excel in intelligence; in the case of a dog, to excel in docility in combination with courage; in that of a lion, to excel in courage only; in that of a sheep, to excel in docility. And of course the activities of the body must be appropriate to the character of 566 the soul, | as has been shown by Aristotle in the *Parts of Animals*, and no less so by me.[8]

So much, then, for methodological principles. But the training which will enable one readily to identify the median within each class of animals, and the median of all, is not something to be undertaken by any ordinary person. It involves an extraordinary degree of dedication, long experience and a great deal of learning in order to be able to find the median in all individual cases. It is by virtue of such a procedure that sculptors in different materials, painters, and makers of images in general, achieve excellence in their various fields, in the representation of each species—producing the most well-formed human being, for example, or horse, or ox, or lion. In each case their aim is the median within the given class.

There is a certain statue which enjoys great fame, known as the Canon of Polyclitus; the name derives from the fact that all its parts are in perfect proportion with each other.[9] Now, this Canon represents something that goes beyond

---

[8] See *The Function of the Parts* I.2, pp. 224–5 below.
[9] 'Canon' was the name of both a theoretical treatise and a statue by the fifth-century sculptor Polyclitus. The statue, also known as the Doryphoros, 'Spear Bearer' (and surviving in later copies) was renowned as a representation of ideal proportions or the perfection of the human form—which

the ideal subject that we have just been considering.[10] For the person who is well-balanced according to *those* criteria will not just be at the median of moisture and dryness, | but will also have the best possible shaping[11]—something 567 which is perhaps a consequence of that good balance of the four elements, but may rather have some higher source of a more divine nature. At any rate such a 'well-fleshed' person will necessarily be completely well-balanced in his mixture; for good proportion in respect of flesh is a product of excellence of mixture. It will also automatically follow that such a body will enjoy optimal function, as well as being in a medial state with respect to hardness and softness, heat and coldness.

[*Book I concludes with some remarks on differences in quality between different parts and substances in the body.*]

BOOK II

[*Chapter 1 begins with a recapitulation, focusing again on the different senses in which the quality terms such as* hot *may be applied.*]

1. ... The human being with the best mixture will be the one whose body is 576 observed to be precisely midway between all the extremes—those of thinness and thickness, softness and hardness, and heat and coldness. Every human body will be found on examination by touch to possess either a good, vaporous heat or one which is fiery and sharp—or neither of these, but the dominance of some kind of cold influence. ('Cold' must here of course be understood as relative to the body of an animal, and indeed of one which is blooded and wet.)

Such are the bodily characteristics of the well-balanced man. His soul, similarly, will be at an exact balance between boldness and cowardice, hesitancy and

---

was also the theme of the treatise. 'Canon' translates *kanōn*; the word can mean both a measuring instrument and a conceptual standard of assessment or regulation, and is elsewhere rendered 'standard'.

[10] There is some doubt over text and interpretation here. It is possible also to understand: 'this Canon is pretty much of the same sort as the subject we are considering', or even 'the subject we are considering is something beyond this Canon'. For full discussion see Singer and van der Eijk 2018, 97–100. No interpretation is entirely without difficulty, but the translation given here (which departs from my previous two translations) does justice to the distinction being made here between levels of composition of the human body—that of the four qualities and that involving divine craftsmanship (on which see also II.6 below)—and to the perception that the invocation of the Canon of Polyclitus should be relevant to that distinction.

[11] *Diaplasis*, also translatable 'formation' or 'construction'. In the biological context, the word refers to both the formative process by which a creature achieves its fully developed structure, and that structure itself. See *The Shaping of the Embryo*; but *diaplasis* and its cognates are also used in reference to the moulding or shaping activity of a sculptor.

rashness, pity and envy. Such a person will have a good spirit, and be affection-ate, generous and intelligent.[12]

These then are the primary and especial features by which the best-balanced man may be identified. But we may add several more features which have the status of necessary consequences of these. Such a person will eat and drink in a well-proportioned manner, and digest his food well, not just in the stomach but also in the veins; his entire | bodily condition will manifest faultless physical as well as mental activities. His perceptive faculties will be in the best possible state, as will the motions of his limbs; his complexion will be good, and also his breathing; he will strike the balance between somnolence and insomnia, between baldness and hairiness, and between black and white [hair] colours. As a child his hair will have inclined towards red rather than black; in his prime the reverse will be the case.

577

[*In the second chapter Galen discusses further differences in mixture due to age, refuting the view that old age is wetter than youth or the prime: for Galen, aging involves a gradual process of cooling, but the view held by some that it also involves increased moisture is based on a sensory illusion. Via a sideswipe at the Sceptics, who attempt to undermine the validity of sense perception, he moves on to discuss the importance of a training of the sense of touch for such enquiries.*]

591   2. ...And let us return once more to the matter in hand, and use the sense of touch to make our primary and especial assessment of the different degrees of heat belonging to different ages. The best sort of assessment is that whereby we use one body only, that of an infant. For it is quite possible to remember the nature of the heat at two years old, and compare it with the state after another two or three years. If a general change is detected in the direction of heat or cold, it is an easy matter to infer the further increase that there will be up to the prime. If, meanwhile, you wish to compare a number of children with a num-ber of people in their prime, you should compare similar types: thin children with thin people in their prime, well-fleshed with well-fleshed, fat with fat. Their complexions, too, and all other features should be as similar as possible. If one is looking for differences due to age, the investigation will be at its most secure if one considers bodies as close as possible in nature. In a comparison between opposite kinds of body there will be a considerable danger of false inference, | as certain differences will arise not because of the age of the bodies in question but because of their innate mixture. One should, moreover, choose

592

---

[12] This is a rare, if not unique, case where Galen connects the theory of the mean which under-lies his physical model with ethical considerations. The understanding of ethical excellence as a mean between two extremes has a clear Aristotelian background, although, with the exception of the boldness–cowardice option, the actual examples given do not feature in Aristotle's *Nicomachean Ethics*. *Euthumos*, here translated 'hav[ing] a good spirit', could also be rendered 'cheerful' or 'confi-dent', and is conceptually related to the *thumos*, 'spirit', in Plato's tripartite soul.

bodies which are similar in terms of general regime and of time at which the examination is made—rather than comparing the well-exercised individual with the man who has been idle, the bathed with the unwashed, the hungry with the full, the drunk with the thirsty, the man who has got hot in the sun with the man trembling with cold, or one who has not slept with one who is well rested. In general, one should avoid all such opposites of nature, regime or circumstance: everything about them should be as similar as possible, with the single exception of age. Indeed, even in the case where one makes the comparison between different stages of the same child, one must take care that all external conditions are kept precisely the same, in order to avoid the false attribution of some difference in heating or cooling arising from these to the change in age.

You may perhaps think that the process of examination which I am recommending is a long one; but it is the one best designed to arrive at the truth, taken as it is from the very essence of the object under enquiry, as discussed in my work on | *Demonstration*. You may prefer to take a short cut, without caring 593 whether it will lead you to the truth or not. But you should realize that the process you embark on will not only fail of the truth, but will be a long one too. For you will not discover what you seek even after three or four years; your ignorance will last all your life. If all one has is opposing arguments between men, nothing can ever be demonstrated properly; in quite general terms, it makes no sense to establish prior propositions on the basis of ones that come later in the argument.

Let us therefore use our perceptive faculties to assess matters of actual as opposed to potential hot and cold in a body, in the first place leaving aside all other kinds of indicator. I leave you to make assessments by means of your own personal testing; but will now give an account of my own assessment. After careful examination by touch of a large number of bodies, children and infants as well as youths and old people, it was my discovery that neither camp was correct—neither those who straightforwardly state that the prime is hotter than childhood, nor those who state that it is colder. If | you take away all external 594 alterations and concentrate on the differences due to age alone, neither state will appear to you straightforwardly hotter.

[*Chapter 3 discusses the method by which one may distinguish also between wet and dry, and describes the relative moisture of different parts and substances of the body; chapter 4 considers the necessary consequences of various mixtures, in terms of their physical characteristics in the body. Chapter 5 begins with a discussion of the hot and dry mixture, and of its connection with hairiness in human beings, proceeding to a detailed account of the production of hair, which is explained as a function of the operation of degrees of heat within the body forcing out a kind of exhalation through the pores, which is then solidified.*]

618 5. ...So much for the generation of hair; we should now pass on to the causes of all the incidental features of the mixtures, as regards the differences of hair according to age, place and nature of the body. The hair of Egyptians, Arabs, Indians, and in general all peoples who inhabit dry, hot places, has poor growth and is black, dry, curly and brittle. That of the inhabitants of wet, cold places, conversely—Illyrians, Germans, Dalmatians, Sauromatians and the Scythian types of people in general—has moderately good growth and is thin, straight and red. Those who live in some land which enjoys good [climatic] mixture, between these two extremes, have very strong hair, with extremely good growth, which tends towards black, is moderately thick, and is neither completely curly nor completely straight. The differences due to age are analogous to these: with regard to the qualities of strength, thickness, size and colour, infants' hair is similar to that of the Germans, hair in the prime to that of the Ethiopians, and the hair of youths and children to that of the people of lands which enjoy good-mixture.

619 And the differences in hair due to the nature of the body are also | in line with these differences due to age and place. Very small children are without hair, since there is not yet a passageway for it in the skin, nor are there yet smoky residues. As they proceed towards youth they grow hair which is short and weak; but as they reach the prime of life it becomes stronger, plentiful, long and black, both because there is now a multitude of pores in them and because they are full of the smoky excretions which arise from dryness and heat. But the hair on the head, in the eyebrows, and in the eyelashes is already present in childhood; for these are generated not in the manner of grass, but in the manner of plants which have been fashioned according to the original plan of Nature; their status is different from that of necessary consequences of mixture (as was also discussed in *The Function of the Parts*).[13] In this case too, however, though their actual existence is a product of the Nature's artifice, their colour and other particularities are necessary consequences of the mixture due to age. They are in general reddish, because the substance lodged in the pores is not yet

620 black. | For there is a great deal of moisture, an easy passage of exit and a weak burning; and the growth is reasonably good because of the abundance of the excretions that nourish it.

[*The chapter concludes with some observations on baldness and other individual differences in hair growth. Chapter 6 begins with an explanation of the importance of considering the mixture of each individual part, rather than generalizing from that to the whole body.*]

---

[13] Galen makes a distinction between features of an organism which are present by design, or by virtue of the 'primary intention' in that organism's construction (*kata prōton logon*) and others which are not directly part of that design, but follow as necessary consequences of some feature of it. See *The Function of the Parts* XI.13, with n. 11.

6. …Different bodies may also have very large heads, or small heads, like 623
birds. Some have crooked or bandy legs, and the extremities of the limbs may
be either thin or stout. Some have broad chests, as mentioned just now; in some
the chest is as narrow as a plank (such people are indeed referred to as 'plank-
like'). When the area of the shoulder-blades, too, is completely lacking in flesh,
bare and sloped forward, in the manner of a wing, such subjects are termed
'wing-form' by the doctors; and the harm associated with this condition, in
which almost the entire space of the chest—which houses the lungs and
heart—is missing, should be quite obvious to all. And there are of course very
many other states of various parts of the body, when that body has deviated
from the natural proportion and fallen into an uneven state of bad-mixture
during gestation.[14] I In such cases, then, one must avoid drawing a conclusion 624
about the whole body from the state of a single part.

Even those who attempt the art of physiognomics do not make simplistic
characterizations of the whole; they too have learned from experience. If someone has a considerable amount of hair on the chest, they will declare him to be
'spirited'; if on the thighs, 'lustful'; but they do not add the reason for these
connections. They may point to the hairiness of chest of the lion, and of the
thighs of the goat; but this is not to uncover the first cause. The question to
which an enquiry of reason seeks the answer is: why is the lion spirited, and the
goat lustful? Those who stop short of this enquiry are merely describing the
facts, without investigating their causes. The student of nature must attempt to
discover the cause of these as of all other phenomena. It is in fact because of the
uneven balance between their different parts that not only the lion and the goat
but many other animals too have parts suited to a variety of different activities.
This area has been very well and fully covered by Aristotle. I   625

The point which concerns us for present purposes has already emerged,
namely that in the investigation of mixtures of human beings one must examine each part individually. One should not, for example, infer dryness and heat
of the body as a whole from a hairy chest; this indicates rather a very high
degree of heat in the heart, for which reason too the subject will be spirited. But
it is also possible that for this very reason the body as a whole is *not* hot and dry,
because it is in this place that the greater part of the heat has been exhaled and
released into the atmosphere. When the mixture of the body as a whole is an
even one, then the entire chest will be very broad, as will the veins; the arteries
will be large and endowed with a very great, powerful pulse; hair will be abundant over the body as a whole, and that on the head will in early years have
extremely good growth, and be black and curly, but baldness will follow in the

---

[14] The 'uneven bad-mixture' (*anōmalos duskrasia*), on which Galen wrote a dedicated treatise, is
that in which the nature of the bad-mixture or imbalance is not the same in different parts of
the body.

fulness of time. The bodies of such individuals will moreover be muscular, with good tension and good articulation, since they have an even kind of mixture; |
626 and their skin will be comparatively hard, black and hairy.

If the nature of the chest is opposite to this, still assuming an even mixture throughout the body—if, in other words, all parts are comparatively wet and cold—the chest will be narrow and without hair, just as the body as a whole will be bare, the skin smooth and white, the hair reddish, especially in youth; there will not be baldness in old age; they will naturally be cowardly, lacking in resolve, fearful, with small, difficult-to-discern veins, and they will also be fatty and weak in their nerves and muscles, with poor articulation of the limbs, and crooked legs. If, however, a mixture has come about which is different through-out the parts, one cannot make any statement about the body as a whole on the basis of one part; one must rather consider each of them individually, and ask, for example, what is the nature of the mixture in the stomach, that in the lungs, that in the brain, and so forth, taking each one an item in its own right.

627   These, then, are matters | which are discerned on the basis of the activities. It is not possible to find out their mixture by touch or sight. And at the same time one must also investigate the bodily states of the parts which surround them, the outermost of which is skin. In our part of the world, where there is a good [climatic] mixture, the skin gives a good indication of the parts beneath, although even here this relationship is not straightforward, the above applying only to those parts which have the same mixture as that of the skin. In northern and southern regions, the [internal] heat is either driven deep within the body, in the former case, being overcome by the cold of the atmosphere outside, or enters the skin, in the latter case, being drawn into it by the surrounding heat. It thus becomes impossible to form a clear impression of the mixture of the internal parts from the bodily state of the skin. For in such regions of poor [climatic] mixture, the mixture of the bodies is uneven, in the sense that the external parts are in a different state from the internal ones. Celts, Germans and all the peoples
628   of Thrace and Scythia have cold, wet skin, | which is therefore also soft, white and bare. Whatever innate heat they have has retreated, along with the blood, into the internal organs; and there the blood churns about, confined in a small space, and seethes; and thus they become spirited, bold and hasty in judgement.[15]

In Ethiopians, Arabs and all other southern peoples the skin has been roasted by the ambient heat and by the effect of the innate heat being drawn outwards; and so becomes hard, dry and black. The body as a whole has very little innate heat, but is hot by virtue of the heat which it acquires from outside....

---

[15] The relationship between anger and the seething or boiling (*zesis*) of the blood in the region of the heart is stated in a famous passage of Aristotle, *De anima* I.1, 403a–b, and also forms part of Galen's physiological account of emotions elsewhere in his work. See *Health* II.9, pp. 324–5 below, and for further relevant passages Singer 2017.

The investigation of mixture should thus always involve an examination of   635
each individual part, rather than a rash inference from one part to the whole, of
the sort that some perform. Moisture is, for example, sometimes inferred from
a snub nose, or dryness from a hook nose; similarly, dryness from small eyes
and moisture from large ones. This last is in fact a point of dispute among such
people: some argue that the eyes are among the wet parts, and therefore that
where they are larger moisture dominates the mixture; others that it is the
strength of the heat which transpires in a concentrated way, and in large volume, at the earliest stage of the shaping, that makes not only the eyes, but also
the mouth, and all other passageways, greater in size; and that it is thus a sign,
not of moisture, but of heat. Both these arguments are wrong, and for the same
reason: that they base a statement about the body as a whole on the state of a
single part. A second mistake is the failure to make mention of the craftsman-
like character of the shaping power of nature ǀ —the power which shapes the   636
parts in accordance with the characteristics of the souls.

This was a point on which even Aristotle raised a doubt: should this power
not in fact be attributed to some more divine cause, rather than just to hot, cold,
dry and wet? Those who rush to make simplistic statements on this greatest of
issues, and explain the shaping purely in terms of the qualities, seem to me to
be in error. The latter are surely only the instruments, whereas that responsible
for the shaping is something different. It is, however, possible even without
engaging in enquiries of this kind to find out whether a mixture is wet, dry, cold
or hot, as has already been discussed. But these people ignore the proper indicators; and then start talking about larger matters, which require a considerable
length of enquiry, and which have up to this day continued to baffle the best of
philosophers. Just because children tend to be snub-nosed, and people beyond
their prime hook-nosed, it does not follow that we should consider all snub-
nosed individuals to be wet and all hook-nosed people to be dry. It may also be
that this kind of feature is the work of the shaping power, rather than of mixture. If indeed it is also ǀ an indicator of the mixture, then only of that in the   637
nose, not of that of the whole body.

[*The book ends with further elaboration of the importance of distinguishing mixture of an individual part from mixture of the whole, and avoiding generalizations
to the latter.*]

BOOK III

[*Book III of* Mixtures *stands in a sense separate from the rest of the work, and is
conceived by Galen as an introduction to his great pharmacological work,* Simple
Drugs. *In it he elaborates in particular the sense in which* hot, cold, *etc., may be*

potential *rather than* actual *qualities of a substance: this is the sense relevant to the identification of the properties of substances used as drugs. Poppy, hemlock and mandragora, for example, are cold not actually, but potentially, which is to say that they have the potential or capacity to cool a body.*]

646   1. It was shown above that each of the terms *hot, cold, dry* and *wet*, as used in the actual sense, is applied to objects in virtue either of an extreme degree of one of these qualities, or of the dominance of one of them, when considered in relation either to the state of good proportion within the object's class or to any other object of comparison. The method by which these states are best identified was also demonstrated. It remains to discuss bodies which have the above qualities in the potential sense; and first we must explain the meaning of the term *potential*.

The explanation is in fact concise, clear and perfectly straightforward. An
647   attribute which | is not yet present in a body, but is of such a nature as to come about in it, is said to belong to that body potentially. It is in this sense, for example, that, even when new-born, a human being is 'rational', a bird 'winged' [*or* 'flying'], a dog 'hunting', a horse 'swift'. We attribute each of these qualities to the object in question on the grounds that it will come to be the case provided that no external factor prevents it. And for this reason we describe those qualities as being present potentially, not in actuality. An actuality is something which is already completed, and present. Potential is something uncompleted, in the future, as it were liable to come about while not yet being present. An infant is not yet rational, but is of a nature to become so; a new-born dog does not yet hunt—it does not yet even have the sense of sight—but acquires the name *hunting dog* from the fact that it is able to hunt if it reaches its final form.

Now, the most proper application of the term *potentially* is to cases where Nature herself will bring about the fulfilment in the absence of any preventive
648   factors. It is also, however, used where | the materials are already close to the substances to be produced. It makes no difference here whether we say 'close', 'proper' or 'specific'. In each case the reference is to an immediacy of change, whereby no means outside the object are required to effect it. One might, for example, say that blood is potentially flesh, as it requires only the smallest change in order for flesh to be produced. Food which has been digested in the stomach, on the other hand, is not a material 'close to' flesh in this sense; it requires the intermediate stage of blood in order to become so....

650   Those substances which have a clear heating effect on our bodies are also easily ignited. How is it, then—some people object—that they do not appear hot to the touch? The relevance of this question is unclear to me. If our claim were that the above substances were hot in actuality, that is, already hot, it would indeed be a cause for surprise that they do not appear hot to the touch. But we are applying the term to them in its potential sense, in respect of their capacity

readily to become hot. | It should therefore surprise no one if they do not in 651
their present state heat the person who touches them. Even wood does not catch
fire until it has been overcome by the fire, and so transformed, and this process
takes a certain amount of time; similarly, drugs do not increase the internal heat
in animals until they have been transformed by this very heat. Now, the manner
in which one is heated by standing in the sun, or in front of a fire, is different
from that in which one is heated by any of the above-mentioned drugs. The
former are hot in actuality, while the drugs are not. Drugs cannot therefore heat
us before becoming actually hot; and this actuality they take from our own bodies, in the same way that dry reeds take it from fire. Similarly, all wood is in its
own nature cold; but pieces of wood which are dry and small are easily transformed into fire, while those which are wet and large require a longer time.

There is therefore nothing surprising in the fact that drugs, too, need first to
be broken down into small, fine parts, and secondly to be in contact with our
bodies for at least a small amount of time, before they will become hot. | If, 652
without having first broken down or heated them, you still expect them to
appear hot, it seems to me that you have forgotten the sense of the term *potentially hot*; you are applying criteria relevant only to actuality. Nor is it surprising
that a substance needs first to be heated itself, in order then to heat another
substance. This phenomenon too may be considered on the analogy of wood.
When a flame is dying out, wood both keeps it going and increases it; but it was
first heated by that flame itself. It is thus not unreasonable to suppose that the
internal heat of living beings uses such drugs for its nutrition, in the same way
that fire uses wood. And this indeed is evidently the case. If you apply any of
these drugs externally, having first made it extremely fine, to a body which has
been cooled down, it is not heated at all; and for this reason we generally massage the cooled parts as much as possible with such drugs, introducing heat in
the process of the massage, and also making porous that which has become
dense through cooling, in order to enable the drug to | enter, make contact with 653
the animal's innate heat, and so become changed and heated. For if the smallest
part of it acquires actual heat, this is then transmitted to the whole by virtue of
its contiguity, just as when one sets a light to the top of a torch with a tiny spark;
there too the fire proceeds to take hold of the whole torch, and has no further
need of the spark.

All substances which are potentially hot, then, do not yet have, in their nature,
a predominance of heat over cold; but they are already close to having such a
predominance, and thus require the assistance of some small external influence
in order to bring it about. In some cases massage is sufficient to supply that assistance; in others fire, or some naturally hot body coming into contact with fire.

It is also unsurprising that some drugs heat the body reciprocally immediately on contact, whereas others require a longer period of time. It is the same

with fire: some things, such as plantain, light pinewood, pitch and dry reeds, are
654   immediately set alight, | others, such as green wood, will not be burned unless
the contact continues for a considerable length of time.

Now, here we must make a distinction, the demonstration of which is given
in the work on *Natural Capacities*, but which for present purposes will be taken
as granted, namely that there are four capacities of the body as a whole: that
which attracts familiar substances, that which retains these, that which transforms substances and that which expels alien substances. These capacities are
those that belong to the substance as a whole of each of the bodies, which substance, as we have seen, is composed of a mixture of hot, cold, dry and wet. But
when the change which a body effects on an object with which it comes into
contact takes place in respect of any one of that object's qualities,[16] it should not
be taken that the action is performed in respect of the whole substance of that
object, nor that the object undergoing the transformation is then capable of
complete assimilation to the body. Soo, too, it is impossible for an object so
changed to provide nutrition to the body effecting that change. It is only when
the body produces a sufficient change, that is, one involving action in respect of
the whole substance of the object, that the body will succeed in assimilating
655   the object to itself, and in being nourished by | the object thus changed. For
nourishment consists in nothing other than a complete assimilation.

2. With this distinction in mind, let us return to our previous argument.
Every animal is nourished by its own proper foods. And the 'proper' ones are
any which may be assimilated to the body being nourished. Now, there must be
some similarity or common element between the substance, considered as a
whole, of the nourisher and the nature of the nourished; and here too, of course,
there are major differences of degree. Some stuffs are more similar and 'proper',
others less so; and therefore some will require a more powerful and longer process, others a weaker, shorter one. The meat of birds, for example, requires a
shorter process, that of pigs a longer one; and cow's meat requires a longer one
still. Wine, which needs least time of all to be transformed and assimilated, is
therefore the quickest to nourish and strengthen. Of course, it still has to come
into contact with the organs of digestion, namely stomach, liver and veins. It is

---

[16] An alternative reading of this passage (Helmreich's, replacing the pronouns of the Greek
manuscript tradition with reflexive pronouns) would give the translation: 'that body's qualities', and
similarly 'of that body' in the next clause and 'whole substance of the body' a few lines below. But
the reading followed here seems the most natural: fundamentally what is at issue is the nature of the
change undergone by the thing coming into contact with the body, and whether this thing is transformed in such a way—'change in the whole substance'—as to be assimilated as food. It should,
however, be mentioned that there is some uncertainty and complexity in the conception of 'change
in the whole substance', which is indeed sometimes conceived in active rather than passive terms;
that is, Galen sometimes speaks of X bringing about change in Y by virtue of *its own*, i.e. X's, substance. See *My Own Doctrines*, ch. 9 and *Simple Drugs* I.3 (with n. 2), V.1, IX.2.1 and XI.24; and for
discussion of the concept Singer 2020.

only after being broken | down in these that it will be able to nourish the body; 656
before this transformation it can never form the nourishment of any animal,
even if it were to remain in contact with the skin all day and all night. And
wheat bread, beet and barley-cake are especially unable to give nourishment
through this sort of external contact.

Now those stuffs which are completely assimilated are called foods; all others
are called drugs. There is, however, a further distinction, within drugs. There is
one type that remains as it is when taken, while transforming and overpower-
ing the body, in the same manner that the body does foods; these drugs are of
course destructive[17] and corruptive of the animal's nature. The other type takes
the cause of its change from the body itself; then undergoes putrefaction and
corruption, and in that process causes putrefaction and corruption to the body
also. These too are clearly destructive. In addition to these, a third type heats
the body reciprocally but does not harm; and a fourth both acts and is acted
upon, | so as to be gradually completely assimilated. This last type, therefore, 657
falls into the category of both drugs and foods.

It should not surprise anyone if some stuffs undergo an enormous change
from their original nature as a result of a very small initial influence. There are
many examples of such phenomena in the external world. In Mysia, in Asia, a
house was once burned down in the following manner. Some pigeon-droppings
had been laid up, and had already undergone a process of putrefaction and
heating; they were emitting a vapour and were quite hot to the touch. Nearby,
almost in contact with them, was a wooden window-frame which had just been
coated with a great quantity of resin. Now, it was the height of summer, the sun
was fierce, and it set light to the resin and the wood. From there it easily spread
to some other nearby doors, and some more window-frames coated with resin,
and the fire reached as high as the roof. Once the flame had taken hold here, it
quickly engulfed the whole house.

The manner in which Archimedes is said to have set fire to the enemy ships
by using firesticks seems to me not dissimilar.[18] | For flax, plaintain, giant fennel 658
and all similarly dry, porous substances are easily ignited by firesticks. Even
stones may give rise to a flame when rubbed together, especially if some amount
of brimstone is rubbed in with them. Medea's poison was of this nature; something into which this has been rubbed will set light to anything, with the

---

[17] I have retained this literal translation of *dēlētērios*, which might more naturally be translated
'poisonous', as Galen mentions other categories of poisonous drugs. See *My Own Doctrines*, ch. 9,
with n. 23.

[18] 'Firesticks' (*pureia*) are usually sticks rubbed together to produce fire; some other mechanism,
involving action at a distance, is presumably what is here attributed to Archimedes. A number of
ancient sources describe Archimedes as devastating the Roman fleet at the siege of Syracuse, and
one, Lucian, describes him, unspecifically, as using craft, or ingenuity, to set light to it. The story
that he did so by the use of mirrors may possibly be what Galen has in mind, but it is otherwise only
attested in much later sources.

introduction of heat.[19] It is prepared from a mixture of brimstone and wet asphalt. This used, in fact, to be performed as a magician's trick: one would extinguish a lamp and then light it again by bringing it into contact with a wall, or with a stone. The wall or stone had of course been covered in brimstone; and once this was realized the thing no longer appeared extraordinary.

So, all these drugs are not yet completely hot, but have a great aptitude to become hot, and in virtue of that are referred to as 'potentially hot'. There should then be no problem with this, nor with the fact that wine has a considerable heating effect on the body when drunk, but no such effect when placed on the

659   skin. As was shown above, wine is not | only a hot drug, but also a proper food causing heat in the living being. Just as the nourishment proper to fire increases a fire, similarly whatever is a proper, natural food for naturally hot bodies will definitely strengthen them and increase their innate heat. This feature in itself is common to all foods; what is specific and unusual in wine is the speed of the change, analogous to that in pinewood, plantain, flax and pitch....

[*The chapter concludes with some observations on stuffs which potentially nourish and warm (wine in human beings, oil for a flame) but which may also cool if applied in excess. Chapter 3 begins with a discussion of the different effects of substances in different places and modes of application—e.g. plasters for the skin—as well as at different times and in different quantities.*]

665   3. ... Is it then remarkable that there exists a drug so hot in potential that it will eat through and burn us if taken in large quantities and when the body is empty, but in very small quantities, and taken in conjunction with substances which control its strength, so far from hurting us will actually have a beneficial heat-

666   ing effect? For example, the juices | known as 'Cyrenaic', 'Medic' and 'Parthian'[20] may not be taken on their own without harm; but if the amount is very small, they are taken with something else and the time is appropriate, they can be of great benefit.

Now those drugs which heat the body, as was stated above, function by taking the principle of their transformation from the body, and then heating it once they have themselves become heated; cooling drugs, on the other hand, such as the juice of the poppy, are not even slightly transformed by the body, but immediately overcome and transform it, even when they are taken hot. For it is their own actual nature which is cold, in the same way that water's is. This, then, is among the many matters correctly discussed by Aristotle, who

---

[19] Medea is supposed to have sent her husband's new bride a garment smeared with poison, which ignited in contact with her skin. The word translated 'poison' here is *pharmakon* (elsewhere translated 'drug'), which in Greek can refer to both toxic and healing substances (not unlike the word 'drug', indeed).

[20] It seems that these refer to the juices of various citrus fruits (see *The Thinning Diet*, ch. 10: the 'Medic apple' is the citron), although the standard Greek lexicon translates 'Medic juice' as 'asafoetida'.

says that among bodies which are hot, cold, dry and wet, some have these qualities in their very nature, others incidentally; water is in its own nature cold, but it will happen sometimes that it is hot, incidentally. This acquired heat, however, is quickly lost, while the innate cold remains. And so just as hot water thrown on to a flame will extinguish it, so too opium, even if it is heated to a high degree before it is given, ⏐ will cool the animal's internal heat, and 667 endanger its life....

The point of particular importance with all drugs which are described as potentially hot or cold is whether they [i] are naturally able to nourish; [ii] take the beginning of their change from the body, before being themselves altered and affecting the body in some way; or [iii] are themselves not altered by the body in any way. Those in the first class, if they are overcome by the body, cause heating, but if not, cooling. ⏐ Those which are to a small extent altered definitely have a 668 heating effect, while those which are not altered at all are strongly cooling.

4. We have stated the importance of distinguishing the essential qualities from the incidental; and this applies not just to hot and cold, but equally to wet and dry. Some stuffs are dry in their own nature, but when melted by great heat acquire the appearance of moisture; this is true for example of bronze and iron. Others, like glass, are wet in their own nature, but in contact with some unmoderated cold appear dry. The assessment of all such substances must be carried out not in a straightforward manner, but—as discussed earlier—in conjunction with an examination of their degree of heat or cold. For if something with a small degree of heat still appears wet, then this moisture belongs to its actual nature; whereas if it appears wet [only] when there is plentiful heat, then it is actually dry. Stuffs which either become fluid in boiling heat or frozen in ⏐ unmoderated cold should not be regarded as wet or dry in their own right. 669 This, then, is the manner of distinguishing the essential from the incidental qualities; and also, by reference to this, of assessing whether a substance is potentially hot, cold, dry or wet. For this latter assessment must be made by reference not to incidental but to essential qualities.

And the one common criterion of assessment in all cases is the speed of the change. And since there are different senses of hot, cold, dry and wet, one of which refers to a domination of one of these qualities, another to an extreme degree of that quality, the object under examination will count as having the quality potentially provided that it changes readily into either of the above states. Olive oil is potentially hot in that it turns easily into flame; and resin, pitch and asphalt are potentially hot in this sense too. Wine is potentially hot in that it easily turns into blood; and in this sense also honey, meat and milk. These stuffs, which undergo alteration in their entire substance, function ⏐ as 670 nourishment to the subject which brings about that change; those which undergo and produce alteration in respect of only one of their qualities are drugs pure and simple, as are those which remain unchanged in their whole substance and affect the body in some way. The last class are also drugs of a kind, but ones which are problematic and corruptive of the animal's nature; therefore they are referred to generically as destructive drugs. Nor should one refuse to classify drugs under this heading merely because in very small amounts they may do no noticeable harm; on that principle fire would not be hot, nor snow cold: in sufficiently small quantities, they too have no clear effect on our bodies. Imagine a spark divided into a hundred parts: the hundredth part obviously still belongs to the class of fire; but not only would it not burn or heat us, it would not even make any impression on our perceptive faculties. A hundredth part of a cold water-drop, equally, so far from harming or cooling us, would not even be noticed.

671 | This, then, is not the criterion to be employed in assessing what is destructive, either; what is to be considered is the opposition inherent in its nature as a whole, and this opposition is evaluated in terms of the need of an intermediate stage for the change. If we take the elements themselves, water does not have the natural potential to turn into fire, nor fire into water; but both do have a natural potential to turn into air, and air into either of them. The change from water to air is an immediate one, and so also is that of fire into air; but any change of fire or water into each other is not immediate. Therefore these two are opposite and hostile to each other. And in the same way the juice of poppy is absolutely opposed to the human body, which is unable to act upon it in virtue of even one of its qualities, still less in virtue of its whole substance.[21]

This, then, is one kind of destructive drug. Another is that which takes the beginning of its change from the internal heat in our bodies, then proceeding to undergo a variety of different alterations, as a result of which our nature is destroyed. All these belong in the class of the destructive, even if in very small

672   doses | their effects may sometimes be indiscernible. Those things which eat through, putrefy and melt the natural state of our bodies are reasonably referred to as potentially hot, those which cool and cause a corpse-like state, as potentially cold....

674   Is it then surprising that opium, a drug so opposite to our nature, is pretty well immediately cooled, even when drunk hot, and thus brings about the simultaneous cooling of the body? It cannot retain its acquired heat because of its own natural cold; but since its substance is not altered by but rather itself alters and transforms us, it does not become in any way heated by us, but itself affects us according to its own nature. Being naturally cold itself, it consequently cools us. There is no further cause for confusion that need arise from this argument. And indeed, the fact that any of these naturally cold stuffs, when heated

---

[21] See n. 16 above; here too there is some uncertainty as to *which* whole substance is meant, that of the body or that of the poppy juice, though I take it that it is the latter.

to a high degree, changes from its own nature, presents no conflict with the above statements; rather, it serves to confirm them. Consider the case of the salamander: to begin with, it suffers no harm from contact with fire; but if the contact is prolonged, it is burned. It is so also with mandragora, hemlock, opium or fleawort: if they are brought into contact with fire for a short time, they preserve their own mixture; | if heated for a longer period, they are at once   675 destroyed, and lose all capacity to perform their previous functions.

The nature of all such stuffs, then, is utterly opposed to human beings; when I say 'nature', I mean the entire substance and mixture from the primary elements, hot, cold, dry and wet. The nature of the stuffs which most readily nourish us, meanwhile, is that which is closest to ours. All others lie somewhere between these two extremes, varying in the extent of their capacity to act upon, and be acted upon by, our bodies. Castor and pepper, for example, act to a greater extent than they are acted upon, whereas wine, honey and barley-gruel are acted upon more than they act. All these, then, do both exert and receive some influence in relation to the body. In general terms, whenever two bodies meet and engage over a considerable period of time in mutual conflict in relation to their alteration, it is inevitable that each of them both acts and is acted upon.

[The chapter proceeds to elaborate on the different degrees to which substances may act upon or be acted upon in particular cases; and to discuss cases of substances which are assimilated by our bodies but still retain the capacity to affect us qualitatively, and so act as both foods and drugs.]

This whole argument thus appears to proceed from this one basic principle.   683 And therefore this principle should be observed consistently; and one should constantly bear in mind that each body possesses some specificity of mixture which is proper to such-and-such a particular nature, but differs from such-and-such another one; further, that if the body alters what is proper to it into its own nature, it will thus increase the amount of substance of the heat within it; and that if it undergoes alteration itself, this will involve either the acquisition of some heat, if the agent of change is a heating agent, or the loss of its own heat, if it is the opposite. Therefore obviously such stuffs must be considered in relative terms; it is in relation to the specificity of the nature effecting the alteration that any substance taken assumes the role of nourishment, | drug or both. Hemlock,   684 for example, is a nourishment for fish, but is a drug [or poison] to men; and hellebore is a drug to human beings but a nourishment for quails. The mixture of quails is able to assimilate hellebore to itself, while that of humans is not.

[In chapter 5 Galen considers further the criteria of assessment of which substances are 'hot, cold, wet and dry' in relation to our bodies, and in chapter 6 recapitulates the different senses in which the quality terms are used.]

The Function of the Parts of the Human Body (excerpts)

The following brief extracts aim to give a glimpse into the content and modes of argument of one of Galen's most important scientific and philosophical works—his seventeen-book *magnum opus* on human anatomy and physiology. The work as a whole provides Galen's strongest statement of the purposive nature of the construction of animal bodies, and of human beings in particular. It also lays out in detail his understanding of the anatomy of the human body, part by part, whereby each anatomical structure is described and analysed in relation to the function for which it has been created.

Greek title: Περὶ χρείας τῶν ἐν ἀνθρώπου σώματι μορίων (*Peri chreias tōn en anthrōpou sōmati moriōn*)
Kühn: III.1–939 and IV.1–366
Edition: Helmreich 1907/1909
Translation: May 1968

BOOK I

III.1   1. Just as we identify animals as individuals by virtue of the fact that each has a clearly manifest boundary of its own, which is not connected at any point to any other animal, so it is too with the parts of that animal. Eye, nose, tongue and brain are considered to be individual parts by virtue of their clearly identifiable boundary. If, of course, these parts had no connection with those near to it, and were completely separated from them, then they would not be parts at

2   all, but actually separate individuals. Those bodies, then, | which neither in all respects possess their own boundary nor are in all respects attached to others, are called parts. It thus follows that there are many animal parts, some greater, some smaller and some in no way divisible into further kinds.

2. And the function of all parts is related to the soul.[1] The body is the instrument of the soul; and the reason for the great differences between parts of animals is that there are great differences in their souls, too. Some are brave, others

---
[1] The analysis given here is Aristotelian in inspiration; see especially Aristotle's *De anima* II.4, 415b and *Parts of Animals* I.1, 640–1.

timid; some wild, others tame; some might be said to form societies and to build, others are loners. In each case, the body is suited to the character traits and capacities of the soul. The body of a horse, for example, is fitted out with strong hooves and a mane, because this animal is swift, haughty and endowed with a certain spirit, while that of the lion—a brave, spirited beast—is fortified with teeth and claws. The case of the bull and of the boar is similar, and these too have their natural weapons, horns and tusks respectively, but the deer and the hare, which are timid animals, have bodies which are swift but wholly unprotected and unarmed. | This, surely, is because speed was appropriate for 3 timid animals, but weapons for brave ones.

Nature, therefore, has neither armed a timid animal nor left a brave one unprotected. In the case of the human being, an animal which is wise and, alone amongst those on earth, godlike, Nature has given hands, in place of all weapons at once: these constitute an instrument which is both necessary for every craft and fitted for peace as much as for war. Human beings did not need the natural endowment of a horn, since they are able to take hold of a weapon superior to the horn, whenever they wish; swords and spears, after all, are bigger and better at cutting than horns. Nor did they need hooves; for both wood and stone can crush more violently than hooves. Furthermore, neither horn nor hoof has any effect at all except at close quarters, whereas human weapons are no less effective from a distance, javelins and darts replacing the horn in this context, and stone and wood replacing the hoof.

But, it may be objected, a lion is faster than a human being. What of it? Human beings have, through wisdom and | use of their hands, mastered the 4 horse, an animal which is faster than the lion, and by exploiting the horse are able both to escape from and to pursue the lion, as well as to use their physically superior position, when seated on the horse, to strike the lion from above. Human beings, then, are not unprotected, nor easily wounded, nor unarmed nor unshod. They may, when desired, be endowed with a trunk[2] of iron, which is harder to pierce than any other bodily part, as well as with every variety of footwear, arms and armour. For it is not breastplates alone, but houses, walls and towers which are his armour. If, on the other hand, human beings were endowed naturally with horn on their hands, or some other such protective armour, it would be impossible for them to use their hands for the construction of houses and walls, or of spears, breastplates and other such items. With these same hands, too, humans are able to weave clothes and to twine nets, fish traps and baskets, as well as traps for birds, so that they are masters not only of the animals of the earth, but also of those of the sea and the air. Such is the defensive or

[2] The word *thōrax* in Greek may refer to a breastplate as well as to the part—the chest area—covered by it.

combative value of the human hand. Yet, since it is at the same time a peaceful
5 and social animal, the human being also uses its hands to ǀ write laws, to set up
altars and statues to the gods and to construct ships—not to mention pipes,
lyres, knives, tongs and all other instruments of the arts—as well as to leave
behind written records of the science or method relevant to each art. By virtue of
such writings—and by use of the hands—it is possible for you still today to consult with Plato, Aristotle, Hippocrates and the other ancient authors.

3. The human being is thus the most intelligent of animals; and thus, too,
hands are the instruments appropriate to an intelligent animal. It is not because
this animal has hands that it is the most intelligent, as Anaxagoras said; rather,
it is because it is the most intelligent that it acquires hands, as Aristotle states,
with perfect understanding of this point. For it was not hands, but reason, that
taught human beings the arts; the hands are the instruments, as the lyre is an
instrument for a musician and tongs for a metalworker. It is not the case that
the lyre instructed the musician, nor the tongs the metalworker; each is a craftsman by virtue of the reason or understanding within him, though he is unable
to practise that craft without instruments.

6   It is exactly the same with the soul. Every soul ǀ possesses certain capacities
by virtue of its own substance, but there is no way of its performing the tasks
which it naturally does perform without instruments.[3] It can be very clearly
seen that it is not the parts of the body that cause the soul to be, respectively,
timid, courageous or intelligent, since newborn animals may be observed
attempting to perform their tasks before the completion of those parts. For
example, I have frequently seen a calf butting before the growth of its horns, a
foal kicking while its hooves were still soft and, indeed, a small piglet attempting to use its jaws aggressively while these were still unprovided with the large
teeth, as well as a puppy striving to bite while its teeth were still soft. Every animal possesses, untaught, a perception of the capacities of its own soul and of
the particular superiorities of its parts. Why, otherwise, would the piglet, when
it is possible for it to bite with its small teeth, leave these idle and desire to use
for the fight those which it does not yet possess? How is it possible to claim that
7 animals are taught the use of the parts by those parts themselves, when ǀ it is
apparent that they know those functions before they possess the parts?
     Take three eggs—one of an eagle, one of a duck and one of a snake—and keep
them at a moderate heat so that they hatch out. Once they are born, you will
observe two of the animals making trial of their wings, even before they are able
to fly, and the third wriggling and eager to crawl, even though it is still soft and
unable to do so. If, further, you rear them to maturity in the same house and
then take them out into the open and release them, the eagle will fly up into the
air, the duck will fly down into some lake, and the snake will slide into the earth.

---

[3] *Organa*, the same word used in physiological or anatomical contexts for 'organs'.

Then, to be sure, the first will hunt, even though it has never learned to do so, the second will swim and the snake will conceal itself. 'For', says Hippocrates, 'animal natures are untaught.'[4] Thus, I believe that it is by nature rather than by reason that all the other animals perform any skill that they possess: moulding in the case of bees, the construction of chambers and tunnels by ants, the spinning and weaving of spiders. My evidence for this is the fact that they are not taught.

4. In the case of human beings, however, it is not just that their bodies are 8 unprotected by armour; their souls are also devoid of any such specialized skill. They have, therefore, been provided with reason in recompense for this lack of specialized skills in their souls, just as they have been provided with hands in recompense for their bodies' lack of protection. These they use both to arm and protect the body in all kinds of ways, and to adorn the soul with all kinds of specialized skills. Just as we saw that the innate endowment of some weapon would entail the permanent possession of this weapon alone, so it is with skills, too. If human beings were naturally endowed with some specialized skill, they would not possess any others. The reason that they have been given none innately is that it is better that they should have the use of all forms of weaponry and all specialized skills. Now, there is an excellent statement of Aristotle, to the effect that the hand is an instrument in place of instruments;[5] and we for our part might do well to produce a parallel statement, that the faculty of reason is as it were a skill in place of skills. Just as, in the case of the hand, although it is itself not one of the individual instruments, its natural excellence at receiving any of those instruments makes it stand in place of all the others, so too the faculty of reason, although it is itself not one of the individual skills, has the natural ability to receive them all within it, | and may so be called a skill in place 9 of skills. Human beings alone of all animals possess a skill in place of all other skills within their soul, in exactly the same way as they possess in their body an instrument in place of all other instruments.

5. Well, then, let us subject this part—the hand—to our scrutiny first of all; and let us consider not simply whether it is useful, or appropriate to an intelligent animal, but whether its construction is, in all respects, such that it could not have been better if it had been brought about in some different way.

[*After this first statement of his view—to be repeated many times throughout the book—that the part has been constructed as well as it could have been for its purpose, Galen proceeds to a detailed discussion, on this basis, of the anatomy and*

---

[4] The quotation is from the 'Hippocratic' *Nutrition*, though the text in the existing manuscripts of that work is slightly different from that cited. (*Nutrition* is now generally considered a post-Hippocratic work, and is not definitely by Hippocrates according to Galen either, but is nonetheless quoted by him quite frequently in support of his own views.) For the argument here, cf. *The Shaping of the Embryo*, ch. 6, pp. 304–5 below.

[5] Aristotle, *Parts of Animals* IV.10, 687a20–1.

structure of the hand. Subsequent books consider the arm (II), the foot and leg (III), the organs related to nutrition (IV and V), the organs related to breathing (VI and VII), the neck, head, brain, nerves and organs of sensation (VIII–XII), the spine and shoulder (XIII), the reproductive and related organs (XV–XVI) and the nerves, arteries and veins (XVI).]

Book VI

[Galen is summing up his views on respiration, heart function and the vascular system, and in particular on the structures of the 'venous artery' (in our terms, the pulmonary vein) and 'arterial vein' (the pulmonary artery), and how their structures are explicable on the basis of their function.[6] The anatomical exposition leads into a more abstract discussion of causes in nature.]

461 11. Indeed, if you put together all the main points of the argument, both those just stated and those written earlier on, it will be apparent to you that the proposition laid out at the beginning has been demonstrated. It would not have been better for the lung to have been nourished rather by some other vein; nor would it have been possible for such an outgrowth either of tunics or of membranes to have arisen from the vena cava. From all of which it is quite evident that it is better that the lung be nourished from the heart. Now, if one vessel, simple in terms of its tunic, is inserted into the heart, while another, which is double, issues from it, it follows necessarily that there must be produced a common space for them, as it were a receptacle to which both are attached, into
462 which the blood is drawn | from the one and sent out by means of the other. This, then, is the right ventricle of the heart; and it has come into being, as our argument has shown, for the sake of the lung. Those animals, therefore, which do not have a lung do not have two ventricles of the heart, either; in such animals there is a single one governing the motion of all the arteries. For the veins have as their source the liver: this too has been demonstrated at greater length in *The Doctrines of Hippocrates and Plato*, and all our arguments in this area are consistent both with each other and with the truth. This, then, brings to an appropriate conclusion our discussion of the right ventricle of the heart, the presence or absence of which in all animals corresponds to the presence or absence of the lung.

12. If anyone wishes to learn the cause of ignorance of those doctors and philosophers who have made false assertions on the number of chambers in the
463 heart, all this has been shown elsewhere, in my discussion of all | disagreement

---

[6] Galen defines as arteries only those vessels which proceed from the left ventricle, and which carry (in his theory) breath (*pneuma*) as well as blood; hence his need to explain why, in the unique case of what we call the pulmonary circulation, the 'artery' (our pulmonary vein) has the structure of a vein, and the 'vein' (our pulmonary artery) that of an artery.

in anatomy. And, just as the demonstrations concerning *activities* precede the discussion before us now, so in turn, the same way, those on disagreement in anatomy, and on anatomical procedures, precede those. We should not, then, in the present work mention the disagreement on the number of tunics of the arteries or veins, nor any other matter which we have previously discussed...except where necessary if what is said is to be useful either for many doctrines or in general terms. Thus, here too, I have decided to make mention of Asclepiades' | incorrect statements about the vessels of the lung, and to show   464 how no one may escape the law of Adrasteia,[7] even someone who is a charlatan and a clever speaker; in fact, such a person will himself in the end admit his charlatanry and become a far more persuasive witness to the truth than anyone else, precisely because he bears witness against his own will.

Now, the first cause of all things that come into being, as indeed Plato showed,[8] is the *aim* of the activity. If, then, someone asks you the cause of your arrival at the market-place, you cannot answer better than by paying attention to this cause. You would invite ridicule if, instead of saying that you had come to buy this or that utensil, or slave, or to meet such-and-such a friend, or to return some item, you omitted that information and stated as the reason for your coming to the market-place the fact that you possessed two feet with the ability both to move easily and to stand firm upon the ground. You would, in that case too, have stated something which may perhaps be called a cause, but not that which is genuinely | the cause, and certainly not the first cause, but   465 rather an instrumental cause, or an account of those things without which it could not have happened—which one should rather not actually call a cause. Plato's understanding in this area of causation in nature was correct; in our account, however, to avoid the appearance of quibbling over words, we shall concede that there are several kinds of cause. The first, and primary, cause is that on account of which something happens; the second, that by which it happens; the third, that from which; the fourth, that through which; the fifth (if you like), that in accordance with which. We should, then, require anyone who is a genuine natural philosopher to produce a response with reference to each of these five, in relation to all parts of the animal.[9]

---

[7] Adrasteia was a mythical nymph, who is associated with Necessity (her name means 'inescapable'). There is a clear verbal echo of Plato here, the identical phrase being used at *Phaedrus* 248c2; but the context there is the passage and fate of souls in their disembodied phase in the supercelestial realm, in relation to their level of ability to follow god and divine knowledge or visions. Galen seems to use the phrase rather to refer simply to an inescapable logical consequence, which leads someone to be refuted on the basis of their own arguments.

[8] In this passage Galen draws on the discussion of causes in Plato's *Phaedo*, esp. 97b–99c; see also *Timaeus* 46c. Plato seems to vacillate, as does Galen here, as to whether certain causes (here the 'material' or 'instrumental'—the 'without-which-not' cause) should really count as causes at all.

[9] Galen's list is based on the well-known Aristotelian schema of the 'four causes' (cf. esp. *Physics* II.3, 194a16–195a3), with certain post-Aristotelian developments. The fifth cause, presented here as optional, is in a sense a Platonist addition related to the Platonic theory of forms or ideas (see

So, when I am asked why the nature of the vessels of the lung has been reversed, so that the vein has been rendered arterial and the artery venous, I offer in response the first cause: namely that it was better, in this organ alone, for the vein to be dense and the artery loose in texture. Erasistratus' response is of a different kind. He states that the vein [sc. pulmonary artery] has arisen at the point where the arteries which are distributed into the whole of the body
466 have their source, I and that it is inserted into the ventricle of the blood, while the artery [sc. pulmonary vein] has arisen at the point where the veins have their source, and is inserted into the pneumatic ventricle of the heart.

13. Asclepiades, meanwhile, bypasses both causes, that from the providence of the Craftsman, which was mentioned as the first cause, and the second, as it were material, cause, and moves straight to the least worthy cause of all—one which someone versed in philosophy would probably not call a cause, without some qualification, but rather a cause in an incidental sense or by consequence. In his complete reliance on this counterfeit currency, as we may call it, he believes himself very persuasive and clever. But he fails to take account of that law of Adrasteia, whereby no other argument will refute the absurdity of his doctrines to the same extent as this very argument of his own, which he has so brilliantly discovered.

[*Asclepiades is criticized for failures both in anatomical observation and in logical argument: he presents the differences in physical nature of the structures merely as a physical consequence of the different levels of exertion carried out by the different parts, but is unaware that there are different numbers of tunics, not just different thicknesses, between the vessels in question, which could not have come about through the causal mechanism he describes.*]

470   We, on the other hand, do not offer one type of cause in our account of every part of the animal, but all of them: one, the first and most important, that it was better this way; next, those concerning the instruments and the material by use of which the Craftsman brings every thing that comes into being into a better form; he has made the arteries of the lung dense and the veins loose in texture for the cause which we have stated; and because it was better to construct it in this way, he has made the veins grow out from the arterial parts of the heart and the arteries from the venous ones; and, since it was necessary to conduct the

---

Seneca, *Moral Letters* 65.4–10, attributing this fifth cause, the *exemplar* or *idea*, by reference to which the craftsman produces his model, to Plato); on the other hand, it is also regarded as equivalent to Aristotle's 'formal' cause—which itself seems to be replaced by the 'instrumental' cause when only four are mentioned. (See also Philo, *On the Cherubim* 125, who uses the same prepositional terminology as Galen's here and, referring to only four causes, substitutes the instrumental for the formal.) Thus, Galen's five causes here are: 'final', 'efficient', 'material', 'instrumental' and 'exemplary' (or—but with a Platonist understanding—'formal'). On Galen's handling of these see also the next note.

appropriate material to each, he made an opening for the arteries into the ventricle of breath and for the veins into the other one. Because it was better for them to be covered | with a physical shape less subject to injury, he made these   471
vessels round; and since he had to craft them from material and through instruments, he mixed the moist with the dry, making a kind of fluid from both, which he then used, as if it were a malleable wax, as a material basis for the vessels that were to come into being. By mixing the hot with the cold, he made these into active instruments, on the basis of the material; and from these, by drying a little of the material with the hot, solidifying it with the cold, and also bringing into being a well-mixed breath arising from the mixture of these, he then blew this breath through the material and extended it, thus constructing a long, hollow vessel, pouring in more of the material wherever it was better for it to become denser, and less, wherever it was better for it to become finer. There you have all the causes included in the account—that from the purpose or end, that from the Craftsman, that from instruments, that from the material and that from the form.[10]

Book XI

[In the context of his discussion of the anatomy of the jaw, Galen inveighs against the folly of those who imagine that such structures could have arisen through random motions of atoms, or without a supervising design; the latter view he attributes not just to Atomists such as Epicurus but, in more general terms, to the influential medical figures Asclepiades and Erasistratus. The following extract may stand as an example of many such rhetorical invectives in the work, and of his championing of the view that 'Nothing is brought about by Nature in vain' (XI.5).]

7. Oh, by the gods!—for it is the part of gods to take pity on madness—why is it   867
that offshoots from the nerves which are above them are inserted into all parts of the face, through a piercing of the bones, but that none of these nerves has wandered off and been implanted in the parts that open the mouth, even though these are nearer? None has even gone up from these to the temples, nor from the temples to these muscles.... How is it, if the | agent responsible for the   868
breaking-open of the mouth were either 'heat unable to be confined', or breath—for this is the level of their ravings—that this agent did not bring it

---

[10] One notes that in this account the Craftsman (conceived here in an apparently anthropomorphic way) has taken the place of the Aristotelian 'efficient' or active cause; and that 'form' seems to be subsumed, in the first sentence, into the concept of 'for the better'. It is also noteworthy that 'instrument' and 'material' are treated simultaneously, and that the account of the material does justice to the Aristotelian notion of the more 'active' elements (hot and cold) and the more 'passive' (dry and wet).

about in the crown of the head? Why was the rupture and the outpouring of breath not made there, in spite of the fact that the natural motion of heat and breath is upward? How is it, indeed, if the construction of our bodies was brought about just by atoms rebounding from and interweaving with each other, that they broke open the head rather than any other part of the body, so that the mouth would come into being there? And if it was through chance that the mouth was broken open, how is it that it should automatically contain the teeth and the tongue?...There is after all no necessity for cleft parts of the body to grow teeth: both the backside and the genitals—especially those of women— also have clefts in them, yet there is no tooth in them, nor indeed any under-lying bone, even a small one.

8. So, according to your view, this too has come about by good fortune,
870 through the atoms?...ⁱ Well, let us grant that all these things have been accomplished—so wisely—simply through some good fortune. Just change their position, alone, and see what then results. Imagine the molars positioned on the outside edge, and the incisors and sharp teeth on the inner: what would then be the function of these ones—and indeed of the others? Is it not the case that everything else related to their function, even though so beautifully ordered by these provident atoms, would have been thrown into confusion simply through this error on their part in relation to positioning? One who directs a chorus of thirty-two dancers in good order is praised as a possessor of skill; shall we not also praise Nature, which so beautifully ordered the chorus of the teeth?

[*Galen moves from his usual topic of the perfection of bodily parts for their func-tion to that of the element of beauty that Nature has included; the discussion leads him on also to a consideration of the difference between the Judaeo-Christian view of creation or design in the universe (the philosophy 'of Moses') and his own (that 'of Plato and the other Greeks'), as well as to the distinction between features due directly to the Craftsman's design and others which 'follow from necessity'.*]

897 13. A good craftsman sometimes produces some superfluous display of his skill, for example on items of furniture, on shields, very frequently on the hilts of swords, sometimes on bowls—that is to say, some adornment or ornamenta-tion which goes beyond the function of the artefact in question—by adding to their design some ivy leaves, vine tendrils, a cypress motif, and so on. In the
898 same way tooⁱ Nature adorned the parts [of animals] through superabundance— and in particular the human being. There are many cases in which this adorn-ment is clearly manifest, but there are also times when it is hidden, precisely because of the brilliance of the function. In the case of the ears it is clearly evi-dent, as indeed in that of the skin at the end of the penis, known as the foreskin, and so too in the case of the flesh of the buttocks. In this last case you will very clearly discern what would be the ugliness of the part, were it to be laid bare, if

you consider the monkey. In the case of the eye, meanwhile, although this part is far more beautiful than all these, the beauty is ignored because of our huge admiration for its function. So too in the case of the nose and the lips, and of many other parts, where their beauty considered in terms of function greatly exceeds the pleasure derived from their sight. If even a small part of the lip, or of the wings of the nostrils, were cut off, the ugliness that would then arise in the entire face is difficult even to express. Yet all these features of Nature have, as stated, come about not through the primary design,[11] but as it were as by-products and for the sake of play. The chief and constant aim in all I is that   899
related to activity and to function. The nature of the difference between an activity and a function has been stated previously, as has the fact that in terms of the construction and generation of the parts the activity is prior, whereas in terms of value the function is prior. And it has also been shown that genuine beauty should be referred to the correctness of function, and that the first aim of all the parts is the function of the construction.

14. I have decided that it would be appropriate for me to say something now about the fact that Nature sometimes also has as its aim proportion and beauty: this, too, is a necessary area of knowledge for those applying themselves to the study of Nature, and has not been discussed anywhere in the book so far. For indeed the hair on the chin does not only provide a covering for the lower jaw, but also contributes to beauty.[12] For the appearance of the male is more digni-fied, especially as he grows older, if he is thoroughly covered by such hair. It is for the same reason that Nature has left the area of the cheekbones and the nose devoid of hair: I the face would in that case have become wild and beast-like,   900
which would be in no way appropriate to a civilized and social animal. Equally, the thickness of the cheekbones itself provides some assistance in the protection of that area, as does the heat of exhaled breath to the nose, so that these too are not entirely unprotected. Moreover, if you touch even the eyes—especially in cold weather—you will very clearly realize the extent to which they are hot; these too, then, are not entirely unprotected or unfortified against the cold, since they possess as a defence the innate heat, which has no need of external layers of protection.

In the case of women, on the other hand, whose bodies are in other respects soft, permanently child-like and unprotected by hair, the bareness of the face was not going to be lacking in beauty; this creature is, in other respects too, lacking in the dignity of character possessed by the male, and therefore does

[11] At a number of points in his causal explanations Galen distinguishes features of an animal which arise directly from the *prōtos logos*—the primary intention or design—from others which come about as necessary consequences; here the contrast is between primary design and adornment.
[12] I so translate *kosmos*, which is however a heavily loaded term, with connotations related to the notion of the designing intelligence which informs the universe, and which in other contexts may also be translated 'good order' or 'design'—or indeed in some cases cosmos.

not require a dignified form, either. For it has already been shown many times—if not, indeed, throughout the whole of this work—that Nature constructs the form of the body in a way appropriate to the characters of the soul. It is also the case that female-kind did not require any especial protective cover-
901 ing against the cold, since they remain at home for the most part; I they did, on the other hand, require a head covered by hair (which they have in common with men), for the purpose of both protection and beauty.

Yet the hair on both chin and head performs another necessary function for us too. When the exhalation of fluids rises up to the head, Nature makes a secondary use of these, especially of the thicker residues there, for the nourishment of the hair. Men, in proportion as they are hotter than women, possess more residues than they do; and so Nature has invented a twofold form of evacuation of these—that through the hairs on the chin and that through those on the head.

Enough, then, on this subject; it remains, however, to state the reason why the forehead, unlike the rest of the head, is without hair, as well as the reason why the skin of this part of the animal alone is capable of voluntary motion. Well, this part too, surely, is protected, to whatever extent we want, by the hair of the head, so that it did not require its own hairs; besides, we would be in perpetual need of a hair-cut if this part too sprouted hairs, in view of its prox-
902 imity to the eyes. I It has been demonstrated elsewhere, not least in the books on the instruments of nutrition, that Nature has taken care that human beings should not have to spend excessive effort upon their bodies, nor be in constant slavery to its needs. It is, surely, appropriate that an intelligent and social animal should expend only a moderate amount of care on its body—unlike the majority of people today, who, if a friend asks them to help in some task, run away, pleading their lack of leisure; then, once on their own, turn to depilating and adorning themselves, and spending their entire life in an unnecessary attention to their bodies, completely unaware, indeed, that they actually possess something greater than their body.

Such people, of course, deserve our pity; for our part, we should discuss the matter before us in a philosophical way, and show how it was reasonable for the skin of the forehead to be not only devoid of hair, on account of the eyes, but also capable of voluntary motion, for the very same reason. For it was necessary that one could open them very wide when attempting to see many external objects at once, and then again draw them together and bind them together,
903 using all the I surrounding parts to close them completely, when we fear contact
904 with some foreign body.... I ... Is it, then, that the Craftsman has instructed these
905 hairs alone [sc. those of eyebrows and eyelashes] I to preserve a constant length, and that they, either through fear of the master's orders, through respect for the god who gives such instructions, or because themselves persuaded that it is

better to act so, do, indeed preserve these hairs as they have been ordered? Well, that is Moses' natural philosophy; and, indeed, it is better than that of Epicurus. The better view, however, is neither of these, but rather that which, while preserving (in common with Moses) a principle of generation, in all generated beings, derived from the Craftsman, adds to that the principle of matter. The reason that the Craftsman has made these hairs in such a way that they require always to maintain the same length is that it was better so; but, realizing that he must produce them in this way, he extended beneath one set of these hairs a hard body, similar to cartilage, and beneath the other a hard skin contiguous, through the eyebrows, with this cartilage. His will that they should become so was not in itself sufficient—any more than it would have been possible for him suddenly to make a rock into a human being, if he had wished to do that.

This is the point of difference between the opinion of Moses and ours, which is also that of Plato and of those ∣ others amongst the Greeks who have engaged 906 correctly in the study of natural philosophy. According to Moses, it is sufficient for God to will the ordering of matter, and matter will immediately be so ordered; for he holds that all things are possible to God, even if he were to desire to make ash into a horse or an ox. Our understanding is different from that: we say that there are some things which are impossible by nature, and that God does not in any way attempt those things, but rather chooses the best from those things which are able to come about. Thus, in the case of the hair on the eyelids, since it was better for them to preserve a constant length and number, we do not say that God willed them so and they immediately came into being; for they could never come into being, even if he were to wish it a million times, by growth out of soft skin. Their erectness, quite apart from any other characteristic, would be quite impossible if they were not implanted in hard skin. We state, then, that God is responsible for both things: the selection of the better, amongst the objects being crafted, and the choice in relation to materials. It was ∣ right for the hairs on the eyelids both to stand erect and to preserve the same 907 length and number; therefore he implanted them in a cartilaginous body. If he had implanted them in some soft, fleshy substance, he would have been worse, not only than Moses, but also than a general who founds a fortification or palisade in a bog.

The uniformity in length of the hair of the eyebrows is similarly related to the selection of matter. For just as grass and plants which sprout on wet, soft ground grow very tall, whereas those which sprout on rocky, dry ground remain small, hard and stunted, in exactly the same way, surely, those hairs which sprout from wet, soft parts of the body have the best growth (those on the head, for example, on the armpits and around the genitals), while those which sprout from hard, dry parts, have small, limited growth. It follows, too, that there are two sources of generation here, as there are also for herbs and plants—one from the

foresight of the Craftsman, the other from the nature of the place. One may
908 frequently observe a field | with wheat or barley coming up, where this looks
just like a short, tender growth of grass, and then some other place equally full
and thick with actual grass. The difference is that this latter thick growth has
been brought about by natural moisture, whereas the field is the product of the
farmer's care. And for anyone unable to distinguish the recently sprouted seeds
from ordinary grass on the basis of the shape of the plants, the order of their
arrangement should provide a sufficient indication. The evenness of the growth,
as well as that of the external outline, which involves straight lines, is sufficient
to indicate the fact that the place has been filled through the operation of some
skill and foresight on the part of a farmer.

In the case of places filled with a spontaneous growth, by contrast, this
growth is not even, nor bounded by definite lines. This is true of the hairs in the
armpits, and of that in other places on the body, which are not organized in
clear lines as are those of the eyebrows, eyelids and head, but rather have uneven
909 edges and are themselves spread in a disordered way. | These are the product,
not of the Craftsman's providence, but of the moisture of the part in question;
and for this reason they grow in abundance in hot natures and very little, if at
all, in cold ones. Those hairs which the Craftsman has taken care of, on the
other hand (in the same manner as the farmer and his field), exist in all
natures—hot, cold, dry, wet—except where these reach the state of a completely
immoderate bad-mixture (which is similar to the case of rocky or sandy earth).

Thus, just as all kinds of earth, except for these very bad ones, are susceptible
to the skill of the farmer, so too every healthy mixture in animals admits of that
of the Craftsman. Only a serious complaint of the part in question would cause
the hair on the eyelids or eyebrows to fall out; so, too, with the hair on the head,
though in that case not such a serious one. Similarly with plants growing in
hard, dry ground: their initial growth is difficult and requires great care, but
their destruction is not easy, for they are securely rooted, held in place and
910 bound in on all sides. By the same token, Ethiopians have | heads which grow
short hair, and little of it, because of the dryness of the skin, but they do not
readily become bald.... It would have been completely impossible to implant
the source of growth of a plant in an actual rock, just as it would be to
implant the root of a hair in bone; but upon the head—a well-mixed place—he
produced, as it were, a fertile field, partly so that it would absorb some of the
moisture flowing into it, which would not then cause harm to the parts beneath
it, and partly to protect the head itself.

Similarly, in the area of the genitals: the hairs have come about by necessity,
for these regions are hot and wet, but also provide a covering, and good order,
to the parts there, in the same way that the buttocks do for the backside, and the
foreskin for the penis. For in many cases our Craftsman makes a secondary use,
for some pressing purpose, of those things which have their generation as a

necessary consequence; for he exceeds in all respects, and is wonderfully invent-
ive in his craftsmanship and in his operation of choice in favour of the better.

BOOK XVII

*[In this last book, Galen sums up the content of the whole work with an 'Epode' or
hymn to the divine intelligence evident in the construction of animals, in particular
in human beings.]*

1. Who would not immediately reflect that some intelligence possessing a won- IV.358
derful capacity treads upon the earth and is extended through all its parts? For
all about us we see coming into being animals which have a wonderful construction. What part of the cosmos could be of less worth than the earthly one?
And yet even here, some intelligence arrives from the heavenly bodies—bodies
whose contemplation leads one l at once to wonder at the beauty of their sub- 359
stance, of the sun, first and foremost, then of the moon, and of the stars. In
these, it is surely reasonable to suppose, just as the substance of their bodies is
purer, there exists an intelligence which is to precisely that same degree better
and more complete. When we see that in slime, in mud, in marshes, or in rot-
ting plants and fruits, there nonetheless come into being animals which provide
a wonderful indication of the intelligence that constructs them, what must one
think is the case of the heavenly bodies? And one may observe the nature of
this intelligence by contemplating the human examples of Plato, Aristotle,
Hipparchus, Archimedes and many other such individuals.

When, then, there arises in such mire—for how else might one characterize a
blend of flesh, blood, phlegm and yellow and black bile—a quite exceptional
intelligence, how much greater should one imagine to be that in the sun, in the
moon or in one of the stars? When I consider this, l it seems to me that a con- 360
siderable intelligence is extended even through the actual air that surrounds us;
and indeed, it would not otherwise be able by nature to partake of the sun's rays
nor of its power. I am convinced that you too will share this belief, when you
consider accurately and properly the skill manifest in animals—unless, as I have
said, some rashly posited doctrine concerning the elements has got in your way.
Anyone who considers the matter with an unprejudiced mind, observing how
some intelligence inhabits even such a mire of flesh and fluids, and above all
seeing the construction of every single animal—for they all present an indication
of the intelligence of the Craftsman—will form a conception of the superiority
of the intelligence in the heavens.

Then, indeed, what seemed previously to be a small thing—the study of the
function of the parts—will be established as in truth the fount of perfect theology,
which is a far greater and more valuable thing than the whole of medicine. This

study of the function of the parts, then, is not just of use to the doctor, but, far
361   more so, to the philosopher | eager to acquire a knowledge of Nature; and into
this Mystery, I am convinced, all human beings should be initiated, irrespective
of race or rank, provided that they honour the gods—a Mystery which has
nothing in common with the rites of Eleusis or of Samothrace. These are
obscure in their revelation of the truths which they wish to impart, whereas
those of nature are manifest in all animals. Indeed, you should not imagine that
the extraordinary level of skill laid out in this work so far is present only in
human beings. Any other animal which you choose to dissect will reveal to you
the same intelligence and skill on the part of the Craftsman; and indeed, the
smaller the animal, the greater the wonder that will arise—just as in the case of
human craftsmen capable of producing carvings in very small physical objects.
Such craftsmen exist even now: one recently made a carving, on a ring, of
Phaethon being drawn by four horses; and each had a bridle, mouth and front
teeth, which were so small that they were actually invisible to me until I turned
the piece around in a bright light....

362   When, therefore, such a great level of skill is apparent in some insignificant
animal, a manifestation of skill which, we might suppose, is performed by the
Craftsman just incidentally, what level of intelligence and power must we suppose to be present in the more worthy animals?

2. This, then, is one—and the greatest—benefit that we receive from this study;
and we receive it not just in our capacity as doctors, but, more importantly, in
our capacity as people desiring to gain some knowledge of the power of a
363   function, | something whose very existence is denied by some philosophers, let
alone its role in providing for animals. A second benefit relates to the ability to
identify those parts within the body which are affected in disease; an under-
364   standing of activity is of value for this too.... | And a third function of this study,
in addition to those stated, is to address those sophists who will not concede to
us that crises are brought about by Nature, and who would deprive animals the
forethought of Nature....

365   3. These benefits—so great and so many—of this work which I have now com-
366   pleted, have been laid out in this last book, as in some fine Epode.... | In the
works of the lyric poets one would find, not just a strophe with its responding
antistrophe, but also a third verse too—an Epode—which, it is said, they would
sing as they stood before the altars, as a hymn of praise to the gods. It is, indeed,
to such an Epode that I liken the present book, and have therefore attached to it
this name.

The Doctrines of Hippocrates and Plato (excerpts)

One of the most remarkable and important works in the history of philosophy and medicine, as well as a crucially valuable source for other ancient philosophers, this nine-book treatise[1] in many ways represents the best exemplification of Galen's scientific procedure and methods of argument, as well as of his relationship with the previous tradition and his intellectual personality. Most centrally, it highlights the importance of his anatomical demonstrations, especially that by which he showed the brain to be the central organ of cognition. It also elucidates his highly influential tripartite physiology of brain, heart and liver, and his understanding of the function of these three organs and their relationship with the three networks of nerves, arteries and veins.

At the same time, it is an extraordinarily rich source for ancient theories of psychology, ethics and the emotions. It presents Galen's own, Platonically inspired but distinctive, account of the nature of the mind, of the relationship between reason and emotion, and of the significance of this model for ethics. But it is also our chief source for the theories of two very important predecessors in those areas: Chrysippus, the foundational Stoic thinker, against whom he polemicizes strongly, and Posidonius, whom he regards as a much more acceptable, 'Platonizing', Stoic, and with whom he aligns his own views.

Finally, the work is remarkable for the way it brings to life the literary culture and argumentative practices of the Roman imperial period. It richly exemplifies a number of fascinating features of that culture: the elaborate and polemical techniques of argument used, in quasi-forensic manner, to prove an intellectual case; the breadth of knowledge of previous literary sources and the way that these are incorporated in the argument; the classicizing attitude to authority, whereby the 'greats' of an era long past—in this case especially Plato and Hippocrates—are treated with extreme reverence, and at the same time exploited, with sophisticated techniques of quotation and interpretation, to support the author's view.

The work was begun during Galen's first stay in Rome (162–6)—according to his account[2] he wrote the first six books during that time, addressing them to his patron Flavius Boethus—though finished later, and seems to have been part of the body of work through which he attracted attention and achieved his spectacular rise to fame and imperial patronage in the 160s.

Greek title: Περὶ τῶν Ἱπποκράτους καὶ Πλάτωνος δογμάτων (*Peri tōn Hippokratous kai Platōnos dogmatōn*)
Kühn: V.181–805
Edition: De Lacy 1978–84 (with English translation)

---

[1] Originally ten-book, but the last is lost: see *My Own Books*, chs. 3 and 5.
[2] See *My Own Books*, ch. 1.

BOOK I

[*The very beginning of Book I, in which Galen gave an account of his anatomical, and especially vivisectional, demonstrations on animals, and their evidence for the brain as the seat of cognition, is unfortunately missing, though parts can be reconstructed on the basis of self-quotations elsewhere, including summaries he gives later in this work, and of some Arabic testimonies. We begin with the first extant passage of extended argument, where Galen attacks Erasistratus' view that the arteries contain only breath* (pneuma), *and also summarizes one such famous vivisectional demonstration.*]

V.184   6. The statement of the followers of Erasistratus, that before being laid bare [the artery] contained only breath, and that it is only when it is laid bare that the blood enters it, is merely the argument of people who have no sense of shame when faced with a clear refutation. Even this shameless statement itself,

185   however, is easy enough to refute. If it were the case that I the blood had entered the pneumatic ventricle of the heart in a way contrary to the normal state, then surely all that organ's normal functions would have been upset: the arteries would no longer pulse in the same way when filled by the air from that region, and moreover a very large number of activities would be destroyed, since their source would no longer exist. (Erasistratus states that this chamber is full of vital breath, Chrysippus that it is full of psychic breath.[3]) In fact, however, the animal suffers no symptom at all. We can teach the truth of this to anyone who is interested, as, indeed we have done on many occasions, to a considerable number of doubters, by making a comparison between two animals—or even sometimes using the same animal—to show the number and variety of ailments that befall the body when a ventricle of the brain is wounded. Nor does it in fact have to be wounded: even without this, the application of pressure to one of the ventricles will immediately result in the animal's being unable to move, perceive, breathe or make sound.

186   The same thing is apparent in humans too, in trepanation. I During the removal of the broken pieces of bone you must, for safety's sake, insert an instrument called the 'meninges-protector'; and if you compress the brain slightly too strongly with this, the person becomes incapable of perception and of all voluntary motion. This does not, however, occur if pressure is applied to the bared heart. Indeed, I once allowed a person to use a smith's tongs to take hold of the heart, since it was actually jumping out of his fingers because of the

---

[3] The 'breath' or *pneuma* in question is an important element in Galen's understanding of the physiology of the major organs and vascular systems: 'psychic breath' was thought to be transmitted from and to the brain through the nerves, in the processes of voluntary motion and perception; vital breath from the heart through the arteries, regulating vital function.

violence of the pulsation; even then, however, the animal[4] suffered no impairment either of perception or of voluntary motion, rather making loud shrieks, breathing freely and moving all its limbs vehemently. It is only the motion of the arteries that is damaged by this handling of the heart; the animal suffers nothing else, but moves all its limbs, and breathes, as long as it remains alive. When pressure is applied to the brain in this way, however, the situation is entirely reversed: the arteries pulse normally, as does the heart, but no limb is moved, nor can the animal breathe or vocalize.

Now, from this something more significant I is apparent, too, namely that the   187
heart does not require the brain for its own proper motion, nor the brain the heart. That, however, is not the reason that I have mentioned this anatomical evidence; it is so that I may show that the psychic breath is contained in the ventricles of the brain. It is on this point especially that I criticize Chrysippus: he agrees that there is some pure, fine breath in the place which is the source of the soul, but he inappropriately locates this source in the heart.

One might, however, make allowance for Chrysippus, who makes the modest assertion that the heart did not grant him the knowledge that it was the source of the nerves, nor, indeed, any other of the points under enquiry in this question. He admits that he is ignorant of anatomy. Aristotle and Praxagoras, on the other hand, may rightly be criticized for their assertion that the heart is the source of the nerves. They observed many other anatomical matters accurately, as one may see from the compositions which they have left us; I but it   188
requires no very long argument to establish that they were either blind, or involved in discussions with blind people, when they wrote about the source of the nerves; one simply needs to turn to the evidence of one's senses. It is evident, as I showed previously, that some of the nerves grow directly out of the brain, while others grow out of the spinal cord, which itself grows out of the brain. Aristotle should not, then, have made the bald statement that the heart is the source of the nerves; nor should Praxagoras have made one which was based on deliberate mischievousness. Praxagoras had never seen a nerve growing out of the heart; yet he had a desire to compete with Hippocrates, and to rule out the brain as their source at all costs. He therefore embarked upon a considerable fabrication, claiming that as they proceed and divide, the arteries become narrow and change into nerves. For the body of the arteries is nerve-like, but hollow; the claim is then that as these progressively divide within the animal, I the tunics   189
collapse upon each other, and that when this first happens the vessel becomes evidently a nerve....

[4] On the basis of evidence elsewhere, Galen seems to be referring to a vivisection performed on a pig.

[*Galen continues to lay out the basics of the anatomy of the brain, heart, nerves and arteries and to point out the errors made by Aristotle and Praxagoras.*]

BOOK II

[*In the first two chapters Galen emphasizes the importance of empirical observation and discusses the various types of argument and evidence used by people in attempted 'demonstrations', pointing to the different levels of rigour or plausibility that these involve.*]

219   3. What kind of premiss, then, should we look for as appropriate and proper to the question under discussion? Certainly, much has been written about this, both by the ancient authors in their works on demonstration (works which give a rather unclear and abbreviated account) and by ourselves, in our books which give clear and lengthy exegesis of these writings.[5] It will be sufficient for the present to give a reminder of the chief point, and to use this alone as our benchmark when we attempt to discover [the truth on] the individual points. This chief point was that it is in the actual essence[6] of the matter under enquiry that we should find the appropriate and proper premisses. So, with regard to this consideration by Chrysippus of the command centre of the soul, we should give an account or definition of the essence of the matter into which we are conducting the enquiry, and use this as a standard and aim in view in our examination of all the individual points.[7]

Now, the command centre of the soul is—as they themselves have it—'the source of sensory perception and volition'.[8] There should, then, be no other basis used to show that that the heart contains this commanding-principle than

---

[5] For a list of Galen's writings of this kind, almost none of which survive, see *My Own Books*, ch. 14.

[6] *Ousia*, here meaning something's definition or what it essentially is; compare *The Shaping of the Embryo*, n. 12, with further passages mentioned there, and for another statement of this criterion of demonstrative argument see *The Soul's Dependence on the Body*, ch. 5 with n. 22.

[7] For 'standard', *kanōn*, see *Mixtures* I.8, with notes. 'Aim in view' translates *skopos*, a word which can also be rendered 'goal' or 'scope': it may mean the goal at which an argument aims as well as the central consideration by reference to which the argument is conducted.

[8] 'Command centre' translates *hēgemonikon*. The term was in standard use by Galen's period, amongst both medical and philosophical authors, to indicate the seat of intelligence and cognition; but it was originally a Stoic term of art, and it seems likely that the form of words he uses here to define it was originally a Stoic one. The use of the term here translated 'volition', *hormē*, is also an example of Galen's adoption of a technical term from a particular philosophical school, which he however uses in his own, non-doctrinaire, sense. In Stoic thought *hormē* (usually translated 'impulse') plays a very specific role in psychology and the account of action, as part of the theory, vehemently denied in this work, whereby rational assent is a precondition for *all* impulsive motions of a human being. But Galen uses the phrase *kath' hormēn*, i.e. 'according to *hormē*', interchangeably with other terms for voluntary motions, and without subscribing to any of the theory Stoics would read into the term.

that it is the source, | for all other parts of the animal's body, of all voluntary 220
motion, and that all sensory perception is brought to it. How, then, will this be
shown? How else than by anatomy? For if the heart does transmit a capacity of
both sense-perception and motion to all the individual parts, there must definitely be some vessel which grows out from it to provide these functions. It is,
then, evident on the basis of the method of demonstration that the approach
that would be of value would be to dissect animals and examine in detail what
kinds of body, and how many bodies, there are that grow out from the heart
and are connected with the other parts of the animal; then, on the basis of their
nature and number, [to show] that this one conducts sense-perception or
motion, or both, and this other one something else; and thus to conclude of
which capacities in animals the heart is the source.

Anything that falls outside this procedure is superfluous and beside the
point; and it is in this respect that a scientific premiss for a demonstration differs from one which is rhetorical, paedagogical or sophistical.[9] In this area,
however, the followers of Zeno and Chrysippus have given us no instruction in
terms of either method or paedagogical approach. So, all these kinds of premiss
are mixed up at random | in their books; very often they start with, say, a rhet- 221
orical argument, follow this with one which is paedagogical and dialectical,
then again one which is scientific, and perhaps then a rhetorical one. They do
not know that scientific premisses have their reference to the essence of the
subject under enquiry, and have this guiding-principle, while all the others have
other sources. Those which a dialectician uses for paedagogical purposes, or to
refute sophists, to make trial of a youth's intellectual 'pregnancy', or to perform
the 'delivery' and lead him towards the discovery of some truth, or to instil
doubt—all these may be called dialectical or, if you like, paedagogical or
consensus-based—I do not care about the particular term. What is important is
to distinguish these from the scientific ones; and as for those which are even
further removed, and make their point through commonplace or everyday
examples, through a form of inductive reasoning based on such examples, or
through reports of personal testimony, to these you may apply the term 'plaus-
ible', or 'rhetorical'—the name does not concern me— | but you should try to 222
recognize their nature. And still further removed from the substance of the
matter under enquiry are the sophistical ones.

The ancient authors have written about all these: in the *Sophistical Refutations*,
about the sophistical premisses, or propositions, if you prefer the term, or

---

[9] The distinctions here made between different types or levels of argument for different intellectual, rhetorical and paedagogic contexts are based on ones developed by Aristotle, especially in his
Topics, *Rhetoric* and *Sophistical Refutations*. The language of pregnancy and midwifery in this context is derived ultimately from a Platonic metaphor, developed especially in the *Theaetetus* and
Symposium.

assertions (this makes no difference for present purposes); in the *Rhetoric*, about rhetorical ones; in the *Topics*, about dialectical ones; and in *Demonstration*, which is also known as the *Second Analytics*, on scientific ones.[10] Therefore anyone who wishes to demonstrate a proposition should first understand the distinction between the types of premiss themselves; and after that should school himself for a long period of time, so that he can recognize which of the above types of premiss is being uttered when anyone is speaking; and so that, in the absence of others speaking, he can himself find them out in a way relevant to each question before him.

[*In the rest of the book, Galen gives examples of the different kinds of premiss and argument, drawing attention to the inadequacy of much argumentation that has been used by various authors in relation to the main topic of the work, anatomy and the structure of the soul.*]

BOOK III

[*In chapter 1 Galen recapitulates the discussion so far and summarizes Chrysippus' arguments that the heart is the centre of cognition and his own objections to it.*]

293   2. The point at issue was not whether the *raging faculty* of the soul is located in the heart, but whether the *reasoning faculty* is located there. It is this latter proposition which he should have demonstrated, without wasting a huge amount of effort on the raging faculty. Nor should he have filled his book with lines of poetry, for example those which he proceeds to cite:

> Sweeter, far sweeter than honey poured down inside,
> It rises high like smoke in the breasts of men;

and again:

> Spirit that raised him, up and out of his mind;

and again:

> Jumping from deep within, his spirit foretold—[11]

294   and countless other such verses, throughout the whole work, which establish that the raging faculty or spirit is in the heart. For the requirement was rather to

---

[10] Galen here mentions several treatises from Aristotle's body of works on logic and on principles and methods of argumentation. The *Second Analytics* is usually known as the *Posterior Analytics*.

[11] The lines quoted are respectively from Homer, *Iliad* XVIII.109–10 and from two unknown sources in Greek tragedy.

show that the reasoning faculty is located there; or indeed, if it was impossible to do that directly, at least to attempt to show that the raging faculty and the reasoning faculty constitute one part. He makes no such attempt in any part of the book, but takes it as an assumption....

All these verses, and countless ⏐ more besides—the vast body that Chrysippus 299/300 cites—state that the spirited part is in the heart. If I were to transcribe them all, I would fill this book, as indeed Chrysippus filled his. Well, as far as Homer is concerned, the above[12] will be sufficient; Chrysippus also transcribes a very large number of verses of Hesiod, and again it will be sufficient to mention two or three for the sake of argument:

> Then from deep down in his breast rose up his spirit

and

> Such spirit-grieving bile she harboured deep in her breast

and

> All the men's proud spirits rose up, then, in their breasts.[13]

Here I am really amazed at Chrysippus' generosity. What he should have done, as a man who had read so many poets, and who realized perfectly well that, as Plutarch showed in his *Homeric Exercises*, they bear witness to any doctrine you like in one or another of their verses, was to choose those verses which actually bear witness to the doctrine which he was keen to prove, ⏐ and to omit those which conflict with 301 it and indeed, in some cases, establish the precise opposite. Yet he mentions all of them indiscriminately. He should have omitted all verses of this latter sort, and assembled only those in which a poet stated that mind, intelligence, intellect and reasoning were contained in the heart, verses such as the following:

> Then indeed from the breast of Athamas Zeus took his mind

and

> Yes, earth-shaker, you know the thoughts in my breast

and

> Always then this thought remained in your breast

and

> No such thought indeed remains in my breast.[14]

---

[12] In the passage omitted before these sentences, Galen has just quoted thirty-eight lines or part lines from Homer which he says were cited by Chrysippus in support of his view.

[13] The first two of these lines are fragments attributed to Hesiod; the third is from Hesiod, *Theogony* 641.

[14] The four lines are respectively a fragment attributed to Hesiod; Homer, *Iliad* XX.20; *Odyssey* XIII.330 and XVII.403 (the last quoted approximately).

The other kind of verse, that which shows the *affections* of the soul in the heart, is extremely abundant amongst the poets; but there is no shortage, either, of this kind just cited, which enable one to show that on the basis of the poets' opinions the reasoning faculty is in the heart.

302 3. It is this latter kind alone that Chrysippus should have chosen—given, that is, that he thought fit to decide the contest on the basis of testimonies. Now, as a matter of fact, if one wanted to represent this enquiry truthfully, it would be fairer to cite more of the others, and fewer of this kind just cited, for that would represent their true relative frequency. But for one wishing to establish Chrysippus' view, of course, this would be self-defeating, especially when it comes to texts which make a clear opposition between reason and spirit, such as the following:

> Striking his breast he upbraided his heart then with these words:
> Brave it, my heart, now; you suffered a worse thing before this.[15]

This is what Homer had Odysseus say to himself when, after he had observed the actions of the serving-women in his house, the heat in his heart had started to seethe and his spirit was about to conquer his reasoning faculty and rush him into a premature attempt to punish the women. For the relationship of reasoning faculty to spirit is the same as that of a horseman to his horse or of a 303 houndsman to his hounds. | It is right in all cases that the naturally greater should rule and be in control—the horseman over the horse, the houndsman over the hounds and the reasoning faculty over spirit—but it does not always happen in reality that the pairing is maintained according to the rule of nature. Sometimes a disobedient horse runs wild and out of control, and carries his rider with him, the latter being unable to win the contest either because of his inadequate capacity or because of his ignorance of the science of horsemanship; and sometimes a strong spirit rushing towards an ill-timed revenge drags a weak or ignorant reasoning faculty vehemently along with it. If they have strength and knowledge, then the reasoning faculty and the charioteer will control the spirit and the horse, respectively. If, however, they lack either or both, then the danger arises that what is lesser by nature will take control over what is greater.

Spirit is greater than the reasoning faculty amongst the Scythians and the Galatians, and amongst many other barbarian peoples; and so it is amongst our own people, in the case of both children and uneducated adults. It is this point that Homer wishes to make by presenting Hector and Achilles, as well as cer-304 tain other such characters, as | youths who are slaves to their spirit or anger, while Odysseus, Polydamas and Nestor control their spirit by their reasoning

---

[15] The well-known lines are from Homer, *Odyssey* XX.17–18; see next note.

faculty—in many instances so strongly that the spirit does not even make a rush towards any non-rational action. In some instances, meanwhile, it does do so, but is held back by the reasoning faculty, as in the lines he writes of Odysseus....[16]

If Homer in these lines is not giving a clear account of the conflict, within a man of temperance, between the spirit and the reasoning faculty, and of the spirit's ready obedience to that reasoning faculty, then there can be no further agreement as to how we might understand the poet. If people are going to cast doubt on such clear statements as these, then there will be no possibility of using the rest of his statements. Odysseus sees the misdeeds of the serving women, is pulled forcibly by his spirit towards their punishment, but is then restrained by his reasoning faculty, which explains to him that the moment is not opportune. And, since the reasoning faculty was not easily able to persuade the spirit to ⎸put off the punishment to a more suitable time, the former engaged the latter with considerable vehemence, like a charioteer forcibly pulling back a horse which is running out of control, and using a strong rein; and thus the reasoning faculty says this to it: 'Endure for the present, my most noble heart, just as you did with the Cyclops, when you saw your comrades being killed by him.' 305 306

Now, it seems to me that Plato's reference to those lines, in book IV of the *Republic*,[17] is extremely pertinent, while Chrysippus' is extremely out of place; and the latter's citation of the lines Euripides gives to Medea, again in a case of the civil war between reason and spirit, even more so. For she knew what an unholy and terrible deed she was doing by murdering her children, and that is why she hesitated and held back, not rushing immediately into the act. But her spirit, like some disobedient horse which has overcome the charioteer, dragged her by force towards the children; then again the reasoning faculty resisted and pulled her away; and then again the spirit pulled her in the opposite direction, then again the reasoning faculty. And so she was repeatedly pulled backwards and forwards by both of them. It is at the moment when she gives ⎸way to her spirit that Euripides has her say: 307

> And, yes, I know what evil I will do;
> But spirit masters all considered thought.[18]

Of course she knows the enormity of the wrongs that she is about to do, since her reasoning faculty teaches her this; yet she states that her spirit is stronger than her reasoning faculty, and that therefore she is drawn forcibly to the

---

[16] Galen proceeds to quote the full passage from the *Odyssey* (XX.5–22), describing Odysseus' inner conflict as he sees the misdeeds in his house, with his heart 'barking' within him and Odysseus rebuking and controlling it.
[17] Plato, *Republic* IV, 441b–c.   [18] Euripides, *Medea* 1078–9.

deed—the opposite case to that of Odysseus, who restrains his spirit by his reasoning faculty. Euripides gave us Medea as an example of barbarians and people untrained by education, people in whom spirit is stronger than reasoning faculty. In Greeks and in people trained by education, on the other hand—whom the Poet has exemplified to us with Odysseus—the reasoning faculty is stronger than the spirit.

Frequently the reasoning faculty is so much stronger than the spirited part of the soul that a conflict never arises between them: | the former rules and the latter is ruled. This is the case with those who have arrived at the goal of philosophy. Conversely, it often happens that the spirit has such control over the reasoning faculty that it constantly rules and leads it; and this is observed in many barbarian people, as well as in children who are naturally spirited, and in a number of wild animals and human beings of the wilder sort. Sometimes, however, neither is so much stronger as immediately to overcome the other, but instead there is an opposition and conflict between them, which is won sometimes by reason, as in the case of Odysseus, and sometimes by spirit, as in the case of Medea. For there are two parts of the soul involved here, or at any rate two capacities. Chrysippus, however, while holding that there are no parts of the soul, nor any non-rational capacities of the soul distinct from the rational one, nonetheless does not hesitate to make reference to these lines of Odysseus and Medea, which manifestly refute his opinion.

[*In the rest of the book Galen continues to argue against Chrysippus' insistence on the heart as the seat of cognition, and on his failure to make a distinction between the rational and non-rational parts of the soul; and he presents further evidence of Chrysippus' erroneous manner of argumentation on the basis of both literary sources and popular notions and linguistic usages.*]

BOOK IV

[*Galen begins the book by blaming his opponents for the length of time he has had to spend refuting false arguments, and by summarizing his opposition to the erroneous views of Chrysippus. He then proceeds to address inconsistencies between Chrysippus' works.*]

365   1. Now, in the first book of his work on *The Soul*, Chrysippus, so far from denying the existence of the spirited and desiderative in the soul, actually gives an exposition of their affections and assigns them a single place in the body. Throughout the whole of his *Affections*, however—that is, the three books in which he considers the enquiry from a theoretical point of view—and also the book on *Therapy*, to which some also give the title *Ethics*, his view is found to be

different. Here, he writes sometimes as it were on both sides of the question, at others as if he holds that there is no such thing as a desiderative or spirited capacity of the soul....

2. ...In the first definitions which he writes of the broad categories of affection, 366 he completely departs from the view of [the ancient writers], defining distress as a *fresh belief that an evil is present*; fear as an *expectation of evil*; pleasure as a *fresh belief that a good is present*. These definitions in themselves involve the mention of the rational in the soul alone, with the omission of the desiderative and spirited; for he holds that this 'belief' and 'expectation' arise in the rational alone. In the definition of desire, meanwhile, which he states to be a 'non-rational urge', I he seems by virtue of this expression to be speaking of the non- 367 rational capacity within the soul. Yet here too he departs from that in his explanation of the term: even the 'urge' included in that definition belongs to the rational capacity. So, indeed, he defines it as a 'rational urge arising in the case of something which provides pleasure to the extent that it should'.

But while in the above definitions he holds that the affections are urges, beliefs and judgements, in some of those that then follow he writes in a way more in agreement with Epicurus and Zeno than with his own doctrines. For he states, in his definition of distress, that it is a *diminution arising from something which it appears should be avoided*, while pleasure is an *elevation arising from something which it appears should be chosen*. 'Diminutions', 'elevations', 'contractions' and 'expansions' (he sometimes uses these terms too) are affections of the non-rational capacity, arising from beliefs. Indeed, it seems to me extraordinary that he is so imprecise in a work which claims to offer both a precise and a logical account.

It is not only here that he manifestly disagrees with himself, I but also when, 368 writing about the definitions of affection, he states it to be a 'non-rational, contrary-to-nature motion of the soul', and an 'impulse in excess', and then both states that he takes 'non-rational' here to mean 'without reason and judgement' and gives as an example of 'impulse in excess' people running energetically. Both these are in conflict with the notion of affections as judgements.

[*In a passage which is a well-known source for the Stoic theory of action, Galen cites at length Chrysippus' analogy between an excessive impulse and legs running out of control.*]

4. ...Chrysippus here manifestly points to the two different meanings of the 385 term 'non-rational' actually in use amongst Greek-speakers: as either opposite to what is reasonable, or in no way partaking of reason. Now, what is opposite to the reasonable is error, or poor judgement. The other sense, that of completely devoid I of reason, is [provided by] impulse and motion in [a state of] 386 affection.... Whatever bad *judgements* someone makes do not involve a

rejection of reason, but rather a mistake within reason, whereas whatever *impulses* are brought about, without recourse to reason, through spirit or desire, these he calls 'non-rational' [*a-logon*] in the other sense, where, as we have said, the letter *a* provides a refutation or denial of the meaning of that to which it is attached. The motion of the soul which is disobedient to reason is non-rational in *this* sense, which includes the complete non-employment of reason.

For if it were the case that we used reason in this motion too, then Chrysippus' statement in the first book of *Affections* would be incorrect, where he says not that one 'is moved through an error, and overlooking something which is in accord with reason', but 'through a rejection of and disobedience to reason'; and

387 so too in the *Therapy of Affections*, | in the passage just cited, where he denies that the sense of 'non-rational', in the definition of affection, is that of opposite to good reason, stating rather that the sense is that of disobedient to and having rejected reason. So, indeed, he adds: 'Such states are, as it were, uncontrolled, as though the person is not controlling himself, but is carried away, just as those who run energetically are carried on forward, unable to control such motion. Those, meanwhile, who are moved in accordance with reason, of whatever kind that is, and steer with this as their leader, either control, or are unaffected by, such motion and the impulses involved in it.'

Here the addition of the phrase 'of whatever kind that is', qualifying 'reason', clearly indicates the distinction of affection from error. For whether this reason is healthy and true or poor and false, one who is moved in accordance with it will never be in a state of affection. In the case of true reason, he is moved appropriately and correctly, in the case of false reason, in a faulty and error-

388 ridden way. When it is reason that leads, either virtue | or error follows, but never affection. For example, to hold that pleasure is the good, as does Epicurus, is an erroneous and false reasoning, and will inevitably produce faulty and error-ridden outcomes in terms of all those actions and individual motions of the soul which faultily aim at pleasure as their goal, but it will not produce affection. The specific characteristic of affection consists, precisely, in the soul's being moved *without* reason....

389 He even adds: 'Therefore | motions which are in this way non-rational are known as affections, and as contrary to nature, inasmuch as they go outside the rational framework'. How, here, are we take 'in this way'? Evidently, in the sense of 'without any reason, and having rejected that reason which Nature has given us as the leader of all individual activities'. In the affections, however, it is not what leads, which is why he states, and quite rightly, that all the motions that take place in affection have gone outside the rational framework. For if the rational framework of a living being has reason as its leader, whereas reason is not what leads or has power over the motions that take place in affection, the person moved by affection has gone beyond his rational nature.

If, however, reason is not what leads in the case of impulse, then the follow-ers of Chrysippus should give us some answer as to what that leader is. It is no use for them to say that it is neither reason nor any other capacity: in that case they would be conceding the notion of an uncaused movement, something that they insist should be absolutely avoided; indeed, they attack Epicurus for his postulation of such a movement. Since, then, in the common view of nearly all the philosophers I —not only Chrysippus, Plato and Aristotle—nothing hap-   390
pens without a cause, they must provide us with an answer to the cause of motion in affection....

6. Chrysippus himself concedes, not just once or twice, but on a large number   403
of occasions, that there is in our souls some capacity other than the rational which is responsible for affection. This we may understand from statements such as those in which he blames 'poor tension' and weakness of the soul for wrongful actions.[19] These are the terms he uses, alongside their opposites, 'good tension' and strength. For he attributes the wrongful actions of human beings either to faulty judgement or to poor tension and weakness of the soul; just as, conversely, right actions are guided by correct judgement along with good tension of the soul. In such cases, though, just as judgement is the task of the rational soul, so good tension is the vigour and excellence of a capacity distinct from the rational, a capacity which Chrysippus himself calls 'tension'. I This tension, he claims,   404
sometimes departs from correct decisions, when the energy of the soul falls short, failing at some point to keep to the instructions of reason and to perform them in full. In such statements he gives a clear indication of the true nature of affection.

Let me actually transcribe a passage in which he expounds this, from the first book of *Affections*:

> It is perhaps in this respect, moreover, that the tensions of the body are called 'poor' or 'good', in relation to that which is nerve-like[20] in body, and in refer-ence to the fact that we either have or lack capacity for the tasks performed through these tensions; and the tension in the soul is described as poor or good.

And then:

> Just as when someone is running or holding on to something, and in other similar activities which are performed by means of the nerves, there is an achieving state, and also a yielding state, in which the nerves have already

[19] *Atonia* ('poor tension') and *eutonia* ('good tension') are derivatives of the word *tonos*, which has a precise physical sense, applied for example to the tension of cords or muscles, but may also be used to indicate various kinds of bodily, or emotional, 'tension' or energy. The distinction between a literal and physical sense and a metaphorical one, applied to the soul, is not always clear, especially in the context of the Stoic theory which understands motions of the soul in a physical sense. See also below, VII.3, with n. 57.

[20] Or 'sinewy'; and similarly 'nerves' (*neura*) later in these quotations could be translated 'sinews'.

been released and relaxed, there is, analogously, something nerve-like in the
soul, by virtue of which we say, metaphorically, that people either have nerves
or lack them.

And he continues, in explanation of this very statement:

405   Some people are unable to withstand frightening events, some I dissolve or
crumple when reward or punishment is meted out, and there are similar reac-
tions to a whole range of similar situations. Each such event overcomes us and
enslaves us, so that we give in to it, betraying friends and cities, or giving ourselves over to all kinds of unseemly actions, as our previous motion has been
dissolved. Such, for example, is Menelaus, in Euripides' portrayal. He draws
his sword and moves towards Helen to destroy her, then sees her beauty and is
bowled over by it, and casts aside the sword, unable even to continue holding
on to it. This, indeed, is the grounds for the rebuke which was addressed to him:

You saw the woman's breast and dropped your sword,
You kissed her, fawned upon the traitorous bitch.[21]

All of which is perfectly correct on Chrysippus' part, but conflicts with the
notion that affections are judgements....

[Galen offers further arguments that the mythological and poetic examples cited by
Chrysippus support the view of an internal conflict between parts or capacities of
the soul, against the Chrysippean model.]

416   7. ...I shall turn now to some of Posidonius' responses to Chrysippus. 'For
example', he says:

the very definition of 'blindness' [atē], like many such definitions stated by
Zeno and written down by Chrysippus, clearly refutes his own view. He states
that distress is a fresh belief that an evil is present to him. Speaking more concisely, they sometimes put it thus: 'distress is the freshly acquired belief in the
presence of an evil'.

Now, he points out that 'fresh' means recent, and asks to be told the cause by
which a belief in [present] evil contracts the soul and brings about distress,
while one which has been there for a considerable time contracts it either not at
all or at least to a lesser extent. This term 'fresh' should in fact not have been
417   part of I the definition, if Chrysippus' view is true. According to this it is not the
'freshness' of the belief that should be stated, but that the belief relates to [the
presence of] an evil which is large, unbearable or unmasterable—the term he in
fact habitually uses.

---

[21] The verse lines were quoted by Chrysippus from Euripides, *Andromache* 629–30.

Here Posidonius counters Chrysippus on two kinds of ground. With regard to this, Chrysippus' second definition, he makes reference to the wise and to those making progress. The former group consider themselves to be in the best possible state, while the latter consider themselves to be in the midst of the greatest of evils; yet neither therefore succumbs to affection. With regard to the first definition, he asks the reason why it is not a belief in the presence of evil, but only a *fresh* belief in it, that brings about distress. And why is it, he asks, that anything for which we are unprepared, and which is strange to us, when it comes upon us all at once, shocks us and removes us from our previous cognitive state, whereas something in which we are trained and to which we are accustomed, and which has been present for some time, either does not have this effect, thus moving us to affection, or has it to a very small extent indeed?

For this reason, he states that we should 'preinhabit' circumstances, and treat future events as though they were present. The term 'preinhabit', for Posidonius, refers to a process of forming | a kind of internal construction or image of the   418 future event, and gradually producing, as it were, a habituation to it. That is why he at this point even mentioned the saying attributed to Anaxagoras, who, on hearing the news of his son's death, responded, with complete self-control: 'I knew that I had begotten a mortal.'[22] ...

Chrysippus in fact himself concedes that affections eventually come to an   420 end, even though the belief remains; the reason for this phenomenon, he says, is difficult to work out....

Posidonius correctly criticizes the following statement of Chrysippus, too: 424

It may happen that the impulse remains, but that what follows from that is not in line with it, because of some other state that arises.

It is absurd, he says, that the impulse should be present but that the activity which accords with it be impeded by some other cause. Chrysippus also says:

So, too, | people weeping cease to do so, and those who do not wish to weep do   425 so, when the circumstances that present themselves produce impressions which are discordant.

Here, too, Posidonius asks the reason why the great mass of people often weep without wanting to, and are unable to restrain their tears, while others, who wish to continue weeping, stop. Surely it is because of the affective motions, in these cases either being so strong that they cannot be controlled by the will, or having ceased so completely that they cannot be stirred up by it. We discover here, then, the conflict and the distinction between reason and affection; and the notion of capacities in the soul is preserved. For the above phenomena

---

[22] At this point Galen proceeds to quote the lines from Euripides about imagining grief in advance which appear also in *Freedom from Distress* (sections 52 and 77).

occur not, for heavens' sake, as Chrysippus has it, because of some sort of cause which reason cannot work out, but because of those causes stated by the ancient authors. It was not only Aristotle or Plato who held this belief; there were others even earlier, such as Pythagoras. Indeed, Posidonius claims that this doctrine was originally that of Pythagoras, but that Plato worked it out and presented it more fully.

This, then, is the reason why it is obviously the case that habits, and in gen-
426   eral, ⎮ the passage of time, have such great power in relation to the affective motions. The non-rational part of the soul becomes 'adapted'[23] in the habits within which it is nurtured and, as has been stated before, in time there is a cessation from affection, as the non-rational capacities of the soul are [sufficiently] filled with the things which they previously desired. Rational opinions, judgements, forms of scientific knowledge and specialized skill, how-ever, do not appear to become difficult to remove simply because of the passage of time itself, nor indeed to change and cease, like distress and other affections. Who ever abandoned, or changed his mind on, the proposition that 'two times two is four' because he became sated with it through the passage of time? Or the proposition that all radii of a circle are equal? So, too, with any other theorem: no one ever put aside his previous opinion through satiety, as people put aside weeping, being distressed, crying, groaning and lamenting and all such states, even when the assumption that the event that has taken place was an evil remains intact....

BOOK V

[*Galen begins the book by summarizing again the argument against Chrysippus' heart-centred, monistic view of the soul, before proceeding to highlight what he takes to be a difference between his position and that of the Stoic founding father Zeno, as well as the rejection of Chrysippus' view by the later Stoic Posidonius.*]

429   1. ...Now, Chrysippus, in the first book of his *Affections*, attempts to demon-strate that the affections are certain judgements of the rational, while Zeno held that the affections of the soul were not the judgements themselves, but the con-tractions and expansions, elevations and lowerings that arise from them. Posidonius, differing from both of them, praises and embraces the doctrine of Plato; and he counters the followers of Chrysippus, showing that the affections are neither judgements nor things arising from judgements, but certain motions

---

[23]   Galen here adopts another Stoic technical term, the verb *oikeiousthai*, connected to the developmental concept of *oikeiōsis*; on this see n. 25.

of different, non-rational capacities of the soul, which Plato termed desiderative and spirited.

[*In the rest of the first four chapters Galen exposes confusions and errors in Chrysippus' account of the analogy between soul and body, in particular in relation to the concepts of the health and disease, and of the beauty and ugliness, of both, and again praises Posidonius for supporting preferable views.*]

5. But let us deal only with those things which are most necessary for the present study, and first amongst these let us address the question of the maintenance[24] of children. It is not possible to say that their impulses are governed by reason, for they do not yet possess reason; nor is it possible to say that they do not experience rage, distress and pleasure, or that they do not laugh and cry and undergo all sorts of other such affections. Indeed, the affections are greater in number and more vehement in children than in adults. But these facts are in conflict with the doctrines of Chrysippus, as well as with the proposition that there is no natural inclination[25] towards pleasure or alienation from pain. All children rush towards pleasures, without any teaching, and they shrink from and avoid pains. Moreover, we observe them in states of rage, kicking, biting, wanting to win and to dominate other children, just as we observe these phenomena in certain animals, although there is no prize offered beyond the conquest itself. Such behaviour is, for example, clearly observed in the quail, the cock, the partridge, the mongoose, the asp, | the crocodile and many others.[26]   460

So, it is evident that children too have a natural inclination to pleasure and victory, just as, at a somewhat later stage of their development, they show themselves to have some natural inclination towards what is fine and noble. It is for this reason that they experience shame at their errors, as they grow older, as well as taking pleasure in fine deeds and laying claim to justice and the other virtues, and performing many actions in accordance with their notions of these virtues, whereas previously, when they were still small, they lived according to

---

[24] By 'maintenance' (*dioikēsis*) is meant here the way that a creature or organism is internally governed or regulated. See also *My Own Doctrines*, n. 14, *The Art of Medicine*, ch. 5 with n. 13 and *The Shaping of the Embryo*.

[25] The word translated is *oikeiōsis*, a key term in Stoic philosophy. It may also be translated 'adaptation', 'familiarization' or 'appropriation', and has the literal sense of 'making [something] one's own'. In Stoic theory it is used to describe the educative or developmental process whereby a child gradually expands his or her sense of belonging, or of what s/he is a part of, beginning with the self and ending with an understanding of one's nature as a social being and one's place in the universe. Galen seems to use the term in a significantly different sense from the Stoic one, to indicate simply our inborn inclinations to pleasure or pain, rather than our natural sense of what is one's own or in one's own interest. And he interprets the Stoics as believing that there is a natural inclination only toward virtue, not towards pleasure. (Compare the similar argument at *The Soul's Dependence on the Body*, ch. 11, with n. 61.)

[26] Galen's point here is that pre- or non-rational creatures (both children and animals) possess not just a natural pleasure-seeking and pain-avoidance instinct, but also a competitive one—that is, they are endowed with (in Platonic terms) both the desiderative and the spirited capacities.

their affections and took no heed of the instructions of reason. There are, then, these three inclinations naturally within us, one according with the form of each of the soul's parts: an inclination towards pleasure, because of the desiderative part; an inclination towards victory, because of the spirited; and an inclination towards what is fine and noble, because of the rational. Epicurus observed only the inclination of the worst part of the soul, while Chrysippus, stating that we are inclined only towards the fine and noble (which obviously is to be equated with the good), observed only that of the best. It was only the
461   ancient philosophers who succeeded in observing all three inclinations. |

Since, then, he overlooks two of them, it is understandable that Chrysippus is at a loss to explain the origin of vice. He is unable to state either its cause or the ways in which it comes into being; nor is he able to discover how it is that children fall into error. For all of this Posidonius—quite reasonably, in my view—criticizes and refutes him. If children have an inclination to the good right from the beginning, then it would have to be the case that vice arises in them not from an internal source—not from themselves—but from an external one. Yet it is observed that even children who have been nurtured in good habits and properly educated invariably make some errors; and indeed Chrysippus himself concedes this. He could, of course, have deliberately ignored the manifest facts and conceded only what was consistent with his own assumptions: he could have claimed that if children are well brought up they invariably become wise men in the course of time. He did not, however, dare to produce such a great falsification of observed reality. In fact, he admits that even when children are nurtured under the sole supervision of a philosopher, and neither see nor
462   hear any example of | vice whatever, it does not necessarily follow that they will become philosophers; for, he claims, there are two causes of corruption, one arising from communion with the mass of humanity, the other from the very nature of things.

I have a problem with both these types of cause. First, with that which comes about from contact with those around one: why would one not hate and avoid any example of vice, if one has no natural inclination towards it? This seems to me a very strange notion; and even stranger that one should be deceived by the things themselves, before having seen or heard them. By what compulsion should children be enticed by pleasure as a good, when they have no inclination to it, or reject and avoid pain, if they are not, also, by nature alienated from it? By what compulsion should they be drawn towards praise and honour, and enjoy these, while they hate and avoid ill repute and dishonour, if they do not, here too, have some natural inclination and alienation in respect of these? It seems that Chrysippus concedes the implication, if not the explicit formulation,
463   of these statements, | that is to say that there is in us some natural inclination and alienation with regard to each of these things. For when he says that

corruption, in relation to matters of good and evil, arises in inferior individuals because of the plausibility of impressions and because of the communion, one should ask him the reason why pleasure produces a plausible impression of good and pain a plausible impression of evil. Also why, if we hear victory at the Olympic Games, or the setting-up of statues, being praised and celebrated by the mass of individuals as good things, or defeat and dishonour discussed as bad things, we readily go along with this. On this point, too, Posidonius attacks him, attempting to show that the causes of all false suppositions in the theoretical realm derive from the pull of the affective,[27] but that this is preceded by false opinions when the rational is in a weak state in terms of its judgement; and that impulse in an animal is sometimes produced as a result of a judgement of the rational, but often as a result of a motion of the affective.

Posidonius also quite reasonably connects this discussion to that of the facts observed by | physiognomists, pointing out that, amongst both animals and 464 men, those which are broad-chested and hotter are all also more naturally inclined to rage, while those which are wide-hipped and colder are more timid. He also mentions that there are considerable regional variations in human beings' timidity or daring, and in their inclination to pleasure or to work, since the affective motions of the soul always depend on the state of the body, which is altered to a great extent by the mixture of the ambient climate. He states, too, that the blood in animals differs in its hotness or coldness, in its thickness or thinness, and in other important respects, which were discussed at length by Aristotle.[28] We shall refer to these at the appropriate point later in our discussion, when we transcribe the actual passages of Hippocrates and Plato on the subject. My present argument is directed toward the followers of Chrysippus, who understand nothing about the affections, and in particular do not understand that the mixtures of the body produce the affective motions appropriate to themselves. | 'Affective motions' is the term that Posidonius habitually used; 465 Aristotle, on the other hand, goes ahead and calls all such states of the soul 'characters', and explained in what way they arise from the different mixtures.[29]

---

[27] De Lacy and others (though not Müller) have taken it that, in order for this to be a consistent assertion of Posidonius' position on the division between rational and affective, some words must be missing here; so, De Lacy's version of the Greek would give: 'in the theoretical realm <come about through ignorance, but in the practical> derive from the pull of the affective'. The need for such an emendation is less clear to me; Posidonius' view may rather be of a complex interaction of rational and affective, whereby the 'affective pull' leads to false propositional views. (Compare the argument at *Affections and Errors* I.5, p. 467 below, on the soul's becoming quickly filled with affections in the absence of the correct precepts.) Such interaction indeed seems to be what is emphasized in the following sentences.

[28] See the passages from Aristotle cited in the *The Soul's Dependence on the Body*, ch. 7, pp. 443–6 below, both on physiognomical matters and on the relationship between qualities of blood and animal characteristics.

[29] 'Characters' (*ēthē*) is De Lacy's emendation of the manuscript reading *ēdē* ('already', 'actually'); if it is not accepted, we should translate rather: 'Aristotle goes ahead and actually calls all such [things] states of the soul.'

This, I suppose, is why the cure of the affections of the soul is easy and straightforward in some, because the affective motions are not strong in them, nor the rational naturally weak and lacking in intelligence, such people being, rather, compelled into a state of affection by ignorance and bad habits, while in others it is difficult and not straightforward, when the affective motions, which arise unavoidably because of the state of the body, happen to be very large and vehement, while the rational happens to be naturally weak and unintelligent. In order for such a person to be improved in his character, the rational part must acquire knowledge of what is true, while the affective motions must at the same time be dulled, by being habituated to good practices.

So, indeed, one should shape a human being with the best aim in view from the very beginning: one should, first of all, exercise care with regard to the
466   actual seeds; I then, with regard to the daily regime that the pregnant mother should follow, in respect of nourishment, drink, exercise, rest, sleep and waking, desire and spirit, and other such matters. Plato gave a very precise account of them all. Chrysippus, on the other hand, failed, not only to make any adequate statement of these himself, but also to leave to his followers any starting-point from which they might proceed to their discovery; for the foundation he laid down for the argument was a faulty one. In this area even Posidonius criticizes him, while also expressing admiration for Plato's statements, both on the shaping of children while they are still in the womb and on their nurture and education after birth. In the first book of his composition on *Affections* he has written what is in effect a summary of these, to the effect that children should be nurtured and educated with a view to making the affective part of the soul well-balanced in its motions, as well as readily obedient to the instructions of reason. The best education of children is that preparation of the affective part of the soul which will make it be as liable as possible to the domination of the rational.[30]

467   For, as he argues, the latter is small and weak to begin with, I but becomes big and strong by about the fourteenth year, by which time it should already be controlling and commanding, like a charioteer, the pair of kindred horses, that is, desire and spirit, which should be neither excessively strong nor weak, hesitant nor headstrong, nor, in general, disobedient, wild or disorderly, but rather willing to follow and obey the reasoning faculty in all respects. Now, the education and virtue of the reasoning faculty itself consists in the knowledge of the nature of reality, as, according the analogy, that of the charioteer is the theoretical knowledge of chariot-driving. Knowledge, however, the argument goes,

---

[30] This sentence is printed in quotation marks by De Lacy, and regarded as a fragment of Posidonius' work by Edelstein–Kidd (fr. 148), though this seem to me uncertain. In general, the precise boundary between Galen's statement of his own views and his transmission of Posidonius', in this passage, is not completely clear.

cannot arise in the non-rational capacities of the soul, any more than it can in horses: these acquire their own proper virtue from some form of non-rational habituation, while the charioteers acquire it from rational instruction.

Immediately following on this is the discussion of virtues; and here too there are two kinds of blunder, one in taking all virtues to be forms of knowledge, the other in taking them all to be capacities. For in the non-rational parts of the soul, the virtues too must necessarily be non-rational, | while that of the rational 468 part alone must be a rational one. It thus seems reasonable to suppose that the virtues of the former alone are capacities, while knowledge is the virtue only of the rational. Chrysippus makes a great blunder here, not in his failure to regard any virtue as a capacity—this is not a major one, and we are not making this a point of issue—but in stating that there are many forms of knowledge and many virtues, but only one capacity of the soul. For it is impossible for there to be many virtues of one capacity, unless, equally, there were many forms of perfection of one thing. There is, in fact, one type of perfection for every thing, and 'virtue' is the perfection of the nature of each—as indeed he himself concedes. (Aristo of Chios, in fact, has a better view, denying that there are many virtues of the soul, and declaring rather that there is one, namely 'knowledge of things good and bad', and thus not giving an account of the affections which is in contradiction to his own assumptions, which is what Chrysippus does.)

6. But we shall return to the virtues subsequently, since Chrysippus attacks Plato on this subject too. Here I have mentioned them simply through a kind of logical consequence, | since one's doctrine on the virtues follows by necessity 469 upon one's doctrine of the affections. Posidonius makes this point, too, near the beginning of the first book of his work on *Affections*; these are his actual words:

> I believe that the investigation of good and evil, that of goals and that of vir-
> tues depend upon the correct investigation of the affections.

The fact that the correct opinion on virtues is indeed bound to that on affections has now, I suppose, been sufficiently indicated; as for the fact that this is true also of the opinion regarding goods and that regarding the goal, I will content myself with transcribing Posidonius' words, which are as follows:

> The cause of affections, that is to say, the cause of the absence of concord, and
> of an unhappy life, is the failure to follow in all things that inborn guiding
> spirit[31] within us, which is of the same nature as the spirit which maintains

[31] The term *daimōn* (translated 'guiding spirit' both here and below, V.2, in a quotation from Plato on which Posidonius is surely drawing) has a traditional religious significance, where it may refer to supernatural beings quite broadly; but in Plato it is used to refer to a very specific kind of entity, one which is intermediate between gods and mortals. The term translated 'evil-spirited' at the end of the paragraph is the derivative *kako-daimōn*. This and the related *eu-daimonikon* (translated as 'good-spirited' in the next extended quotation) would more usually be translated in terms

the whole universe; and instead at some time to fall in with and be dragged along by the worse spirit within us, the beast-like one. Those who ignore this neither give a good account of the cause of the affections nor arrive at the correct opinion regarding the good life and concord. For they do not see that the

470   primary element of such a life | is to avoid being dragged along by the non-rational, evil-spirited and godless part of the soul.

In these words Posidonius gave clear instruction on the extent of the error of the followers of Chrysippus, not only in their reasoning on the affections, but also in their reasoning on the goal of life. This is 'to live in concord with nature', but in the sense that Plato taught, not in the sense that they mean it.[32] For, since there is a better and a worse part of the soul, the person who follows the better may be said to live in a way which is in concord with nature, while the one who tends rather to follow the worse may be said to live without that concord. The latter lives a life of affection, the former one in accord with reason. Not content with this, Posidonius makes a still more manifest and vehement assault on the incorrect account of the goal of life given by followers of Chrysippus. The passage is as follows:

Some, overlooking this, contract the notion of 'living in concord' to that of doing everything admissible for the sake of those things which are 'first by nature'—thus making it similar to the establishment of the goal as pleasure, freedom from disturbance, or some other such object. This displays an incon-

471   sistency | in the very way of stating it, and nothing fine or good-spirited at all. For such things follow as necessary consequences of the goal, but are not themselves the goal. Now, once this distinction too has been correctly made, it is possible to use it to remove the confusions which the sophists put forward, but it is not possible so to use the notion of 'living in accordance with the experience of what happens in the whole of nature'—which has the same force as that of saying 'to live in concord when this does not conduce to the achievement, in a small-spirited way, of indifferents.'[33]

of 'unhappiness' and 'happiness', but in the present context a close connection with the notion of the actual *daimōn* within us seems clearly intended.

[32] The phrase quoted, 'to live in concord' (*homologoumenōs zēn*) was the classic formula offered by the early Stoics for the goal of life; it sometimes appears also in the form 'to live in concord with nature' (*phusei*).

[33] The passage is difficult to follow, possibly contaminated by textual errors, and full of technical Stoic jargon. The phrase 'living in accordance with the experience...' is supposed to have been put forward by Chrysippus as an equivalent to 'living in concord with nature', and it is this equivalence that Posidonius is attacking. 'Indifferents' is technical term of Stoic philosophy, referring to things which may be worthy of choice or rejection in general terms or other things being equal, but are not in themselves of ethical significance (I here read *adiaphorōn* for the MSS *diaphorōn*). A 'preferred indifferent', such as good health, would be roughly equivalent to something 'first by nature'. The thrust of Posidonius' argument is that there are some Stoics, including Chrysippus, who have understood the fundamental tenet of 'living in concord (with nature)' in such a way that it looks more like the pursuit of pleasure—an interpretation which is to be rejected.

Now, this might be sufficient to indicate the incongruity of Chrysippus' statements about the end, in his account of how one may achieve this 'living in concord with nature'. Still, I think that it will be better to add also the following passage of Posidonius, which is as follows:

> Once the cause of the affections was discerned, it removed this incongruity, showing the sources of the corruption that arises within the domain of things that are to be sought or avoided. It also distinguished the relevant modes of training and clarified the confusions regarding that [form of] impulse which is due to affection.

These, then, are not trivial or random benefits that he claims we shall derive from the ǀ discovery of the cause of the affections: we have been helped by this 472 discovery to an accurate understanding of what 'living in concord with nature' actually is. A person in the grip of affection does not live in concord with nature; a person not in its grip does live such a life. For the former is following that which is non-rational and unreliable in the soul, the latter that which is rational and godlike.

As regards the first sentence in the above quotation: some mistakenly believe those things which are appropriate to the non-rational capacities of the soul are appropriate in absolute terms; such people do not realize that to take pleasure and to dominate one's neighbour are the things sought by the beast-like [part] of the soul, while wisdom and all that is good and fine are the things sought by that which is rational and godlike.

As regards the second sentence: we prescribe routines involving different rhythms, harmonies and practices for different people, as Plato taught us; we should nurture those who are dull, sluggish and lacking in spirit with the use of strong rhythms and harmonies which move the soul vigorously, and in practices of a similar sort, and those who are too spirited and who rush about in an over-excited way with the use of the opposite kind.[34] Why on earth was it, after all—we should address this question too to the followers of Chrysippus—that Damon, the musician, when he came upon an *aulos*-player who was playing in the Phrygian mode to some youths who were drunk and behaving over-excitedly, instructed her to play rather in the Dorian mode, whereupon the youths immediately ceased their uncontrolled motions? Obviously it is not that people adopt the views of the reasoning faculty of the soul because of the playing of the *aulos*; it is through the affective [part] of the soul, which is non-rational in its nature, that they are either stimulated or calmed, by means of non-rational motions. Benefit or harm to the non-rational in the soul comes

---

[34] The point is elaborated by Galen in practical terms at *Health* I.8, pp. 322–3 below. The clearest Platonic background to this notion of a musically based training for the soul, differentially applied to different characters, is found at *Republic* III, 411a–412a.

about through non-rational means, benefit or harm to the rational through knowledge or ignorance.

It is not this benefit alone that Posidonius claims we shall derive from an understanding of the cause of the affections; he also states that this 'clarified the confusions concerning that impulse that is due to affection'. He continues to explain the nature of these confusions, as follows:

> Surely you have observed long ago how people, even when convinced by rea-
> 474   son that there is some evil | present or imminent, nevertheless do not experi-
> ence fear, but that they do experience it when they form a mental image of such
> an evil. For how could the non-rational be moved by reason, unless you present
> it with some sort of picture, similar to an actual perceptible picture? Thus, for
> example, people sometimes experience desire [for someone] as a result of a
> vivid description, or experience fear of an approaching lion on the basis of a
> very clear encouragement to run from it, even without actually seeing either.

... He then offers the reason why in the course of time affections become calmer
475   and weaker—a question to which Chrysippus, by his own admission in | the sec-
ond book of his *Affections*, had no answer. I said something on this point at the end of book IV, and will add just a little more here, by way of summary of Posidonius' rather long statement on the subject. The affective [part] of the soul over a period of time both sates itself on its own desires and tires of very long-lasting motions, and thus reaches a state of comparative calm, with moderate motions, at which point the reasoning faculty is able to take control of it, rather in the manner of a rider who has been carried off by force by a runaway horse; here too the horse both tires of running and becomes sated of its desires, so that the rider is able to take control again. This is very frequently observed; and those whose job it is to train young animals allow them to tire themselves out and sat-isfy themselves with their wild motions, before then taking them in hand.

Chrysippus has no account to give of all this, since he was not able to refer the cause to the affective in the soul. Moreover, as Posidonius also shows in his
476   remarks that follow, Chrysippus is here at odds not just with observed fact | but also with Zeno and Cleanthes. He uses the following lines of Cleanthes to dem-onstrate the latter's view on the affective [part] of the soul:

> —What is it that you want, o spirit? Tell me that.
> —I, Reason? To do all I want.
> —A lordly wish; but say it once again.
> —Whatever I desire—that that may be.

Posidonius claims that these exchanges clearly indicate the opinion of Cleanthes concerning the affective [part] of the soul, since he makes the reasoning faculty address the spirit as a separate individual.

But Chrysippus does not think the affective is different from the reasoning faculty, and he also refuses to allow that non-rational animals have affections, though they are clearly maintained by desire and spirit, as Posidonius discusses at length. Those animals which move with difficulty, those which are attached to rocks or other surfaces in the manner of plants, he states to be maintained by desire alone, while all other non-rational animals are maintained by both capacities, the desiderative and the spirited, and it is human beings alone that are maintained by three, having acquired a rational source in addition....

[*In the final chapter of the book Galen gives a detailed analysis and defence of Plato's proof, in book IV of the* Republic, *that there are three parts of the soul responsible for our different impulses.*]

BOOK VI

[*In chapter 1, Galen distinguishes different senses of the terms* energeia *and* pathos, *with particular reference to Plato's discussion of the soul and its appetites in book IV of the* Republic. *In particular, a* pathos *maybe understood either as a motion which a body undergoes which is due to another body rather than being the proper motion of that body itself, or as a pathological or abnormal motion or state.*]

2. Therefore it would be good not to skirt over these passages, but rather to go over[35] the whole argument devoted by Plato in the fourth book of the *Republic* to the proposition that there are three forms within in our souls. Here, too, particular attention must be paid to what is said, and one should begin by going back to the actual words, and not believe that Plato has forgotten his own statements when, having said that our soul has three *forms*, he then also states that it is divided into three *parts*. The rational, spirited and desiderative may correctly be termed both forms and parts, just as one may say that vein, artery, nerve, bone, cartilage, flesh and so on are forms, but then proceed to discuss them as parts. One may truthfully say that these are parts of our bodies, for the whole is composed of them, but, equally, that they are forms of the body. For it is only with the uniform parts that differences [in part] do not correspond to differences in form. Examples would be different parts of the flesh, of a vein, or of fat: in these cases | it would not be true to say that the whole [flesh, etc.] is composed of such-and-such a number of *forms*. In the case of the non-uniform parts, the number of different forms is the same as the number of different parts.   514

515

---

[35] The verb, *analambanein*, can also mean 'to learn by rote'.

Plato states our soul to be some such thing, composed of three parts; and so he likens the desiderative part to a multifarious and many-headed beast, the spirited to a lion, and the rational to a human being. This image is more appropriate than that in the *Phaedrus*, in which he states that two of the forms are horse-like in shape while the third is the charioteer. But he gives the former image too, in the ninth book of the *Republic*, to indicate more clearly the nature of each of the forms of the soul.[36] Since, then, he holds that they have separate places in the body, and are extremely different from each other in their substance, Plato naturally gives them both appellations, 'forms' and 'parts'; Aristotle and Posidonius, on the other hand, do not call them forms or parts, but state that they are capacities which come from the heart; and Chrysippus reduces spirit and desire not only to

516   a single substance but also to a single capacity. | Now, the extent of this last individual's departure from the truth has already been sufficiently indicated above; the blunder of Aristotle and his followers, too, in their belief that they are three capacities of a single substance, has been shown sufficiently in the previous books, and will be demonstrated equally by the subsequent one.

We shall first establish, on the basis of his own statements, that Plato himself calls the rational, the spirited and the desiderative both forms and parts of the soul. In the *Timaeus*, discussing the desiderative soul, of which he says plants also partake, he writes as follows:

> What we are referring to now partakes of the third form of soul, which, it is said, is situated between the diaphragm and the navel.[37]

In the same book, too, discussing the rational, he says:

> We should form this conception of the sovereign form of soul within us: that the god has given it to each of us as a guiding spirit—that form which, indeed, we say inhabits the highest part of our body, and lifts us up from earth towards our natural kinship with the heavens.[38]

517 | Again, in the same book, he calls the two—spirited and desiderative—together a form of soul, in the following statement:

> They constructed another form of soul in it, the mortal one, which has within it terrible and unavoidable affections.[39]

Equally, within the same *Timaeus*, he again uses the appellation 'forms' for the three parts of the soul, in the following account:

> As we have said many times previously, he established three forms of soul in us.[40]

---

[36] The two passages meant are *Phaedrus* 253c–254a and *Timaeus* IX, 588c–d.
[37] *Timaeus* 77b.   [38] *Timaeus* 90a.   [39] *Timaeus* 69c–d.   [40] *Timaeus* 89e.

In the same way in the fourth book of the *Republic*, too, after having stated, of the spirited, that it is distinct from the desiderative, he proceeds to consider whether it is also distinct from the rational, and says:

> Is it, then, different from this too, or is it a form of the rational, so that there are not three but two forms within the soul, the rational and the desiderative?[41]

And he writes similarly in the ninth book, in the following statement:

> When someone has calmed the two forms, but has stimulated the third, in which thinking arises...[42]

and also in this one:

> Since, then, I said, the pleasures, and indeed the life itself, of each form are in dispute, not just on the question of how to live a nobler or uglier life, or a worse ǀ or better one, but also of how to live a more pleasurable or pain-free life, how are we to know which one of them speaks truest?[43]   518

Why then transcribe still more passages? These are sufficient to show the man's opinion, that is to say that he holds that these three, the rational, the desiderative and the spirited, are forms of our souls. Indeed, he states that they exist independently of each other—the desiderative in plants and the rational in gods. (The reason why the spirited is not able to exist alone in any body will be demonstrated by the subsequent argument, when we set down the quotation from the *Timaeus* in which he explains the function for which it came into being, stating that it was as an assistant to the rational soul, like a dog to be used against the wild, many-headed creature which is desire.)

It is quite reasonable, then, that he calls them forms of soul, both in the passages which I have already transcribed and in many others, too, which it would be superfluous to mention, since his opinion is already clearly understood on the basis of these. That he should also call each of them parts of the soul is also unsurprising. ǀ For he has himself explained to us, first of all, that   519 anything which is a form may legitimately also be called a part, but that not every part is automatically also a form; secondly, that it is not legitimate to refer to any composite thing as uniform, as if it were a whole continuous with itself; for it consists of a definite number of parts, and it is not legitimate to delimit something uniform in terms of a number of parts. Plato, then, with very good reason, terms these both forms and parts, of the soul; and this fact requires no further argument.

3. Now, the fact that one of these is located in the head, one in the heart and one in the liver was the proposition before us from the beginning. In the previous

---

[41] *Republic* IV, 440e.   [42] *Republic* IX, 572a.   [43] *Republic* IX, 581e–582a.

books this has been shown for two of the parts. There remains the desiderative part, which requires a specific demonstration of its own. This we shall give in the present book; but we must state this first, right at the beginning of the argument: that this demonstration will not proceed from equally manifest [propositions], nor directly from the nature of the subject under enquiry, as was the case with the previous ones. Rather, it will proceed from its specific attributes.[44] For

520 when the nerves ⎸ were constrained by a ligature or cut it was apparent that the parts contiguous with the brain preserved their original capacities, while those beyond the ligature immediately lost both sensation and motion; and similarly in the case of the arteries, that those contiguous with the heart continued to pulse normally, while those cut off by the ligature became completely devoid of pulse. It was clearly observed, too, that those affections of the soul that take place in rage and fear caused the heart to depart from its normal activity. We discussed also all the ways in which, if the brain suffers pressure or puncture in the ventricles, this harms the entire body, and the fact that this proves clearly that it is the source of motion and sensation.

In the case of the liver, on the other hand, we have no demonstration of this kind to make, either by exposing or compressing it, or by constraining the veins with a ligature; for it is not the source of a manifest motion, in the same way that the heart is of the pulsing motion and the brain of that of sensation and volition. Nor is it the cause of immediate harm, as both of those are: rather, the animal suffers harm over a period of time, in respect of both good nutrition and

521 ⎸ good colour, when the liver's energy is impaired. So, too, if you constrain a vein with a ligature, or indeed cut it out altogether, the part to which it leads will be seen to become worse nourished and worse in colour in the course of time, but will not undergo any notable damage immediately.

For the liver is the source of the same kind of capacity that exists in plants. We may call it a capacity for present purposes; but in due course we shall give a more precise account whereby it will be shown that the liver is the source of many capacities; and it is preferable to refer to what is contained in each of the three organs as a *substance* rather than a *capacity* of the soul: the rational in the brain, the spirited in the heart and in the liver the desiderative—or, in Aristotle's terminology, the nutritive, the vegetative or the generative, each of these terms being derived from one aspect: 'vegetative' from growing, 'nutritive' from nourishing and 'generative' from the process of generation. Plato, on the other hand, uses the term 'desiderative', on the basis of the plurality of desires in it; and the Stoics do not refer to this, which maintains plants, as soul at all, but as nature.

522 Well, let each of them use the term ⎸ which they prefer, but as regards the factual distinctions themselves, let them rely on demonstration, in the same

[44] That is, from attributes specific to the part/form in question, the desiderative, rather than from its actual essence. The terminology *sumbebēkota idiai* is Aristotelian in origin; cf. p. 242 above.

way that we have already done in the case of the brain and the heart, and are setting out to do in the present book in the case of the liver. We shall start from those things which are more evident. Thus, having been schooled in these, we may more easily discover some of those which are less clear; and we may also be well provided with premises when it comes to those. The clearer area, then, from which to start is that of the veins, and of the question, whether the liver is the source of these in the same way that the heart is the source of the arteries and the brain of the nerves or whether, as some think, the heart transmits the natural capacities not only to the arteries but also to the veins. For this enquiry it will be best to consider first the generation and maintenance of plants; for it surely seems reasonable that, since they are endowed with this capacity and no other, they may provide evidence of the part from which it proceeds.

When any seed is thrown on to the ground, if the latter is dry the seed will not itself bring about any further action towards the generation of the plant, I since the earth draws towards itself all the seed's innate moisture; if, however, 523 the earth is moderately wet, the seed becomes soft, and the natural covering which surrounds it, which is like its skin, swells up, and first of all, when the moisture within the seed has been turned to air, then, after that, a fine, soft shoot is extended through the break in both directions: upward towards the air and down into the earth. And these are clearly seen both to produce a continuous growth and to move constantly in the same direction in which they started. As time goes on, then, if the seed is that of a large tree, that part which moves into the air becomes its trunk, and that part which leads into the earth its root; and each splits into many divisions, if it is a seed of a tree of that kind.

Now, one source of generation and growth, for all parts of the plant, is that place from which the trunk goes up and the beginning of the root goes down; and it is obvious that the capacity which maintains the tree starts out from there as it were from a central hearth. I This, then, has opposite kinds of motion: one 524 which goes downwards into the earth, as well as involving a splitting of the first roots into many divisions and the increase of the resultant ones; the other, upward, which produces certain offshoots from the trunk, then divides these into others, and so on up to the final, finest outgrowths. And it seems that it shapes the entire upper part, that is to say the tree, for the sake of the tree itself and for that of the fruits, while it shapes the lower one for the sake of the provision that takes place through nutriment. For the ends of the roots seem really to be something like the mouth in animals: the many mouthlets draw from the earth the nourishment which has been crafted by nature.

Let us then transfer this image to animals. First, consider the largest artery: this, like the trunk, splits after growing out from the heart, with the smaller part then leading up to the brain and the larger extending down the spine. Then, observe all its outgrowths which lead to all the parts of the body, in the manner stated in the first book, I and another artery leading out from the same ventricle 525

of the heart, this one splitting into the lungs in a similar way to the part of the root that goes down into the ground. For, just as plants pull in all their nourishment from the earth through the roots, so the heart pulls in the air from the lungs through these arteries. These two arteries grow out from the heart and constitute its two main outgrowths. And, just as in the plant the trunk is the broadest of all the branches, and the part which splits into roots is the broadest of all the lower parts, while that in the middle is the source of the plant, in the same way the trunk-like artery is the largest of all those in the animal, that which grows into the lungs is the largest of those in them, and the heart itself is in the middle, between them, and is the source of the capacities that maintain them. To a man versed in matters of nature, it is quite evident, even apart from these considerations, that larger things are the sources of smaller, as, for example, a water source is greater than the channels into which it is divided. Yet some are so illogical as to suppose
526   that I what comes after a source is greater than the source, deceived by the example of rivers, which are very small at their springs but increase as they proceed. This, however, is not necessarily the case: some receive tributaries, and so quite naturally increase in size; others diminish, as they are split into channels. No river proceeding from only one spring has its head smaller than its subsequent extension; where, on the other hand, it is the result of a confluence of many springs, it stands to reason that the whole is larger than each of these.

But even apart from this example, if we were to make the smaller vessels the sources of the larger in the body, the argument would contradict itself, by being compelled to concede that the source of the three major organs, of artery vein and nerve, is in every part of the body, so that, for example, the heel or finger would be the source of the largest artery, or of the vena cava and of the spinal cord; for we have here, as it were, the trunks of, respectively, arteries, veins and nerves. So perhaps the person who brings forward this
527   argument will also have the temerity to suggest I that the outgrowths of trees and the ends of the roots are the sources of the plant. Now, indeed, the ends of the roots may be termed sources—sources of nourishment of the tree, and this is similar to the situation with the veins that connect with the stomach and the arteries that divide into the lungs. Yet to call all the ends of the veins sources *tout court* is ridiculous; for none of them, except for those just mentioned, is the source of nutrition, nor is any the source of the internally organizing capacity. If it were so, every part would be a source. If, on the other hand, the suggestion is that some ends are sources but others are not, this is a hypothesis without any possibility of demonstration. For why would certain ends be considered sources and others not? Why, for example, those in the brain rather than those in the lungs, or why those in the liver or spleen rather than these—or indeed why these rather than those in some other part or organ? Even as a youth, when I heard my teacher Pelops attempting to

show that the brain was the source of all the vessels, I did not agree with it, nor on later examination did I approve it....

[*In the next chapters Galen argues on the basis of anatomical observations for the proposition that the liver is the source of the veins, against rival views, and against confused understandings of the nature of a source.*]

8. ...Now, indeed, let us complete the proof of the proposition before us. The 572 first origin of blood which is wet in its mixture and red in its colour is in the liver, and the channels which carry and distribute it to the whole body are the veins. The first origin of blood which is yellow, hot, fine and aerated is in the left ventricle of the heart, and the arteries distribute and carry this kind of blood to the whole animal. I This has been shown at greater length also in our work on 573 *Natural Capacities*. The material which was deferred in the previous books, then, on the blood in the heart, has now been given; and at the same time the mistake of those who state the heart to be the source of the veins has been shown. These individuals concluded from the fact that the heart was the source of *some* blood that it was automatically also the source of the veins—as if it were not the case that the arteries, too, contain a kind of blood (namely the finest and hottest kind). The heart, then, is the source not only of the arteries but also of that blood which is aerated and seething, and this indicates that the spirited part of the soul is located there, too. It is in relation to this, then, that Plato spoke of the heart as 'fount of the blood which is borne vehemently through all the limbs'. For it is not the same thing to say, simply, 'fount of the blood', and to add 'which is borne vehemently'. The blood which proceeds from the liver is not borne vehemently, for, indeed, neither is it aerated nor do the veins containing it have any pulse. The blood proceeding from the left ventricle of the heart is hotter I than this, and significantly aerated, as its vessels do pulsate. 574

However, this kind of vessel, just like the other, is also referred to as 'vein' by the earliest doctors and philosophers; it is the later ones who refer to the pulsating vessel as 'artery' and the one without pulse as 'vein'. That this was indeed the earlier terminology has been previously shown by many, as also in other writings of our own. For the present I shall mention only what is helpful for our immediate purposes. When the motion of the artery in the elbow, especially the left elbow, is from birth swift, great and energetic, this indicates that the spirited capacity in the heart is strong, and that the hot in it is at its peak and seething; this is usually termed 'passionate' and 'quick-tempered'. Hippocrates, terming this artery a vein, writes like this in the second book of the *Epidemics*:

The person in whom the vein in the elbow pulsates is passionate and quick-tempered, the person in whom it is calm is sluggish.[45]

---

[45] *Epidemics* II.5.16.

The fact that the terms 'pulsate' and 'pulse' were used by early writers to refer to
575   a motion of the artery so vehement[46] | that it was perceptible to someone even
before contact was made by touch, has been demonstrated in other works, and
indeed is obvious here, from the antithesis with the terms 'calm' and 'sluggish',
which evidently refer to someone who is not prone to anger, and thus the
opposite of 'passionate' or 'quick-tempered'. In this explanation of the use of the
term 'vein', then, we have incidentally accomplished something of considerable
importance, namely to show that Hippocrates, before Plato, placed the source
of the spirited capacity in the heart. I shall, however, return to this point later.

Now, however, I shall go back to the verbal formulation which Plato makes
in relation to the arteries (referring to them as veins): 'the heart, fount at once
of the veins and of the blood which is borne vehemently through all the limbs'.[47]
Since at that time pulsating vessels were not yet termed 'arteries', as they are
now, this term being applied only to those vessels which more recent doctors
have termed 'rough arteries' [tracheiai], Plato quite reasonably added also that
576   it was the fount 'of the | blood which is borne vigorously through all the limbs',
in order to distinguish the category of 'vein' of which he takes the heart to be
the source. The blood which proceeds from the liver, on the other hand, has
been prepared as nourishment for all parts of the body. This, I believe, is why
Plato in speaking of it said: 'in this whole region crafting as it were a manger of
nourishment for the body'. Moreover, from the fact that he states the part of the
soul in the liver to be 'desiderative of food and drink',[48] but makes no such addition in the case of the heart, it is evident that he takes it that the nourishment is
borne from the stomach to the liver, and that from there some part of it goes to
the heart for the purpose of generation of the blood in the heart.

Now, the fact that the transfer of nourishment from the region of the stomach to the heart is not immediate, but takes place via the liver, has been sufficiently demonstrated elsewhere, in my Natural Capacities, and I do not need to
rehearse that argument further. It will, however, be useful to make at least this
addition to the argument. It is necessarily the case that the spirited organ is sig-
577   nificantly hot, but this is not so | of the desiderative: this latter, in the case of
plants, will be very much less hot than the spirited, while in the case of animals
the difference will not be as great, but will nonetheless be considerable. It would
not produce a fluid which is as hot as it is if it did not have this quality itself;
nor, on the other hand, would it keep the veins devoid of pulse if it were the
source of a seething heat. It is, then, to indicate this that Hippocrates wrote:

---

[46] Galen is pointing to an apparent linguistic connection between the word for pulse (sphugmos,
verb sphuzein) and the word 'vehement' (sphodros).

[47] Timaeus 70a–b; the text of Plato as we have it reads rather 'knot of the veins and fount...', but
the manuscripts of Galen read 'at once' (hama) for 'knot' (hamma), and it seems that the latter reading represents the text of Plato as Galen knew it.

[48] This and the previous phrase quoted are from Timaeus 70c and 70d respectively.

The root of the veins is the liver; the root of the arteries is the heart; from these blood and breath travel to all parts, and heat moves through them.[49]

He means that blood travels from the liver, breath from the heart, and heat from both.

It therefore made no difference whether they spoke of the liver as source of blood or as source of the desiderative soul; but it was in a way more appropriate for a doctor to base his instruction on bodily organs and a philosopher on the capacities of the soul. But once one proposition has been shown, the other follows from it. Indeed, Hippocrates and Plato were clearly writing about them in this way; it is just that the former produced a longer argument in relation to the bodily organs, the latter in relation to capacities of the soul.

| It is for this reason, then, that Hippocrates says: 'the root of the veins is the   578
liver', and continues with the following anatomy of the veins:

The hepatic vein is in the lower back, as far down as the great vertebra...[50]

Plato, on the other hand, talking not in terms of the veins but of the capacity   580
which maintains them and which has its origin in the liver, proceeds with the argument roughly as follows, in the *Timaeus*:

What in the soul is desiderative of food and drink, and of those things which it requires because of the nature of the body—this they located in between the diaphragm and the boundary in the region of the navel, in this whole region crafting as it were a manger of nourishment for the body; and they bound it there, like a wild animal, but one that it was necessary to feed conjointly, if there was to be a mortal race at all.[51]

And, a little further on, he adds: 'To guard against this very thing, the god put together the form of the liver.'

In the case of this organ, then, the two of them have as it were distributed the arguments between them, the one speaking of organs and the other of the capacity which maintains them. In the case of the | heart, meanwhile, both of   581
them have treated of both aspects. Plato, first, says in the *Timaeus*:

the heart, the fount at once of the veins and of the blood which is borne vehemently through all the parts, they established as a guardhouse, so that, when the passion of the spirit seethes on receipt of some report from the rational— when, for example, some unjust act assails them from without, or, indeed

---

[49] *Nutrition* 31. It is striking that Galen here without comment quotes from a Hippocratic text which seems to contain the very distinction between arteries and veins which he has just denied to be present in earlier authors. (In fact, *Nutrition* is now thought to belong to a considerably later period than that of Plato and the core works of the Hippocratic corpus.)

[50] Galen proceeds to quote a lengthy passage from this text, *Epidemics* II.4.

[51] *Timaeus* 70d–e.

from the internal desires—then every part of the body endowed with sensation, quickly sensing the injunctions and threats through all the narrow channels, will become obedient and follow it in all respects, and thus allow that
which is best to be the leader throughout all the parts.[52]

Plato thus combined both arguments in one, those regarding the spirited soul and
those regarding the heart and the vessels which grow out from it. Hippocrates
himself, for his part, does not refrain from making some statement about this
kind of soul, especially in the passage which I transcribed a little earlier, in which
he made an inference from the pulse in the elbow to the character traits of the
soul, but also in his account of the treatment of lack of colour and of feebleness in
582   cooled | conditions of the body. For there he says: 'Make it your habit to instil
quickness of temper, for the restoration both of colour and of fluid.'[53]

Indeed you may feel that Plato is providing a commentary on this very passage when he says of the heart: 'so that, when the passion of the spirit seethes'.
His philosophical successors in fact went so far as to give this as the definition
of spirit, or of rage, stating it to be a 'seething of the hot in the heart'.[54]
Hippocrates, meanwhile, when speaking of the origin of fever, says: 'For, while
cooling the feet, it increases, being lit from the chest and sending out as it were
a flame to the head':[55] he is aware that the heart is the source of the innate heat.

It is not my task now, however, either to assemble all the statements of these
men, or to provide a commentary on them, especially when I intend to produce
such commentary in separate, specialized treatises. Here, as I said at the outset,
my purpose is merely to examine and assess their doctrines from the point of
view of whether or not they agree with each other in every respect....

BOOK VII

[*Galen begins with an apologia for the length of the work so far.*]

587   1. ...Now, since, even after the first books, certain individuals still went so far
as to vindicate the truth of the arguments put forward by Chrysippus and
others on the command centre of the soul, my followers (for whose sake I have
mainly been writing this) thought that one should add the solutions to those
objections. It thus became necessary either to lengthen the treatise or to give
the appearance of not having completely demonstrated the proposition that
animals are maintained by three sources; and it seemed preferable to extend the
length. Now, the end result shows that we made the right choice, namely to

---

[52] *Timaeus* 70a–c.   [53] *Epidemics* II.4.
[54] Galen here refers to the well-known definition of anger in Aristotle's *De anima*, I.1, 403a–b.
[55] *Regimen in Acute Diseases*, spuria, 7.

refute *all* the arguments which were put forward. There is now no Stoic nor Peripatetic philosopher who is as bold as they were previously; and some have even openly changed over to the true position, doctors admitting that the capacity of perception and motion flows from the brain and philosophers that the reasoning faculty of the soul is there. For they were ashamed when one of their premisses was manifestly refuted by anatomy. | By proceeding logically 588 on the basis of this false premiss, in conjunction with another, which is agreed by all, they produced a false syllogism. This latter premiss is the one stating that 'where the source of the nerves is, there is the command centre'—which is indeed true. The proposition used for the former premiss should have relied on the findings of anatomy; when, then, the proposition that they held, that the nerves proceed from the heart, was shown to be wrong, then of course this rendered the conclusion of the whole syllogism false....

In fact, most of Chrysippus' statements are true, especially those in that book 590 in which he shows that the virtues are qualities. Since, however, the statements in that book are in conflict with the views of one who takes there to be a single capacity in the soul, a capacity called both 'rational' and 'evaluative', and who denies the existence of the desiderative and spirited, as Chrysippus does, one might criticize him on those grounds. The fact that he correctly defeats Aristo's position, on the other hand, is not something for which he could be criticized. Aristo believes that there is one virtue, which is called by many names according to its particular relationships. Chrysippus actually shows that the plurality of virtues and vices arises not from any relation, but through the relevant substances being modified in | their qualities; this is consistent with the view of 591 earlier authors, and it is this, too that Chrysippus expounded, slightly adapting it and using different terminology, in his work *That the Virtues are Qualities*, where he uses arguments that ill befit one who has proposed the rational as the only part of the soul and denied the existence of the affective part.

How, then, am I responsible for the length of these books, when I am compelled, now, to show that Chrysippus has used the arguments of a sect other than his own in order to refute—quite reasonably—the opinion of Aristo?...

I am not to blame for the length of the arguments in these areas; the blame 592 lies rather with those who have never been trained in the demonstrative method and who do not love the truth. It is the same with the question of the number of the virtues: the scientific account is brief indeed, while those that originate in ignorance and competitiveness are many. | Which, then, is the scientific 593 account? It is, of course, that which proceeds from the essence of the matter, as was shown in my treatise on *Demonstration*. For one should start from the *notion* of virtue, proceed from there to the discovery of its *essence*,[56]

[56] For the distinction between the 'notional' and 'essential' account, compare *The Art of Medicine*, Preface, with n. 2.

investigating whether there is one essence of virtue in the soul or more than one. Here, as stated in *Demonstration*, we take 'essence' in the most general of its senses, which is that of 'existence'. Virtue is said to be the best state, or perfection, of each individual's nature. Now, if virtue is indeed something of this sort, there will be one virtue for each individual thing. If what is best or what constitutes perfection is a single thing, then as far as the rational part of the soul is concerned, it necessarily follows that its virtue be knowledge; and if this reasoning faculty is the only one in our souls, one should not look for a plurality of virtues. If, on the other hand, there exists also a spirited part, there

594   must arise a virtue of this part too; and if | there is also a third part, the desiderative, there will be these three separate virtues; and then a fourth arises from their relationship with each other.

That is hardly a long argument. Nor, indeed, is any scientific argument long. But we are compelled to produce long ones by those who utter great nonsense. Here, for example, it was necessary to rehearse an admittedly not extremely long, but still moderately long, argument on the virtues of the soul. For if there are separate faculties of reasoning, desire and spirit, as was shown to be the case earlier, then there will be some single virtue for each of them. So, then: call the one in the reasoning faculty wisdom, or moral judgement, or knowledge, or whatever you wish, and that in the spirited faculty, in turn, courage, or whichever term you prefer (the precise terminology does not concern me, merely that it must be a single item); and call the virtue that arises in the remaining part, the desiderative, self-control. (We will consider later the difference between Aristotle and Plato concerning the virtue of this part, which is not a great one.)

595 | Thus, when each part of the soul possesses the beauty which accords with its level, one may reasonably call the soul as a whole 'just'. Now, in the non-rational parts of the soul the virtues are simply certain conditions or capacities, while in the rational the virtue is not merely a condition or capacity, but also knowledge. For this part of the soul alone partakes of knowledge; the others are capable of acquiring better or worse capacities or conditions, but cannot partake of knowledge, any more than they can of reason. This, then, is how brief the truth is.

[*The view of Aristo of Chios is outlined, that virtue is a single thing, knowledge of good and evil, this knowledge acquiring different names (courage, justice, etc.) in different contexts; and Chrysippus is attacked for refuting this view, which seems to rely on the same view of the soul as his own.*]

600   3. ...It has been shown that the maintenance of the animal once born is carried out by three sources. One, located in the head, has the following functions: in itself, mental impressions, memory, intellection and discursive thought, and relationally, the guidance of sensation in respect of the sensory parts of the animal and of motion to those parts capable of voluntary motion. The second,

situated in the heart, I has these: in itself, the tension[57] of the soul, its constancy   601
in respect of the commands of the reasoning faculty, and its unyielding quality,
and, in states of affection, the seething, as it were, of the innate heat, in cases
where the soul desires revenge upon one who it thinks has done the person
wrong (this state being called 'rage'); relationally, to be the source of heat for the
individual parts of the body, as well as of the pulsatory motion of the arteries.
The remaining capacity, situated in the liver, has as its functions everything
concerned with nutrition in the animal, of which the most important element
for all blooded animals is the generation of blood. The enjoyment of pleasures
belongs to this capacity, too, and when its motions are greater than they should
be it brings about lack of restraint and indiscipline.

Now, the demonstration that shows the source of the nerves to be in the head
at the same time also shows the particular part of the head in question. For
there are two premises in the argument, one being that which is intrinsic to the
notion, essence or nature, or however one wishes to term it, of the question
under discussion, the other being that which is apparent through anatomy. I It is   602
through a precise knowledge of this latter that one also acquires knowledge of
the part of the head from which the source of the nerves derives, namely that
this is the brain, not the meninges. For each of the nerves that grows out from it
is threefold in substance: there is the interior part in the middle, which is analogous to the pith in trees, and this has its source of generation in the brain;
enclosing this all round there is, first, the outgrowth of the fine meninx [*pia
mater*] and secondly that of the thick one [*dura mater*].

Erasistratus for a long time saw only the external part of the nerve which
proceeds from the thick meninx [*dura mater*], and so thought that the whole of
the nerve grew from there; and most of his compositions are full of statements
that the nerves grow from the meninx that envelops the brain. Later on in his
life, however, when he had time to devote exclusively to the observations of the
art, and performed his anatomical procedures with greater attention, he
acknowledged the pith, as it were, of the nerves too, and the fact that this grows
from the brain. His statement on this is as follows:

> We also observed the nature of the brain. Now, the brain was I bipartite, like   603
> that of other animals, and there were long ventricles lying within it, connected
> to make one through a point of contact between the parts. From this point
> there was a connection to what is known as the *epenkranis* [*cerebellum*], and
> here there was another small hollow. And each of the parts was separated off
> by the meninges; the *epenkranis* was separated off individually, as also the

[57] The word is *tonos*, usually applied to a physical state or quality, for example that of strings or
muscles, or to the 'intensity' of exercise, but here unusually characterizing an ethical or affective
state. See the similar usage attributed to Chrysippus above, IV.6, with n. 19.

enkephalos [brain or *cerebrum*], which is similar to the jejunum, having many folds; and indeed the *epenkranis* even more so, constructed with many complex twists. It was thus possible to learn from these observations that, in human beings just as in other animals (deer, hare and all those which are superior to most in running, through being well provided with muscles and nerves for this purpose), this part is large and multiform. There were also outgrowths of the nerves, which were all from the brain, and, in summary, the brain appears to be the source of the nerves in the body. For the sensation that arises from the ⏐ nostrils has been connected by passages to this part, as have those from the ears. And there were outgrowths from the brain leading to the tongue and eyes, too.

604

In this passage Erasistratus admits that at this point he has clearly seen the fact of which he was previously ignorant, namely that each of the nerves grows out of the brain. He also writes accurately of its four ventricles, which in previous time he had also not seen. If he had carried out the test on living animals which we have done (not once or twice, but on very many occasions), then he would have gained a secure understanding of the fact that the hard, thick meninx has come into being for the protection of the brain, while the soft, fine one has come into being both for this purpose, but even more for the purpose of binding together all the vessels in the brain, arteries and veins.

It is stated at length in *Anatomical Procedures* which observations I claim should be made in anatomy in order to reach such doctrines as these; but I shall mention here too such of them as are most relevant to the present discussion. ⏐ If the bone of the head is removed while the animal is still alive, and the thick meninx is laid bare, and you then stretch this back with hooks on either side of the straight line in the middle at which it descends into the brain in a double fold, and either simply make a cut in it, or excise it altogether, the animal does not lose either sensation or motion; nor does it do so even if you either cut or completely excise that part of it which protects the whole of the hind part of the brain. Even if you cut out the whole brain itself in some way, the animal will still not become motionless or without sensation until the cut reaches one of the ventricles. The hinder one harms the animal most, and next after that the one in the middle; each of the front ones causes less harm, but more in older and less in younger animals. The same effect as that of such cuts into the ventricles is produced by compression of them, which we sometimes see—not because it is applied deliberately, but because it happens even when people are exercising extreme care—in persons undergoing trepanation, when the bones of the head are broken.

605

From these observed facts, then, one might form one of two conceptions about the ⏐ breath in the hollows of the brain: either, if the soul is non-bodily, that this breath is its first habitation, as one may put it; or, if the soul is a body, that this breath actually is the soul. Since, however, after the ventricles are

606

drawn together again, the animal soon regains both sensation and motion, it is not possible to say that this soul is <either> of the things mentioned. It is therefore better to suppose that the soul inhabits the body of the brain, whatever this soul is in terms of its actual substance (for the investigation has not yet reached that point); and that this kind of breath is the soul's first instrument for the purpose of all forms of sensation, and also of deliberate motion, in the animal. This is why in the period during which it is removed from the brain, before it is gathered within it again, it causes the animal to lose sensation and motion, but does not deprive it of life. If it were the substance of the soul, the animal would immediately die on its departure.

It is thus reasonable to suppose that this kind of breath is generated in the ventricles of the brain; that it is for this reason that a considerable number of arteries and veins terminate there, from which are generated what are known as the choroid | networks; and that, as I have said, this breath is the first instrument of the 607 soul. It is yet more likely that this breath will be produced in the process of the vessels, especially the arteries, breathing it out into the ventricles of the brain, since one observes the net-like web[58] which arises from the arteries which go into the head, when first they enter the cranium and reach the point inside it known as the base of the brain. Nature has prepared there a considerable space, like a chamber for this netlike web, a chamber surrounded by the thick meninx; and to this space go a substantial number of the arteries known as 'carotid', one vessel on each side, with many divisions, making the web too a multiple one, with in fact many webs lying one upon the other, as well as being connected and entwined. From this web, then, a further pair of arteries grows out, similar in size to that which originally came from the carotids, and leads up to the brain, both weaving through the other parts of it with a very large number of offshoots and producing the plexuses at the ventricles. | Now, the breath in the arteries is, and is known as, 608 vital breath, while that in the brain is the soul breath—not in the sense that it is the substance of the soul, but in the sense that it is the first instrument of the soul, which itself (whatever its actual substance) inhabits the brain.

And just as the vital breath is generated in the arteries and in the heart, the material of its generation coming from the inhalation of breath and from the vaporization of fluids, so the generation of the soul breath comes from the further processing of the vital breath; this, more than any other substance, obviously requires a complete change. If one considers that Nature required a complete processing for semen and milk, which fall far short of soul breath in their power, and therefore engineered a long period for them in the organs of

---

[58] Or 'retiform plexus': a thick network of blood vessels which Galen believed to be at the base of the brain. His observation here is based on animal rather than human anatomy; the closest equivalent to this network of vessels in human beings is the Circle of Willis. See also *Affected Places* III.12, p. 389 below.

coction, thus preparing for the semen the spiral before the testes and for the milk the length of the vessels which lead into the breast, it is reasonable enough that for the production of soul breath from vital breath Nature crafted the net-like web, which is a kind of labyrinth next | to the brain.

609

This much we have been taught by the indications given by construction of the parts; the fact that the soul breath is neither the substance of the soul nor its habitation, but its first instrument, we have been taught by the fact that when it is released through wounds the animal becomes as though dead, but revives when this breath is reassembled. In short, all that has been stated or that is about to be stated has been discovered either from the construction of the parts or from what arises from incision or compression. Even amongst the channels within the brain, some lead down through what is known as the 'funnel' to the palate, while some end at the back of the nostrils and others are apparent in the optic nerves. There is also one, unpaired channel leading to the first formation of the spinal cord; and if the thick meninx is cut at this particular point, the entire channel is laid open, along with the extremity of the posterior ventricle.

This, indeed, was a major reason for Erasistratus' error in thinking that animals lose motion immediately on the cutting of the meninx; for he observed that | this happened immediately on the severing of the meninx in the case of oxen pierced at the first vertebra. But this results not from the injury to the meninx but from the laying bare of the posterior ventricle....

610

611   4. Is it the case, then, since the whole animal loses sensation on the emptying of the breath from the ventricles of the brain, and we therefore stated that this breath has a role in the sensory function and motion of the parts, that one should therefore take it that there is some breath in every nerve? Should we, further, take it that this breath is local and innate to the nerves, and is then struck by that breath that comes from the source, as though by some messenger? Or rather that there is no such thing innate to them, but that it flows from the brain at those moments when we make a deliberate choice to move a part? I am not readily able to make a definite assertion on this point. Let us rather set ourselves both these possibilities, to be investigated together, as well as a third,

612   namely that of qualitative alteration by contiguity. It is this possibility, | it seems to me, to which people are gesturing when they speak of a flow taking place *in virtue of some capacity, without substance*. For the transmission of qualities to contiguous bodies is referred to by these people as the flow of capacity, just as is the case with light of the sun in the ambient air: some transmission of quality proceeds from the former and arrives at every part of the latter, while the substance of the sun remains where it is (this was shown in my work on *Demonstration*). It is thus not possible immediately to assert whether a capacity flows from the brain through the nerves to the limbs, whether the substance of the breath reaches all the way to the perceptive or moved parts, or whether it enters them only up to a certain point, in the process bringing about a

vehement alteration, and it is this alteration which is then transmitted up to the limbs which are moved.

Certainly something of this kind takes place in the case of visual sensation, as was shown in *Demonstration*. The fact that a ray-like breath is carried in those nerves is observable through the anatomy of the larger animals, where one sees that they have perforations both in their source higher up and in the juncture with the eyes....| ...Here, the structure indicates to us the fact that 614 some breath is carried through these channels to the eyes, as does the fact that when one of them is closed the pupil of the other becomes wider, and when the first one is opened again that immediately returns to its normal size....| ...Is it then the case that, just as some breath reaches the eyes through 616 the optic nerves, it is so too with all the others, and that there is some pathway within each one of them, although this is invisible because of its size; or is it, rather, impossible that this be the case with the nerves of the finest fibres in the body? For in this latter case we would have to conceive of the body of the nerve as something which encircles that channel, while itself being finer than a spider's web, so that this would itself be very easily severed, while the channel within would be very easily blocked, pretty much at the slightest event.

For this reason | I take it that there are not channels in all the nerves. Perhaps, 617 then, someone may say: 'If it is possible that *any* nerve is able to conduct the capacities from the source to the parts below even though it is not hollow, it must be possible that *all* the nerves do that.' But why, in that case, is the channel at the outgrowth of the spinal cord visible, in the same way as that in the optic nerves? Surely it is because transmission of capacities by contiguity is a weak phenomenon, especially where the part receiving the transmission is either a large or a hard one, whereas if a fine substance enters the part up to a certain point, in a violent impact, the effects of the alteration are increased? As already stated, this phenomenon commonly known as transmission of capacity is a passing-on of the alteration, as happens to the air by the agency of the light of the sun. It is therefore reasonable to suppose that the breath that comes to the eyes is, on first entering them, made one with the ambient air, in the process altering it to its own specific nature, but that it does not extend out further than that.

[*There follows a detailed account of the theory of vision; of the anatomy of the eye; and of the other senses.*]

BOOK VIII

[*The book again begins with a recapitulation of the previous argument, which Galen claims could have been completed much more quickly were it not for the argumentative inadequacies, sophistries and confusions of other people.*]

655   1. ...The true account is, indeed, so short that I shall show you how it reaches its conclusion within a few syllables. As follows:

> The location of the source of the nerves is that of the command centre;
> but the source of the nerves is in the brain;
> that, then, is the location of the command centre.

This, then, is one argument, and it has a total of thirty-nine syllables—the equivalent, that is, of two-and-a-half lines of hexameters. There is another, which consists of five such lines in all:

> The place where the affections of the soul more manifestly move the parts
>   of the body is the location of the affective part of the soul;
> but it is apparent that the heart is involved in a great change of motion in
>   cases of rage and fear;
> this, then, is the location of the affective part of the soul.

If you were to put these two arguments together, the resultant total would be no longer than eight hexameter lines.[59]

656   Who, then, | is responsible for five books having been written on matters which admit of a scientific proof occupying eight lines of heroic verse? It is certainly not I, but rather those philosophers who refuse to employ geometrical demonstrations. These philosophers, as I have said, are a source of shame to me. Who, furthermore, is responsible for a sixth book having been written, in addition to these, about the third source—a source which, to be sure, requires a longer discussion, but certainly not one that ought to fill up a whole book? It is those who lack the training to follow geometrical demonstrations; for the demonstration of this investigation also consists of a few main points. It was shown both that in the case of plants the thickest parts are the ones that grow out from their source and that in the case of the two sources that were the subject of the previous demonstration, that of the nerves and that of the arteries, the equivalent of the trunks are next to the sources and the parts analogous to branches are generated as the trunks proceed.

This one premiss was demonstrated through evident facts; and a second, too, namely that the veins are the instruments of the vegetative capacity in us, which we share with plants; fine veins descend into the stomach and the intestines in 657   the same way that the roots of trees descend into the earth, | all of them growing

---

[59] The assessment of the length of a passage of prose in terms of numbers of lines of hexameter verse may sound odd, but this seems to have been a standard way of measuring the lengths of texts. The traditional Homeric hexameter line has a minimum of twelve and maximum of seventeen syllables, and can be taken fairly reliably to average sixteen; it seems that this length of sixteen syllables could also be regarded as the standard length of a line in a papyrus manuscript. See also *Freedom from Distress*, n. 16.

out from one vein, the one at the gates of the liver. Further, then, a very large vein grows out from the liver: the one known as the hollow vein; and what seem like branches split off from this and travel throughout the body. From these considerations it was concluded that the source of the veins was the liver; and from this conclusion in turn it followed that this organ was the source of the capacity which we share with plants—that capacity which Plato calls the desiderative.

This is one demonstration of the liver's being the source of the desiderative capacity and of the veins; another is taken from the fact that no other part is found in the animal to which all the veins are joined. Some say that the vena cava, which grows out from the convexity of the liver, actually grows out from the right ventricle of the heart. If, then, the veins in the whole of the body split off from this vein in a way analogous to branches, the heart would be the source of all of them. But the veins which go out from the concavity of the liver, like roots, into the stomach, the jejunum, the small intestine, the caecum, the colon and what is known as the rectum, | as well as the spleen and the omentum, do   658
not grow from this; rather, there is another vein which is the source of all these, located at the gates of the liver. How then will the right ventricle of the heart be the source of the veins, when neither the veins mentioned nor, moreover, those in the concavity of the liver, are connected with the heart? The liver, on the other hand, is connected both with all of these and, through the one which grows out from its convex part, with those throughout the whole body. This latter is the vein generally known as 'hollow' (cava) because of its size, though Hippocrates and those who revere his works call it 'hepatic', from the organ from which it grows out. This, then, in any case, is your second demonstration of the fact that the liver is the source of all the veins and because of this also of the nutritive capacity.

There is even a third, extra demonstration: if we take the right ventricle of the heart to be the source of the vena cava, this will be opposite to the observed finding in the anatomy of fishes. For, indeed, none of them has a right ventricle of the heart, since those | animals also lack lungs. (The reason that the existence   659
of the right ventricle is dependent on that of the lungs has been shown in my treatise on *The Function of the Parts*.)

The argument just stated gives, as I said, considerable extra credibility to the doctrine; we may add another too, similar in status, from our consideration of the straightness of the vena cava.... If the vena cava grew out of the heart, | then   660
surely this, just like the [great] artery, would split, with one part going up to the throat and the other down to the liver.

These four demonstrations were given in the sixth book of the present treatise, for the benefit of those who understand the nature of a sufficient demonstration. There are other statements in that book, too, to add to the credibility of the doctrine; yet these do not have a scientific demonstration, like the first two arguments. Some counter-argument, furthermore, was given to those who hold a different opinion. For my part, then, the proposition before us could have been demonstrated very quickly indeed; and for the length of the argument one should blame not us, who are refuting the erroneous arguments which those people have written, but rather the authors of those arguments.

[*Most of the rest of book VIII is occupied with discussion of Plato's and Hippocrates' views on element theory and related matters of the causes of diseases and physiology of the body.*]

BOOK IX

[*Galen aims to complete the discussion of areas of agreement between Hippocrates and Plato. A large part of the book is occupied with their views on similarity and difference, and related dialectical issues; the central point of the importance of making correct distinctions and advancing arguments that proceed from secure logical starting-points leads Galen into digressions, on the mistakes made by philosophical sects, on the limitations of knowledge and on the argument from design.*]

779   7. ... The enquiry into things which have no relevance to character or to everyday activities, then, is consistent only with the approach of those philosophers
780   who I have chosen to engage in theoretical philosophy: for example, whether there is anything beyond the cosmos: if so, what is its nature; whether this cosmos is self-contained; whether there are more than one, and, indeed, whether there are a very great number; similarly, whether this cosmos is generated or ungenerated; and whether, if it did come into being, some god was its craftsman, or whether it was no god, but by a non-rational, unskilled cause, which, by a process of chance, made it just as beautiful as if a supremely wise and powerful god had supervised the construction. Such enquiries as these, however, are of no value for the purposes of good management of one's own household, appropriate attention to the affairs of the city, correct and generous behaviour towards one's relatives, fellow-citizens and guests.

Some, however, have come to these enquiries even while taking the goal to be a practical one: they have proceeded gradually from enquiries with a clear useful purpose, as if making a transition to similars. For, indeed, it is not equally useless to enquire into the question of providence and the gods as it is to
781   enquire into the question whether the cosmos had a beginning or not. I It is good for all of us to enquire into the existence in the cosmos of something greater than human beings in capacity and wisdom; but the enquiry into the nature of the gods' substance—whether they are incorporeal, or have bodies

like us—is unnecessary. This, and many similar enquiries, are completely without value for the virtues and activities known as ethical and social,[60] just as they
are for the cure of the affections of the soul.

On these matters an observation of Xenophon's is particularly pertinent: he
not only expresses his scorn for their lack of utility but claims that Socrates
shared his view. Socrates' other followers agree with him on this, too—including
even Plato, who, when adding to his philosophy a theoretical enquiry into
nature, attributes the speech on this to Timaeus, not to Socrates (just as he
attributes the extended dialectical enquiry to Parmenides and his pupil Zeno).[61]

It is because of a certain similarity between those amongst the theoretical
enquiries in logic and in natural philosophy which are useful and those which
are useless that the latter have also been added; for it is impossible wholly to
ignore natural philosophy and logical theory, even in a theoretical enquiry into
| ethics and politics; but you will find that these, too, belong amongst those   782
which are not useful. Many false arguments are very similar to true ones, both
in the starting-points of their demonstrations and in all the subsequent legs;
and sophistical arguments are composed on the basis of a similarity with true
ones. The people who know how to distinguish and separate them from each
other are those who have a schooling in that subject-matter with which the art
is concerned, as well as, of course, being endowed with a natural mental aptitude. This latter feature ought to be assessed in childhood by the most intelligent elders in each city, so that each person then proceeds to learn the art which
is appropriate to his nature. Now, however, we observe that many people engage
in the rational arts without even being able to follow their own utterances.

8. The fact that the demonstration of every doctrine must rely on rational[62]
starting-points has been shown by us in practically all our treatises; but I shall
add an example here as a schooling exercise, since at the beginning we set ourselves the investigation into the capacity to separate matters from each other
and to analyse | accurately the similarities and dissimilarities in each case. We   783
should, after all, not content ourselves with the proof of the proposition that
one must school oneself in individual matters, but rather show that in practice
too. Neither did Plato himself, nor Hippocrates, content himself with a general

---

[60] The Greek word is *politikos*, which could also be translated 'political', but which also has a
broader sense of 'everyday'; the present translation attempts a compromise between the two senses.
For a similar usage see *My Own Doctrines*, chs. 8 (with n. 21) and 15.

[61] Galen refers to Plato's major and influential work on cosmology, the *Timaeus*, in which the
'plausible account' of the creation of the cosmos is put in the mouth of an apparently fictional character, Timaeus, and to his *Parmenides*, in which the philosophers Parmenides and Zeno are the
main interlocutors. For this interpretive distinction on the basis of the different characters to whom
Plato assigns different arguments, compare *My Own Doctrines*, ch. 8, with n. 20.

[62] Here and in the previous sentence the word translated 'rational' could also be rendered
'logical': the sense of *logikos* is that of involving reason or logical argument.

exhortation in this area: they actually schooled us with many individual examples. Let us choose, then, as the material for this enquiry the nature of the providence towards us of the Craftsman, and let us take our starting-point from the structure of the body. For some state that it is shaped not in accordance with the providence of a wise Craftsman, but by some kind of chance which is devoid of either skill or rationality. These are using a faint similarity to bolster the credibility of their statement, namely that there are some events in life that happen in a similar way to those that are produced by the exercise of skills. They say, for example, that the outline or shape of certain mountains is similar to the face of a lion, and that of certain others to that of a serpent, or to that of some other animal; or that it has been known to happen that someone in strik-

784   ing a rock has broken off | just the right amount so that the remainder resembles the shape of a lion.

In making such statements about events which have happened once in the history of the known world, they are completely failing to take account of the assessment that is naturally made by all human beings about the products of the arts, and of the very great similarity of our own shaping to those—and this in spite of the fact that they see many people working with materials who are *not* called shoemakers, carpenters, or sculptors until such time as it is apparent that everything crafted by them has come into being for some useful purpose. For there is no other indicator of a skill than the function of each of the parts within the thing crafted. Now, if the person cutting, sawing and joining the wood makes a couch in which all the parts turn out to be fitting for the function for which it was constructed, this person is said to be a skilled craftsman. If, however, he makes the feet on the right unequal to those on the left—of a different thickness, length or shape—or if it is apparent that he has made a blunder of this sort with the back-rest, or with the pieces of wood which run the length of

785   the couch, or one of the vertical parts, then we say that he is unskilled. | ... And all think that [this kind of success] is indicative of a specialized skill, not because they have been taught to make this assessment, but because they have an innate conception of skill as something distinct from chance. That which is correctly completed in all respects we are convinced is a product of skill; but

786   that which is so only in one or two respects, | we are convinced is a product not of skill but of chance.

It is by virtue of this same conception that those amongst the doctors who engage in anatomy have all been in awe of the skill of Nature. For the body is not in reality, as it appears from the outside, composed of ten, or perhaps twelve, or even twenty, parts. It is composed of more than two hundred bones, and very many more than two hundred muscles; and to each of the bones there comes a vessel which nourishes it, which people call a vein, and to each of the muscles not only one of these but also an artery and a nerve; and those on the right-hand side of the animal are exactly equal to those on the left, bone to bone, muscle to muscle, vein to vein, nerve to nerve and artery to artery....| If 787 you enumerate the aims of the structure, then discover that each of them is correctly executed, his greatness will be apparent to you; I mean that of the Craftsman....|...Just as we make an assessment of those amongst human beings 789 who shape objects, then, so we should amongst divine beings; thus we should be in awe of the Craftsman of us, whichever of the gods he may be. If we conclude from the fact that we cannot see him that he does not exist, then we are no longer being true to our assessment of the similarity to the case of the products of artistic skill; for | we do not form our assessment of the skilled nature of 790 the production of a ship or a couch by observing the person assembling them, while omitting the investigation into the function of each of the parts. It is, rather, this latter investigation which we take to be the central one....| 791

9. Plato, however, also made an assertion as to the cause of our actual construction; he stated that the Craftsman god of the cosmos commanded his children, in words, to shape the race of men, taking from him the substance of the immortal soul, but adding to it the generated part.[63] But this much we should realize: there is not the same mode of demonstration and proposition involved in the statement that we have been constructed in accordance with the providence of some god or gods, as there is in the knowledge of the substance of that constructing agent, or indeed of the substance of our souls. That the construction of our bodies is a product of the ultimate wisdom and power, | has been shown by 792 what I said a little earlier. What is said by Plato about the substance of the soul, however, and about the gods who have shaped us, and even more so all that he says about our bodies, does not claim to go beyond the level of the plausible or likely; and Plato himself makes this clear in the *Timaeus*, before even embarking upon the natural-philosophical account, and then also adding such a declaration in the course of the exposition. Thus, Timaeus himself, in whose mouth Plato puts the whole account of the nature of the cosmos, says something like this:

> If, then, Socrates, we find that we are not capable of presenting accounts which are in every way completely self-consistent and accurate, with regard to many things concerning the gods and the generation of all things, do not be surprised; rather, we should be happy if we provide accounts which are not exceeded in likeliness by anyone else's, for we must bear in mind that I who produce them and you assess them are human in our nature, and that it is therefore reasonable for us to accept a likely tale on this subject, without seeking more than this.[64]

---

[63] The account referred to is at *Timaeus* 41a–d.   [64] *Timaeus* 29c–d.

He states that his writings on the soul, too, are within the bounds of the plausible and the likely, in the following words:

793   Now, this account | of the soul—how much it has that is mortal, and how much divine, and where, with whom, and by what agency the parts were separately located—all this we could only confidently assert to be true if a god were to speak with us; we may, however, dare to state the likelihood of what we have said, and ever more so the more we consider it; and let us indeed make that claim.[65]

In the same way, then, that he prefaced these statements on the soul with the assertion that our understanding extends only to the point of the plausible and likely, for this reason I too do not have the confidence to make a bold assertion in this area; I do, on the other hand, state that I have demonstrations that there is a plurality of forms of the soul, that it has a threefold location, that one of the forms is the divine one, by which we reason, and the other two are affective: one by which we experience rage and one by which we desire the pleasures of the body, this last one existing also in plants; and further, that the first of these is located in the brain, the second in the heart and the third in the liver. For there are scientific demonstrations on these matters, too, and I set out the case for them in the first six books of this treatise, without making any statement about

794   the substance | of the three parts of the soul, nor about its immortality, nor, indeed, making any enquiry at all as to whether he is using the term 'mortal' literally in relation to the two parts of the soul, or whether he applies this appellation to them in spite of the fact that they are in fact immortal, on the grounds that they are inferior to the rational part and act only in relation to the mortal parts of the animal.

That the forms of the soul have a threefold location, as well as the number and nature of the capacities of each, are facts which are valuable for the art of medicine and for that branch of philosophy known as ethical and social, and are therefore a reasonable subject of enquiry for both Hippocrates and myself. The enquiry, on the other hand, as to whether the spirited and the desiderative are in fact immortal, as many Platonist philosophers hold, or whether the statement in the *Timaeus* that they are mortal is a literal one, has no value at all for medicine or for that branch of philosophy known as ethical and social, and has thus quite reasonably been put aside by doctors and by many philosophers.

[*The treatise concludes with some further discussion of different kinds of argument and levels of epistemic certainty.*]

---

[65]   *Timaeus* 72d.

The Shaping of the Embryo

In this work, thought to have been written very late in his career, Galen lays out his views on embryology, and the relationship of these to the findings of anatomy, on the one hand, and to questions of causation in biology, on the other. In particular, he addresses the problem of how information is transmitted to the embryo and growing organism—how it is that it 'knows' both how to develop in the womb and how to perform its motor functions from birth. It contains some of Galen's strongest statements of his belief in intelligent design, but at the same time some striking and original arguments addressing the problem of *how* goal-directed activities arise in animals, and of how genetic information is passed on in conception and gestation.

Greek title: Περὶ κυουμένου διαπλάσεως (*Peri kuoumenou diaplaseōs*)
Kühn: IV.652–702
Edition: Nickel 2001

1. Both doctors and philosophers have addressed the subject of the shaping[1] IV.652 of the embryo, without providing any anatomical basis for their statements. And it is really little wonder that these people miss the truth, as well as disagreeing amongst themselves. In this field even careful dissectors have remained ignorant of certain matters; how much greater will be the errors of those who trust in their own conceptions without any reference to the evidence of anatomy.

Hippocrates was the first we know of to give a | truthful account of the shaping 653 of the embryo; and he conducted his enquiry on the basis not of theoretical suppositions, but of the observations of sense perception—and a substantial number of these, too, unlike some who make absolute pronouncements on the strength of something noticed on one or two occasions. One doctor, for example, having seen an embryo aborted at thirty-two days, and observing that the outline of its construction was already clear, has declared this to be the case with all embryos—having failed to read either Hippocrates' writings or any of the works of others who have described these matters. For there is no one

---

[1] *Diaplasis*, also sometimes translated 'formation' or 'construction', refers to both the structure of an organism and the process by which it achieves that structure; the same word is used for the moulding or shaping activity of sculptors. In Galen's biological analysis, *diaplasis* represents a level of organization and complexity beyond that present in either the elements or the uniform parts. See *The Art of Medicine*, especially ch. 19, 26, 29 and 33; *Mixtures* II.6 , *Health* I.1.

determinate time-frame for all embryos, within which they achieve either clear shaping, motion, or birth. In fact, this whole subject was accurately dealt with in the writings of Hippocrates, and in those of the most reliable of his successors. The writer of the treatise on *The Nature of the Child*—whether that was Hippocrates or his pupil Polybus—gives the following account, which is both clear and accurate, of an aborted six-day-old foetus[2] which he observed:

654   I myself saw a foetus which had remained in the womb for six days | and was then aborted; the appearance of this foetus, as I judged it then, I take as evidence for the rest. Let me explain how I came to see this six-day-old foetus. A lady had in her service a highly-valued musical entertainer, who used to go with men. Now this entertainer had to avoid becoming pregnant on account of the consequent lowering of her value. She had heard, in the course of women's gossip, that if a woman is to become pregnant the seed[3] does not come out, but remains inside. With this warning in mind, she always took care on this point. On one occasion she realized that the seed had not come out, and told her mistress; and word reached me. On hearing what had happened, I instructed her to jump up and down so that her heels touched her buttocks. After the seventh jump, the foetus poured out onto the ground with a noise; seeing it she was amazed. Let me describe it: it was as if the shell of a raw egg were removed, and through the membrane beneath it was visible the fluid within. This sufficiently sums up its basic appearance. It was also red and round; and within the membrane were clearly present a number of thick,

655   white fibres | pressed in with thick red liquid; around the outside of the membrane was some bloody substance; in the middle a fine protrusion, which I took to be the navel: through this it at first both expelled breath and took it in, and it was from this point that the entire membrane extended which surrounded the foetus.

2. In this text the membrane surrounding the foetus should be understood to be what is known as the chorion, containing within it the thick, white fibres, together with thick red fluid, which are an outline of the veins and arteries in the process of generation. Thus, as the embryo grows, it is always observed to be surrounded by the chorion, which is full of veins and arteries. There is in fact nothing apart from these three things that makes up its substance: there are

---

[2] 'Foetus' here translate *gonē*, whereas 'embryo' is the translation used for Galen's more usual term, *to kuoumenon* (literally, 'that in the process of gestation'). There seems no significant semantic difference in this context, *gonē* being the term used in some Hippocratic texts (see also next note); but I have preserved this difference in translation

[3] Again the noun is *gonē*, which has a considerable semantic range; here it seems clearly to refer to semen. (An alternative suggestion has been made that it here refers to the male member, the practice recommended to avoid pregnancy thus being coitus interruptus, but this seems less plausible on linguistic grounds. See also *Simple Drugs* X.1, with n. 17, which again seems to confirm this.)

a very large number of veins and arteries, extending alongside each other, themselves surrounded by and in contact with a continuous, white, membrane-like body.

There is then a distinction amongst animals which bear an embryo. There are those which are not far from the nature of humans, such as goats, sheep, | pigs, 656 oxen, horses and donkeys; here the chorion is observed to be conjoined to the womb of the pregnant animal, through the arteries and veins. And these vessels take the source of their generation from the arteries and veins of the womb, the extremities of which feed into the internal space of the womb; it is by these vessels alone that the embryo is connected with the bearer of the embryo. For there is no other perforation of the chorion: the embryo is not conjoined to the womb anywhere else. The rest of its interior form, while extended within the womb, is merely in physical contact with it without any actual join.

Now, the vessels within the chorion have extremely narrow origins, by which (as I said), they are united with the ends of the vessels of the womb; as they move further from the womb, however, they join together with each other at a single point, in very much the same way as do the roots of plants. In the case of plants, a large number of very fine root-ends come together to form other, thicker roots, which in turn meet to form others, and so on up to the base of the trunk. | In the same way the arteries and veins of the chorion come together to 657 produce others which are thicker, and these in turn give rise to yet others; and after this has been repeated a very large number of times, the concourse of all the individual vessels comes to a head in two arteries and two veins, between which is formed a channel leading straight into the base of the bladder of the embryo (the part which anatomical virtuosi have named the urachus). The other mouth of this channel grows gradually wider as the four vessels become separated, and gives rise to a fine membrane similar in outline to a sausage, which is extended over the outside of another such membrane, that which contains the embryo. The anatomists have given names to these two membranes: the one is called after its shape, 'sausage-shaped', while the other, containing the embryo, is known as the amnion.[4]

These are on the outside; the parts specific to the embryo itself are: first of all the skin, brought about by its Craftsman as a covering or garment that grows along with it; then | in addition the parts inside the skin that are continuous 658 with the four vessels. None of these parts is able to be generated before all the vessels in the chorion acquire their connection with the aforementioned four; for, obviously, each part of the embryo requires the appropriate nourishment, both for its original generation and for the whole of its subsequent

---

[4] 'Sausage-shaped' translates *allantoeidēs*, which gives us the modern anatomical term allantois; amnion literally means 'lamb's'.

maintenance;[5] and there is no other material to nourish it apart from that which is supplied from the animal which bears it. There is, therefore, no part of it capable of being generated without this bloodlike substance.

Now, those parts, on the other hand, which are white and without blood cannot be generated from blood itself, as can the substance of the liver. This is why the liver is generated very quickly, from blood, since its corporeal substance is extremely similar to that of blood. If you cut an animal's vein and allow the blood to flow into fairly hot water, you get a coagulation which is very similar to the substance of the liver. So this organ is the readiest to acquire solid form, and does so simply by being physically surrounded by the womb itself.

659   Of the other | parts, those composed of both flesh and blood require longer for their generation; and the actual body of the vessels, arteries and veins, which is itself entirely devoid of blood, may reasonably be assumed to acquire its first generation from the substance of the semen,[6] when this comes into contact with the extremities of the vessels which lead into the womb; for the sperm may very readily and easily produce such a type of part from its own substance, which has so much viscosity.

Now, since the first rudiments of the vessels are generated at the mouths of those vessels leading into the womb, it is natural to suppose that the semen which shapes them provides them with nourishment, by drawing blood from the womb, and so gradually broadening the parts thus first generated, increasing their length, and both augmenting and gradually bringing together the finer parts in the generation of the broader ones. This, then, appears to be the way in which the vessels and membranes are produced, deriving their initial constitution, and also their subsequent increase in length and breadth, from the sub-

660   stance of the semen, | in the same way as it may be observed with trees that the rest of the tree is formed with the trunk as its origin, both in its upward extension and in its division into branches. Let this, then, be laid down as the foundation of the argument that follows.

3. Let us now consider how it appears that the entire subsequent shaping of the embryo is carried out by the power within the semen; and let us again take as the starting-point for this discovery the observations of anatomy.

Of the four vessels that we have been discussing, which, along with the channel in the urachus, form the navel, the first pair is observed to be unified as soon as it passes through the skin of the embryo, forming one great vein which

---

[5] On 'maintenance' (dioikēsis), see *My Own Doctrines*, n. 14; *The Art of Medicine*, n. 13; *The Doctrines of Hippocrates and Plato*, passim.

[6] *Sperma* may also be translated 'seed', the same word being used also for plant seeds and for the 'female seed' which exists as a counterpart to sperm in ancient theories of conception. In contexts such as the present one, however, where the clear reference is to the substance produced by the male in coition, I have preferred the more readily comprehensible 'semen'.

is inserted into the liver. Now, when I say 'inserted', I am communicating the appearance that arises in dissection. It is not actually that this vein inserts itself into a pre-existing liver; rather, the opposite seems to be the case: when the vein at the navel divides internally, like the trunk of a tree, it first of all splits into two, each part producing a number of outgrowths | analogous to the tree's 661 branches; then, from one part of this division of the veins there develops as a growth the flesh, already mentioned, which is the substance of the liver, while from the other, that which gives rise to the mesentery, there develop the stomach and spleen, the entire coiling of the intestines, the omentum and the part known as the rectum. These too do not pre-exist, but are produced simultaneously with the division of the veins, in the same way that the substance of the liver develops as a growth around each of the veins individually and thus achieves its shape as a single organ connected with them all together on the outside.

The arteries, however, do not acquire this extra substance growing out from them immediately after their division below the skin, nor are they subdivided into many parts. They remain for a long time two only; they surround the embryo's bladder and, with that as their support, proceed downward, to the lower end of the body, until they reach the so-called 'broad and holy bone',[7] in which may be observed two arteries, which go down, one on each side, to the legs, the great artery of the spine, which | is observed to connect with the left 662 ventricle of the heart, being divided into these two.

Now, it is not the case here, as it is with the generation of the liver, that no further point remains for enquiry. It was from the multiple division of one part of the vein leading from the navel that the liver acquired its outgrowth and its further elaboration. The material of the heart, meanwhile, from which this organ is generated, must be supplied from the mother either through the arteries or through the liver, in the latter case by means of the vein which leads up from it for the purpose of generating the parts above this organ. This would take a long time, and not happen immediately in the first days, during which the liver—which is only a short distance away from the body of the womb—has its initial generation. The object described by Hippocrates as appearing round and red, within the chorion of the six-day-old foetus, must be the liver, as yet in an unarticulated and unshaped state. In foetuses aborted after thirty days, these three parts of the body—liver, heart and brain—appear clearly, alongside each other, the liver being bigger than either, | with the heart and brain far behind.   663

It is not, however, possible to determine the exact time of the first shaping of the heart: nothing clear can be learnt from abortions which take place in the

---

[7] Or 'sacrum'; the modern anatomical term is a Latin translation of that used by Greek anatomists (*hieron*), just as 'rectum' above is a translation of *apeuthusmenon*.

first month, nor does the dissection of animals which are similar to humans yield any secure conclusion, so long as the embryo remains unarticulated. Once the articulation has started, most of the other parts have no clear definition, but, as already mentioned, those three—heart, brain and liver—can be observed, in close proximity to each other.

Originally, when, in writing my treatise on *Semen*, I was compelled also to give some account of the chronological order of the shaping of each part, I stated that the heart, like the liver, has as it were the foundation of its generation in the first few days after conception. What led me to this reasoning was the extraordinary importance of this organ's function in the fully-grown creature. When, however, I realized that all other doctors and philosophers were of the view that, until the point of clear articulation, the embryo is still maintained in
664   the same way as plants, | it appeared to me more plausible that the heart had no function at all in the initial stages of generation, and that its shaping must definitely take place subsequently to that of the liver. And I set about enquiring how this comes about.

Now, one of two procedures must be in operation: either the heart is produced from the liver, by blood coming up from it at the same time as the generation of the vena cava,[8] or by means of the great artery—for this too contains blood, not just air, as Erasistratus believes. It is understandable that most people have been deceived in this matter, especially the philosophers, since they have no knowledge of the observations made in animal dissections—most useful amongst which are those made in dissections skilfully performed on living animals, whereby their internal parts are laid bare. From this point of view too, then, a long explanation is needed for those who desire to learn everything thoroughly and scientifically. I have written one treatise investigating *The Function of Breathing*, and another, in addition to that, on *The Function of Arteries and their Pulses*. One who is schooled in those works will know that the
665 | embryo has no need of the function of the arteries in the first stages of its generation, nor of the pulse, nor of the heart—any more than do plants. We should perhaps have made some enquiry into the generation of plants earlier. From a consideration of the conditions necessary for plants, we shall be able to learn exactly what needs the embryo has during the period in which it is still maintained by one soul in the same way as plants are.

Now, in discussions where this is not the precise subject of our investigation, we refer to this kind of soul as 'nature', using the term which is generally applicable to all kinds of being. This term is preferred by Chrysippus and his followers in their precise investigations, too, whereas Aristotle and Plato depart from this

---

[8] Although Galen usually refers to this vein as *koilē phleps*, 'hollow vein'—of which, again, the modern anatomical term is a direct Latin translation—he here uses the term *hēpatitis* ('hepatic vein'), which, as mentioned below, he takes to be the older, Hippocratic term for the same vein.

usage, employing the term 'soul', Aristotle with the addition of the epithet 'nutritive', Plato with the addition of 'desiderative'.[9]

Since, then, our present discussion is not a passing one, as when the enquiry centres on some other topic, but one which aims diligently at the utmost precision, let us first remind ourselves of the generation and maintenance of plants. As their soul is a non-composite, single thing ∣ —for they have neither a spirited 666 nor a rational element—there is some hope that we shall find the maintenance of plants to be a pure, unadulterated thing too.

And let us begin our discussion of the generation of plants by recalling the phenomenon of seed being placed in earth which is moderately moist and warm. Have in your mind the case of a tree, or some other large plant: the activities of the nature which maintains it will be more easily observed in a large body. Immediately a double outgrowth is seen to arise from the seed: downwards into the earth and upwards into the air, each part of roughly the same size. Initially these growths are fine ones, then, as time goes on, they mature and are extended in length, and on reaching a reasonable size, divide into further outgrowths. These too divide into others, and so forth. The plant is nourished and grows simultaneously in all these parts at each point in time; and it fruits at each extremity once the plant has reached its maturity.

∣ Since, then, the maintenance of the embryo is, in the first stages of its gener- 667 ation, the same as that of plants, it is obvious that its growth in the first phase will be very little. But once it begins to be clearly articulated, growth will be greater; and greatest of all in embryos which are already articulated, as the Nature which maintains them is now at work in many parts simultaneously.

What, then, is the limit of this early period in which the embryo still has no need of the heart? It seems to me that it is the point at which the whole division of the veins takes place at the liver. And I say 'whole', since this division is two-fold (I am not the first to have observed this fact: it is a matter of agreement among all anatomists). The vein from the navel, on first reaching the space inside the skin which envelops the embryo, immediately splits into two (in the same way as we observe that the trunks of many trees split into two major branches). Then further veins grow out—like branches—from each of these two, and from these yet others, and so on, until they terminate at the extremities; it is around each of the two parts of the division that the ∣ substance spe- 668 cific to the liver, which was discussed earlier, grows out, both encircling them and filling up the spaces between the divisions, rather in the manner of a broom. Thus the outgrowths from the lower part of the vein arise in the

---

[9] Compare the argument of *My Own Doctrines*, ch. 3. Here and in what follows the Platonic doctrine of the tripartition of the soul (into the rational, spirited and desiderative) forms the essential background to Galen's thought, as it does also in *The Doctrines of Hippocrates and Plato* and *The Affections and Errors of the Soul*.

concave parts of the organ, which partially envelop the right side of the stomach, while those from the higher part of the vein arise in the convex parts, where it touches on the diaphragm. It is for this reason that these two 'gates' of the liver arise in the embryo; for all the veins of the body are parts or offshoots of the great vein which can be observed to pass through the navel, the higher gate coming into being for the production of all those veins in the region of the liver, the lower for that of those leading to the stomach, spleen, omentum, and all the intestines. And when the liver is completed, the largest vein is gathered together from the veins in its convex parts, in the same way that the trunk of a tree is gathered together from its roots. This vein is called the 'hollow vein', the term being applied to it as hollow par excellence, to indicate its greater size
669   in relation to the other veins. Hippocrates, | observing its origin in the liver, called it the hepatic vein [hēpatitis].

This vein, then, extends the whole length of the animal: one part of it is conducted downwards, being fixed in the middle of the spine, the other upwards through the middle of the chest to the neck. This latter produces, first of all, sizeable outgrowths into the diaphragm, then, proceeding from them, very fine outgrowths into the membranes which divide the chest and into the pericardium; and, after, these, into the right ventricle of the heart, and the chest.

We may reasonably suppose that the veins from the lower 'gates', which are subdivided into all the parts around the stomach, cause the generation of the latter at the same time. So, while the upper part of the vena cava is conducted upwards to the heart, the part which is conducted downwards simultaneously produces outgrowths to the kidneys (for these are the organs nearest to the liver) and to the regions around the spine at the lower back. In the same way it is reasonable to suppose that the part of the spine and chest above the diaphragm, which takes outgrowths from the vena cava as this is conducted upwards,
670   derives the material for its generation | from them, simultaneously with the shaping of the heart.

For the previously mentioned pair of arteries, too, which are brought together in a single artery, is at this point already capable of reaching it: we observe this single artery to be fixed in the middle of the spine, up to the point at which it approaches the heart. It is thus plausible that it is by drawing blood from this artery—blood which is much hotter than that in the veins—the heart acquires its greater heat than that of the liver: the difference is the same as that between the two types of blood. The heart has two ventricles: into the right ventricle flows the blood from the liver, which is moderately hot; into the left ventricle flows the much hotter blood from the arteries. And once it has acquired both the ventricles and the two types of material, since then the substance of both has been completed, the heart itself pulses and at the same time moves the arteries with this same motion. At this point the embryo is no longer maintained merely as a plant but now also as an animal—an animal such as a clam, trumpet shell, pen shell, oyster or shellfish: these require very little | 671 motion of the pulse, if any at all. For it has been demonstrated that pulsation is a characteristic of hot bodies; and no bloodless animal is clearly hot, nor is any clearly hot animal bloodless.

Now, even without the heat from the heart, there was already an innate heat, of a lukewarm sort, in venous blood, and therefore also in the liver. But the heart is to the animal a kind of hearth or furnace. Without it the heat of blooded animals is like that of a house in summer: just as the house will become hotter if a fire is lit in it, in the same way the animal's body derives from the heart a heat greater than that which is innate to the veins and liver, and of course also to the blood within them.

Erasistratus is of the opinion that the arteries do not contain this fluid at all. Our view—which accords with the observed appearance—is that a hotter kind of blood, of finer consistency, is present in them: this is the nature of the blood which flows out of an artery when perforated. I believe that Plato, too, was alluding to this fact in the *Timaeus*, when he said:

> The heart they set up in the position of watchman, as the fount at once of the
> veins and | of the blood which is borne vehemently through all the limbs.[10]   672

For we note that he does not here say that it is the fount of blood in general, but only of that sort 'which is borne vehemently through all the limbs'. Now the blood in the veins properly so called is not of that kind; but the ancients applied the term 'vein' indiscriminately to both arteries and veins.

In the same way that it was reasonable that the heart be formed after the liver, and it is for that reason that the liver was placed closer to the womb of the mother, so too it was appropriate that the brain be placed still further from the womb: its construction was to take place later, since the embryo has no use for a brain, having no need to see, hear, taste, or smell; nor to carry out activities with its limbs, nor, quite generally, any other type of voluntary activity, or to be provided with the faculty of touch, with the ability to form impressions, with reasoning or with memory. Therefore the brain, and the whole region of the face, acquire their shaping later, in a third phase. It is at this time too that the | limbs are articulated, and all the parts mentioned above which conduce to 673 the completion of its construction.

---

[10] *Timaeus* 70a–b. According to the standard version of Plato's text, we would translate 'the knot of the veins and the fount…', reading *hamma*, 'knot', rather than *hama*, 'at once'; but it seems that the translation given may reflect the version of Plato's text that Galen actually read. See also *The Doctrines of Hippocrates and Plato* VI.8, with n. 47.

It is obvious, too, that the bone in the head becomes solid after all the other bones; this is why it is so fine and fragile in the front top part that in new-born babies the motions of the brain may be perceived not just by the sense of touch but by sight alone. This then constitutes a fourth phase after the initial conception, that in which those parts which were shaped later on in the gestation are strengthened. It follows then that the most vigorous activities in infants are those of the nutritive soul, and second after them those of the heart, while the brain-functions are quite feeble, to the extent that they are unable not only to run or walk with their legs, but even to stand; still less to engage in reasoning as to what is in their own interest, to learn, to recollect a sensory experience or verbal lesson. It is at a later time that both the bone in the head is strengthened and the teeth appear, and also that hair grows on the head, so that new-born 674 children are clearly incomplete both in their bodies and ⏐ in respect of the best part of the soul, namely the rational. For the capacities of the soul are activated at the same time that their instruments are brought to completion. This may also be learned from the book in which I show that the soul's capacities follow the mixtures of the body.

4. Why then did Chrysippus and many other Stoic and Peripatetic philosophers see fit to make these pronouncements about the heart, that it comes into being first of the animal parts, and that the other parts are generated by it? And that since it is the first to be shaped it must necessarily be the source of the veins and arteries as well? For it is not evident that it is generated first; and moreover it has already been demonstrated that, within all the arts, the same artist produces both the first part of the object being crafted and all the subsequent parts up to its completion, and that it must be the case that the arteries and veins are produced first of all, from the substance of the semen, as was shown in our treatise on *Semen*.

Thus, even if someone else produces some statement similar to these pro- 675 nouncements about the heart, claiming for example that the chorion, or the ⏐ liver, is the source of all the activities of the animal, we shall not be persuaded, since we know that the source of generation of every created body is different from the source of its maintenance. For example, one set of people builds cities; another maintains them. The same is true of ships, or indeed of any product of craftsmanship: the people who construct them are not the same as the people who make proper use of those constructions.

Amongst the capacities that maintain our lives, reason, which comes into being and reaches its completion last of all, nevertheless is in charge and maintains human affairs—for the good, when the soul as a whole is in its correct, natural state, for the bad, when it is perverted into an unnatural state. But it is not my present purpose to investigate the actual performance of the activities. The subject before us in this work is the shaping of embryos. It is a subject of great value in itself, not only to the philosopher but also to the doctor. The enquiry was also necessary because of people who take premisses for their demonstrations from sources from which they should not be taken. For there are those who omit to use as the starting-point of their demonstrations the proper nature of the actual subject under discussion, | resorting to non-evident   676 matters instead.

It is of considerable value to doctors in cases where either half of the body, or nearly all of it, becomes paralysed, and incapable of motion by means of voluntary activities, and also in cases where it is either completely devoid of perception or with very unclear perceptions, to know to which part of the body to apply the remedies. But this is impossible to ascertain before the enquiry is carried out as to whether all the animal's parts derive from themselves both perception and the type of motion mentioned; whether some capacity flows to them through the nerves from the brain, as is the common view of all anatomists; or whether, as some say, from the heart.

The Stoics—in spite of the fact that it seems strangely irrelevant to the discovery of that goal whose achievement they say constitutes happiness—have not only attempted this enquiry but have also done so without recourse to the findings of anatomy, which would have made possible its solution. If in this case they insist, as they have insisted in so many others, on pursuing the investigation into a matter of no use to them, they should have used manifestly observed facts | as the starting-points of their demonstration, following the practice of   677 those doctors versed in anatomy.

Instead, they assert that the heart is the first part to be shaped, without being able to adduce any anatomical evidence that they have used as the starting-point for that discovery, nor any theoretical demonstration; and then, conjoining one piece of ignorance to another, that the other parts are formed by the heart, and that it is in charge, not only of their generation but of their maintenance too.

Now, in earlier times, when the state of anatomical knowledge was not so well advanced as it is now, there would naturally have been some confusion regarding the source which supplies perception and motion through the nerves to the parts of the animal. But now that long and consistent clinical experience has moved doctors universally to share the well-established view of the anatomists, and no one confronted with cases of *mania* without fever, of melancholy, of any kind of damage to the faculties of memory or reason, of phrenitis with fever, of lethargy, epilepsy, or apoplexy, would refrain from | applying treatment   678 to the head, they alone are still conducting an enquiry into matters which are already clearly known to anyone who wishes to find them out.

Enough of this for the moment. We have shown elsewhere how certain philosophers have addressed themselves to considerations of no value for their purpose, involving themselves in long enquiries without being able to discover even a plausible pretext for their enquiry, in the way of those who approach the study of either philosophy or of happiness on a theoretical basis.

5. It will be appropriate at this point, however, to make a crucial addition to the foregoing—a statement of another matter that is unknown to our venerable philosophers, just as is all evidence derived from anatomy. Let us begin with a statement of Herophilus. He asserts that anatomical demonstrations, which tell us, for example, that such-and-such a part grows out of such-and-such another, cannot be used as the basis for any direct inference towards our actual doctrines, although they are so used by certain individuals who misunderstand the issue. Other evidence is needed in order to discover the capacities that maintain 679 us, not inspection of the parts alone. I Our argument now requires certain distinctions—distinctions which were set out more fully in *The Doctrines of Hippocrates and Plato*, but which we shall recapitulate here, insofar as they are necessary for our present purposes.

The first distinction is amongst arteries, veins or nerves when cut or constricted by a ligature; some are observed to maintain their activities beyond the point at which the ligature is tied, others to lose them completely. The same thing may be manifestly observed in the case of the spinal cord, too: if it is severed at a given point along the spine, those nerves which grow from above that point clearly retain the functions of motion and perception, while those below lose these immediately. From this it is obvious that these capacities flow into the spinal cord from the brain. On the same principle, if any artery is ligated, everything above the ligation—everything, that is, which retains its connection with the heart—is observed to pulse as before, but the other parts lose pulse immediately; so that it is obvious here too that the source of motion for the arteries is from the heart.

680   This, then, I is the best and clearest way of determining the source of the bodily activities; next after it is the substance of the bodies in question—whether it is the same throughout, or of a completely different nature. Now, the substance of the spinal cord and the nerves is in every respect the same as that of the brain, just as that of the casements which contain them is the same as that of the meninges which contain the brain. That of the arteries, however, is nothing like that of the heart, nor is that of the veins like that of the liver. In those cases, then, where it is observed to be the same, it is obvious that the finer bodies are offshoots of the thicker ones, the former requiring the latter for their production just as surely as the branches require the trunk. But in the other cases, where the substance of the vein is clearly different from that of the heart and the liver, then on the basis of these data it is not obvious whether the vena cava grows out from the heart, and subsequently acquires its in-growth to the liver, or whether its source is in the liver, and from there it develops up to the

heart—or neither of these, the source of the vein in question being some third part of the body. It is understandable, then, that, | while agreeing on the source 681 of generation of the nerves, anatomists have continued to enquire into that of the vena cava; and even if it is established that the liver is the source of generation of the vena cava, it would still remain unclear, on this basis, whether it takes on the role of source of maintenance in fully-developed animals, in the same way that it is prior in generation, or whether this source comes to them from elsewhere.

We must also make the distinction as to whether the larger veins are sources of the smaller, or vice versa; for some doctors have erred here too. It is, for example, an error to state that their extremities are the source of the veins leading into the stomach and intestines. The generation of these extremities cannot even be conceived of without the fact that the vein coming from the chorion sends an outgrowth of itself which is then distributed into those extremities. On the basis of this observed fact it seems reasonable to conclude that the vein-sources that are in the womb are like the extremities of the tree's roots, while the one which arrives through the navel corresponds as it were to a trunk. Thus, all extremities of veins that are observed in an animal have a position analogous to branches, not | to roots.   682

On a previous occasion I attempted to investigate also the argument as to the sense in which it may be said that first of all to be produced from the semen are the walls of those two vessels which in the foetus and in the fully-grown animal alike appear the largest—that is, the great artery and the vein between the navel and the liver—and that, once these divide, those in the chorion are produced, and then the extremities of these are similar to the extremities of a tree's roots. On this account, too, however, it is still evident that neither the liver nor the heart is generated first; for their generation clearly requires bloodlike substance, which comes to them from the womb, through the vessels.

So one will again conclude, as stated previously, that the semen must have the role of craftsman,[11] and that the vessels by which blood is distributed from the mother for the generation of the organs must be the first thing to come into being, followed by liver and heart—in the same way as the foundations of a house or the keel of a ship. But at the same time that the | power in the semen is 683 shaping them, we may reasonably suppose that certain other parts are being shaped too, parts adjacent to these and between them and the womb. For it could not reasonably be thought that the power that carries out the shaping of

---

[11] An alternative translation would be 'must contain the rationale of the Craftsman' (the Greek words are *logos* and *dēmiourgos*). Whether one prefers the translation given or this alternative, the central point, one indebted to an Aristotelian approach to the subject, is that the semen provides the form, or formative principle (as distinct from the material), in the development of the embryo. Galen elaborates this point in greater detail in *Semen*.

plants and animals would stand still at any point, but rather that the whole of this power causes some outgrowth and increase to all the parts simultaneously. So the nature which shapes animals will not refrain from the construction of the other parts, but will develop the veins and arteries, in a continual process of subdivision, and will cause the growth around them—in the way that the liver and heart were explained to grow around the vessels—of the other organs, at the same time also bringing about the correct shape and position, and all the other attributes appropriate to the parts.

And so the hasty assertion that the other parts are produced by the part which is shaped first is in every way refuted. The cause of the construction of this first part does not somehow then depart from the embryo, commanding its own creations to produce the rest; if this were the case, then the arteries and veins, which are the first to be produced, would actually be responsible for the production of the remaining parts. Nor does it evidently appear that the bodies 684 of arteries and veins are outgrowths of the substance of liver and heart, I in the same way as the spinal cord and nerves are of the brain and its meninges. The most plausible solution, if one is to make an assertion in the domain of the non-evident, is that that which is responsible for the production of arteries and veins also subdivides them and brings them on into every part of the embryo, and shapes the parts around these vessels, in their proper places. It is also most plausible that once the parts have been shaped, and have achieved their final completion, they begin to perform their own proper activities by means of their own proper substances; and that the kidneys, for example, have no need of any other organ for their own specific activity, and that the same applies to the womb, spleen, intestines and in general to every natural organ. Since, however, the substance of the parts remains constant neither in quantity (for there is con-siderable outflow from them every day) nor in quality (this too is subject to manifold alteration), it requires assistance from the other parts so that what is lost may be replaced and any qualitative alteration corrected. The nature of this assistance, in terms of all its varieties and qualities, has remained undiscovered not just by all philosophers but also by those doctors who have embarked upon the enquiry without recourse to anatomy.

685   I The heart, then, which some claim to be alone responsible for the mainten-ance of the animal, ceases its motion when deprived of breath, and when that happens the whole animal dies. Such deprivation of breath takes place not just in cases of strangulation, or where the channel of breathing is blocked by inflammation of the parts around the larynx, but also through damage to the nerves which move the chest (by cutting, compression or ligation), the spinal cord being the source of all these nerves, and the brain in turn of it. Thus, the brain is of importance to the heart for the latter's preservation: it moves the chest by means of the nerves, and it is by the dilatation of the chest that

inhalation takes place; by its compression, exhalation. In the same way, the heart provides some service to the brain, and the liver to both of these. All this has been shown in my works devoted to these matters.

But it is not just the case that all these three organs alone derive benefit from each other; all other parts do so too. For the present, then, let a single reminder suffice of all the other individual points that were made in *The Function of the Parts*. It is on account of the liver that the kidneys and the two bladders come into being, I that which receives bile growing out from the liver itself, and that 686 which receives urine being attached to the kidneys, and also the spleen, which cleanses the slimy excretions of the organ. It was also shown in my writings on *The Function of the Parts* that the stomach performs a preparatory digestion of the nourishment for the liver, and that the intestinal tract comes into being for the purpose of distribution of this nourishment to it—as was every other individual matter regarding each part of the body. And yet doctors and philosophers who have not even the slightest acquaintance with this work still have the effrontery to make these dogmatic pronouncements, attributing everything to the heart.

Perhaps I have prolonged this argument further than is justified by the subject in hand; but it is no wonder that doctors versed in anatomy become enraged at the behaviour of certain individuals who not only pronounce on matters they do not understand but even have the audacity to charge those who do understand them with arrogance. Those who believe that the part first shaped by Nature goes on to shape the others, and that this part is the heart, are deceived on both counts; but even if these points were conceded—not just that the heart is I shaped 687 first of all, but also that it shapes the others—it would not necessarily follow that the activities of the fully developed animal are the responsibility of that organ. To be the source of generation is not the same as to be the source of maintenance.

6. In turning, then, to the principal subject of this treatise, we shall show, not only that those people have not seen fit to inform themselves about enquiries which have been properly conducted by doctors, but also that they believe that in describing the embryo as shaped by nature they are making some utterance which amounts to more than a commonplace. No one, surely, is so stupid as not to understand that there is such a thing as the cause of generation of the embryo; and it is this cause and that we all call 'nature', even if we do not know what this entity is.[12] Now, I have shown that the construction of our bodies

---

[12] 'Entity' translates *ousia*, more usually translated 'essence' or 'substance'. The word has a range of meanings, some of them informed by the post-Aristotelian philosophical tradition. It can mean both the physical material of something's composition, and what something, including a non-material thing, is in its true nature or by virtue of its definition. See also the discussion of the 'substance of the soul' later in this chapter, and also in *My Own Doctrines* (see ch. 2 with n. 8, and chs. 7

manifests to an extraordinary degree the intelligence and power of the one who made it; and so I could wish that the philosophers might, for their part, show me the identity of its maker. Is it a wise and powerful god, who has, first of all, conceived how each animal's body should be constructed and, secondly,

688 endowed each one with an appropriate power I in accordance with that plan? Or is it some other sort of soul, distinct from that of the god?

Of course, those who do not believe that the entity corresponding to this 'nature' (whether that entity is something incorporeal or corporeal) has any intelligence at all will not agree that it manifests an extraordinary degree of it; nor, then, will they be persuaded that it acts in this skilful manner in the shaping of the foetus. Such is the argument of Epicurus and those who hold that everything happens without Providence; but this is not convincing. It would be necessary either that the shaping of the foetus achieve its beneficial goal by virtue of some motion devoid of reason or design, or that what happens is like the case of those who construct magical devices;[13] they provide the first impetus of the motion and then depart, so that their constructions continue to move, by design, but only for a short space of time. It could be that in the same way the gods, once they have constructed the seeds of plants and animals in such a way as to be able to perform this enormous range of transmissions of motions, no longer act themselves.

The former proposition needs no refutation from me, being as it is held in contempt by those persons to whom the present work is chiefly addressed.[14]

689 The latter requires closer examination. Is it feasible that the kind of fluid I that is found in the act of generation makes no error right up to the point of achieving the desired goal, in a process involving the transmission of such a large number of motions? Just as it is incredible to imagine that, within such a great multitude of parts, it happens by chance that no error arises, so too it is rash to assert that the succession could be accomplished in a skilled manner by some non-rational entity—which is the claim of these individuals. But what is even more remarkable is the phenomenon that we observe throughout our lives, namely that none of those who pretend to a knowledge of natural philosophy has ever taken

---

and 14), and in *The Soul's Dependence on the Body*; and see further *Health*, n. 14 and *Simple Drugs* I.3, with n. 2.

[13] *Thaumata*: the same word in Greek may refer to 'tricks' and 'wonders'. What are meant here are especially certain kinds of automata that impressed the spectator by continuing their motion for some time without any external input.

[14] It is not clear to whom, specifically, the present work is addressed. As we see in *Prognosis*, many in the intellectual milieu to whom Galen appealed had an Aristotelian outlook; and a providential world view was shared also by the Stoics. If Galen's implied claim here is that Epicurean or Atomistic views were not taken seriously by respectable intellectuals amongst his contemporaries at Rome, it is not clear whether such a view is supported by the facts, but nevertheless it is of interest that he makes such a claim.

account of or enquired into this process. What is actually at work in the activities of the parts? We shall bring this argument to conclusion with one or two examples for the sake of clarity.

Let us consider first the extremity of the hand, which has fingers composed of three bones each, connected to each other by joints. I believe that those who intend to discover the nature of the heavenly bodies and the entire universe would do better first to verse themselves in this study: by which organs motion takes place in them; how at times they may be extended through | their joints, 690 either many of them at once or each individually; how they may be turned to the side in one of two ways, towards either the thumb or the little finger. For if they realized that all this takes place through the muscles—a fact which we are not aware of until they are laid bare in a dissection—they would wonder how it is that not only we but also small children can immediately stretch or bend a given finger on request, without any knowledge of the muscle in operation. This is even truer of the tongue, in the case of which not even anatomists agree about the number of muscles that move it, so far are they from a secure knowledge of the muscle responsible for each individual type of movement.

But this too has been a subject of enquiry on the part of the more conscientious among the doctors; and it was suggested by one that each muscle functions like an animal, which becomes aware of our volition, and so retracts the tongue and moves it about accordingly, to form the shape appropriate to the sound which is to be produced. This explanation, however, has not seemed plausible to any of the other doctors. It does seem remarkable that a | small 691 child who hears that such-and-such an object is named 'bread' is able to utter that sound without knowing how the tongue must be shaped for that, nor which muscles are involved in each individual movement, and indeed can even utter a whole line, in the course of which the tongue undergoes many changes, in accordance with each sound.

Since, then, there are more than three hundred muscles in our bodies, it is not plausible that each of them is an animal. On the grounds of that implausibility I therefore abandoned that view, and adopted another, which is held in repute by a different group: that the nerves, by pulling the muscles towards their own source, cause the lower part of the bones involved in the joint to follow, the extremity of the muscle being implanted in this part. Even here, though, in addition to the fact that we do not know which of the muscles is to be contracted in each case, considerations of size, too, indicate the contrary, since extremely small nerves are implanted in very large muscles—nerves which are not observed to move during voluntary motions while the animal is still alive, as the muscles are, and which even in a dead body, when activated manually, do not appear to draw in the muscles in the way that the muscles | do the bones in 692 the joints.

And yet the very fact that each of the muscles is moved in a motion proper to a volition makes it implausible that semen is constructed in the same way as those theatrical effects, without any realization or awareness of its own actions. The argument of those who claim that the soul shapes the body around itself, which appears plausible on the basis of certain observed facts, is contradicted here too. The basis of such an argument is the fact that the ability to use the parts of the body is present at the moment of birth. Thus, each animal is observed to defend itself with that part of the body in respect of which it is superior to others: the calf, for example, attempts to lock horns before those horns have grown; the foal will kick before its hooves are hard; the puppy will attempt to bite even if its teeth are not yet sufficiently strong; and birds attempt to fly before they are able. Now, these considerations would seem to indicate that the soul which employs the parts has an understanding of their employment, as would be the case if it had made them itself rather than using parts made by some other. But why, when we wish ⏐ to move a part in whatever manner, it moves immediately, without our knowing the muscle responsible for that movement, is among the most baffling of enigmas. Anatomists have only with great difficulty discovered the specific activity of each muscle, by dissection. And so some have been persuaded that there is one soul which constructs each of the parts, and another which provides the impulse to voluntary activities. According to this argument, apparently, the soul which shapes the parts would continue to remain in the animal's body, for it would not be possible that the present one uses each part correctly, while that responsible for the actual construction absents itself.

We thus see that the subject of the soul which shapes the parts is problematic from every angle. One point alone seems to be clearly established, namely the skill of the one who constructed us, which no one considering the matter with an open mind could possibly attribute to the workings of chance without rational input.

There are in our bodies many more than three hundred muscles, by which the parts are moved in voluntary motions; and each of these possesses the appropriate shape, ⏐ size, beginning and end, position and implanting of nerve, vein and artery, which are adapted to the individual muscle in both size and place of implantation. And in all that great number you will find nothing to criticize (this has been demonstrated in *The Function of the Parts*). Yet if we assume the existence of three hundred parts, each with ten purposes in its construction, and it is observed, further, that everything functions correctly, then the total number of purposes would be three thousand. And I have not yet mentioned the most wonderful aspect of their construction, which is that the muscles on the left side are exactly equal to those on the right side, as is also the case with the arteries, veins and nerves; and so this figure of three thousand may be doubled. The same is also true of the bones, which number more than two hundred. And indeed the purposes of these are in each case many more than ten; when doubled the figure will therefore be in excess of four thousand.

The same level of skill is manifest in the organs, too, and in all the parts quite generally, so that if one were to enumerate the purposes of the whole construction, the result would be some number, not of thousands, but of tens of thousands— | each one functioning perfectly. As I have said, I could never be 695 persuaded that these have come about without an extraordinarily wise and powerful Craftsman. As to the identity of this Craftsman, I had previously hoped to learn this from the philosophers who make pronouncements on the cosmos and the generation of the universe; for I should have thought it a much easier matter for these people to find out the manner in which their own bodies were constructed. And so I presented myself as a pupil to one of these people, in the hope of hearing from him demonstrations of the same sort that I had learned in geometry. But when I realized that, so far from producing geometric-style demonstrations, he could not even utter rhetorical proofs, I moved to another; he too began from his own personal assumptions, proceeding to assert views opposite to those of the previous philosopher. I tried a third, too, and a fourth; and from none of them, as I have said, did I hear a flawless demonstration. Much grieved at this, I have continued up to the present time to seek, on my own resources, to find some secure argument concerning the construction of animals. But I have found none. I admit this fact in the present work; | and I 696 call upon those clever philosophers engaged on this matter, if they find some wise solution, to share it with us without jealousy.

For when I observe that children utter whatever sound we instruct them to— smyrna, as it might be, or smilē, or smēgma,[15] without any knowledge of the way in which the muscles move the tongue in the way appropriate to that sound, still less of the relevant nerves, then it seems most plausible that the one who shaped the tongue, whoever that was, either himself remains in the parts that he has shaped, or has constructed the parts as animals which recognize the will of the command centre of the soul. When, however, I find that it is a consequence of this that there is one soul in our command centre, and a number of other souls in each of the parts of the body, or indeed one common soul which maintains all the parts, I reach an impasse, unable to discover anything about the artificer who shapes us even in terms of a possible conception, let alone secure understanding. When I hear some philosophers assert that matter, which has been endowed with soul | from eternity, structures itself by contem- 697 plation of the Ideas, then I come even more strongly to the conception that

---

[15] The words mean respectively 'myrrh', 'knife' and 'soap'.

there must be only one soul, which both shapes us and continues to employ each of the parts. But again, against this is the fact that the soul that maintains us has no knowledge of the parts that obey its impulses.

Those who have addressed the subject of elementary sounds have progressed to such a level as to be able to assert that one particular sound is produced by attaching the tongue to the teeth known as incisors (those in the upper jaw or in the lower), another by raising it to the roof of the mouth, or to some other part; also that the breath which is brought up from the larynx sometimes reaches the passages in the nose, but is at other times emitted by the open mouth, and that this is sometimes done in a large amount, all at once, at other times in smaller quantities and gradually. And yet none of them has said anything at all on the subject of which muscles bring about these motions; and there is as yet no firmly established discovery in this area even on the part of those most experienced in anatomical observation.

698   Nevertheless, individuals who have discovered none of these matters, | nor indeed made any enquiry into them whatsoever, rush to make not just one pronouncement, but a whole succession, for which they take as their first assumption something unknowable to the senses, and undiscoverable to reason, namely that the heart comes about first of all, then proceeding to add a second one on top of that, namely that it is the heart that shapes the other parts—as if its own shaper, whoever that may be, had ceased to exist. Then they adduce, as if it were a consequence of this, that the deliberative part of our soul is situated there. And if (they proceed to argue) the deliberative part is there, then so will be that which desires food, drink, sex and possessions, and of course also the part concerned with anger and competition. None of the above is a necessary truth; in fact, even if they appear possible to some on first impression, they have subsequently been refuted by many observed facts.

The first phase of the shaping points us—if we consider the matter logically and with the help of anatomical data—to arteries, veins, chorion and liver, not 699 to the heart. The second and third phases are as | discussed above, and we have also given an account of the developments which take place after birth, involving both the addition of parts not yet in existence and the completion of parts which were not yet fully developed.

A particular cause of wonder might be how the similarity between offspring and parents comes about. For again, it appears that the soul which shapes the body comes from the parents to the embryo, as though contained in the semen. What its substance is, I cannot say; for I have heard the discourse of some who are convinced that the soul is incorporeal, but comes together with the semen, using it as the appropriate material for the purpose of shaping the embryo in gestation. Some of them, on the other hand, say that the semen is not its material, but its instrument, for the material is the mother's blood. Others again contradict this, and hold that the semen (either the whole of it, or, as some think, the breath contained in it) is the artificer himself. I have addressed this subject specifically in a work in which I consider the statements of Chrysippus in his writings on *The Soul*, and also in another work, in which ⏐ I investigate the   700 apparent self-contradictions in Plato's writings on the soul.[16]

As already stated, however, I have found none of these beliefs to be scientific-ally demonstrated, and so I admit my puzzlement on the subject of the sub-stance of the soul, about which I am not even able to reach the level of a plausible statement. I confess, then, that I am at a loss as to the cause respon-sible for the shaping of the foetus. For I observe in this shaping the utmost intelligence and power, and I cannot allow that the soul in the semen—that soul which Aristotle calls vegetative and Plato desiderative, and which the Stoics consider not to be soul at all, but nature—shapes the foetus, since this kind of soul is not only not intelligent, but entirely devoid of reason; nor, however, can I entirely distance myself from that opinion, in view of the similarity of the off-spring to the parents; and I am disinclined to the rational soul that remains after birth throughout our lives, because of the fact that we do not know, before anatomical research, either the parts of the body or the functions of those parts.

One of my Platonist teachers told me that the soul that extends through the entire universe ⏐ shapes the embryo; my reaction was that the skill and power   701 involved would be worthy of that entity, but I could not tolerate the conclusion that scorpions and venomous spiders, mice and mosquitos, vipers and worms, helminths and ascarides were constructed by her, for such a doctrine appeared to me verging on blasphemy.[17] Nor do I think it reasonable that the soul of mat-ter could reach the appropriate level of skill.

Only the following, then, do I believe myself able to declare definitely about the cause of shaping within animals: that it involves an enormous degree of skill and intelligence; that after the shaping the entire body is maintained through-out its life by three sources of motion; that from the brain through nerves and muscles; that from the heart through the arteries; and that from the liver

[16] Not all the positions summarized by Galen in the foregoing are easy to assign to particular historical figures. The notion of seed as instrument as opposed to mother's blood as material would seem to be Aristotelian, that of the breath (*pneuma*) in the soul as having a formative role appar-ently Stoic (see also *My Own Doctrines*, chs. 7 and 11); neither Chrysippus' work on *The Soul* nor Galen's dedicated response to it have survived (though *The Doctrines of Hippocrates and Plato* con-tains extensive fragments of it, in other areas); nor has the work mentioned on Plato. For the argu-ment regarding naturally evil creatures, compare *The Soul's Dependence on the Body*, ch. 11, pp. 453–4.

[17] With the phrase 'the soul that extends through the entire universe' Galen refers to the doc-trine of the 'world soul', derived from Plato's *Timaeus* and a prominent feature of Platonist, and especially Neoplatonist, thought; which Platonist teacher is meant is unknowable. Elsewhere, Galen specifically identifies only two such individuals in his account of his education, 'a Platonist pupil of Gaius' in his home town of Pergamum (see *Affections*, ch. 8) and Albinus at Smyrna (*My Own Books*, ch. 2).

through the veins. The manifest starting-points on the basis of which I have ventured to state these opinions have been made clear in a number of treatises, especially in that on *The Forms of the Soul*; but I have nowhere presumed to declare the identity of the substance of the soul. Even whether it is entirely |
702   incorporeal, whether it is something bodily, whether it is completely immortal, or perishable—I have yet to find anyone who has employed geometric-style proofs on any of these questions, a point I discussed also in my treatise on *The Forms of the Soul*.[18]

---

[18] Galen mentions a work of this title also at *The Doctrines of Hippocrates and Plato* IX.9, and it may be the same as one mentioned in *My Own Books*, ch. 16; but it has not survived.

IV

HEALTH, DIET AND LIFESTYLE

The Best Constitution of our Bodies *and* Good Condition

This pair of short treatises is mentioned several times by Galen as occupying a position in the curriculum of study immediately after those on physical theory and the composition of the body and before those on physiology and clinical practice, and thus contributing to the basic understanding of health and its maintenance in human bodies. They give a synoptic view of some important conceptions and categorizations regarding health, disease and the functioning of the body.

Kühn: IV.737–55
Edition: Helmreich 1901

The Best Constitution of our Bodies

1. What is the best constitution of our bodies? Is it the same as that with the IV.737 best mixture? This was the opinion of many of the ancient doctors and philosophers. Or is it rather the case that, while the optimal constitution necessarily has optimal mixture, optimal mixture does not in itself necessarily entail optimal constitution? For the health of our uniform parts consists in a well-balanced mixture of hot, cold, dry and wet; but the shaping of the animal on the basis of all these parts | consists in the position, size, shape and number of the compo- 738 nent elements. And it may appear possible that a body composed of parts which are all, or for the most part, well mixed may nevertheless have some defect in respect of their size, number, shaping, or relationship with each other.

Let us then attempt to give an account of all these matters in order; and let us begin with the terms which are necessarily used in this discussion, since these too are the subject of some dispute. Some talk of the best constitution (*kataskeuē*) of the body, others use the term state (*diathesis*), or condition (*hexis*), disposition (*schesis*) or nature (*phusis*), and so on, according to their individual preferences. Now, I have no objection to people employing whatever terminology they wish; but I do think it wrong to make objections to other people's choice of terminology; for I believe that one's greatest concern should be with the actual matters under discussion, not with the words attached to them. Let one, then, posit whichever terminology one prefers—that of best constitution,

state, condition, disposition or nature of the body, or indeed any other such term,
739   provided one starts with the agreed notion | and proceeds from that towards
the discovery of the essence, conducting the enquiry in accordance with some
sort of order and method. One who adopts such a procedure will be far more
deserving of our praise than one who displays a virtuosity in the use of terms.

Let us indeed follow this procedure ourselves: let us begin from the shared
notion, methodically apply to it the relevant distinctions, and thus proceed to
what follows in the enquiry.

2. What, then, is the conception which all people share of the best constitution
of the body? For it is possible that, although one hears people use different
terms, the underlying conception is the same for all these people. Everyone,
without exception, is in favour of the 'healthiest' body, as also of that with 'best
condition'; and in both cases they are looking at the same object, and applying
their intellect to that; but their conception is not a fully articulated one, nor do
they have the capacity to communicate it clearly. Moreover, people think it
good both that the activities of all parts of the body should be vigorous and that
the body should not be readily susceptible to morbid influences. The fulfilment
of the first of these conditions, that one's activities be in their normal state, constitutes health (*hugieia*); and the addition of a certain degree of vigour makes it
good condition (*euexia*). And not being readily susceptible to diseases is a common feature of both.

740 | Thus, the state of good condition is certainly the healthiest, and is the goal
of all human beings; and it possesses also the incidental properties that the
activities function correctly and that the state is not readily destroyed. It is for
this reason too that the term good condition seems appropriate for it. This
notion of stability and indissolubility is implied in the term condition itself, and
even more so in the term good condition, which suggests the best possible condition.[1] With regard to the best constitution of the body, then, the application
of either epithet, 'healthiest', or 'of best condition', is perfectly correct; and the
criterion of such a state will be that the activities function correctly, and that
this good functioning is not readily altered.

Now that this has been clarified, we must next enquire, what is the essence of
such a condition of the body? And here our starting-point must be an enquiry
as to the state of our bodies in which we enjoy this optimal functioning of the
activities. At this point we must make reference to matters that have been demonstrated previously in other works. First, that our bodies are a mixture of hot,
741   cold, dry and wet, | which was shown in our treatise on *The Elements according
to Hippocrates*; secondly, the distinction between the mixtures of the parts, as

---

[1] In Greek the word translated 'good condition', *euexia*, is formed from the addition of *eu*
('good' or 'well') to the noun *hexis*, 'condition'; in Galen's usage *hexis* is a stable or firmly
established state.

discussed in our work on *Mixtures*. Then, too, that for each organic part of the body there is a single cause of activity, governing all the parts which it contains, and that everything else that goes to make up that organ as a whole comes into being for the sake of that cause. These matters have been adequately shown in *The Function of the Parts*. The best constitution of the body will thus be that in which all the uniform parts (this, of course, is the name given to those which appear to the senses as simple bodies) retain their own proper mixture, while the composition of the organic parts, on the basis of these, has the best-balanced constitution, in terms of size, number, shaping and relationship with each other. That body which is in the best state in respect of all its activities will readily be found to be the least prone to illness. The part which functions best is a product of both good-mixture of the uniform | parts and well-balanced constitution of 742 the organic ones; and that is the nature of the body already described. It is therefore evident that it is this kind of body that will function best of all. The fact that it is also the least prone to disease may be gathered from what follows.

3. Damage to our bodies arises in two ways: from external causes or from the residues of our nourishment. External causes are those which affect people through excessive heating, cooling, moistening and drying. Fatigue, sleepless-ness, distress, worry and all other such items, should also be placed in this cat-egory. Within those arising from residues of nourishment, there is a twofold distinction in class, since the manner of their disturbance is twofold: through either quantity or quality. The specific distinctions within both are numerous.

Now, the insusceptibility of the body which is in a well-balanced state is already evident on the basis of that very good-mixture, which, by virtue of the fact of its maximal distance from all the extremes, will not readily fall into a bad balance of mixture. | Moreover the fact that it enjoys good function, too, pro- 743 vides the best basis for its immunity from illness, since such a body is the least prone to the ill effects of exertion. It is this body, too, which enjoys the best humoral fluid of all, enabling it more easily to withstand the negative influences of distress, anger, sleeplessness, worry, rain, drought, plague and, in short, all pathological causes. It is bodies with bad humoral fluid that readily succumb to such causes, being in themselves already close to a state of disease.

The state mentioned, then, is not readily destroyed by harmful external effects upon the body. Its insusceptibility to diseases arising from residues of nutrition may be seen from the following consideration, namely that no build-up, nor poor quality, of humoral fluid will readily accumulate in such a nature or, hav-ing accumulated, cause harm to the living being. For the correct balance of the natural activities in relation to each other, and the individual excellence of each, have | the twin effects of preventing the build-up of such residues and facilitat- 744 ing their speedy expulsion; and, even if some such substance does remain in the body for a longer period, this kind of body will be the least susceptible to its effects. Susceptibility to pathological causes is a property of weak natures, those with bad-mixture, while the ability to withstand them over a long period is a property of strong ones, those which enjoy good-mixture; these are the natures which we have described as the best.

The indicators of such a nature, considered in terms of its good-mixture, are available to you in my work on *Mixtures*; and, considered in terms of the correct balance of the organic parts, in the seventeenth book of *The Function of the Parts*; I will nonetheless give a reminder of them in what follows here too. We have shown, in our writings on the subject of health, that it is not a narrow, single or indivisible item, but rather involves a considerable spectrum. It therefore seems to me appropriate, if the present discussion is to be of value to practitioners of the art, for me not just to produce a conceptual construction of that kind of body that will be rarely found in its practice—an example of the Canon of Polyclitus,[2] as it were—but also to make reference to that which deviates 745 from that kind in certain respects, but whose I defect is not, so far, large or blatant. It will thus be possible easily to recognize both the best constitution of the body—even if its appearance is rare—and all the others which we encounter on a daily basis. (For the body which is in an absolutely correct state in all respects, with no imbalance in either the uniform or the organic parts, is by no means a regular occurrence, but rather a somewhat infrequent one, whereas that which deviates from it slightly may be constantly observed.)

4. Now, the perfectly well-mixed body is at the midpoint between soft and hard, hairy and bare, broad-veined and narrow-veined, and between largeness and smallness of pulse. The body which is perfectly well balanced in terms of the organic parts will be, to summarize it simply, similar to the characterization given of the Canon of Polyclitus.

Those which are hotter than they should be, but not by much, as also those 746 which are colder, drier or wetter, I but only to a moderate degree, and those which have some one part which is not correctly shaped, may all, in some respects, appear actually superior to the state of good balance. For example, a harder body will be less susceptible to all external influences, a softer one to all internal ones. Similarly, a denser body is less susceptible to external influences, a more porous body to internal ones.

So, Hippocrates' statement in *Nutrition*, that 'porousness of body is healthier for transpiration in those bodies in which more is removed, and unhealthier in those in which less', refers to the effects of residues of nutriment on health and disease. It is not Hippocrates' purpose in that book to consider healthy and morbid bodies in general terms; rather, his discussion there addresses all good and bad effects of

---

[2] See *Mixtures* I.9, with n. 9.

nutrition, and thus naturally also makes mention of healthy and morbid bodies, insofar as these states are related to their residues. It is in relation to their residues that more porous bodies are healthier and denser ones more morbid. Conversely, the more porous type is more prone to all external influences, | while the denser   747 type is less so. It is, then, a yet further advantage of the well-balanced body that it cannot be stated to be either porous or dense; just as it is at the midpoint with respect to the other excesses, so too with respect to these.

Yet each of these excesses is superior in some particular respect. The denser body is less susceptible to external influences, the more porous one to internal ones. No body may be found which is perfectly immune to both types; but that which is at the midpoint between all excesses will be moderately so, and this is precisely the one that we claim to be the healthiest of all. So, too, a body drier than the well-balanced one is less susceptible to moistening influences, while a wetter one is less susceptible to drying ones. As has already been stated, then, the medial body is not the least susceptible in all respects; rather, it is worse than each other type *in one particular respect*, but is nevertheless preferable to all these.

Nor is it necessary that such a body be either large or small, or medium-sized. This point was made in *Mixtures*; but let us recapitulate it here too. A large body is so by virtue of the large amount, and a small one by virtue of the small amount, of material of which it is made up, | in the same way that a large   748 statue is made from a large quantity of bronze, and a small one from a small quantity; but nothing is to prevent either type from being well-balanced in terms of its parts. The body with the best mixture will be that which is neither markedly dense, porous, hard, soft, hairy nor bare—whatever its size. If, in addition, it enjoys a good balance in terms of the internal relationship of the organic parts, such a body will also be the most beautiful to behold, and perfect in its constitution. Bodies which are larger or smaller than the norm have become so for one of two reasons. These are: in the case of largeness, excess of either moisture or matter; in the case of smallness, dominant dryness or lack of moisture. For growth continues until the bones become hardened; and when this takes place when the size is still small, this is a result of either dryness or lack of moisture. Cessation of growth, then, also comes about for one of two reasons. Largeness is not, therefore, straightforwardly a sign of moisture, nor smallness of dryness; in cases where the large body is also soft, and the small one hard, then the former will be wet and the latter dry. | Since these features   749 always occur together, it is superfluous to consider largeness or smallness. The specific indicators of mixture are sufficient; and the distinctions relevant to these have been laid out more fully in *Mixtures*. If, then, the above account is accurate, the best constitution of the body should be taken to consist in two things: good-mixture of the uniform parts, and good balance of the organic ones.

Good Condition

IV.750 The term 'condition' is customarily applied to any state which is stable and not readily destroyed, and may be used equally as a positive or negative term. The terms 'good condition' and 'bad condition', on the other hand, distinguish the nature of the condition under discussion. Now, a condition which is described as good without qualification arises only in a body endowed with the best constitution of the body; one which is described as good with qualification may occur in every type of body. Bad condition, meanwhile, may arise in every 751 | bodily constitution, whether one means bad condition without qualification or in relative terms.

Now, if one wishes to know the precise nature of good condition in the unqualified sense, one should call to mind our statements on the subject of the best constitution. As has been shown frequently elsewhere, there is a considerable spectrum within health; its intensification is termed 'good condition' by both philosophers and doctors of old times; its looser version is not given any specific name, but rather referred to by the same general term as the whole category, 'health'. Good condition is an optimal form of health, and thus arises in bodies with the best constitution. A body without such a constitution would not admit of optimal health, and therefore also not of good condition.

Now, 'good condition' is also used in relative terms, that is to say by reference to the individual nature. One may thus add a qualification, and speak of 'Dion's good condition', or of 'Milo's good condition'; of course, Achilles' good condition, or Heracles' good condition, would also count as good condition without 752 the addition of the qualification, in the same way that | Achilles is 'fine' without any qualification, while a monkey is not fine in this sense, but only fine for a monkey. Also requiring the addition of a qualification is the good condition of athletes, about which Hippocrates made a very apt comment when he said: 'Amongst people who take exercise in the gymnasium, peaks of good condition are dangerous.'[3] Hippocrates is not here saying that the good condition which is so called without qualification is dangerous when it reaches a peak; indeed, its peak consists precisely in the fact that it is the most stable of all states of the body. But the good condition of athletes, or gymnasium practitioners (or whatever other term one may wish to use), which is *not* good condition in the unqualified sense, naturally does become dangerous when it is taken to a peak. As Hippocrates says: 'The athletic state is not natural; better a healthy condition.'[4] Now the perfection of the healthy condition is good condition; but that of the athlete's state is only termed 'good condition' with the addition of a qualification, in the same way as one may speak of 'a beautiful monkey', 'a long

---

[3] *Aphorisms* 1.3.   [4] *Nutrition* 34.

cubit', a 'false quart' or a 'counterfeit drachma'.[5] For a cubit which is long is not, then, ⎮ a cubit in the unqualified sense: the phrase 'long cubit' must be under-   753
stood as a whole; and so too with the expression 'false quart'.

So, quite generally, something to which a term is applied without the add-ition of a qualification is not of the same nature as something to which it is applied with a qualification; and it may sometimes be the case that the former kind of object is a highly desirable one while the latter is to be avoided—as indeed is the case with the athletes' good condition. So far is it from being desirable that it is in fact quite rightly condemned, not just by Hippocrates and the other doctors of old, but also by the best philosophers, including Plato, who in the third book of his *Republic* shows its complete uselessness for the pur-poses of the normal performance of one's activities and explains the danger it represents to health. For its exponents aim at the acquisition not just of good-mixture of the body but also of physical bulk, and this cannot take place with-out an immoderate filling of the body.

In order to arrive at a correct understanding of genuine good condition, ⎮ we   754
should make a comparison between this and the athletic version, investigating the points of contact and opposition between the two. Good-mixture of all parts of the body is common to both. So too is excellence of the activities; and it follows from these points that good humoral fluid is a common point too. So much for the shared features; the points of opposition are as follows. Genuine states of good condition involve good balance of the blood, as well as of the mass of all the solid bodies; athletic states involve a poor balance of these, and especially of the fleshy ones. When such a state reaches its peak, a dangerous situation necessarily obtains. When such individuals eat under compulsion, and their stomachs digest vigorously, and distribution of the food results readily from the digestion, with the further consequences of blood-production, addition of matter to the body, further growth, and nutrition, there is a risk that the condition becomes overfilled, so that there remains no natural place for the addition. In this case the veins become immoderately filled with blood and the innate heat is smothered and extinguished, being deprived of the possibility of ⎮ transpiration. Even if the subject withstands this, there will still occur some   755
rupture of the vital vessels situated in the region of the liver, lungs and chest.

---

[5] These examples of counterfeit currency and false measure (the quart, *choinix*, was a standard unit, taken to correspond to the daily allowance of corn for one person) make Galen's point against athletic 'good condition' particularly forcefully: after all a counterfeit drachma is not just 'not a drachma except in a qualified sense'; it is simply not a drachma. It is noteworthy also that Galen has made a transition in his examples from cases where the sense of the *adjective* is qualified by its rela-tion to a noun ('fine monkey') to ones where the sense of the *noun* is qualified by its relation to an adjective (or possessive): 'long cubit', 'athlete's good condition'. (The former linguistic feature, that adjectives, in particular quality terms such as 'hot', 'dry', etc., must be understood in relative terms, is essential to much of Galen's argumentation on perceptible properties, especially in *Mixtures*.)

These vessels, indeed, have softer membranes than those in the limbs, and receive nutrition earlier; and it happens as a result of the quantity of natural heat, in conjunction with the continuous nature of the activities, that the blood undergoes something similar to fermentation, and so ruptures their tunics, in the same way that wine jars are sometimes broken by young wine in the process of fermentation.

These consequences, then, all follow of necessity from immoderate filling; and the demonstrations relevant to them follow from the arguments[6] of natural science. The fact that the innate heat is extinguished when the veins are over-filled with blood was stated in my *The Function of Breathing*, and the fact that the veins are ruptured, in my anatomical works. It would appear that Hippocrates, too, is aware of this, not just from his statement that 'Amongst people who take exercise in the gymnasium, peaks of good condition are dangerous', but also from another text: 'In cases of sudden loss of voice, stoppages 756 of the veins | cause the harm.'[7] Here Hippocrates is using one particularly vital example to indicate the sudden paralysis of any activity; by stoppages of veins he means the overfilling, as a result of which they are unable to receive cooling through transpiration.

---

[6] By *logoi* here Galen may also (as suggested in what follows) be referring to his own actual works of natural science, rather than, or as well as, to the arguments of the science in a more general sense.

[7] For the first quotation see n. 3 above; the second is from *Regimen in Acute Diseases*, appendix, 4.

Health[1] (excerpts)

Galen's major work on healthy lifestyles and health maintenance extends over six books, and covers topics as varied as the precise nature of the baths, foods, wines and exercise regimes, including massages, recommended for different bodily constitutions; the early care of children; recipes for home preparations; and age-related differences in physique and lifestyle.

The following very brief extracts are taken mostly from the first book, which has as its main theme the nurture of children, and takes as its starting-point the optimal case of a child with the best possible bodily endowments and life opportunities. They aim to give an overview of Galen's conceptual understanding of the nature of health and the principles underlying a healthy lifestyle (*diaita*), and also an insight into his views on the extent to which psychological factors can affect health, both positively and negatively. A theme that runs through the work is the requirement of freedom from work obligations—that is, that one must have the leisure to devote as much time as needed, and whenever it is needed, to the care of the body—if one is to achieve optimal health outcomes. Galen does, however, acknowledge the need to provide prescriptions for people with suboptimal life circumstances, too, and is reasonably optimistic about the version of health that these can aspire to, even if this will not be in every way optimal. Indeed, another central tenet of the work is that there is a spectrum of health: one may legitimately be called 'healthy' even if one does not enjoy perfect, or perfectly stable, health.

Unlike a number of more technical works, this treatise is avowedly intended for a non-specialist readership—people interested in medicine but who are not themselves doctors. Though its dating is controversial, it may belong late in Galen's output; at any rate the sixth book seems to have been written considerably later than the rest, and certainly after the death of Marcus Aurelius (AD 180).[2]

Greek title: Τὰ ὑγιεινά (*Ta hugieina*)
Kühn: VI.1–452
Edition: Koch 1923
Translation: Singer 2023

---

[1] The title has also been translated as 'Hygiene' or 'The Preservation of Health' (the latter being an English version of the title *De sanitate tuenda*, adopted by Thomas Linacre for his 1517 Latin translation of the work, dedicated to Henry VIII).
[2] On the date see Singer 2023: 68–79.

BOOK I

VI.1   1. As we have shown elsewhere,[3] there is one single art that concerns the body, which however has two primary and essential parts. These are known respectively as 'healthfulness' and 'healing'.[4] They have opposite functions: the former aims to preserve the bodily disposition as it is, while the latter aims to alter it. Health comes before sickness, both in time and in importance, and so it makes sense that we should consider the preservation of health first, before moving on

2   to the | cure of sickness. Both however share a common method, in terms of their discovery: the analysis of the bodily state which is properly called 'health'. After all, we will neither be able to preserve an existing state of health nor to recover one which has been lost unless we have some idea what health actually is. This has been discussed elsewhere, too.[5] It was shown that the health of the 'uniform' parts consists in a balance of cold, hot, dry and wet, while that of the organic ones derives from the composition, number, magnitude and shaping of those. It is the person who is capable of preserving these features who will excel at the preservation of health. And this will be accomplished by first discovering all the ways in which they may be lost. There would be no need of an art to take care of[6] the body, if the body in question were in no way vulnerable to being affected. Since, however, it is so vulnerable, and in many ways, it requires some art to supervise it—an art which will both identify those various

3   kinds of harm and be capable of protecting it from them. |

2. There are two kinds of harm and decay in our bodies. The first kind is unavoidable and biologically innate to us, from the moment of our conception; the second is not unavoidable, and does not arise from us internally, but is still no less destructive of the body than the other kind. Let us distinguish these. Blood and semen are the sources of our generation, blood being the appropriate material, malleable by the Craftsman,[7] and semen, performing the function of the Craftsman. Both consist of the same basic elements, namely the wet, the dry, the hot and the cold—or, to refer to them by substances rather than qualities: earth, water, air and fire. (This was all demonstrated in *The Elements according to Hippocrates*.) The differences that arise are in the quantities in that mixture. Semen contains a larger amount of the fiery, airy substance, blood

4   more of the earthy, watery substance | ... but semen too is fluid and watery. On

---

[3]   Galen refers to his polemical treatise *Thrasybulus* (translated in Singer 1997a and Singer 2023).

[4]   The Greek words are *hugieinon* and *therapeutikon*: the former is related to the English 'hygiene', and sometimes so translated.

[5]   See *The Art of Medicine*, chs. 1 and 2. The distinction of levels of analysis of the body that follows is essentially Aristotelian.

[6]   'Take care of' translates *pronoeisthai*, the verb cognate with *pronoia*; see *The Best Doctor is Also a Philosopher*, n. 1, *My Own Doctrines*, n. 9 and *Affections and Errors* I.4, with n. 11.

[7]   *Dēmiourgos*; see *The Shaping of the Embryo*, especially chs. 2, 5 and 6, and *The Function of the Parts of the Human Body*, especially VI.13, with n. 10.

both sides, then, we are generated from a wet substance. This must lose its wetness, if it is to be turned into nerves, arteries, veins, bones, cartilage, membranes and all other such things. Right from the start, in fact, something which dries must be a fundamental element....

Later, as the embryo becomes gradually more and more dried out, it acquires the faint outlines and patterns of the individual parts; and when it has been still further dried out, it acquires also the precise form of each. Once born, it continues to I become drier and stronger until it reaches the prime.[8] At that point 5 there is no further increase; the bones, having achieved their full hardness, cease to grow; the vessels have all achieved their full extension; and all parts are at their peak of vigour and strength. From then onward the organs begin to become drier than their optimal state and perform their functions less well; and the creature becomes less well-fleshed and thinner. At a further stage of drying-out, it is no longer just less well-fleshed, but actually shrivelled, I while the limbs lose vigour 6 and become less stable in their motions. This is the state of old age, which is analogous to withering in plants. Withering is the old age of plants, and it arises from excessive dryness. This innate form of change, then, is the first unavoidable cause of decay in every generated body. The second, which obtains in the case of animals, is a flowing-away of their whole substance, which is due to the innate heat.

Such damage is in itself inescapable; but it is possible with foresight to avoid further forms of damage which will otherwise follow from it.... Since the substance of which all creatures are composed is in constant flux, the whole body will in this way be destroyed and dissipated if one does not introduce into it something similar to that which has flowed away. This surely is why Nature has endowed both animals and plants, at the very outset, with innate tendencies I that draw them towards what is needed in each case. No one has taught us to 7 eat, drink or breathe; but we possess within ourselves, right from the start, the capacities that accomplish all these activities without any instruction. Through eating we replenish the drier part of the substance that has been lost or voided, and through drinking the wetter part; through both we restore the previous state of good balance. And we preserve the balance of the airy and fiery substances through respiration and the pulse....

3. Since, then, in all creatures a great deal of substance is lost in this way every day because of the innate heat, and we require food, drink, respiration and the pulse in order to preserve the state of good balance, there unavoidably arises the generation of residues. The ideal would be if it were possible to introduce, throughout the body as a whole, stuff which was exactly the same in kind as the substance evacuated; I that would be the most healthful outcome. But 8 since what flows out from each part is of precisely the same nature as that part,

[8] For Galen there are four main phases of life: childhood, the prime, the post-prime and old age.

whereas nothing eaten or drunk is of precisely that same nature, it is necessary that Nature first subject them to a preliminary transformation and coction,[9] to render them as close as possible to the composition of the body being nourished. Anything which is not thoroughly processed and assimilated at this stage is not added to the body; it is superfluous, or residual, and moves around the spaces within the body. This indeed is why the name 'residue' has correctly been given to it by our predecessors. Since, then, eating and drinking are necessary, and the generation of residues is a necessary consequence of them, Nature has provided us with organs for their separation, and endowed those organs with capacities by which they either attract, move on or expel the residues.[10]

   In order to keep the body constantly clean and free from residues, then, it is important that one have no internal obstruction and that one not become feeble in
9 the operation of one's bodily functions. | The two first and fundamental aims in view in the construction of the healthful daily regime,[11] then, have now been explained: the replenishment of things evacuated and the separation of excess products. A third, that is the avoidance of the creature's premature aging, follows automatically from these. If one correctly performs both the replenishment of what is evacuated and the removal of the residues from within, the creature will be healthy, and will maintain itself in peak condition for a very long time....

[*In the following extract Galen moves from consideration of psychological and ethical qualities in relation to the nurture of children to discussion of the significance of psychological factors for health more broadly. In this context he gives a rare insight into the activities of, and his attitude towards, the temple medicine practised at the Asclepieion of Pergamum: it is prescriptions given in that institution that are meant by the reference to the 'instructions' of the god Asclepius.*]

39 8. The kind of child presently under discussion is that which is best in all
40 respects. | Such a child will require the preservation of, rather than any adjustment to, its character traits; one must avoid their being destroyed. The same kinds of factor—in terms of their basic category—are responsible for things being preserved and things being destroyed. In the case of the soul, character traits are destroyed by bad habits in food, drink, physical exercise, things watched and heard, and music in general. So the person who occupies himself

---

[9] *Pepsis*, literally 'cooking'. On Galen's understanding the nutritive process is closely analogous to a process of heating or cooking, during which the stuffs ingested are gradually transformed in such a way that they ultimately become the stuffs of which the body is composed.
[10] Galen refers to his view of the four natural capacities or faculties (*phusikai dunameis*)—those of attraction, repulsion, assimilation and expulsion—which he takes to be fundamental to the functioning of plants and animals; see *My Own Doctrines*, ch. 3, with n. 14.
[11] *Diaita*: the term, from Hippocratic times onward, includes diet, but also exercise, baths and environmental and other lifestyle factors.

with the art of health must have experience of all these: it should not be thought that the shaping of the character of the soul belongs within the domain of the philosopher alone. It does belong within that domain: the philosopher is concerned with the greater aim of the health of the soul itself. But it also belongs within the doctor's domain, insofar as he is concerned to prevent the body from succumbing to illness. For we find that rage, weeping, anger, distress, excessive worry and the poor sleep which tends to result from these provoke fevers, and may lead to serious diseases.[12] Conversely, an idle intellect, lack of intelligence, and complete lack of spirit in a soul are frequently observed to give rise to poor complexion and poor absorption of food, through the feebleness of the innate heat. It is vital that our innate heat be kept within the healthy range: | this is   41 achieved by a good balance of exercises of both body and soul. The wrong level of motions, in the area of desire, argument and spirit,[13] make a creature either too bilious (when these motions are excessive) or too cold and phlegmatic (when they are deficient). In the former case there may also arise fevers, and the kinds of ailment related to heat; in the latter, obstructions in the liver and internal organs, as well as epilepsy, apoplexy and other such illnesses—those involving catarrh and the flow of liquids.

I have myself frequently restored people to health by correcting such imbalances in their motions—people who had suffered for many years as a result of their psychological characteristics. And our patron god Asclepius bears witness to the same point: he often instructs patients to write poems or comic sketches, or to compose particular kinds of song, in cases where the spirited in them has become too vehement and has thus made the mixture of the body excessively hot. Conversely, he equally often | instructs people to engage in hunting with   42 hounds, horse-riding and armed fighting. He even specifies the precise form of hunting or of armed fighting in each particular case. When the spirited has become feeble, his intention is not simply to stimulate it: he actually stipulates the type and level of the physical exercise required. The hunting of wild boar, of bears, of bulls and of similarly fierce beasts does not sharpen the spirit in the same way as that of hares, of deer and of similarly timid ones; and there are parallel differences between light and heavy armour, between swift running and moderate motion, and between competition with others and exercise on one's own. There is also a considerable difference between loud, vocal encouragement and silence....

---

[12] See *Freedom from Distress*, section 7, for such—in some cases fatal—consequences of emotional distress.

[13] The trio 'desire, argument, spirit' reflects Galen's Platonically based tripartite understanding of the main intellectual/ethical faculties or capacities in the soul: the rational (the domain of argument), the 'spirited' (that concerned with competitiveness, shame and anger), and the desiderative (that concerned with the bodily appetites for food and sex). See further *The Doctrines of Hippocrates and Plato* and *The Affections and Errors of the Soul*; also *The Shaping of the Embryo*, ch. 3.

To return, then, to our subject, that of small children endowed with the best bodily mixture: these require considerable care in order to avoid any unbal-
43   anced motion arising in their souls. ⏐ For when not yet able to communicate through language they must indicate their discomfort by crying, shouting, raging and disorderly motions. In such cases we are compelled to guess what they require, and to attempt to provide it, before their distress grows to the point where it plunges both soul and body into a motion which is excessively vehement and disordered. Small children cry and move in a chaotic manner, as though struggling, whenever they experience some irritation internally, when- ever they are caused discomfort by some external factor and whenever they want to defaecate, urinate, eat or drink. It may also be that they are expressing a desire for warmth, when disturbed by the cold, or for cooling when disturbed by immoderate heat—which may also be because of the amount of clothing that has been put on them. This too can be a major source of discomfort, lead- ing to the contortion of the whole body and motions of the limbs. Remaining still for too long, however, can also be a source of distress. All creatures desire an optimal state of balance and are pained by its opposite....

[*The remaining books deal with healthy lifestyle recommendations for a variety of bodily conditions and ages, with books II and III focusing on exercise and massage especially, and book V containing a dedicated discussion of care in old age. There is a loose structure throughout, whereby the discussion moves from the consideration of the optimal natural bodily constitution in conjunction with optimal life circumstances, to deal successively with various suboptimal cases in both areas.*]

BOOK II

[*In the context of a discussion of exercise, and its tendency to increase the internal heat, Galen digresses to consider other factors related to heat. In the process he gives a brief but striking account of the physiological nature of a number of emotional states.*]

138   9. ...In exercise, there is an increase in the innate heat in living beings which arises internally to their own bodies. That is a common feature of all exercise, but it is not specific to exercise alone: there is also an increase of the innate heat that takes place in states of rage, anxiety and shame. Rage, in fact, is not simply an increase in heat, but a kind of seething of the heat in the region of the heart. It is for this reason that the most distinguished philosophers even say that this is what the essence of rage is; the appetite for retribution is an attribute of rage, not its essence. The innate heat is increased in states of shame, too; in this

case it first moves swiftly inwards, then collects deep within the body, and finally increases because of this accumulation and because of its constant motion. For the breath [*pneuma*] does not remain at rest in persons suffering from shame; it churns about inside, all over the place, in conjunction with all the blood—as is also the case in anxiety. I shall say more about such affections of the soul later on in the book.[14]

BOOK VI

[*In this extract from book VI Galen gives an unusual glimpse into the daily life, and exercise practices, both of the emperor and of those in his immediate entourage. The passage is also of interest for its discussion of Roman timekeeping. Greek and Roman sundials and water-clocks measured seasonal hours: the total period of daylight on any day is divided into twelve equal 'hours', which are therefore significantly longer in the summer than in the winter. As is clear from Galen's account here, while these seasonal hours are the standard ones in use, at least some people would mentally carry out the conversion from such hours to regular (equinoctial) ones, thus gauging how much actual time was expended in work, exercise, sleep, etc., on any given day.*]

5. Let us consider the following case first: that of one who enjoys a flawless 405 bodily constitution, but has a slave-like existence, having to attend all day upon a monarch or other powerful person, but being allowed to leave at the end of the day. Here, however, we must make a distinction, as to what is meant by 'the end of the day': our discussion will lead to misunderstanding on the part of the reader if we do not add the appropriate specifications. It is not enough, when one is aiming to provide appropriate health instructions, to say that someone is released 'at sunset' on a certain day, to attend to the care of his body; one must also specify the nature of the day in question—whether it is close to the summer or winter solstice, or to one of the equinoxes, or at some point between these. In Rome, for example, the longest days and nights both have a length equivalent to just over fifteen equinoctial hours, and the shortest a length of just

---

[14] In this passage Galen adopts Aristotelian terminology and indeed bases himself quite closely on a well-known passage of Aristotle, *De anima* I.1, 403a–b, while significantly distorting its content: Aristotle presents 'seething of the blood' and 'appetite for revenge' as two aspects of one phenomenon (the accounts of the 'natural philosopher' and the 'dialectician'), and certainly not the former as definitionally prior to the latter. On *ousia* (either 'essence' or 'substance') see also *My Own Doctrines*, n. 8 and *The Shaping of the Embryo*, n. 12 (with further references). *Agōnia*, here translated 'anxiety', is the experience of a competitor or artist in anticipation of the performance. The promise in the last sentence is not fulfilled; further on Galen's account of the physiology of emotions see Singer 2017.

under nine, whereas in the great city of Alexandria the longest have a length of fourteen and the shortest ten. During the shortest days and longest nights, then, one who was dismissed from his service at sunset would quite comfortably be 406 able to take his massage, his bath ⎮ and a decent amount of sleep; but one who was dismissed at that time on the longest days would not be able to do so.

Still, I have never yet encountered someone who had such unfavourable life circumstances as that. Indeed, of all the emperors I have known, Marcus Aurelius Antoninus was the most assiduous in the care of his body, going to the gymnasium at sunset on short days, and on the longest ones at the ninth or at the latest the tenth hour;[15] it was thus possible for those who accompanied him in his daily activities to leave at that point, to attend to their bodies in the remaining part of the day, and still go to bed at sunset. And, since the shortest day is equal to nine equinoctial hours, they would get enough sleep even then....

412 6. Let me mention my own habitual practice on days when I was compelled to bathe late either because of consultations with patients or because of some other professional obligation. Say that the day on which this happened was one of thirteen equinoctial hours in length, and the expectation was that the care of the body could start around the tenth hour. In such a case I would take the simplest food possible, namely bread on its own, around the fourth hour.[16] (There are those who cannot bear to eat bread on its own without some relish, such as dates, olives, honey or salt, and others also take a drink at the same time; but I never drank anything as an accompaniment to such nourishment, confining myself to the bread alone.) The amount of every such nourishment should be such that it will have been completely digested in the stomach before the tenth hour; in that case one may even take exercise if one wishes to, without suffering harm.

---

[15] Sunset on the shortest day in Rome would be about 16:40; on the longest day, the ninth hour would be about 16:55, the tenth about 18:10.

[16] The fourth hour at the time of year Galen mentions would be around 11:00, the tenth around 17:30.

The Thinning Diet

This treatise presents the principles and details of a form of diet which Galen considers an important one in health care, indicated for many individuals and conditions. He often refers to the work itself (for example in his major treatise *Health*), sometimes while also mentioning his much larger, three-volume, work, *The Capacities of Foodstuffs*. Since, however the latter is never mentioned here, we may conclude that the present work pre-dates that larger one. The 'thinning' of the title is not primarily slimming in the modern sense, but rather a thinning or refining of excessively thick or dense humoral fluids in the body, considered to be the cause of certain sub-optimal states of health. At the same time, there is at least a strong causal connection understood between the concepts of 'thin' and 'thick' as used here and those of thinness and fatness as we would understand them. The word translated 'diet', *diaita*, is the same as that also sometimes translated 'regimen' or 'daily regime': it may refer—as usually throughout this text—to diet in the narrower sense, but also to the broader repertory of lifestyle prescriptions central to the Galenic approach to preservation or improvement of health, including exercise, bathing, massage and attention to the physical environment and other lifestyle factors.

Much of the treatise is devoted to the listing of plant and animal foodstuffs; and much of its interest lies in the evidence it gives for the varieties of plants and animals available in the ancient world and for their culinary and medicinal use. Here it should, however, be mentioned that there are considerable difficulties and imprecisions in our identification of, in particular, many of the plants in question. There is no certainty in the modern equivalences for ancient Greek plant names given in dictionaries or herbals, some of which represent no more than plausible conjectures; and matters are complicated by the changes in the flora and agriculture of the Mediterranean region over the last two thousand years. While in general the characteristics of the plant meant, and the family to which it belongs, are reasonably clear, it should be understood that the precise allocation of a modern name in many cases represents an approximation or best guess, rather than a secure identification.[1]

Greek title: Περὶ λεπτυνούσης διάιτης (*Peri leptunousēs diaitēs*)
Kühn: not present
Edition: Kalbfleisch 1923 (marginal page numbers are those of this edition)

1. The thinning diet is indicated for the majority of chronic illnesses, which   433
can, indeed, frequently be put right by such means alone, without recourse to

---

[1] There is a growing body of research on these questions, both on the basis of ancient and medi-aeval botanical texts and from the perspective of archaeobotany. Useful reference points for the description and uses of plants in the ancient world, and (with the caveats given here) for their modern equivalents, are L. Beck's (2005) translation of Dioscorides' *De materia medica* (2005) and M. Haars (2018) (in German).

drugs. It will therefore be desirable to give a more precise specification of this diet; for wherever a result can be achieved purely by regimen, it is preferable to refrain from pharmacological prescriptions. Even with complaints of the kidneys and joints (provided the patient is not yet presenting joints full of 'stones'), I have known many cases where the thinning diet led either to complete remission or at least to a lessening of the pain. I have also known quite a few sufferers from chronic breathing difficulties derive such benefit from it that they returned completely to normal, or else suffered very few attacks over a long period. Among its other effects is to counteract enlargement of the spleen and hardening of the liver; and it will completely cure minor or incipient cases of epilepsy. Even the more chronic and ingrained cases will be considerably ameliorated.

Doctors have named this type of diet 'thinning', and its opposite 'thickening',[2] in accordance with the fluid produced in our bodies in each case; and the diet has stood the twin tests, over a long period, of experience and reason. The senses of smell and taste alone present sufficient evidence of it to the intellect, before each type of food has even been put to the test. Any food which is irritating and biting to the senses is obviously acrid and endowed with the ability to cut through thick fluids; and if taken to excess it will cause biting and considerable discomfort to the stomach. Such stuffs give off acrid smells, too, when they are vomited or 434 excreted; | most of them also give rise to urine and sweat which is acrid and of an unpleasant odour. Some will even remove abscesses or growths on which they are placed, eating through them easily; and some will perforate the skin. Many bring up a sort of scale on the skin, and a sort of ulceration, especially the type known as scabs. All these facts constitute substantial indicators that the fluids within the body, similarly, will be thinned by the acrid, cutting capacity of such foodstuffs; and indeed experience confirms this. All bodies which are full of thick, viscous, cold fluids are observed to be considerably benefited by foods of this kind.

2. Of course, as in any other area, the doctor must act as supervisor, in order to determine the correct time and the correct amount. Inexpert use of such food brings the risk of poor humoral fluid. That part of the instruction, however, is beyond our scope here: we are merely considering the foods themselves.

Vegetables

No one could fail to have noticed the thinning power of garlic, onions, cress, leeks and mustard, such is the strength of this capacity within them. Next in

---

[2] The adjectives from which these two verbs are derived, *leptos* and *pachus*, refer to the physical consistency of stuffs, or of parts of the body. In certain physical contexts, for example that of the skin, the latter is conceived as opposite to *araios*, 'porous'. The two adjectives may also be translated 'fine' and 'dense', and the verb related to the latter 'densify'; in the present work I have preferred the more natural English terminology.

capacity after these are Cretan Alexanders, pellitory, oregano, catmint, watercress, pennyroyal, savory and thyme, when these are taken fresh rather than dried; in their dried state they are drugs rather than foodstuffs.

In general, all dried plants are stronger in effect than fresh ones. By the same token, among plants which are not dried, the more mature ones are more powerful than the younger; and plants that have grown on hill-tops or places lacking in water are stronger than those which have grown in fertile plains, gardens or marshland.

These observations apply to plants in general. But to return to the list: next come the fruit of the caper and of the terebinth; and then varieties of rocket, water parsnip, celery, parsley, basil, radish, cabbage and beet. Mallow, blite and orach, incidentally, in spite of their close similarity in appearance to beet, are dissimilar in their capacity; these are watery, bland plants, quite without any acrid capacity. In fact, they are very similar to bottle gourds, water melons, melons and plums.[3] These types of plant are all wet, cold and productive of phlegm, and even more so those which are eaten raw: apples, pears and snake cucumbers.[4] For this reason some people actually I boil the harder specimens of snake   435 cucumber, in the same way they do bottle gourds. Apples and pears, too, cause less harm when cooked; if they are raw, those which are most suitable for preservation are less bad. But I digress.

3. Let us return to where we left off in our enumeration of those foods which have a thinning effect on the fluids within the body; but at the same time let us begin with a little more precision in our definitions.

All young succulent plants have a gentleness in their capacity due to the moisture which they acquire so long as they are still in the process of growing, as was mentioned above. For this reason many plants normally used as drugs can at this stage be eaten as foods: the stalks of laserwort and mustard, for example, and also of pellitory, golden thistle and eryngo, and countless others,

---

[3] The cucurbit family constitutes a particularly problematic area for clear or secure identification in modern terms. (See Janick, Paris and Parrish 2007.) It seems clear from descriptions and images that the main cultivars were varieties of *Lagenaria siceraria* (bottle gourd or calabash) and *Cucumis melo* (melon), while the evidence overwhelmingly suggests that the cucumber, *Cucumis sativus*, was not yet cultivated at this time—in spite of this word frequently being given in both dictionaries and texts as the translation of *sikuos*, which is here instead translated 'snake cucumber'. (The snake or Armenian cucumber is in fact a long variety of *Cucumis melo*, Flexuosus, which is similar in taste to the cucumber.) It also seems clear that the genus *Cucurbita* (squashes, pumpkins), native to the New World, was unknown in the ancient Mediterranean. The varieties of melon grown were in general not sweet, the breeding of sweet varieties being a later development. But uncertainty remains: *kolokunthē* (here 'bottle gourd') could arguably be translated rather 'colocynth' (or 'bitter melon', *Citrullus colocynthis*) and *sikuos* might then refer to bottle gourd.

[4] *Mēla* ('apples') may also refer to quinces; the word covers a range of orchard fruit, which are sometimes then further specified by the use of adjectives; see also nn. 19 and 20 below. The phrase 'apples, pears and snake melons' may be an interpolation, in which case we should rather translate: '...cold and productive of phlegm, and even more so those of them [i.e. of those just mentioned] which are eaten raw.'

which indeed are commonly referred to as wild vegetables, because of the fact that at a slightly later stage they all become prickly and inedible even for animals. It is important to realize that all plants of this type are strongly cutting when they are fully grown, but moderately thinning when still in the process of growing. Thus, the stinging nettle, for example, before it dries out, is just as edible as mallow or beet; fennel, rue, coriander and dill belong to this type too, in addition to having a noticeable heating power.

There is another kind of wild vegetable which is less cutting than those mentioned; this kind appears to belong between the two, having neither a definitely cutting nor a thickening effect. The general name for these is *seris*;[5] but the individual species are given different names by rustics, for example varieties of lettuce, chicory, the pepperworts of the Syrians and countless similar ones in every region. The Athenians use the term *seris* indiscriminately for all of them; for the ancients did not allot any names to the individual species. There is no species of them which is universally known, since none is grown in every place; so one must learn the general indicators of their capacities, and not rely on species names nor on individual descriptions. If, for example, the
436 taste or smell, or both, give an acrid, biting, hot impression, | you may expect that the plant will have a cutting, thinning capacity; and even if it has a pleasant smell, imparting to the taste the quality of a spice, it will still be hot in its capacity, but less so than those which bite and eat through and have a clear heating effect. Plants with some salt or natron[6] in their taste have a certain cutting quality too; and most of these also purge the stomach. Bitter ones have an equally thinning capacity, and therefore are generally eaten cooked. However, it makes a considerable difference whether such foods are taken with honey-vinegar, with vinegar, with salt or with olive oil; their effect is intensified by vinegar and honey-vinegar, but neutralized by olive oil. (It is not just that olive oil contains nothing which would have a thinning effect on thick fluids; it actually destroys the thinning power of substances which naturally possess it.)

So these foodstuffs, and any others with watery or bland tastes—which most vegetables, especially cultivated ones, possess because of their excessive moisture—are all eaten with vinegar. Those which are best eaten raw are mixed with garum,[7] those cooked are taken with olive oil; and some are eaten with

---

[5] *Seris*: a standard translation of this is 'endive', but the Greek word was clearly used for a wide variety of more or less similar leaf vegetables, and it is difficult to find even an approximate English equivalent for this broad category term.

[6] Natron (Greek *nitron*) was a naturally occurring deposit, consisting mainly of carbonates of sodium, which was found predominantly in areas of the Near East, and harvested for medicinal and other purposes.

[7] Garum was a fermented paste or relish made from a variety of fish products, and in widespread use as an accompaniment to savoury food in the Roman world.

various kinds of relish,[8] all of which contain vinegar; some also with honey or mustard, and with the possible addition of dill, lovage, cumin, celery, caraway seeds or similar things. For Nature herself points the way, teaching the correct course of action not only to those with some degree of expert knowledge but also to the lay person. I myself would frequently have recommended constant use of such relishes to those who required the thinning diet, were it not for the fact that some cooks add a considerable quantity of date to their mixtures. One must, therefore, gain a basic understanding of relishes too. Some are made largely from acrid and hot ingredients; those just mentioned belong to this type, as do those prepared with onion, garlic or coriander. All these are thinning in their capacity, while those which have a smaller proportion of these ingredients and a larger proportion of thickening ones are mixed in effect.

4. Since my first aim was to discuss foods of a vegetable nature, most of which are thinning, I should therefore now consider those known as asparagus, both the marsh variety and the *myacanthus*; as well as *chamaedaphne* and bryony, chaste and elder, and similar varieties. To this type belong also the tendrils of vines and brambles, and any other edible shoot or leaf of a tree. That of the *myacanthus* has a medium capacity, | while that of the marsh asparagus and   437 *chamaedaphne* deviate from it slightly in each direction, the former being wetter than it by the same amount that the latter is drier. Equally beneficial for the mouth of the stomach are those of bryony, chaste and elder; and still more so those which are markedly tart and astringent, such as bramble and vine. Elder cleanses the lower stomach. But cleansing power can only be ascertained by trial, while other effects may be conjectured on the evidence of the taste. Astringent ones are all good for the mouth of the stomach, and in general medium in capacity. The 'brain' of the date palm belongs in this class: this is the name given to the succulent growths at the top of the tree; the ones that grow at the side are known as the 'oars'.[9] The latter actually manifest some bitter quality; and to the extent that they do so are more cutting than the others; and if they bite or heat the tongue perceptibly, they should be placed in the class of the definitely thinning.

Seeds

5. We have given sufficient consideration to foods consisting of the vegetables themselves, and will proceed to discuss seeds.

---

[8] *Hupotrimma*: a relish or condiment consisting of foods grated together, and, as here indicated, with a predominantly sharp or sour taste.
[9] By 'brain' is presumably meant either the inflorescence or the clustered fruits of the date palm; meanwhile it is easy to see how the shape of the spathe suggested oars.

In general terms, the effects of seeds are similar to those of the plants from which they come, but they are drier than these and therefore also more thinning. Not all of them are edible, just as not all the plants from which the seeds are taken are edible. But those seeds which are eaten are, as I have said, of the same nature as their respective plants, but drier and hotter. Thus, the seed of the poppy, for example, is much more moderate than the poppy itself, and is therefore considered harmless, and put in the mixture for bread and many other baked foods; but it does have a cooling effect, as is clear from the fact that it causes heaviness and somnolence. But the poppy is stronger than the seed in its cooling effect, to the same extent that that the juice is stronger than it. The seed of the lettuce is also soporific, for this plant too is wet and cold. These seeds should therefore be avoided by those on the thinning regime. Sesame seeds, too, produce thick, sticky fluids in the body; but the seeds of celery, parsley, 438 cumin, caraway and dill, as also | those of lovage, stone parsley, ajowan, hartwort, wild carrot and Cretan hartwort, and all fragrant, acrid and hot seeds are definitely indicated for users of the thinning diet. Some of them have such a strong capacity that it is equal to those of drugs in the most proper sense. The seed of rue is one such, being among the very strongest, with a considerable thinning power. The seed of the chaste tree, and that of hemp, too, not only have medicinal effects but also give rise to headaches. These should only be used for one purpose, namely for the purging of blood through the urine. But it is not my purpose here to lengthen the treatise unnecessarily by a digression on drugs.

6. Let us return to the other kind of seeds, which some call cereals.[10] A more common usage among the Greeks is to call this class as a whole pulses; but some call them harvest-grains; while others refer to the class as a whole as pulses [ospria], reserving the name of harvest-grains [chedropa] for those which are harvested by hand, and calling those which are reaped with the scythe grains [sitos]. Some refer to wheat alone when they use the word grain; others apply it to barley too. Well, let everyone choose the names they wish; I shall begin my account with a discussion of the effects of these pulses.

Wheat is a highly nutritious food, and one which produces a viscous, thick fluid in the bodies. If one were to take it without preparing it in the usual way, one would acquire a markedly thick, viscous fluid. Nor should one eat wheat simply boiled—a practice which I have observed to be widespread among

---

[10] Dēmētria spermata, literally 'seeds of Demeter', that is of the goddess of fertility and the harvest. There is some variation and unclarity, not just in the general usage of the terms that Galen goes on to discuss, but also in his own usage. The terms here translated 'pulse' and 'harvest-grain', ospria and chedropa, are also sometimes used to refer to grains more broadly. They are more usually applied to legumes only (as indeed Galen makes explicit, defining ospria—which he regards as a subset of cereals—as 'those that are not used to make bread', and going on to list varieties of pulse under that heading, at The Capacities of Foodstuffs I.16); but, as indeed emerges from the end of this paragraph, there is also some fluidity in his usage, and e.g. barley may be treated as a kind of osprion.

peasants in Asia, who season it with a little salt; nor boil the flour in either water or milk to make a thick soup. All such preparations are difficult to digest and give rise to bad fluid. The only suitable method of preparation is also the only one which, quite rightly, nowadays enjoys a good reputation, namely that involving leaven, salt and an earthen pot.[11] Baking in an oven, though, is an only slightly inferior method. But none of the other methods is even worth mentioning.

And there are considerable differences between types of wheat, too. Those which are heavy, dense and yellow to the base are the most nutritious, and also give rise to thick, viscous fluids. Those which are light, fine-textured and white inside are both less nutritious and less productive of these fluids. Semolina and groats are also significantly nutritious, productive of thick fluids, and viscous. The former should not be part of the thinning diet; the latter may be enjoyed in moderation, both on its own, boiled and mixed with honey-wine, or with a   439 wine which is sweet, but yellow and light—that is, basically similar in capacity to the Falernian. It can also be mixed with a variety of other foods, especially grated beet and soups made from birds. Anyone wishing to make a thick soup or gruel from groats should not only mix it with dill, but also add a little leek, mallow, catmint or hyssop. The addition of pepper also contributes substantially to the thinning effect, as in the case of many other foods. Barley-gruel in itself has a cleansing effect, and therefore does not need hyssop; if one wishes to intensify its capacity, one may add a little pepper. There is no need to take honey with barley-gruel, except for the purpose of cleansing the chest and the lungs. Such a mixture is not suitable for ailments of the liver or spleen; these organs are better treated by a gruel made of groats, either on its own or, especially, prepared with honey. But we shall consider the whole subject of honey and its uses below.

Let us return to barley—for its use is not confined to gruel alone. In many parts of the world it is used for bread. It is made into flour and cooked with milk; or ground and made into cakes; or cooked with water, like groats, and served with sweet wine or *siraion*.[12] Barley bread has the following characteristics: low nutrition, and very little tendency to thickness of humoral fluid or to wind, however it is prepared. Barley cakes: low nutrition, like the bread, but a greater drying effect because of the grinding. Barley flour has greater wetness than either of these, and a greater tendency to the production of residues and of wind; and it is best prepared with milk in the same way as groats. When taken with something sweet, barley is much more efficacious in regard to the regime we are considering than are groats, which produce thick, viscous fluids. But one

[11] The *klibanos* or *kribanos* was a small earthenware or terracotta vessel heated from the outside by burning embers; the oven (*ipnos*) of the next sentence was a large baking oven.
[12] New wine, boiled down.

should try to take barley, too, with honey, or with some wine of the same type as Falernian, not with *siraion*, nor with foodstuffs which contain a considerable degree of thickness. In the same way one may use einkorn, and oats, except for those types which are both less digestible and more productive of residues than barley-gruel and groats. Many such seeds are grown in Mysia, in Asia, where they are made into bread; but this sort of bread too is indigestible and product-

440 ive of poor humoral fluid. *Olura*, as it is | called, exists in large quantities in Asia, and belongs midway between these types of grains and wheat: it is worse than wheat to the same degree that it is better than those which we have just mentioned; and it is used in the same way.

One should not seek any other edible form of one-grain wheat [*zeia*] apart from these, as far as the Greek-speaking lands are concerned. I cannot be certain which of the two the ancients referred to by the name *zeia*, but there is no third kind similar to these two; the name was applied either to einkorn [*tiphē*] or to *olura*. Mnesitheus applies these two terms, *tiphē* and *olura*, to the same seed, regarding *zeia* as a third type inferior to these. I believe that by *zeia* he refers to what we now call *tiphē*, or to something even worse than this.

This seed requires to be made into gruel, in the same way as barley, *olura* and oats. When the husk is removed it is much denser and smaller than wheat, *olura* and barley; it is yellow, like wheat, not white like barley. In some places—Cappadocia, for instance—there exists a 'bare barley'; this is the name actually given to it by the people of these parts. It is excellent in all respects, and best taken boiled in water like spelt, with some kind of sweet wine.

7. Broad beans, too, no less than barley, have a cleansing effect; but they are difficult to digest and markedly flatulent.[13] Peas are greatly preferable, being in all respects superior to broad beans. Yellow, long and green beans are considerably worse even than broad beans. However, lentils are not bad in all respects, in spite of the thick fluid which they produce. They may be used as substitutes, in the absence of some more suitable food. Lupines, too, are similar to lentils, but have less of a drying effect. Chickpeas are a flatulent, indigestible food, greatly productive of residues; but they are useful for their diuretic properties, as well as having a cleansing effect. Bitter vetch is more a food for cattle than for men, but has a cutting capacity, and can be used in the preparation of a

---

[13] By *kuamoi* are meant fava or broad beans, or a similar variety, an important staple in the ancient Mediterranean diet. In relation to the list that follows precise identification is impossible, and indeed Galen himself elsewhere acknowledges variation and uncertainty in the applications of some of the terms. He does however clarify that the 'long bean' (*dolichos*) is the only one of which the entire fruit, rather than just the seeds, may be eaten when fresh, though he also says that this same variety is called by some the 'pod bean' (*lobos*); he further remarks that some say that the *phasēlos* (here translated 'green') bean is the same as the *lathuros* (not mentioned in this text), which some would identify with *Lathyrus sativus*, the grass pea or chickling vetch. (See *The Capacities of Foodstuffs* I.28 and II.1.)

medicine which cleanses the chest more than any other. *Boukeras* or *tēlis*[14]—both names are used—may sensibly be taken before meals, too, together with garum, for the emptying of the stomach from below. Some people also take the juice of this with honey, because of its heating and cleansing powers. But excessive use should be avoided, as it may cause headaches. In fact, all foodstuffs which are taken in this way to cleanse the stomach must be used in very small doses; most of them are flatulent and indigestible, as are | lupines, yellow beans   441 and green beans. Better to take Damascene plums as a starter, cooked in a mixture of honey and water, if one needs a thinning diet. And those from Spain have an even greater cleansing power.

In addition to these, sea urchins, and soups made from mussels and similar items,[15] as also from old cockerels, cleanse the stomach and cause no harm to one who has chosen the thinning diet. Millet, Italian millet and any other such seeds have poor fluid and cause wind and indigestion; but such seeds do dry to a considerable degree not only the moisture of the stomach but indeed the whole body. A thick soup is also made from the so-called pod beans—these too are cultivated—in a way similar to that made from broad beans. It is important to be aware that this too tends toward fluid and phlegm, although pod beans are less flatulent than broad beans, and do not have their cleansing quality. I need hardly add descriptions of all the other bad seeds, which are universally avoided anyway, without my having to warn against them. Suffice it to say, in summary, that barley is the grain preferable to all others, and freest from ill effects, in the context of the thinning diet; that wheat loaves baked in earthen pots have second place; and that one should endeavour to abstain from all others, except perhaps from peas, lentil broth, or groats, of which one may, if one wishes, partake sparingly.

Meats

8. Your greatest and most abundant source of food for the thinning diet is provided by rock-fish[16] and small mountain birds. Birds of the marsh-meadows, lakes and plains are wetter and more productive of residues. Animals that live in the hills are invariably drier and hotter in mixture, and their flesh is the least phlegmatic and sticky. Those that live in the mountains are, in general, far better than those lower down; and mountain birds, in particular, are in my opinion

---

[14] Both are apparently names for fenugreek.

[15] Literally, 'from all the *koncharia*', where *koncharia* probably corresponds roughly to bivalve molluscs.

[16] The term seems to correspond roughly to 'freshwater fish', except that, as becomes clear from the argument, altitude (i.e. being found in mountainous, rocky areas), not just the freshness of the water, is a major positive consideration.

infinitely superior to those of the marsh-meadows and plains, not just because of the fineness of the air but also because of the nature of their nourishment. One should therefore eat starlings, thrushes, blackbirds and partridges, along with other mountain birds, but steer clear of ducks and all birds of the marsh-meadows. So too one must avoid bustards, geese and the other large birds which are also known as 'bird-camels',[17] and all birds of this kind, if one is at all interested in the thinning diet. All these have flesh which produces residues.

442   Furthermore, those known as tower-birds, too, | and those that live around vines, and pigeons from towers, are better than those from ordinary houses. Similarly, wild pigs are better to eat than the domestic variety. It is in fact a general rule that exercise, the consumption of drier rather than wetter foods, and the breathing of fine, clear air rather than its opposite make animals better to eat. The flesh provided by domestic pigs is the most nutritious of foods; but at the same time it is very sticky because of the idleness of the animal and its plentiful consumption of wet foods. This, then, should be completely avoided by the user of the thinning diet, except perhaps for its extremities—and even these should only be used if one is taking a reasonable amount of exercise. In that case one may eat the ears, snout and feet of the animal, and try the stomach too, and the womb if it is well cooked. People whose lifestyle is comparatively slow and idle should refrain altogether from eating not only the meat of domestic pigs, but that of the mountain variety too. They should confine themselves to mountain birds and rock-fish—all those, in short, which have soft, friable flesh. (Examples are a number of varieties of the wrasse.) Those with hard or sticky flesh should be avoided absolutely. Now, the meat of cod is soft but less friable than that of rock varieties, while that of red mullet is friable but not also soft. These two indicators should be to the fore in the consideration of all animal flesh. If it has both qualities, the meat may be eaten in plenty; if neither, it should be abstained from entirely. Meats that have one but not the other may be eaten in the absence of the other types, but excess should be avoided. Thus, one may take cod, red mullet and other kinds of sea fish in the absence of fresh-water fish—especially if they are eaten with mustard, as is the scorpion fish.

Some kinds of animal possess one of the characteristics mentioned but should nevertheless be avoided in view of their excessive nature in respect of the other. Eels, for example, and most of the cephalopods and cartilaginous fish,

443   in spite of the softness of their flesh have a sticky, phlegmatic | quality which

---

[17] *Strouthokamēlos* is the standard word for an ostrich. It seems at least possible, however, that Galen is here referring rather to some kind of wading birds: these would be found in the marshy or wet habitats under discussion here, whereas the ostrich's habitat is arid or semi-arid. (The etymology of the word, with its reference to the appearance of a camel, certainly also seems consistent with long-legged waders.) Otherwise, Galen is indeed referring to the ostrich, but is poorly informed about its habitat; ostriches were prized at Rome, including for displays in the circus, but were doubtless seldom seen in the wild.

causes considerable harm to users of the thinning diet. So too do most kinds of bivalve. Goats and cows have the least wet, phlegmatic, sticky flesh, but they too cause a lot of harm because they are extremely hard and difficult to break down. Most testaceans and crustaceans, too, should be avoided, as they possess either both these qualities, or at least hardness of the flesh. The only cartilaginous seafoods which are suitable are the torpedo and the stingray; and these too may be used in the absence of rock-fish, but should preferably be prepared with grated beet or clear broth, with a generous addition of leek and a little pepper. Similar to these in their capacity are sole and turbot.

Turning to the other land animals: he-goats, rams, and indeed sheep and goats in general provide unsuitable nutrition. Only kids may sensibly be used; the meat of sheep should be avoided as excessively wet. The horse and the ass would only be consumed by someone who was himself an ass; and to eat leopards, bears or lions you would have to be a wild beast. But the meat of deer is close in nature to that of the ass, and so this too should be avoided. Hare meat is in other respects appropriate for a drying diet, but is useless for present purposes, as it produces quite thick blood.

Consumption of the blood of any animal should in fact be avoided, but especially, for the purposes of the thinning diet, the blood of hares. Similarly, all internal organs should be avoided, for these too are indigestible and productive of residues and poor fluid. As for dogs and foxes, I have never tasted their meat, since it is not the custom to eat it either in Asia or in Greece—nor indeed in Italy. But I understand that there are many parts of the world where they are eaten, and I would infer that the capacity would be similar to that of hare meat; for hare, dog and fox are all equally dry. Now, just as we allowed the use of pigs' extremities, so too the wings of cockerels. Their testicles and internal organs, though, are unsuitable for the user of the thinning diet. As for the meat of their actual bodies, I would not forbid this, provided the person using it is well exercised and the bird raised in the mountains. Those who are not well exercised should only take the meat of cockerels in moderation, and the same applies to pigeons and I turtle doves. The turtle dove, however, does have a drier nature, 444 especially the mountain variety. This kind may be eaten without ill effect. But both the turtle dove and the partridge, and all other animals with moderately hard flesh, must not be eaten immediately, but hung[18] for at least one day. The ring dove, though, as well as having harder flesh than the pigeon, turtle dove or partridge, is also indigestible and productive of residues. Partridges and turtle doves do not have this extremely hard quality, nor are they indigestible or productive of poor fluid. In fact, their hardness is readily transformed if their

---

[18] This word is not certain, but the reading (based on the Latin translation *suspendendo*, corresponding to a hypothetical Greek *kremasmenon*) seems more likely than what appears in the Greek manuscript.

bodies are left for a day, and they become friable and perfectly digestible. They are also a source of useful nutrition for the body, and produce the least sticky blood—blood, in fact, which is midway between thickness and fineness, which is, indeed, the most appropriate outcome of a healthy diet.

Roots

9. We have said enough on this subject; let us now turn to the remaining foodstuffs.

Roots of vegetables are practically all productive of residues, and indigestible. For our present purposes, however, the roots of the wild carrot and of caraway contain nothing harmful, though nothing useful either. Turnips, on the other hand, are completely contra-indicated, and even more so grape hyacinths; and mushrooms are worst of all. Thus, one must be suspicious of all roots, unless there is something biting, acrid or hot in the taste of them; even the roots of beet, for example, are to be avoided. In spite of the fact that this vegetable is not at all phlegmatic, its roots should not be eaten. As for the mallow, in this case it is not only the roots or the stems that produce phlegmatic fluid, but even the leaves, although these are less harmful. From the point of view of the thinning diet, the wild ones are better than the cultivated. Truffles belong in the same class too, except to the extent that they are found in sandy land, which is less wet, and in this respect they are less harmful than mushrooms. In brief, all roots should be treated with suspicion, as they are likely to be indigestible; and the only ones one should try are those which are hot and acrid, such as garlic, onion and radish—and even these should be taken rather as medicine than as food.

Fruits and Nuts

10. We have now said enough about roots, too, and should turn to the fruits of trees.

Many of these are wet and cold, especially those which cannot be preserved. The least harm is done by those which empty the gastric cavity, for example 445 | blackberries, and next after them plums, cherries and figs. Fruit which are slow to pass through the system are the worst of all, especially if their bodies are also hard. None of these should be taken, except for those suitable for preservation, which include several kinds of pear, apple and grape. And one should eat the softer specimens rather than the hard ones. None of these fruits should be eaten in excess, nor should peaches, nor apricots,[19] which the Romans call *praecocia*;

---

[19] More literally, 'Persian apples and Armenian apples': both were regarded as varieties of *mēlon*, usually though approximately translated 'apple'.

nor, above all, those known as jujubes.[20] Furthermore myrtle, nettle-fruit and any species similar to these are not appropriate; the sorb apple and medlar, too, though fine in other contexts, are not indicated for the thinning diet, especially the medlar. In general, fruits which are extremely tart and sour are bad for this diet, and are only of use for the fluids in the gut, or for a loosened stomach.

Among fruits which can be preserved over the winter, the most suitable are dried figs and filberts (which are good for other purposes too). Pistachios, too, are good for our diet, and slightly bitter almonds are not bad. Hazelnuts[21] are harder than these and have no power to cleanse out the residues in the internal organs. Chestnuts and acorns are very bad when raw, and fairly bad even when boiled, baked or ground. The position of olives is a medium one in the context of the diet under consideration, and so I have nothing of note to say either for or against them. The same applies to dried grapes. Those, on the other hand, which are preserved in masses, or branches, or whatever one wishes to call them,[22] are quite useful for weaknesses of the stomach, but not very good for our present purpose; and this is even truer of those steeped in wine. Raisins, provided they are not actually sour, are bad for an enlarged spleen or liver, but quite good for ailments of the chest and lungs. Sour pomegranates, on the other hand, are bad for the latter purpose but good for weaknesses of the stomach.

All other fruits of trees may be judged on the basis of the above: those which are hard and sour are always bad; others may be taken in moderation, and if they have a number of different qualities in different parts, one should take only the parts which are sharp and acrid, avoiding the others. There are many of this kind, such as the 'Medic apple', which we call the citron; | its skin is acrid, while 446 the inside is sharp, and the flesh is productive of thick and phlegmatic fluid.

11. With fruits that are preserved in vinegar or brine, bear in mind that they lose their original capacity to the extent that they are altered by the preparation; and, as we all know, vinegar and brine belong to the category of things which cut and thin. Thus, even preserved fish have a marked thinning and cutting effect on thick, viscous fluids; but here one should still choose only those with soft flesh, avoiding the cetaceous, and especially whales themselves. One may, however, try these too, either in the absence of anything better or if one desires to for some other reason, provided that one adjusts them either with an acrid relish, such as one composed of mustard, or of olive oil and vinegar. It should indeed be realized that with all foods, quite generally, preservation or preparation with the above-mentioned condiments has a very great influence on their

[20] In Greek 'Seric apples', where 'Seric' originally referred to a place or people in the far east of Asia—those from whom silk was originally derived. (See also *Affections and Errors*, n. 23.) The jujube is a small date-like fruit of the buckthorn family.

[21] Literally, 'the so-called Pontic nuts'.

[22] This apparently refers to the mass of grapes left over from a winepress.

thinning effect. Every person for whom the thinning diet is indicated should make efforts to have most of his food prepared with vinegar or with honey-vinegar, and to have them preserved in advance wherever possible. Even pork meat may safely be eaten if it has been preserved in this way; otherwise it must be avoided for the thick, viscous fluid it will produce.

Honey, Wine and Milk

12. We have covered this topic adequately too. Let us move on to honey, wine and milk.

Honey is virtually unique among sweet foods (or for that matter sweet drinks) in being productive of fluid which is genuinely fine in its consistency. Sweet wines, for example, all have a marked tendency to produce thick blood (they are themselves black, and thick in their consistency), and even more so the wine which is called *siraion*, which is fresh wine boiled for a long time. Some people also apply this name to the liquid that comes from boiling dried figs; this is similar in effect to bad honey, and has some cutting capacity, though a considerably lesser one than honey. The dried figs themselves have a lesser cutting capacity still, and fresh figs a lesser one again. These last do not in fact belong within the thinning diet.

447 Now, sun-ripened figs | constitute an item in a middle position; one cannot attribute to them either a substantial thinning or thickening effect on the fluids. All others are below this midpoint; for those which are not yet ripe are cold, thick in their fluid, indigestible and flatulent, as is fresh wine. They do have only one good quality, namely that they go through the system quickly, thus causing little damage. Sweet grapes are similar in their nature, and dates even more so. In Alexandria, Cyprus, Phoenicia and Lycia dates will not even survive preservation, and are only eaten fresh: their excessive moisture makes them too prone to putrefaction. Those which are preserved are less harmful; yet here too the fluid is thick, and one must avoid eating them in the case of the ailments mentioned.

Amongst sweet[23] wines, one may with the greatest confidence take those which are clear and translucent, and yellow or pale yellow. A wine will of course not be both sweet and colourless; nor, indeed, will a yellow wine be *very* sweet.[24]

---

[23] I follow Kalbfleisch in reading 'sweet' (with the Latin manuscripts) for the 'thick' of the Greek. (However, the Latin versions also give a different sense for the main verb: either 'one will not taste' or 'one will not find', rather than 'one may with...confidence take'.)

[24] The colour words used by Galen in relation to wines are not straightforward in translation, and in some ways surprising to modern conceptions. The picture seems to be of a spectrum from transparent or colourless, through pale yellow (*ōchros*) and yellow (*xanthos*) to black (in our terms, red), with the darkest red or blackest ones being the sweetest. (Note that 'colourless' renders *leukos*,

All these kinds of wine produce a fluid of a medium consistency. Thick, black, sweet wines fill the veins with thick blood; colourless, thin ones cut the thick fluids and cleanse the blood through the urine. But wines which are yellow, sweet and translucent, being somewhere between these types in their appearance, lie between them in their capacity too. They neither thicken the fluids, as do the black wines, nor have the diuretic effects of the colourless ones. There are many such wines amongst every people, the best-known being the Ariusian, Lesbian, Falernian, Tmolite and Theran. On the basis of these you should be able to choose other similar wines. All such wines give rise to good blood and to fluid which is well balanced in terms of its thickness. Most of them, however, are also highly fragrant, and hotter than the norm, and thus naturally affect the head; they should therefore be avoided by sufferers from headache, *hēmikrania*, or indeed complaints of the head in general, including epilepsy or *mania*. All chronic ailments of the chest and lungs, however, provided they do not involve fever, I are greatly ameliorated by these kinds of wine, especially those ailments 448 which are purged by coughing. This is because, in order to be properly expectorated, the stuff needs not only to be cut and heated, but also moderately wetted. Where dry, viscous mucous persists for too long, the forceful attempt to eject it will give rise to vehement coughing, and there will be the risk of a vessel being ruptured.

Thick, sweet wines, then, which have a constant level of moisture due to their thickness, are, when taken in conjunction with thinning drugs, good for ailments of the chest and lungs. These should not be hard, sour or at all astringent, but should tend rather to be like honey in smell, taste and overall capacity. The Pamphylian wine, known also as Skybelites, is one such, and can be used as a kind of yardstick by which to assess similar ones. The Skybelites is the best of its kind, but failing this the Theran, *protropos, siraion*, Therenos or Karuinos can also be used.[25]

An example of a dark wine which is both sweet[26] and tart is the Cilician wine known as Abates. This wine is of no use for the ailments of the chest and lungs which were just mentioned; and even worse would be any wine which was noticeably sour, and either totally or almost totally lacking in sweetness. Such wines are not held in high regard, and so people tend to be unaware of their existence, in spite of the fact that they are in fact quite widely produced. This is because they are not profitable wines for the merchants, nor will a person who

which would usually be translated 'white': the latter translation would make no sense here, where clearly the 'yellow' and 'pale yellow' wines are also, in our terms, white wines.)

[25] Most of the wines here mentioned (which are discussed at greater length in *Health*, V.5) are from parts of Asia. *Protropos* apparently refers to a 'pre-treading' wine.

[26] I follow the manuscript reading here, but 'sweet' looks out of place and should perhaps be replaced with 'thick'. If 'sweet' is correct, the sense is presumably that such a wine retains some element of sweetness alongside the tartness.

owns such a wine take much note of it. After all, no one is going to serve a sour, thick, dark wine at a drinking party, at a wedding, at a religious festival, or indeed at any other kind of celebration. Such a wine is filling and slow to pass through, and inhibits both kinds of excretions, those from the stomach and equally those from the bladder; it also remains for a long time in the lower abdomen, and readily becomes sharp and leads to vomiting. The only thing it is suitable for is fluids in the stomach, and even for these it should not be taken in excess. A wine of this kind is produced quite plentifully in the plains of Aegae, 449   in Aeolia; and a similar one | in Pergamum's neighbouring city of Perperena. The people of those parts drink it without ill effect, because of their habituation; but even so their consumption of it is moderate. Anyone who is not used to it, and anyone who drinks it to excess, will suffer ill effects. Such wines very clearly provide nourishment to the body of the drinker; and I have seen young men who frequented the places of public training in those parts take it to build up the good condition of their bodies, just as they would pork.

Anyway, those wines are completely contra-indicated for the diet which we are considering. Still, I should not be criticized for enlarging on a subject other than the one I have announced; for anyone who is determined to make successful use of the thinning diet must not merely seek out thinning foods, but also avoid thickening ones. Indeed, the whole of medicine is defined as the knowledge of things unhealthy as well as things healthy, and the latter kind of knowledge is no less important. It does no less damage to partake of unhealthy things than to abstain from healthy ones. If, then, one is to make proper use of both these classes, one must have knowledge of all, though primarily of the healthy ones, since these are to be chosen in their own right. There is also a third class between these two, which produces neither benefit nor harm; and this too must be properly evaluated, as neither healthy in a way which makes it worthy of selection nor unhealthy in a way which is actually harmful. If, then, such an item is present, we should not make pointless efforts to avoid it as if it were something dangerous; nor, if in its absence, should we pointlessly seek it out as something which might do us some good. Indulgences that a doctor may allow to the patient fall within this class. If a patient asks for something harmful, no one will accede to the request, any more than if he tries to avoid something beneficial. But if a patient wishes to omit or to include something which is neither, he should be humoured. In this case, unlike that of things healthy and unhealthy, all that one has to take into account is the fulfilment of the patient's desire, not any benefit or harm.

The sense, moreover, in which the nature of foodstuffs, drinks and other items is healthy, unhealthy or neither is not a straightforward or single one; it is always a relative sense. For example, it is only in relation to the diseases that I mentioned at the beginning of this treatise that the thinning diet is healthy and the thickening unhealthy, and that the diet which has no particular effect in either direction, but leaves things in the body as it finds them, is between the two.

Having established this, let us return to the matter in hand. In general terms, it should be understood that, while in the context of the chest and lungs sweet wines taken with some thinning medicine purge the thick, viscous and phlegmatic fluids, so, in cases of enlarged liver or spleen, the harm done by such a treatment will outweigh the benefit. For there is a concerted pull from these organs ǀ upon the stuffs drunk down into the gastric cavity, whereby they can   450 quickly become wedged in the extremities of the vessels, especially in the liver, where the veins coming from the portal meet those coming from the vena cava. Therefore all sweet foods are unsuitable for cases of inflammation or hardening of these organs, or of obstruction in the narrow mouths of their vessels. This applies even to honey, in spite of its cutting capacity; but the excess sweetness of may be corrected by combining it with vinegar.

Both theoretical considerations and the results of your own experience should thus lead you to the conclusion that a mixture of honey-vinegar is the most suitable thing of all for the thinning diet. The drug-like character that belongs to some of the efficacious substances is not present in this case; nor is it productive of bad humoral fluid, nor indigestible, nor unsuitable in any other way. If, moreover, one uses squill vinegar, then this will be the most cutting not only of foods but also of drugs; vinegar or wine of this sort should thus be used by anyone wanting an extreme cutting and thinning effect on those thick, sticky or phlegmatic residues which the body produces.[27] I know of many cases where people who in other respects followed a regime which was not at all healthy were made healthy all the same, just by virtue of this vinegar or wine with squill. This is no reason to neglect everything else; rather, one should employ the right physical exercise, and keep careful account of the qualities and quantities of foods as described. It is after all preferable to subject oneself exclusively to the beneficial influences, and so arrive more quickly at the goal, rather than to mix bad practices with good and so be in danger right up to the end.

The whey of milk is a thinning substance, too, and also evacuates the stomach. It is best to use it frequently, but at certain intervals. Milk itself, however, has something of a thickening effect, and cheese even more so. Those on the

---

[27] The addition of sea squill (*Drimia* or *Urginea maritima*) to wine or vinegar was a traditional medicinal recipe. It is notable in this passage that Galen explicitly mentions *oxos* ('vinegar') and *oinos* ('wine') as interchangeable. The former Greek word may refer both to vinegar and to a form of cheap, diluted sour wine, *posca*, which was very widely drunk by the poorer classes in the Graeco-Roman world, including in the Roman army, and considered to have both refreshing and health-giving properties. Though I have translated *oxos* as 'vinegar' throughout, the reference may sometimes be to this form of 'vinegar-wine'. The frequently mentioned foodstuff 'honey-vinegar' (*oxumeli*), too, may be a mixture of honey with this sour wine, not with vinegar proper.

thinning diet should avoid consumption of cheese, which is in fact among the most thickening of all foods, on a level with grape hyacinths and snails,[28] and brains, and among internal organs liver, spleen and kidneys. I strongly recommend avoidance of these foods, as also of mushrooms, and of boiled eggs; eggs which are scrambled,[29] as it is called, have a moderately thickening effect, as does the porridge of groats when taken without the addition of dill or leek, and also of some seriously cutting substance such as hyssop, mallow, savory, pepper and thyme. (The pepper should be sprinkled on lightly at the end, the other items cooked with it.) If it so happens that one actually needs to take milk, this
451   too should be boiled with some of the above. I Milk mixed with honey is quite useful for ailments of the abdomen; but it is extremely harmful to the parts in the region of the liver and spleen, when these require a thinning diet. (One must always bear in mind what I said at the very beginning, and not think that this statement holds without qualification in relation to those parts, with no reference to the nature of the illness—as discussed above.) Now, the thickest sort of milk is that which is most like cheese, such as cow's or pig's milk, and the thinnest is the most whey-like, for example ass's milk. Goat's milk lies halfway between the two. Boiled milk, however, is the thickest in fluid, since boiling removes the thinner, more whey-like part of the milk. If, however, one adds honey, salt or both, it will be much thinner. It is thus clear that ass's milk taken with salt or honey is the least productive of thick fluid; this will in fact do no harm to the user of the thinning diet. All other sorts of milk should be avoided.

[28] At this point the Greek manuscript also has 'and all *ospria*'—the term for cereals used above (see ch. 6 with n. 10). Since a blanket veto of these seems to make no sense, on the basis of that earlier discussion, I have omitted this phrase. It is possible that what Galen wrote was rather *ta ostrea panta* ('all bivalves') or *ta ostrakoderma* ('testaceans').

[29] The precise sense is not clear, but Galen seems to refer to an alternative and preferable way of cooking eggs.

The Exercise with the Small Ball

The precise identity of the game described here is difficult to ascertain; but the short treatise shows Galen's interest in, and attention to the detail of, the exercise regimes appropriate to his patients, and the relationship of these to his broader theories on the preservation of health, including on the role of psychological factors and the relationship of exercise for body and for 'soul'.

Greek title: Περὶ τοῦ διὰ μικρᾶς σφαίρας γυμνασίου (*Peri tou dia mikras sphairas gumnasiou*)
Kühn: V.899–910
Editions: Marquardt 1884; Schäfer 1908

1. The great health benefits of physical exercise, Epigenes, and the fact that it should precede food, have been very well established in the past, by the best philosophers and doctors. Yet the great superiority of the exercise with the small ball has not been sufficiently discussed by anyone. So it seems right to me to state what I know on the subject; you, who have a better training in this art than anyone, may evaluate my account, which may then be found useful by any others with whom you may wish to share it. V.899

In my view the best exercises of all are those ⎮ with the capacity not only to exert the body but also to delight the soul. Those who hit upon hunting—hunting with dogs and all other kinds—found a way of combining exertion with pleasure, delight and competitive spirit; they were wise men who well understood human nature. The motion of the soul here involved is so powerful that many have been released from their disease by the pleasure alone, and many have been found to be cured. No bodily ailment is so great that it can dominate those of the soul. One should not, then, neglect the motions of the soul, nor fail to consider what their nature should be; in fact, one should take much greater care of them than of the bodily motions, for a number of reasons, but especially because of the degree to which the soul is more important than the body. This is a consideration common to all forms of exercise that involve pleasure; but there are others which apply particularly to the exercise with the small ball, which I shall now enumerate. 900

2. First, there is its accessibility. If you consider how much preparation and leisure are necessary for hounds and all other hunting equipment, ⎮ you will clearly realize that no one in public life, nor any practitioner of the arts, can 901

possibly take part in such exercise. It requires considerable resources and a great deal of free time. The form of exercise we are considering here, on the other hand, is the only one which is so democratic that anyone, no matter how small his income, can take part. You need no nets, no weapons, no horses, no hunting hounds—just a single ball, and a small one at that.

It is, moreover, adaptable to the other activities of life, so that none of these need suffer as a result of it. What practice could be more convenient than one which is suited to every level of human fortune and to every human activity? The ability to engage in the exercise afforded by hunting is something which the individual cannot determine; it requires money for the provision of the equipment and leisure to enable one to await the right moment for the hunt. The provision of the equipment required for our exercise, on the other hand, is accessible to the means of the poorest of persons; and the time of its employment may fit into the schedule of even the busiest of individuals.

So much, then, for its benefits of accessibility. Our exercise is also the most
902 sufficient of all. | This fact can best be apprehended from a consideration of the capacity and nature of each of the other kinds of exercise. It will be seen that they are all either vehement or mild in their nature, and that they move the lower body more than the upper, or some part to the exclusion of the rest, such as the lower back, the head, the hands or the chest. The capacity both to move all parts of the body equally, and also to be practised in either an extremely vehement or an extremely mild form, is something found in no other exercise except for that with the small ball. It may be partially very swift and partially very slow, or partially very vehement and partially very gentle, in accordance with the individual's wishes and the evident needs of his body. So too it may, if this is thought beneficial, move all parts equally, or alternatively some more than others.

When the competitors square up, attempting to prevent each other from taking the space between, this exercise is a very heavy, vehement one, involving much use of the hold by the neck, and many wrestling holds. The head and neck
903 are exerted by these holds, and the sides, | chest and stomach by the clenches, shoves and constrictions as well as the other wrestling-style holds. The lower back and legs are also subject to great strain in this kind of activity, which requires great steadiness on one's feet. Advancing, retreating and leaping to the side, too, represent a considerable exercise for the legs; in fact, these are really the only actions in which all their parts are moved in the correct way. The act of coming forward exercises one set of nerves and muscles to a greater extent, the act of retreating another; and that of dodging to the side another still. The concentration on a single type of motion of the legs, on the other hand, as is the case in running, provides an uneven, unequal type of exercise.

3. And as with the legs, so with the arms too, the exercise with the small ball is the best, as its practitioners tend to move them in every possible orientation as

they take hold of the ball. Here again the variety of forms which the exercise takes means that different muscles are extended more vehemently at different times; thus all, in turn, are exerted equally, | one group rests while another is active, and in this alternation between activity and rest no muscle remains idle throughout, nor does any become strained by constant exertion.   904

The sense of sight is also exercised; this becomes clear when we consider that anyone failing accurately and quickly to anticipate the trajectory of the ball must miss his catch. The mental faculties, moreover, are sharpened by the mental exertion involved in the effort not to drop the ball and to prevent the opponent from taking the middle ground, or to seize it himself, if he is in that situation. For although mental exertion on its own leads to thinning, when combined with some exercise which is connected with competitive spirit and is able to cause pleasure, it is of the greatest benefit both to the health of the body and the intelligence of the soul.

In fact, this very capacity to assist both body and soul towards their respective excellences is one of the great qualities of this form of exercise. It is fairly easy to see that it has the power to give both of them the most important types of training—those which the rulers or laws of a city would especially command their generals to undertake. | The task of a good general involves attacking at   905
the right time, doing so by stealth, seizing one's opportunity, appropriating the enemy's possessions either by force or by unexpected attack, and defending those already acquired. In short, a general should be a skilled guard and thief; there, in a nutshell, is the whole of his art. I can think of no other exercise which provides the same degree of practice in defending what one has already gained, recovering what one has lost, or anticipating the enemy's intentions; and I should be very surprised if anyone else can. Most exercises, in fact, have the opposite effect on the mental activities, rendering them idle, sleepy and slow; and indeed the kind of physical exercise practised in the wrestling school[1] promotes rather the quantity of flesh than the cultivation of virtue. Many have become so stout that as a result they suffer from breathing difficulties. The products of such training will hardly become great generals, or experts in kingship or political affairs; one would be better off placing such matters in the charge of a pig.

It might be thought that I would approve of running, or other such exercises which thin the body. But this is not | the case. For imbalance is in all cases to be   906
deplored. Good balance is the aim to be cultivated by every art; any deviation from this is a defect. The practice of running can therefore be recommended

---

[1] *Palaistra*, also translatable 'gymnasium', the area for sports activity, typically in the Roman world attached to a bathhouse complex. A variety of exercises, not just wrestling, was performed there; and Galen sometimes gives a more positive account of some of these than he does here; however, he is hostile to the usual practices of athletes and their trainers (on this see *An Exhortation to Study the Arts*).

neither for its propensity to thin the bodily condition nor for its failure to provide any stimulus to courage. Victory belongs not to those who can run away
quickly, but to those with the capacity to win in hand-to-hand combat; it was
not their extreme fleet-footedness which enabled the Spartans to achieve so
much, but their confidence to stay and fight. If one examines the matter purely
in terms of health, too, such activity fails, to the extent that it provides an
unequal exercise to the different parts of the body: some are bound to be
overstretched while others remain entirely idle. Neither of these features is
beneficial; in fact, both are causes of the germination of the seeds of disease, as
well as the production of an enfeebled capacity.

4. The form of exercise most worthy of our approbation, then, is that which is
sufficient to bring about bodily health, harmony of the parts and virtue in the
soul; and all these things are true of the exercise with the small ball. It is able to
907   benefit the soul in every way; | and it causes equal exertion in all parts of the
body. At the same time it is extremely beneficial for health, and brings about a
well-balanced condition, without any disproportionate accumulation of flesh or
excess thinness. It is adequate for the purposes of actions requiring strength
and also well-suited to those which require speed.

Now, the most vehement manifestation of this exercise is equal to that of any
other exercise; but let us also consider its most gentle manifestation. There are
times when this too is required, either because the individual is at an age where
he is not yet—or no longer—able to undergo heavy labour, wishes to reduce the
level of his exertion, or is recovering from illness. In this context too I believe
that our exercise is superior to all others: if one engages in it gently, then no
other is equally gentle. In this case, then, one must use the middle space, stand
a modest way off, and alternate between gentle advances and remaining in the
same place; and after a fairly short period of exercise take a soft massage with
olive oil and a hot bath.

908 | This is the gentlest form of all, so much so that even for those in need of rest
it may be highly recommended, has great power to restore an enfeebled
capacity, and may be of very great benefit to the old and to children. But other
forms of exercise may also be practised with the small ball, which are stronger
than these but still gentler than the most vehement type. These too should be
known to anyone who intends to learn the correct practice in its entirety. If,
moreover, as frequently happens as a result of the performance of some necessary task, one has exerted either the upper or the lower parts disproportion-
ately, or only the hands or feet, this exercise will enable one to rest the parts
which were previously exerted while providing a compensatory degree of exertion to those which were previously idle. If, for example, one throws energetically from a considerable distance, one is using the legs little if at all; and thus
one rests the lower parts while giving vehement exercise to the upper. If, on the

other hand, one runs more, and throws quickly, from greater distances, but less often, one will exert the lower parts to a greater extent. And that part of the exercise which involves urgency | and speed without great intensity exercises 909 the breath more, while the vigorous part, that is that involving holds, throws and catches, but not speed, tends rather to tone and invigorate the body. If the movements are both intense and urgent, then there will be great exertion of both body and breath; this is the most vehement of all possible exercises.

The degree of intensity and relaxation indicated for each circumstance cannot be written down here, for the quantity applicable in an individual case is not something which may be stated. It is, however, possible to discover and teach this in the context of one's actual practice. And this is, indeed, the point of utmost importance; for the right *type* of exercise is of no use if the *amount* is wrong. This is a matter for the instructor in charge of the exercises.

5. Let us move to the conclusion of our argument. I should not like to omit from my account of the positive attributes of this exercise the fact that it is free of risk. This is not true of most other sorts of exercise. Running, for example, has frequently killed people, through the rupture of a vital vessel; and similarly the phenomenon of loud, violent sounds being produced all at once has been known to cause very great harm in a number of cases. Energetic horse-riding can cause ruptures in the region of the kidneys, as well as damage to the chest area, or even sometimes to the spermatic channels—not to mention, of course, the mistakes that may be made by the horse, as a result of which it often happens that the rider is thrown and immediately killed. The jump, the discus and the exercise involving turning have also caused many injuries. I need hardly mention the numbers injured in the ring, all of whom seem to have suffered a maiming no less than that of Homer's Prayers. For the Poet says of them:

Limping, all shrivelled up, deprived of sight.[2]

And so it is with those who have competed in the ring. They may be observed to be lame, disfigured, crushed or at least mutilated in some part or other. Since the exercise with the small ball has, in addition to those already listed, the advantage that it does not involve any danger, then surely it must be the most beneficial exercise of all.

---

[2] Homer, *Iliad* IX.503.

V

DIAGNOSTIC AND CLINICAL PRACTICE

The Pulse for Beginners

In this introductory work, written during his first stay in Rome, Galen explains in outline his views on the pulse, summarizing a complex area of physiological theory and diagnostic practice which is expounded fully in four much longer treatises, which together constitute his great study of the pulse. The diagnostic importance of the pulse is a theme that runs through Galen's clinical work; see for example the case histories recounted in *Prognosis*.

A remarkable feature of Galen's clinical medicine, and of his pulse theory in particular, is the extraordinary range of variables which his theoretical model identifies, and which he claims—after long and painstaking training—to be able to distinguish in practice. Galen is here building on a substantial previous body of work on the pulse, by his famous predecessors Herophilus, Erasistratus and Archigenes amongst others.

One important aspect of Galen's physiological understanding of the pulse should be noted at the outset. On his view there is a simultaneous diastole or expansion of both the heart and the arteries, followed by a simultaneous systole or contraction of both. Thus, the expansion, or increase in tension, perceived in the artery during pulsation corresponds to a simultaneous outward or pumping motion of the heart, rather than, as in modern medical understanding, to the heart's contraction or systolic motion. The role of diastole and systole (terms which Galen usually applies to the pulse, rather than to the heart) are thus in effect reversed, in relation to our understanding of them. In what follows, partly to avoid confusion between the ancient and the modern model, I avoid those terms, translating *diastolē* as 'expansion' and *systolē* as 'contraction'.

Greek title: Περὶ τῶν σφυγμῶν τοῖς εἰσαγομένοις (*Peri tōn sphugmōn tois eisagomenois*)
Kühn: VIII.453–92

1. In what follows, my dear Teuthras, I shall set out the points which are useful VIII.453 for the beginner to know regarding the pulse. You have available to you another work of mine which covers this art as a whole.[1]

---

[1] What is meant is Galen's main body of work on the pulse—*The Distinct Types of Pulse, The Discernment of the Pulse, Causes in the Pulse* and *Prognosis by the Pulse*—which he sometimes refers to in this way collectively as a single treatise. (These treatises are now available in translation in Johnston and Papavramidou 2024.) But, as we learn elsewhere (see e.g. *Freedom from Distress*, section 35), Teuthras died before Galen's second arrival in Rome, well before the presumed date of composition of those four major treatises. We are thus left with a problem in understanding the references to them here and elsewhere in this work (see also chs. 8 and 12 below). Either these references must have been added to the text later, in which case presumably by another hand, or,

The pulse is the same in all the arteries and in the heart; thus one may infer the nature of the pulse throughout from a single example. The perception of this motion in the arteries, however, is not equally possible in all cases. It is clearer in those arteries situated in the parts with less flesh, and comparatively fainter in those in the parts with more. The motion of those arteries that are concealed

454   beneath thick flesh, that are within bones, | or that have other bodies in front of them, is not perceptible, at least in normal states. When the body is highly ema-ciated, the motion of the artery in the spine is frequently evident to one touch-ing the upper abdomen; some have even succeeded in perceiving those which were previously unclear within the limbs. The motion of those in the temples, the instep of the feet, and the inside of the wrist is always perceptible. Less easily perceptible than these, but still not hidden, are those in the head behind the ears and those on the inside of the arms. There are certain others too, which are not completely concealed by the quantity of flesh; but there is none easier to find, better formed or more useful in practice than those in the wrists. The lack of flesh in that part makes these the most manifest; one should consider also the fact that one need not strip any part of the body to examine them, as is the case with many other arteries, and that these arteries are arranged in a straight line, which is of considerable importance to the precision of one's discernment.[2]

455   2. On touching an artery, it will become apparent to you that it is distended in every dimension. There are three dimensions in every physical body: length, depth and breadth. When the living being is in a normal state, the artery will be found to be very well-balanced in its distention; in abnormal states it will have a deficiency here or an excess there, in one or other of these dimensions. At this point you have to remember the nature of the pulse in its normal state; if, then, the abnormal pulse appears broader, you should term it 'broad'; if longer, 'long'; if deeper, 'high'.[3] Conversely, if it appears of less than the normal dimension in any of these respects, it should be termed 'narrow', 'short' or 'shallow'. If the abnormality affects all three dimensions equally, that which is diminished in all these respects must be termed 'small', and that which is augmented, 'large'. These, then, are the quantitative distinctions in the expansion of the pulse.

3. There are then the distinctions specific to motion: quickness and slowness,
456   the former being a hurried kind of motion, the latter | a relaxed kind. These too are to be assessed by comparison with the normal state. The vehemence or faintness of a pulse, meanwhile, consists in the quality of the impact; the

perhaps more likely, Galen is referring to an early or informal draft of the longer treatises that may have been available to students or associates even during his first stay. I am grateful to Clarine Rijpstra-van Daal for drawing my attention to this issue.

[2] *Diagnōsis*, also sometimes translated 'diagnosis', but with the broader sense of distinguishing or discerning; see also *The Art of Medicine*, n. 4 and *My Own Doctrines*, n. 30.

[3] The terms 'high' and 'deep' are used interchangeably for this dimension.

former pushes back the sense of touch violently, the latter weakly. Smoothness and hardness are qualities of the tunic of the artery; in the former case the artery appears as it were fleshier on impact, in the latter drier and more leathery. Now, this type of distinction in the pulse is discerned at the same time as the motion; it is not, however, a type specific to motion, as are the three previously mentioned. For within those three, quickness and slowness are a matter of the quality of the motion; vehemence and faintness, of the quality of the impact; largeness and smallness, of the quantity of the expansion; and the expansion too involves motion. The smoothness or hardness of a body, on the other hand, is not dependent for its nature on any motion. These, then, are the four types of distinction within the pulse that you will discover during the beat.

4. There is also a fifth, which consists in the interval between beats. | 'Interval' 457 is the term habitually used by doctors for the space of time between two beats, during which the artery undergoes both expansion and contraction. The training of beginners should be conducted on the basis that the contraction is not itself perceptible.[4] We refer, then, to a 'beat' and an 'interval', the former being the impact upon the sense of touch due to the motion of the artery, the latter the period of rest between two beats. It is in respect of this interval that a pulse may be 'frequent', 'infrequent' or 'medium'—which is the normal state for a pulse. You will recognize these, too, by the quantity of time: the frequent pulse is that in which the period of rest is a short one, the infrequent pulse that in which it is long. The terms 'rest', 'interval between beats' and 'contraction' are equivalent.

5. There is then the distinction between 'even' and 'uneven', which applies within each of the above distinctions. Evenness consists in the continued equality of any of the above characteristics. If, for example, the size is the same continuously, then the pulse is said to be 'even in size'; if the speed is the same, then it is 'even in speed'. And so also for vehemence, frequency and faintness. Unevenness, meanwhile, is | a loss of equality arising within any of the above 458 distinctions. One pulse may be uneven in size, another uneven in speed, another in vehemence, and so also in faintness or in frequency—or indeed in any of the other respects.

6. It may also happen that one unequal pulse occurs within a series of equal beats, but in a regular manner; and there are many varieties of this phenomenon. There may be three equal pulses with the fourth unequal, in a continually repeated manner, or four with the fifth unequal; and so too with any other number. Quite frequent is the case where five equal pulses are followed by an unequal sixth, or six equal pulses by an unequal seventh. In these cases

---

[4] On works for beginners, see *My Own Books*, Preface. The more advanced level of training, whereby the contraction also becomes discernible as a diagnostic sign, is vividly described in *The Discernment of the Pulse* I.1.

evenness has been lost, therefore the pulse is 'uneven'; but a certain regularity has been preserved, therefore it is 'regular'. The single unequal pulse that destroys the equality always comes at the same numerical interval; and thus the pattern represents the preservation of regularity of a kind. If however there is no such pattern, such a pulse is termed 'irregular'.

459   7. There is also the unevenness that is found within a single pulse, both in the sense of the parts of the artery being different from each other in terms of position and motion, and in relation to the motion of each individual pulse in itself. Unevenness in position of the parts consists in the fact that the artery appears to move up and down, forwards and backwards, to the right and to the left; unevenness in motion in the fact that it moves more quickly or slowly, earlier or later, more vehemently or more faintly, for a longer or shorter length or time, or all the time, or not at all. Unevenness within each part consists in a clear interruption (as for example with the 'gazelling') or in a recurrence (as with the 'double-striking').[5] Then there is the case of inequality of speed, as for example when it starts more quickly but ends more slowly, or the reverse; or where similar differences arise in terms of vehemence and faintness, or smallness and largeness. And in these contexts the motion may be divided not just into two periods of time, but into several—in accordance with the possibility of discerning these with the senses. These, then, are the types of simple unevenness within a single pulse.

460   8. Then we have the composite types, which represent all possible combinations of one type with another; here it may be that one type is combined with one other, or one with many, or many with many. Some of these have their own specific names, such as the 'worming', the 'anting' and the 'hectic'.

In the worming, the impression is given of a worm winding its way through the artery, and surging in the manner of a wave, so that the entire artery does not undergo expansion at the same time. The term 'worming' is used for this phenomenon in the context of a small expansion; if the expansion is large it is simply referred to as 'wave-like'. Of course, the worming is also faint and frequent. When, however, the pulse is reduced to extreme faintness, frequency and smallness, this is called 'anting'; here the pulse appears quick but is in fact not. The term 'hectic' is applied (as also to fevers) to a pulse which does not undergo any great change, but remains much the same, but is complicated and never dissolved, the bodily condition as a whole having become pathological. This description applies to both the fever and the pulse.[6]

---

[5] As with the worming and anting varieties of pulse below, the gazelling takes its name from its supposed similarity to the characteristic motion of an animal, in this case the leap of a gazelle, which seems to stop for a moment in mid-air before starting again.

[6] The term 'hectic' is derived from *hexis*, that is a 'condition' or stable state, and refers to a phenomenon observed constantly as part of such a 'condition'. (It is through its frequent use as applied

The above account of the distinctions in pulse should be sufficient for the beginner. One who | wishes to examine the matter in greater detail may consult 461 an entire treatise which I have devoted to *The Distinct Types of Pulse*. There is therefore no need now to discuss the 'full' and 'empty' pulse, nor 'rhythms', as these matters having been treated in detail in that work; and the argument will in any case be unclear to the beginner. Let us then recapitulate what has been said so far, before turning to the next subject.

A large pulse arises from a substantial distention of the artery in length, breadth and depth; a long one from distention in length only; a broad one, in breadth only; a high one, in depth. A vehement pulse is one which strikes the sense of touch vigorously; a soft pulse is one in which the tunic of the artery is smooth. A quick pulse arises when the distention of the artery takes place within a short time span; a frequent pulse, when it takes place at short intervals; an even one, when the pulse is continuously equal; a regular one, when the periodic pattern of the pulse remains equal. (If there is inequality in one beat alone, then the pulse is referred to as 'uneven in one beat'.) And the opposites of the above types should be clear enough: the small, short, narrow, shallow, faint, hard, slow, infrequent, uneven, and irregular. It should be obvious, too, that while all the other pairs of opposites involve the existence of | a midpoint, there 462 is no midpoint between even and uneven, nor between regular and irregular. By the same token, the normal state in all other cases is that corresponding to the midpoint; in this latter case, the only normal state is the even, both uneven and irregular being abnormal.

9. There are many ways in which the pulse may change; indeed one can hardly find any cause of change in the body which does not involve the pulse in its effects. The varieties of change may—according to the most fundamental mode of distinction—be divided into three. Let me enumerate these before turning to the specific consideration of individual types.

First is the category of natural change; second, that of that which is not natural, but nevertheless not unnatural; third, that of unnatural.[7] All these arise

---

to a particular type of fever—one which is constantly present—that it eventually acquired its everyday sense in modern English usage.)

[7] The Greek term *kata phusin*, literally 'according to nature', and elsewhere translated 'normal', is here translated 'natural' (so too, *para phusin*, literally 'against nature', above 'abnormal', here 'unnatural'). In the context of states of the body, the terminology of 'normality' seems more appropriate: what is at issue is what is normal for the individual in question. In the context of the discussion of *causes*, meanwhile, I have preferred 'natural', 'unnatural' and 'non-natural' (or 'not natural'): the point here is whether a given cause is 'in accordance with nature', in the sense of conducing to health, or not. This division of causes became a canonical one in later medical thought, with a prominent role for the category of the 'non-naturals', understood as the six types of 'necessary' factor for health (such as motion and rest, things taken into the body). Each of these is in itself neither in accordance with nature nor contrary to it; their health impact differs according to the particular form they take and the individual case. See *The Art of Medicine*, ch. 23 with n. 21; but the three categories seem to be treated rather differently in the present text from that 'classic' statement.

from differences in nature; for the arteries move differently in different individuals. These differences must first be understood by one hoping to recognize the cause and the extent of a pulse's change; and what is specific to each individual may be precisely learned by examination. The artery must be touched on a number of occasions, most particularly when the subject in in perfect health and resting | from all vehement activity, but in other bodily states too. Since, however, it is not possible for the doctor to have carried out such a test on all patients—for it frequently happens that a doctor is called to the bedside of a patient whom he has never met in a state of health—it is best for the expert to be superior to the layman in this context too. And this superiority may be gained by acquiring knowledge of those features which apply generally to the majority. For there is something which we may broadly term the common nature of men; and also that of women. There is also a common nature of people whose mixture is on the hot side, and another of those on the cold side; and the same applies to thin people as a whole, or to stout people. Within each of these common natures, it is rare to find something which is not similar to the majority. It is therefore also rare for one with a clear understanding of this common nature to make a mistake.

Men in general have a much larger pulse than women; it is also much more vehement, slightly slower and considerably less frequent. Those with a hot mixture have a pulse which is much quicker and more frequent, but only slightly more vehement. | Those who are thin by nature have a pulse which is much larger and more infrequent, but only slightly more vehement.

The above, then, are the differences in nature. The changes according to time of life are basically as follows. The pulse of a newborn is comparatively frequent, while that of an old man is infrequent; the natures of those in between depend on their proximity to childhood or old age. By the same token, the pulse in childhood is very quick, while that in old age is slower; and the other ages lie between the two. The difference in frequency, however, is much greater than that in speed. As regards size and vehemence at different ages: the largest pulse occurs in the prime and the smallest in old age, while that in childhood lies between them, but is slightly on the larger side; the most vehement is also that in the prime, while the faintest is that in old age, and that in childhood is midway between them. Such, then, is the pulse at different ages.

As regards seasons: mid-spring is the time of the largest and most vehement, which are also well-balanced in terms of speed and frequency. | The same applies also to mid-autumn. As spring proceeds, there is a loss of size and vehemence, but an increase in speed and frequency. Finally, as summer comes in, the pulse becomes faint, small, quick and frequent. As autumn proceeds, there is a loss of all qualities: size, vehemence, speed and frequency; and so at the onset of winter it has become small, faint, slow and infrequent. The pulse at the beginning of spring is similar to that at the end of autumn, and vice versa; that at the beginning of summer to that at the end of summer; that at the beginning of winter to that at the end of winter. Thus, the position of equidistance from both midsummer and midwinter corresponds to a similar change. Midsummer is in one way the same as, but in another different from, midwinter. The pulse is small and faint in both seasons; but it is swift and frequent in summer, and slow and infrequent in winter, nor is it as small in summer as in winter, nor as faint in winter as in summer. | These, then, are the changes in pulse due to the seasons of the year.   466

The changes due to place are analogous to those due to season. The pulse in very hot places is similar to that in midsummer; and that in very cold places similar to that in midwinter. That in well-balanced places is similar to that in mid-spring; and those in places between these differ proportionately. As for other states of the ambient air: if it is hot, this is similar to a hot season, if cold, to a cold season; if it is medial, this state is similar to the season of mid-spring.

In pregnancy the pulse is larger, more frequent and quicker; its other features remain in accordance with nature.

Sleep, too, ought to be in accordance with nature, if anything is; but it also gives rise to changes in the pulse. At the onset of sleep the pulse becomes smaller, slower, more infrequent and fainter; as it proceeds, the slowness and infrequency are intensified, especially when nourishment is taking place; and it becomes larger and more vehement. In the course of time it changes again in the direction of the faint and the small; but preserves its slowness and infrequency. | On transition from sleep to wakefulness, the pulse first of all   467 becomes large, vehement, quick, frequent and involving a certain degree of agitation; after a short time it returns to the well-balanced state.

Acquired states of the body affect the pulse in the same way as natural ones. A naturally thin person, on becoming well-fleshed, will acquire a pulse of the same kind as one naturally well-fleshed, and vice versa. And obviously the examination of this difference due to thinness or fleshiness must be made in isolation from any change in capacity. So too in every other context, so that the change arises in the one respect alone which is under discussion in each case. The above remarks about the well-fleshed should be taken as applying equally to the stout, the latter being a more intensified case of the former. Acquired mixtures of the body, too, affect the pulse in the same way as natural mixtures.

10. Let us now, then, turn to the other kinds of change resulting from non-natural causes.[8]

---

[8] It seems not entirely clear whether this is meant as the start of the section on the non-natural causes (in which case we should insert a comma and 'those' after 'kinds of change' in this sentence), or its continuation. According to the 'classic' understanding of the non-natural causes (see previous note), the ambient air and sleep come under this heading; so we may think that their discussion

468 Exercise, | in the early stages, and as long as it is practised in moderation, renders the pulse vehement, large, quick and frequent. Exercise in large amounts, or exceeding the capacity of the individual, makes it small, faint, quick and extremely frequent. In cases of great excess, whereby the subject is scarcely still able to move, and only at great intervals if at all, and there is a considerable dissolution of the capacity, the pulse is rendered very small, faint, slow and infrequent. If a state of complete dissolution of the capacity is reached, then the pulse will be that specific to this state; the nature of this pulse will be discussed in due course.

Hot baths, so long as they are kept within the bounds of moderation, make the pulse large, quick, frequent and vehement. If they exceed this, it becomes small and faint, though still swift and frequent. If they go still further, they make it small, slow, infrequent and faint. The immediate effect of cold baths is to make the pulse small, slow, infrequent and rather faint. The subsequent effect depends on the precise details, but in all cases leads to either numbing or

469 vigour. | Those which numb and cool down an individual make the pulse small, faint, slow and infrequent; those which heat and produce vigour make it large and vehement, and well-balanced in speed and frequency.

Food taken in such quantities as to burden the natural capacity renders the pulse uneven and irregular—and also, according to Archigenes, fairly swift and frequent. Taken in good proportion it makes the pulse large, vehement, quick and frequent. Food taken in insufficient quantities to provide proper nourishment does not cause change in the same way as that taken in the right proportion, but rather one which is smaller and less long-lasting. The effect of wine is similar to that of food, except that the change is immediate, and the effect ceases earlier; also, that it increases speed and size more than it does vehemence and frequency. One might say that wine raises the size to the same degree that food taken in the right proportion renders the strength more vehement and more long-lasting.

470 | Of all things taken, water has the briefest effect on the pulse; yet it does have an effect, the same in kind as that of food. And everything else changes the motion of the arteries to the same extent that it has the capacity to provide nourishment, heat or cooling. The above, then, are the effects of the so-called 'non-natural causes' on the pulse.

11. We turn now to the changes due to unnatural causes. Here we should first remind ourselves of those points relating to the unnatural causes which have already been covered by our previous discussion. States of the air or quantities of food which burden the natural capacities, as well as ill-proportioned use of exercise, baths or sleep, are all unnatural; for the quantitative excess of those same causes

must have begun at the end of Kühn p. 465, with the account of seasons. But no explicit indication of that change of category is made there, nor is it made explicit that we have been considering non-natural causes before the present sentence.

which we term 'natural' and 'non-natural' renders them 'unnatural'. Both those causes which are unnatural in this quantitative sense, and those which are unnatural in kind, are infinite in number, and therefore cannot be fully comprehended in any account. Even here, however, the role of the art consists in organization and division of this infinite expanse, as far as that is possible, into genera and species.

It is, in fact, not unreasonable to state that every unnatural cause does, broadly, one of two things: | either it dissolves and dissipates the vital capacity or   471 it compresses and burdens it. The capacity is dissolved by a lack of food, by the ill effects of diseases, by the strength of affections of the soul, by pains of a vehement or long-lasting nature, and by immoderate evacuations. It is burdened by large quantities of matter and by ailments of the organs, such as inflammations, indurations, lumps, abscesses and all kinds of decay. Now, the dissolution of the capacity renders the pulse very small, faint and frequent; while its compression, and what we have termed its 'burdening', render it uneven and irregular in every respect, especially those of vehemence and size. These latter are the particular forms of unevenness specific to the compression of the capacity, and to the heavy burdening of the capacity, which comes about in a larger number of distinct types, and of slight burdening, which comes about in fewer. Where the harm is slight, there is a greater tendency to large rather than small pulses, and to vehement rather than faint ones; where it is great, the opposite holds. Sometimes a motion is lost completely, and sometimes an additional one occurs, in this kind of bodily state. In the latter case a smaller | degree of harm   472 appears; in the former, a greater. This, then, is the general nature of the changes common to all forms of dissolution and compression; each individual type then has its own specific features, depending on the effective cause in each case.

The kind of dissolution of the capacity which comes about through lack [of food] involves a change, initially towards faintness, smallness, quickness and frequency; at the next stage, towards faintness, smallness, slowness and infrequency; and finally, towards extreme smallness, faintness and frequency; and towards a false impression of speed. This is what is known as the anting pulse. The worming pulse also arises from the dissolution of the capacity, but in cases where this still retains some degree of resistance. The difference between the worming and the anting lies in the fact that in the former there has not yet been a contraction to an extreme state of faintness and smallness, and that the unevenness is manifest within one beat, an unevenness which arises through the parts beginning to be moved earlier or later. Therefore it is less slow than small; sometimes, in fact, it is not slow at all. And for this reason it is the least bad. When a collapse[9] takes place in the context of a fatal, acute fever, this is not

---

[9] The Greek term is *sunkopē* (or *syncopē*), a disease category which involves the notion of a sudden loss of strength, including stoppage of breath and in some cases, as suggested a few lines later, some kind of cardiac event.

473   associated with the worming pulse, | while other types of dissolution of the capacity do for the most part result in a worming pulse, especially in cases where there is no fever, or very little. By the same token, collapse of the heart results in an anting pulse; *cholera*,[10] severe fluxions of the gastric cavity, haemorrhage, female flux[11] and all those ailments that involve acute evacuation for the most part cause a worming, but in very extreme cases an anting, pulse. And when these complaints occur without fever, you will find an even greater tendency towards the worming, which will be both marked and of long duration. Such, then, are the most common forms of change due to unnatural causes.

12. Let us now give an account of their individual types.

In rage the pulse is high, large, vehement, quick and frequent. In pleasure it is large and infrequent, but not especially vehement. In distress it is small, slow, faint and infrequent. In cases of sudden, vehement fear it is quick, disrupted,

474   irregular and uneven; in cases where fear has been present for a long time, | it is like that in distress. In all these affections, where they are present for a long period of time, the same kind of pulse results as in cases of dissolution of the capacity. For indeed, all these have the effect of dissolving the capacity, quickly in severe occurrences, more slowly in mild ones.

Pain of the sort which affects the pulse—and this happens in the case of severe pain or pain in the most important bodily parts—acts in the same way as inflammation. In the early stages, when it is still small, it renders the pulse fairly large, vehement, swift and frequent; once it has become larger and more severe, so that it is already causing harm to the vital tension, it makes the pulse fairly small and faint, and also quick and frequent. And in cases where it remains for a long time, or becomes more vehement, each of these features is intensified. Pain which actually dissolves the capacity brings about a change towards faintness, smallness, a false impression of quickness, and excessive frequency.

The pulse which is common to all cases of inflammation is like a saw. Here the artery, which obviously takes on a hard appearance, appears to be partially

475   distended and partially not. This pulse has a certain | disrupted quality about it, too. It is also quick and frequent, but not always large. The features specific to different cases are as follows. At its inception the pulse is more vehement, swifter and more frequent than the norm; as it grows, all these features increase, and it now also becomes clearly harder and more disrupted; at its peak, it is clearer, harder and more disrupted, but now smaller than before, though not fainter, except in cases where the ailment exceeds the patient's capacity; but it also becomes more frequent, and quick. In cases where it remains for a long period, and the hardness reaches a point similar to that of an induration,

---

[10] An illness involving discharge of bile (*cholē*).
[11] On 'female flux' see *Affected Places* VI.5, p. 401 and *Prognosis*, ch. 8, p. 59.

thinness and hardness of the pulse are added to the above features. These things come about in cases of inflammation which change the pulse of the living being as a whole, either because of the size of the inflammation or because of the importance of the part in which it arises.

Where the inflammation does not affect the whole living being, the pulse will be as already described, but confined to the part in question. And each of the above features is intensified or diminished according to the degree of inflammation and the nature of the organ which it affects. The parts with more nerve in them, for example, give rise to harder, more saw-like, smaller | pulses. The 476 parts with more vein or artery have the opposite effect, those with more artery having the larger pulse of the two, which is also liable to become uneven and irregular.

It should by now be obvious what will be the nature of the pulse in those suffering from inflammation in the liver, in the spleen, or in the kidneys, bladder, stomach or colon, as also of those suffering from pleuritis, peripneumonia or any other disease in which a fever follows from the inflammation of the part. The pulse will, however, undergo alteration as a result of the particular effects arising from the nature of the symptoms—both those which are necessary consequences of these inflammations and those which happen to arise concurrently with them. The effect will thus be a mixed one, arising from the characteristics of inflammation itself, from the nature of the part affected and from that of the symptom present. Inflammation of the diaphragm, for example, is apt to lead to spasm; inflammation of the lungs to suffocation; that of the mouth of the stomach to collapse; that of the liver to lack of nutrition; that of the stomach to poor digestion; that of the kidneys to retention of urine. Those parts which are more sensitive affect the pulse because of the pain experienced; | those which are less so affect it by virtue of their bodily state alone. 477

All these phenomena, then, give rise to the wide variety of alterations of the pulse in cases of inflammation. The method of distinguishing them has been fully discussed elsewhere; here I shall give a summary for the use of the beginner.

In pleuritis the pulse is quick, frequent, and not particularly large. It may also appear to be vehement, but in fact, though not faint, it is not actually vehement either, as far as the ailment itself is concerned. In all cases it must be borne in mind that we must examine the change due to the thing itself, and distinguish this from any incidental change due to some other cause. What happens with the pulse in pleuritis is that it has the effect of making the artery as it were more nerve-like, and harder, a change which is similar to an increase in vehemence. This tends to deceive the untrained, who are unable to distinguish a hard beat from a vehement one. Here, as with many other distinct types of pulse, the majority of doctors are unable to make the distinction, and are thus apt to cast

aspersions on our writings. Their own ignorance makes them contemptuous of
478 what is actually the correct analysis. But I we need not prolong our present discussion on account of them; we have written a specific work on *The Discernment
of the Pulse.*

I therefore urge the student to train both his faculties of reason and his sense
of touch, in order that he may be able to recognize pulses in practice, not just to
distinguish them in theory. The starting-point for this practical experience is
the theoretical instruction. Yet the actual degree of frequency is not something
that can be expressed in words, even though there is a great difference between
what exceeds the usual level associated with pleuritis and that which falls short
of it. For there will necessarily be excess when there is a change to peripneumonia, or a threat of collapse; while deficiency inevitably leads to *kataphora* or
damage to the nerves.[12] Similarly with the type of unevenness which is as it
were saw-like, and which is specific to pleuritis in particular: the relaxed version of this indicates a soft pleuritis which may be readily resolved,[13] while the
intensified version indicates a problematic one, which is not thus readily
resolved. In cases of weak capacity, this latter kind is acutely dangerous; in cases
of strong capacity, it will be gradually resolved, converted into an abscess, or
superseded by a process of wasting and withering.[14]

479 When a pleuritis is I in the process of being resolved, the pulse very quickly
loses any unnatural change it has undergone. When it is in the process of
becoming an abscess, the pulse becomes that specific to abscess; by the same
token, that which is being consumed by a withering will have that specific to
withering. The pulse in abscess is at first similar to that of an inflammation at its
peak; for that is how the abscess itself begins. Sometimes it is uneven and
irregular; in all cases hectic. Once the pus is ready, it is similar in other respects,
but more even; when it bursts it is fainter, broader, slower and less frequent. The
pulse in cases of withering undergoes more than one type of change. As far as
possible, one must specify these on the basis of evident distinctions. Patients
who have in a short space of time contracted a withering in connection with an
inflammation which has not yet been dissolved have a pulse which is faint,
fairly quick, very frequent, and tapering in size within one beat. Archigenes
refers to these as 'sloping down' or 'sloping away', by which expressions he
clearly wishes to indicate the fact that the pulse is brief in its expansion, with a

---

[12] For *kataphora* see *Affected Places* III.6 with n. 2.

[13] The Greek term for 'resolved' here is the verb *pettein*, the standard term elsewhere for 'coction'
or 'digestion'.

[14] 'Withering' translates *marasmos*, a technical clinical term for Galen, to which he devoted a
treatise. Though the cognate marasmus exists in modern medicine, the sense of the term in Galen is
rather that of a wasting of the flesh or body understood as due to lack of moisture and analogous to
the withering of plants.

kind of falling-off at either end. I For the contraction comes about not from an   480
overall reduction, but from a curtailment at either end, causing it to taper in
length at both. And this applies not only in these cases, but also in the majority
of cases of withering of any kind; it applies in all cases of withering due to
inflammation, but in the majority of other cases of withering too—unless,
indeed, it is the case that these too are caused by some hidden inflammation. If
so, this will then be the pulse specific to withering due to inflammation, and
will not occur in any other cases of withering.

The pulse is hectic in all cases of withering. This is the single feature which is
most widely shared by all occurrences; secondly, there is the tapering unevenness in size of the expansion, which is also present in most cases. Thirdly, there
is the frequency: this too is an inalienable feature of all cases of withering due to
inflammation; but it also obtains in cases where a patient is in acute danger as
a result of a state of the heart or collapse associated with the mouth of the
stomach, and has taken wine to remove that danger, but then suffered withering
sometime later. (But it may be that this type of fatality too is best regarded as
resulting from some small inflammations which we cannot perceive.) I Some of   481
these patients, too, have the 'sloping down' pulse; but again it may be that it is
only those whose withering results from an inflammation that have this, while
the others are those who suffer from withering without inflammation. This
point is uncertain. In any case, such patients have a pulse which is hectic or
faint, extremely frequent, and in some cases also the nodding pulse. This, then,
is the second distinct type of pulse in withering.

The third is that of those who have an infrequent pulse. In these cases too,
however, the preceding fever has made it more frequent; and the extreme state
of dissolution of the capacity also has a significant effect in this direction. But in
between these two states, when all fevers have been cooled down, but not yet
eliminated, we have this change in the direction of infrequency. This type of
withering is specific to old age, arising especially when the part affected is in the
region of the chest or lungs. Such patients retain the feverish hardness of the
pulse, even if it is infrequent. In very few cases of withering does the pulse
acquire any other unevenness than that already mentioned, pertaining to
the size.

The pulse of those suffering from the complaint known as 'wasting' is small,
faint, soft, moderately quick, and hectic. I That of sufferers from peripneumonia   482
is large, with a somewhat wave-like character, faint and soft; it is similar to that of
sufferers from lethargy, except in cases where it approaches a state of unevenness—
both unevenness within one beat and what is known as 'systematic' unevenness. In the former case, it sometimes becomes as it were interrupted and
turbulent, and double-striking; in the latter, it has the other distinguishing features, but also missed or extra beats. Since all peripneumonics have acute fever,

and also have a certain degree of *kōma*, the frequency of the pulse will depend on which of these two predominates: if the peripneumonia is more feverish, the pulse will be very frequent; less so if it has more *kōma* in it.[15]

The pulse in lethargy, then, is similar to that in peripneumonia, in size, faintness and softness; but it is fainter, less uneven, and subject to missed beats rather than extra ones. Sometimes it also becomes double-striking. It is, however, always wave-like, at least in the deep *kataphora* to which this discussion refers. For we are here setting out the nature of the pulse in diseases in their 483 full-blown form, with all their proper indicators; | on this basis it should also be possible to recognize the extent of a disease which is not yet full-blown and lacks some feature or the other, and to decide how far it is developed and what other symptoms may still occur.

Now, since we have mentioned unevenness frequently, and irregularity only a few times, the general point should be understood that irregularity tends to follow as a result of unevenness. It is in fact quite rare to find an uneven pulse which is regular. Less serious illnesses may give rise to an uneven but regular pulse; more serious ones will cause both unevenness and irregularity.

In phrenitis the pulse is small (in very rare cases it has been observed to be large), and moderate in tension. It is also hard, nerve-like, frequent and very fast. It has a certain wave-like quality too; and will sometimes appear to manifest a slight tremor, at other times to be spasmodically cut short. That specific symptom of fever which relates to speed is clearly present at both ends of the expansion, especially the external one.[16] One may also sometimes observe a vehement occurrence of unevenness in relation to position. Indeed, the whole 484 | artery frequently appears to leave its proper place and move upwards in a disrupted manner, with a motion more like a sudden surge than the expansion proper to pulses; similarly, it will move downwards as if dragged downward in a spasm, rather than undergoing a normal contraction. Excessive frequency is a warning sign of imminent collapse.

There is also another ailment, which must either be described as neither lethargy nor phrenitis, but halfway between the two, or as belonging to both types; for it is a mixture of the features of phrenitis and lethargy. Let us consider this ailment specifically and proceed now to discuss its pulses. To avoid giving the appearance here of the sort of riddle which is set as a question for public discussion, I shall make clear its nature through its attendant signs. In most cases the eyes are closed; the subjects are sleepy and snore. Or alternatively, there is an intense, unblinking stare, similar to that in *katochē*. If one asks these persons a

---

[15] For *kōma* see *Affected Places* III.6 with n. 2.
[16] That is, the final moment of the expansion, that where it reaches its greatest 'external' extension.

question, or compels them to conversation, they are difficult and slow in their responses. They frequently also make confused utterances, answer questions wrongly and talk random nonsense. Such is the nature of this ailment: my present purpose is to make its nature clear by means of its attendant features, since it lacks a name of its own. Its pulse $^|$ is quick and frequent, in the manner of 485 phrenitis, but less so; its strength is also less than that in phrenitis. It is broad and short; it does not have the overall curtailment of the external part of the motion, but it happens in a different way, whereby the pulse rushes to conceal itself inside, causing the contraction to be speeded up and the expansion to be muffled. It is in this respect different from that of phrenitis, which does not have this feature of curtailment.

The pulse in people suffering from *katochē*—this is the traditional Greek term, whereas doctors of more recent times refer to the ailment as *katalēpsis*—is similar to that in lethargy in most respects, especially in size, slowness and infrequency. The two ailments as a whole are in fact not greatly different. The pulse in those suffering from *katochē* is however not weak, nor soft; and this represents a marked difference, as does the fact that the whole condition of lethargic patients is subject to relaxation and swelling, while in *katochē* it is subject to tightening and being drawn inward. They also differ from each other in the degree of evenness: the pulse in *katochē* is even, $^|$ that in lethargy uneven. 486 Archigenes claims, further, as a specific feature of the former that the place of the artery is found to be hotter, as also in patients about to undergo spasms with *kataphora*.

In people suffering from spasms, the actual body of the artery appears to be drawn inward and wedged in on all sides, not in the manner of something being compressed by someone, or forced into a narrow passage; nor, however, does it appear tremulous, as is the case in fever, especially at the paroxysm; nor incapable of distension, as may happen over a long period of time, especially where there is some fault, or some damage to the organs. It rather resembles a hollow body endowed with nerves, such as the gut, or something similar, being subjected to tension simultaneously from both ends. And so too the motion is uneven, as the artery is moved up and down like a string. Here one does not get the impression of an expansion or contraction; it is more like a disruption, in which the artery appears to leap outwards and then again to be drawn inwards; and this happens without any clear distinction in the motion: at one and the same time one part appears to move to the surface, as if being shot out, while another is borne inwards, as if being pulled by someone; and also one part $^|$ appears to 487 move quickly, another slowly.

The pulse in people undergoing spasms also appears vehement and large. In fact it is neither faint, nor small, nor as vehement or large as it appears: one is deceived by the beat, which because of the tension appears strong, and because of the disruption appears to leap out. This also sometimes gives it the appearance of depth; the sense of touch encounters what seems like a harsh sound. In fact, this pulse is unmistakeable to anyone with experience. It is quite unlike any other, both in the tension in either direction and in the spasmic nature of the motion. When this pulse is combined with that of *kataphora*, the motion is difficult to detect; only one who has trained himself meticulously to recognize each pulse by its individual features will also be able to identify this combination.

In paralysis the pulse is small, faint and slow; in some cases it is also infrequent, in some frequent, but with an irregular missing of beats. The pulse in epilepsy and in apoplexy is of a similar nature: the following remarks about
488 epileptics may be taken as applying also to apoplectics, | but in more intensified form. So long as the disturbance is still moderate, and the ailment not sufficiently strong to dominate the patient's nature, one will find no significant change, in size, vehemence, speed, frequency or hardness. The only feature is that the artery is subject to tension in both directions, as in spasm. When the ailment becomes strong enough to burden the capacity, there is a certain unevenness and a strong tension and the pulse becomes smaller, fainter and less frequent. When it causes great compression and completely overcomes the capacity, the pulse is rendered faint, frequent and quick.

The pulse in sore throat presents a degree of tension, not unlike that in spasm, but is large and wave-like, as in the case of peripneumonia. By determining which of these features predominates, one may predict the course of the illness. If peripneumonic characteristics are to the fore, the sore throat will end in peripneumonia; if spasmic ones, in spasm. In patients who suffer violent suffocation, the pulse is small and infrequent in the final stages, frequent and uneven.

489 | In acute cases of *orthopnoea* the pulse is uneven, irregular and with missed beats. In moderate cases it is frequent; in extremely violent ones, slow and intermittent; in the terminal phase, frequent and faint. In hysterical suffocation[17] the pulse is extended as in spasm; in terminal cases it is frequent, irregular and with missed beats.

Illnesses of the *stomachos*—let us for present purposes follow the general usage, whereby this term is applied to the mouth of the gastric cavity—affect the pulse in a variety of ways. If it is inflamed only, then the change will be of the same kind described in the case of the inflammation of a nerve-like body. If there is compression, biting, relaxation, vomiting, nausea, lack of appetite, or pain, the pulse will again be in accordance with that particular type of symptom. Biting sensations, vomiting, nausea, hiccups, disturbance and feebleness

---

[17] See *Affected Places* VI.5, with n. 32.

have a powerful positive effect on the frequency of the pulse, at the same time as making it small and faint. I In some cases it also becomes somewhat quicker. 490 Compression on its own, without any of the above symptoms, makes the pulse infrequent, slow, small and faint. Such compression arises from the consumption of heavy foods of a kind which do not possess any powerful capacity of their own, but cause difficulty by their sheer quantity, and because of certain fluids that flow in, without themselves having any biting quality. This kind of pulse will arise particularly in cases where cooling also results from these causes. It is also similar in cases of ravenous hunger.

Now, all bodily states which cause greater frequency lead in chronic or vehement forms to the worming pulse. Those which cause greater infrequency not only intensify the distinguishing features stated, but also engender a similar type in terms of the unevenness within a single pulse. This makes it seem as if the body of the artery has been pierced in many places, and has lost its continuity; one has the tactile impression, in the expansion, of contact with sand.

In dropsy the pulse is large, frequent, slightly hard and with a degree of tension, in the *askitēs*[18] variety of the disease; in the 'drum-like' it is I fairly large, 491 not without strength, fairly quick, frequent, slightly hard and with a degree of tension; in the 'throughout-the-skin' variety, it is wave-like, fairly broad, and soft. In *elephantiasis* the pulse is small, weak, slow and frequent. In jaundice without fever it is fairly small, fairly frequent, fairly hard, not faint, nor quick.

In subjects who have taken hellebore, the pulse just before the vomiting, while they are undergoing compression, is broad, infrequent, fairly faint and fairly slow; as they are vomiting and retching it is uneven and irregular; as they recover, it is regular, but still uneven, though less so than before; when they are close to the normal state it is even, larger than before, and more vehement. Those who in these circumstances suffer collapse, spasm and hiccups have a pulse which is small, faint, irregular, quick and very frequent. In those who experience suffocation it is small, faint, I irregular and uneven, but not frequent, 492 nor quick; rather, it tends to slow down. It also manifests a certain wave-like quality, broadness and sometimes also a certain brief tension in the artery.

---

[18] The term was a standard one for dropsy, or for a variety of dropsy; it is etymologically connected with *askos*, a hide or wineskin. The 'drum-like' terminology suggests that in this case the belly was drawn tight like a drum.

Affected Places (excerpts)

This six-book treatise is one of Galen's most significant and influential works in the area of diagnosis and clinical practice. It was probably written late in his career, and introduces a number of concepts and clinical perspectives not found in other works.

In the course of a 'head to toe' account of the body and its pathologies, it develops a sophisticated analysis of the bodily location of disease, and of the relationship between parts primarily affected—by 'protopathy' or 'idiopathy' (*prōtopatheia, idiopatheia*)—and those affected secondarily or by sympathy (*sumpatheia, deuteropatheia*); much of the first book is devoted to these concepts. The third book contains some of Galen's most detailed accounts of mental disorders and of the pathology of the brain, and of the particularly important ancient disease category of melancholy (*melancholia*); the extracts below begin with the most significant passages from that book.

The focus on the original bodily source of diseases has some unexpected consequences, in terms of the order of topics. Our extract from book IV, one of Galen's most vivid accounts of the mental disturbance known as phrenitis, appears as a digression from the discussion of the eyes. (And there is further material on phrenitis in book V, because of the aetiological connection that complaint was thought to have with the diaphragm.)

The last of our extracts comes from book VI, where the context is the ailments of both female and male reproductive organs. Here Galen gives his most comprehensive account of another ancient disease category of enormous historical importance: hysteria (or more precisely, 'hysterical suffocation'). The extract also sheds considerable light on ancient gynaecology and on the relationship between female and male practitioners, as well as containing some of Galen's reflections on the nature and physiology of sexual desire.

The tone and content of some passages in the work suggest that it was a work intended for the use of students or close associates of the author, rather than for wider distribution.

Greek title: Περὶ τῶν πεπονθότων τόπων (*Peri tōn peponthotōn topōn*)[1]
Kuhn: VIII.1–452
Editions: books I and II: Gärtner 2015 (with German translation)
　books V and VI: Brunschön 2021 (with German translation)
Translation: Siegel 1976

---

[1] This is the form of the tile which became standard, in both Greek and Latin (*De locis affectis*); the full form of the title was rather 'The Discernment of Affected Parts' (Περὶ διαγνώσεως τόπων πεπονθότων). It also became known through mediaeval Latin translations as 'On Internal Parts' (*De interioribus*).

BOOK III

6. It is conceded by all doctors, through the actions they actually perform in VIII.160
all cases of ailment of the rational capacity, that the home of this capacity is
the head. We should, then, consider the nature of the bodily state in each such
ailment—impairment of memory, for example, since I have undertaken to
give an account of this. Such impairment is often observed to be accompanied
by some impairment of the reasoning faculty, just as the latter is often
observed to be accompanied by the former. This is because the bodily state is
the same in both cases, but intensified in cases where the reasoning faculty is
lost at the same time as that of memory, a phenomenon known as stupefaction
[*mōrōsis*]. | Both are also lost in cases of lethargy and in all ailments involving 161
karos,[2] and so the state must belong to the same class in all these. The most
fundamental class in question here is that of bad-mixture; this, as previously
shown, is a state common to the uniform parts, which are those to which action
primarily belongs. The second distinction in terms of class is that they are
clearly cases of a *cold* bad-mixture: such a mixture is observed to numb the
activities of the soul, as shown by those animals which are compelled by the
cold to hibernate, as well as by all cooling drugs and cold foods. Lettuce, for
example, produces kataphoric slumber, if taken in large quantities. All heaviness of the head, too, when this comes about in the absence of biting pain,
involves a kataphoric tendency to sleep, and is of course greatly alleviated by
the extraction of phlegm.

The same conclusion is also indicated by the phenomena of burning and
cooling of the head: burning leads to sleeplessness, while cooling is kataphoric.
Moreover, diseases which involve bile, and which are hot, clearly bring about
derangement and phrenitis, while those opposite to these, involving phlegm
and cold, bring about sluggishness and *kataphora*. | The primary capacity, then, 162
relevant to the production of diseases of both sleeplessness and *kataphora* is
that involving either hotness or coldness of the bad-mixture; but a secondary
factor is the wetness or dryness. Baths, for example, render everyone sleepy by
moistening the head, as does the drinking of well-mixed wine, and all moistening forms of nutrition. Soo too with times of life: children are more prone to
sleep because of their moisture, old men less so because of their dryness. Let
these facts, then, stand as evidence of the fact that abnormal moisture has the
second place in relation to inactivity of the soul, while cold has the first place.
This is why excessive moisture on its own brings about long, deep sleep, and

---

[2] I leave *karos*, *kōma* and *kataphora* (with the related adjective 'kataphoric') untranslated, though
the first could in some contexts simply be translated 'unconsciousness'; all three terms refer to an
unconscious or semi-conscious state arising in certain bodily conditions.

similarly dryness on its own brings about sleeplessness, in the two states mentioned by Hippocrates in the line:

Sleep and sleeplessness: when either is greater than the norm, it is bad.[3]

Where cold is present in conjunction with significant moisture, then we find
the ailments related to *karos* and *kataphora*; where such moisture is absent we
find impairment of memory and stupefaction. Since, however, there is great
variation in the degree, not only of moisture and cold, but also of dryness and
163 heat, there is a very great variety | in the causes of impairment to the activities
of the soul.

(In the interests of clarity of exposition, let us call the activities of the rational
in the soul 'commanding' and those of the non-rational ones 'character-based';
the latter are not our subject now, no more than the ailments of the heart or of
the liver.)[4]

Since, then, immoderate sleep and immoderate sleeplessness arise because
of, respectively, moisture and dryness of the mixture, so too different degrees of
sleeplessness or sleep follow from different degrees of moisture and dryness.
Furthermore, as has been previously shown, such bad-mixtures come about in
two ways; therefore each bodily state, too, will have two versions, one arising
from the wet or dry fluids, the other from the bodies themselves, when the solid
bodies reach the same state of bad-mixture as the wet.[5] In addition to the bad-
mixtures mentioned, there is also a third, which is a combination of the two, as
occurs for example in the case of *kōma* with sleeplessness, where there is an
excess of both the phlegmatic and bilious fluids.

Within the opposition of hot and cold, analogously, there arise both simple
164 bad-mixtures and those which are a combination of both. | When bile—I mean,
of course, yellow bile—is mixed with phlegm, we get the state which is a mixture of hot and cold. And if it is accepted that the state which is a combination
of opposites may occur also in the solid parts themselves, then on this assumption there will be three primary bad-mixtures within each opposition. All such
ailments, then, arise in the brain, but they differ from each other not just in
the variety of combinations, nor just in the degree of both the simple and
the combined states, but also in the fact that the bad-mixtures sometimes arise

---

[3] This statement appears in very similar form at *Aphorisms* 2.3 and 7.72.

[4] The Greek terms are *hēgemonikos* (literally 'leading', the same word which appears in noun
form as *hēgemonikon*, the 'command centre' of the soul or brain) and *ēthikos*, more usually translated 'ethical'. (On this word and this connection between 'character' and 'ethics' in its translation
see *The Soul's Dependence on the Body*, ch. 9 with n. 54.) For the theory of the location of the non-
rational capacities in the heart and the liver see *The Doctrines of Hippocrates and Plato*, passim. In
the final remark here Galen is making a connection between the ethical analysis of the capacities
and pathologies of the 'soul' and those bodily locations.

[5] In other words, the fluids in the body: Galen sometimes uses the terms 'wet' or 'moisture' to
refer to the fluids or humours (*chumoi*).

within the ventricles of the brain and sometimes within the vessels that run through it, or in the moisture dispersed throughout the body of the head. There is then a fourth case, too, where the body of the brain itself suffers from bad-mixture.

7. One should pay close attention to sleep in patients who have suffered loss of memory or intelligence (for stupefaction is a loss of intelligence): is the patient significantly prone to sleep, or moderately so, or not prone to sleep at all, I but in his normal state in this respect? Through this enquiry you will discover the predominant bad-mixture. One should consider, further, whether there is expulsion [of fluids] from the head through the nose and mouth, or whether these parts are observed to be dry; from this, too, you will be able to make an estimate of the state, just as you may in the case of catarrh or discharge of mucus: in these, too, the quality and quantity of the fluids expelled, in conjunction with consideration of the preceding causes,[6] indicates the state of the head, which is either hot, as happens in cases of burning, or cold, as in the case of cooling. Without having made all these distinctions, it is impossible to discover the appropriate treatment for each state. So, for example, in the case of great impairment of memory, the bad-mixture will definitely be a cold one, and it will be appropriate to heat it; it will not, however, necessarily be appropriate to dry it, nor, indeed, to moisten it. If the bad-mixture involves moisture, then one should dry it; if dryness, one should moisten it; if the state is midway between these, one should preserve this as it is.

For example, I know of one case where a person had almost totally lost his memory, and had also suffered impairment of his reasoning faculty, through devotion to work and through lack of sleep arising from his I studies; and another of a vineyard worker who suffered the same as a result of his labours, in conjunction with a thinning diet. Obviously both these individuals would be harmed by all drying and heating factors, and benefited by those which moisten and heat. Impairments of the commanding activities may be accompanied by fever, too, as in the cases of phrenitis and lethargy; or they may arise without fever, as in *mania* and melancholy; and also in both sympathy and protopathy of the brain.[7] Those which are identified precisely on the basis of their own specific symptoms, are constant and have not been preceded by others arise through protopathy; those which are not thus precisely identified, do not persist, and arise from other symptoms, are the result of sympathy. Here we should also bear in mind that there is one kind of sympathy which consists in a

165

166

---

[6] The distinction between 'preceding' (*proēgoumenai*) and 'antecedent' or 'procatarctic' (*prokatarktichai*) causes is a technical one in Galen's system: the former are internal or predisposing causes that have arisen within the patient's bodily constitution, the latter external factors or triggers; see also *The Art of Medicine*, ch. 18 with n. 19.

[7] i.e. both in cases where the brain is affected as a consequence of a pathology elsewhere in the body (sympathy) and where it is the organ first or primarily affected (protopathy).

process, and disappears at the same time as the causes that produce it, and another which reaches the status of a stable state of those parts which suffer the sympathy, and persists even after the causes that produced it cease.

Now, the fact that all ailments of the commanding activities arise in the brain 167 | is agreed by all doctors—provided, that is, that they do not think one thing in their mind but say something different, because of the argumentative competitiveness of a sect. To discover the nature of a bad-mixture, however, is not a trivial task. For this the doctor must have both a devotion to work and a capacity for enquiry, not a compulsion to investigate how he may contradict what has been correctly stated by previous authors on the command centre of the soul—a matter so manifest that even people without education are convinced that it is in the brain.

One might, perhaps, forgive armchair philosophers[8] for being mistaken on this point; but in those with long experience in medical matters such argumentativeness—one might rather call it shamelessness—is unforgivable. After all, they bathe the head in all cases of infirmity arising from sleeplessness, as also in all cases of delirium, phrenitis and lethargy. Even Archigenes applies medicaments to the head in cases of impairment of memory, and the treatment he undertakes in the case of stupefaction is also applied to the head. What doctor with any experience will heal sufferers from apoplexy, epilepsy, *opisthotonos*, 168 *emprosthotonos* or *tetanos*[9] in any other way? | Or, for that matter, those suffering from paralysis of half the body? Do not all doctors address the main part of their therapy to the first vertebrae, in cases of spasmodic ailments, since experience leads them to this part immediately—and so too in cases of paralysis of half the body, where they at the same time also heat the brain? The cure for sufferers from apoplexy follows the same procedures, as does that of sufferers from epilepsy. When the ailment arises from the mouth of the stomach or some other part, then they treat that part especially and primarily, while at the same time also preparing the brain, to protect it against being affected. This, then, should be the focus of the enquiry, rather than the question of [the location of] the command centre of the soul, which is abundantly obvious to all those who are not warped in their judgement; nor that of the source of the nerves, an enquiry which is not to be pursued by turning to the gods for prophecy, but by acquiring an education from men versed in anatomy.

8. Many have convinced themselves that the source of the nerves is the heart because of their inability to distinguish a ligament from a nerve—a confusion to which an ambiguity in linguistic usage contributes, since many doctors refer

---

[8] Literally, 'philosophers sitting in a corner'.
[9] *Opisthotonos*, *emprosthotonos* and *tetanos* were understood as varieties of muscle spasm or convulsion.

to ligaments as I 'connective nerves'.[10] I have no quarrel with them over that   169
terminology, provided it is understood that [in the present context] they are
talking of the *voluntary* nerves (as they themselves call them), which, we state,
have their source in the brain, and *not* of these 'connective nerves'. They themselves, after all, do not claim that spasm or paralysis is an ailment of the connective nerves, but of the voluntary ones. Where, then, the whole body is
perceived to be in spasm, it may be taken that the entirety of this kind of bodily
part has been affected simultaneously; it is, as it were, the trunk of all the nerves,
like the central branch from which the offshoots grow in a tree. It is not like a
branch with a few offshoots in one particular part, as would be the case where a
leg or a single arm is in spasm. Spasm of a whole limb indicates that the source
of the nerves leading into that limb has been affected, and this would be analogous to the case where some single branch of a tree is affected; when the entire
body is affected by the ailment, one should conclude that it is the common
source of all nerves below the face which is affected, in a way analogous to the
tree's trunk.

This source is the upper part of the spinal cord,[11] and it is for this reason that
all doctors with any experience apply their remedies to this, I without paying   170
any attention at all to the heart in such a case. If, on the other hand, the face is
observed to be in spasm along with the whole of the body, we then treat the
brain itself, not just the outgrowth of the spinal cord. Spasm of the lips, for
example, is quite frequently seen, as is that of the eyes, of the skin of the brow,
of the whole area of the cheeks and of the root of the tongue. Since, then, we
have learned from anatomy that all these are moved by muscles which take
their nerves from the brain, we are convinced that in such cases it is the brain
which has been affected. In a case, however, where we see that these parts are
unaffected but all the others are in spasm, we will be convinced that it is the first
part of the spinal cord that has been affected.

We should, as I have already said, learn these matters at the outset, before
proceeding to consider the different states. Some doctors, however, do not even
attempt to make an enquiry into the states, but argue about matters which are
manifestly apparent, wasting our time, which should not need to be spent in
refutation of those who try to overturn the correct statements of previous doctors, but rather on the discovery of the matters which they overlooked—that is,
certain matters on which they either made no assertion at all, I or on which they   171
made assertions without demonstration or appropriate specification, or simply
with omissions. This, for example, is the case of Hippocrates when he states that

---

[10] The term *neuron* had a wider reference, especially in earlier medical Greek, than simply
'nerve', and even more so in everyday usage; in classical literary texts for example it is sometimes
translated 'sinew'.

[11] The term Galen uses here is *muelos*, which also refers to 'marrow'.

spasm arises as a result of filling. The statement is true, but he had obviously been persuaded by someone to make the assertion in this way for the benefit of men of understanding, who had already learned the fundamentals of medicine, not for all and sundry. I myself, for example, had received this fundamental education, and so was able to understand to which causes Hippocrates was attributing spasm.

For since all voluntary motion is observed to take place through a process of drawing-in of the muscles into the parts to which they are joined, and it is observed further that such drawing-in cannot take place without the drawing-up of the muscle towards its own source, then it is only by virtue of the fact that the spasm takes place without our volition, in the parts which undergo such spasm, that this motion will differ from the normal motion.[12] So, just as, in the normal state, that volition which is extended through the source of the nerves in the brain provides the source of motion first to the nerves, and through them to the muscles, so, if we find the cause by which the nerves can be drawn in 172 without this source, | we will have reached an understanding of the origin of spasm.

To one who has observed how the nerve-like bodies which are the strings of a lyre sometimes undergo such a degree of tension, merely from the mixture of the ambient air, that they break, it is no hard matter to conceive that the same state may arise in the nerves of a living animal. What state of the ambient air is it, then, which leads to such tension and to the breaking of the strings? It happens both when this becomes extremely dry and when it becomes excessively wet. Moisture will soak them and thus cause them to swell up to a greater bulk than normal, causing tension; dryness, as in the case of the sun tightening hides as it dries them, also has the effect of pulling on the cords and increasing their tension. So too, we observe for example that leather straps, when dried by fire, contract and are tightened. Once this has been understood, it will not be difficult, in a case of spasm, to discover whether it has come about through dryness, that is to say an insufficiency of wet substance, and evacuation, or through a build-up of moisture, that is to say the effect which is the opposite of insufficiency, and is referred to by Hippocrates as filling. When the spasm arises from labour, lack of sleep, lack of food, mental exertion, and dry and burning fever, 173 as is the case with phrenitis, | one should take the cause to be dryness and evacuation; in the case of one who is drinking plentifully, filling himself constantly and living an idle lifestyle, it is reasonable to suppose that it is the opposite kind of state that has produced the spasm; and this is filling.

---

[12] The argument depends on the conceptual and linguistic connection in Greek between 'spasm' (*spasmos*, with cognate verb *spasthai*) and 'drawing-in' (or 'contraction', *epi-spasthai*): Galen's point is that the *spasthai* that takes place in spasm is a special case of the (*epi-*)*spasthai* or 'drawing-in' or contraction that is the normal activity of a muscle in voluntary motion.

9. Epilepsy, too, is a spasm of all the parts of the body; it is not a continuous one, like *emprosthotonos, opisthotonos* and *tetanos*, but one which occurs at intervals; and it differs from the previously mentioned forms of spasm not just in this respect, but also in the impairment to both intellect and sensation. From this it is evident that the origin of this ailment is somewhere higher up, within the brain itself. Since, however, it tends to cease quite suddenly, it is reasonable to suppose that the ailment is brought about by thick fluid in the actual ventricles of the brain, which impedes the paths of exit of the breath, so that the source of the nerves agitates itself in an effort to push out the offending substances, and perhaps also that the spasm of epilepsy comes about through the outgrowth of each nerve becoming soaked, in a similar way to that whereby spasm has its origin in the spinal cord. The suddenness of both onset and dissolution indicates I that this ailment never arises through dryness and evacu- 174 ation, but always through thickness of fluid. An obstruction of the channels may come about suddenly because of a thick or viscous fluid; but for the brain or the fine membrane [*pia mater*] to reach such a level of dryness that it undergoes something similar to a leather hide is something that could not happen in a short period of time. In addition, we have here the inability of the patient to see or hear, or indeed to perform any action of sensation, as well as the lack of awareness of what is happening; the reasoning faculty is impaired along with the capacity for memory. From all these facts it is reasonable to suppose that the ailment has arisen in the brain, through a fluid blocking the paths of exit of the soul breath within that organ's ventricles.

The reason for the term 'soul breath', and the capacity of this entity, have been shown in my work on *The Doctrines of Hippocrates and Plato*.[13] There we followed the observed facts of anatomy; and in doing so it seemed to us reasonable to suppose that the soul itself resides in the body of the brain, within which rational processes take place and the I memory of sense impressions is stored; 175 and that the breath in the brain's ventricles, and especially that in the hindmost one, is the first instrument of the soul for the purposes of all forms of sensation and of voluntary activity. One should not, however, discount the middle ventricle as less important, for there are many plausible considerations that lead us towards it, and indeed also away from the front two. A precise knowledge of these matters is however of no benefit for treatment: it is sufficient for correct treatment to understand that the affected place is the brain, and the viscous or thick fluid accumulated within its ventricles. These are the considerations of value for the purpose of the cure—which is, after all, the purpose for which we conduct this enquiry into the affected places and their states. The consideration

---

[13] See *The Doctrines of Hippocrates and Plato*, passim, especially VII.3–4, pp. 276–9.

of different types of thick fluid, in particular whether they are phlegmatic or melancholic, is also of such value.[14]

Here we should remind the reader again that the term 'phlegmatic', when used on its own, is applied to all persons in whom moisture and coolness predominate in the mixture, and the term 'melancholic' to all those in whom dryness and cold predominate; but there are, to be sure, great individual differences 176 | within both the phlegmatic and the melancholic. So, for example, the phlegm which is expelled in the daytime by many, by coughing or vomiting or through the nose, is full of vaporous breath, so that it is not uniform even in its appearance; but there is another kind of phlegm which does appear uniform; to this kind belongs the raw fluid which is present in the urine, as well as that referred to by Praxagoras as 'glassy'. Saliva which is not extremely moist or watery appears to be of this kind too. Yet even saliva, if we judge it according to the sense of taste, does not appear to have one single quality; still less, then, the category of phlegm as a whole. Sometimes we perceive the saliva in our mouth as salty, sharp, or briny, and also sometimes as without any quality, as it were watery, the latter being the case when our daily regime is without fault. Melancholic fluid, too, has clear differences in its consistency: that which is, as it were, the sediment of blood has a clearly quite thick appearance, like the sediment in wine; but there is another type, much finer than this in its | composition, which appears sharp both to those who vomit it up and to those who smell it.

This type is abrasive to the ground, too; it rises, froths and produces bubbles, like those which arise in fermenting leavens.[15] The type which I likened to the thick sediment will not produce this frothing when poured on to the ground, except in the case of someone at that moment suffering from a burning fever, and it has very little sharpness of quality; in this case, indeed, I usually call it melancholic fluid or melancholic blood, for I do not think it correct at this point actually to call it black bile. In some people this fluid is produced in great quantity, either because of the mixture they possess from birth, or because of a habitual diet which transforms the food into such a fluid in the process of coction within the veins. Like the thick fluid of phlegm, this thick melancholic fluid too sometimes gives rise to epilepsy, if it is retained within the paths of exit of the ventricles of the brain (either the middle ventricle or the hindmost one).

---

[14] 'Melancholic' here has its literal or physical sense, i.e. that of containing or consisting of black bile (*melaina cholē*). Galen habitually uses the adjective in this way, to refer to a quality of the fluid in the body, whereas the noun *melancholia*, 'melancholy', refers to a syndrome with a complex range of physical and psychological manifestations, as we shall see below.
[15] Kühn's text (*zeousi zōmois*) would rather be translated as 'boiling soups'; but the present translation (which requires a slight emendation, to *zeousais zumais*) seems to make better sense in the context, especially since both the verb translated as 'froths' in the previous clause (*zumō*) and the noun translated as 'frothing' in the next sentence (*zumōsis*) are cognate with this word for leaven (*zumē*), and would themselves naturally be taken to refer to a frothing due to the action of yeast.

When, however, it becomes excessive in the body of the brain itself, it produces melancholy, in the same way that the other [kind of] fluid of black bile,
that which | arises through the roasting of the yellow bile, produces bestial   178
derangement, both with and without fever, when this fluid becomes excessive
in the body of the brain. It is for this reason that there are two types of phrenitis, a more moderate one which has its origin in pale yellow[16] bile, and a more
vehement one which is the result of yellow bile; and there occurs, further, a
bestial and melancholic derangement, from the roasting of the yellow bile.
Those derangements, which occur during the peaks of fevers, affect the brain by
sympathy, not by idiopathy; and this is why they are described, not just by doctors but by laypeople, as delirium, derangement and alienation, but not as phrenitis; for a phrenitic derangement will not subside along with the peak of the
fever. Just as the fever of phrenitis, then, is one of the symptoms of the state of
the brain, so too derangement is one of the symptoms of burning fever, as here
many hot vapours are carried up to the brain.

Similar to this, too, is the origin of symptoms similar to cataract, arising from
the states of the stomach; there is a two-way exchange of ailments between the
gastric cavity and the head, | because of the magnitude of the nerves which go   179
down from the brain to the mouth of the stomach, which also explains the
exceptional level of sensation that exists in this part of the body. This is the reason, too, why vomiting of bile occurs as a consequence of those fractures of the
head which make contact with the membranes of the brain; why upset and a
biting sensation in the mouth of the stomach sometimes occur as a consequence of any type of head pain; and why melancholic despondency occurs as a
consequence of those ailments known as hypochondriacal[17] or gassy—for this
too belongs in this category. Similarly, derangement may arise from acute
fevers, and the state which involves symptoms similar to cataract may arise
from certain states of the mouth of the stomach and the gastric cavity. So, too,
those who are suffering inflammation in the nerve-like parts are more prone
than others to derangement, which occurs sometimes through the heat itself
alone rising up to the head, by contiguity, and sometimes through the vaporous, smoky or sooty breath doing so.

10. Just as there are considerable differences in ailments of the head which hap-
pen through sympathy, so too | in those which happen through protopathy   180
themselves. So, for example, when thick fluids become excessive within the
actual substance of the brain, they cause that organ harm, sometimes in its

---

[16] The adjective is *ōchros*: here Galen seems to work with a colour range, from *leukos* (white or
colourless), through *ōchros* (pale yellow, tawny, straw colour), to *xanthos* (a warmer yellow), with
red conceived as a point still further along the same range.

[17] i.e. of the *hupochondrion*, that is the upper abdominal region (literally, that 'under the cartilage' of the breast).

capacity as an organic part, sometimes in its capacity as a uniform one. The former is the case with blockages of the channels, the latter with alteration of mixture. It is for this reason that the following statement appears at the end of the sixth book of the *Epidemics*:

> Melancholics habitually also become epileptic, in most cases, and epileptics melancholic. The tendency towards one or other depends on the direction which the infirmity takes: if it turns its course rather toward the body, they become epileptic; if toward the intelligence, melancholic.[18]

In this passage he indicates, first that the transition from the one ailment to the other takes place in a majority of cases, but not in all; for, since epilepsy is brought about not by the melancholic fluid alone, but also by the phlegmatic one, what arises from the melancholic fluid sometimes makes the transition into melancholy, but what arises from the phlegmatic one makes the transition to another ailment, which I shall discuss shortly, but does not produce melancholy.

181   There is another | important observation which is also contained within this Hippocratic statement. Since the soul is either a mixture of the active qualities, or is altered by the mixture of these,[19] he is stating that the bile which is injurious to the brain in its function as an organic part has turned its course towards the body[20] (and this happens in the case of blockages), but that the mixture which does harm to it in its function as a uniform part has turned its course towards the intelligence. A distinction however needs to be made here which has, it seems to me, been overlooked by doctors: just as there is sometimes observed to be a single mixture throughout the observable parts of the body, for example in jaundice, in the ailment known as *elephas*, in dropsy, and also in bad-condition, as well as in poor colour arising from liver or spleen, while on other occasions a single part alone is altered in its mixture by having received a bitter-bilious, phlegmatic or melancholic fluid, so too it is possible sometimes that the brain, when all the blood within the veins has become melancholic, is itself also damaged in accordance with this common principle of damage; but also possible for another mode of alteration to take place, wherein

---

[18] *Epidemics* VI.8.31.

[19] Cf. *The Soul's Dependence on the Body*, where Galen also seems to entertain both these possibilities. For Galen's understanding of the hot, cold, wet and dry as the fundamental 'active qualities' in bodies, see *My Own Doctrines*, ch. 9, and see also *The Elements according to Hippocrates*. However the precise formulation 'mixture of the active qualities', as applied to the soul, seems to be unique to the present text.

[20] The Greek text reads 'the body of the brain' here, but I have omitted the last three words, which I suggest have been added in error through a half-copying of the phrase 'to the brain' on the previous line. According to the binary distinction being made here, it does not seem correct for the 'body of the brain' to appear on this side of the divide: the activities and pathologies of the *body* of the brain seem rather to be those corresponding to the brain in its capacity as a uniform part.

ǀ the blood within the human body as a whole remains unaffected and only that   182
in the brain is altered.

Further, there are two ways in which this may come about, either through
the inflow of the melancholic fluid from elsewhere, or through its generation in
that place itself. The latter occurs as a result of great local heat, which roasts
either the yellow bile or the thicker and blacker part of the blood. This specification makes a considerable difference to treatment. When the whole body has
melancholic blood in it, it is appropriate to begin the treatment with venesection; when this is the case only of the blood in the brain, then the patient does
not require venesection—not, at least, on the basis of this state: it is possible
that he may need it on some other grounds.

You should carry out your determination as to whether the whole body contains a melancholic fluid or whether such a substance has collected in the brain
alone on the following basis. First, I recommend that you consider the nature of
the bodily condition, bearing in mind that those who are soft, white [in com-
plexion] and fat have the least melancholic fluid, while those who are thin,
darker and endowed with broad veins, have the greatest tendency towards ǀ the   183
generation of this kind of fluid. Those who are very red in complexion, too, are
sometimes prone to a sudden transition to the melancholic mixture; next after
these are those with a yellow colour, especially if they happen to have previously followed a daily regime involving sleeplessness, excessive labour, mental
exertion and the thinning diet.

In the case of such persons, the following kinds of indication also belong
within the same class: whether some flow of blood has been stopped, or, indeed
whether there has been some other habitual evacuation of blood or, in the case
of women, menstrual flow; then, what kind of nourishments have been used,
whether those which produce melancholic blood or the opposite kind. By 'those
which produce melancholic blood' I mean the eating of the meat of sheep or
cows, and even more so that of the males of those species, but most especially
that of asses or camels (for there are those who eat the meat of these animals, as
there are some who even eat that of foxes and dogs). The eating of hares, too, is
highly productive of this kind of blood, and even more so that of wild boars.
Snails also produce melancholic blood, if eaten in excess, as do all meats of ter-
restrial animals when preserved in salt; and amongst water creatures, tuna,
whale, seal, dolphin and shark, ǀ and all the cetaceous animals. Of vegetables,   184
cabbage is practically the only one which naturally produces this kind of blood,
along with the shoots of various trees prepared with brine or brine-vinegar
(I refer here to those of the mastic, terebinth, bramble and wild rose). Amongst
pulses,[21] lentils are by far the most melancholic food; after this, the variety of

---

[21] See The Thinning Diet, ch. 6, with n. 10; the word *ospria* may be used to refer both to pulses
and to grains more generally.

bread known as bran bread, and that made from einkorn and from the poor-quality grains which some peoples use instead of wheat; we have classified these in the first book of our work on *The Capacities of Foodstuffs*. Of wines, those which are thick and black[22] are the most apt to produce melancholic fluid, if one drinks them in excess and then for some reason or other has to keep one's body at an excessive heat. Mature cheese also very readily produces this kind of fluid, if ever it becomes overheated within the body. Now, if a person has been following this kind of regime before falling ill, one may make some further con-jecture on this basis; if the regime has been one involving foods of good fluid, then one should investigate the person's exercise, as well as | the factors of dis-tress, sleeplessness and worry.

185

There are some who even experience the production of melancholic fluid in the context of fever-based diseases, as has been said. For the purposes of more accurate diagnosis, the time of year, the previous and present climatic condi-tions, and also the place, and the age of the patient, are of considerable import-ance. If you have already considered all these thoroughly, and on that basis think it likely that the melancholic fluid is contained in the veins throughout the body, you may proceed to the most reliable diagnostic test, by cutting the vein at the elbow. It is better to cut the middle one, since it is joined both to that known as the shoulder vein and that which runs through the arm-pit to the hand.[23] If it is then observed that the blood that flows is not melancholic, then stop immediately; if, however, it is observed to be so, remove as much as you take to be sufficient for the condition of the patient's body.

There is also a third type of melancholy, as in the case where epilepsy has its beginning in the gastric cavity; the same state is referred to as hypochondriacal or gassy disease by some doctors. It will be sufficient here if I set down the symptoms as described by Diocles as accompanying this illness, in his book entitled | *Ailment, Cause, Treatment*, where he wrote as follows (these are his actual words):

186

> There is another that occurs in the gastric cavity, which is similar[24] to those previously described; some call it melancholic, some gassy. In such cases eating—especially the eating of indigestible and burning foods—is followed by: frequent spitting of wet substance, acidic belching, wind, burning in the hypochondriacal region, 'splashing' which is not immediate, but delayed, and sometimes powerful pain in the gastric cavity, which in some cases extends to

---

[22] See again *The Thinning Diet*, ch. 12, with n. 24; 'black' wines are some subset of (in our terms) red ones.

[23] What are apparently meant are, in modern terms, respectively the median cubital vein, the cephalic vein and the basilic (or, higher up, the axillary) vein.

[24] In the translation I am following the reading of the Arabic tradition and of some of the Greek manuscripts, whereas Kühn's version would rather give the translation 'dissimilar'.

the broad of the back. Once the food has been digested these things are diminished, but they occur again after eating; and the disturbance frequently occurs both in cases of fasting and after a meal. Where people vomit, they vomit undigested food, as well as phlegm which is rather bitter, hot and sharp, so much so that it causes discomfort to the teeth. Most of these things begin from a young age; but they are long-lasting, whatever their origin.

After this preamble, Diocles proceeds immediately to add the cause. He writes as follows:

> One must take it that people who are called 'gassy' have more hot than they should have in the veins which receive nutrition from the stomach, and that in these people the blood had been thickened. The presence of an obstruction   187 in the region of these veins is indicated by the fact that the body does not receive the nutrition, which instead remains unprocessed in the stomach, whereas previously these channels received this nutrition, separating most of it off into the lower part of the gastric cavity, and also by the fact that on the second day they vomit, unable to draw down the food into the body. The fact that their degree of hot is greater than normal may be most clearly realized from the burning that they experience, and from what is administered to them. For these people are observed to derive benefit from cold foods, which in general tend to cool and dissolve the hot.

Diocles then continues to complete his account, in the following statement:

> Some say that in such ailments the mouth of the stomach, being contiguous with the intestines, undergoes inflammation, and that as a result of this inflammation an obstruction is formed in it which prevents the food from descending to the intestines at the appropriate times; and that, when this happens, by remaining in the stomach longer than it should, the food produces lumps, burning sensations and all the other things already mentioned.

Now, this is Diocles' account. | He has omitted, in his list of symptoms, those   188 most crucial to the syndrome as a whole, those, that is, which are the distinctive features of melancholy and of this gassy and hypochondriacal ailment. I believe that the reason for this is that they are already implied, indicatively, by the name of the disease itself—if, that is, we have learned Hippocrates' dictum:

> When fear and despondency continue for a long time, this is melancholy.[25]

It is, however, worth enquiring why in his presentation of the cause Diocles put down the causes of the other symptoms but not that of the actual impairment of

---

[25] This classic characterization of melancholy (the end of which, more literally translated, reads 'such a thing is melancholic') is from *Aphorisms* 6.23.

the intellect. The explanation as to why melancholic symptoms follow as a consequence, either in cases where there is greater heat in the veins in the stomach or in cases where there is inflammation of the parts in the region of the pylorus, has been omitted. It would be quite obvious, even if Diocles failed to mention it, that the stomach is filled with gassy wind, which is then alleviated by the belching of this wind, as well as by the type of vomiting which he mentions. But it was difficult for him to give an account of the specific features of melancholy at the same time as describing that state of the stomach. Let us then supplement 189 his account, ǀ clearly communicating the nature of the state of the stomach that arises in such ailments.

It seems that there is some inflammation within it, and that the blood contained in this inflamed part is rather thick and melancholic. It is similar to the case where some sooty or smoky exhalation, or, generally, vapours of some kind, are carried up from the stomach to the eyes and produce symptoms similar to cataract.

It is by exactly the same principle that, in this case, a melancholic exhalation, like some sooty or smoky exhalation, is carried up to the brain, and so the melancholic symptoms arise in relation to the intellect. The most constant head pain which we observe is that arising from yellow bile contained in the stomach; by the same token, this pain is immediately removed when the bile is vomited. Further, these kinds of pain are biting and corrosive, in the same way that others are observed to involve a sensation of weight, and still others one of tension or suspension. Moreover, it is agreed by the best doctors that the head suffers through sympathy with the stomach not only in these cases, but also in epilepsy.

190 Now, ǀ fear is always present in melancholy, but the same kind of abnormal impressions are not present in every case, those whereby, for example, a person thinks that he is made of terracotta, and therefore avoids contact with others, in order not to be shattered, or, on seeing cockerels crowing, flaps his arms against his sides, just as they flap their wings before they crow, and imitates that animal with his voice. Then there is the case of the person who feared that Atlas, who holds up the cosmos, might tire and drop it, causing himself to be crushed and the rest of us to be destroyed along with him; and there are countless other impressions of this kind.

Yet there are differences between melancholics. They all share the characteristics of fear, despondency, a negative attitude to life and hostility to other human beings; yet not all desire to die. Indeed, a chief characteristic in some melancholics is, precisely, the fear of death. Yet there are also some who, in an apparently very strange way, combine the fear of death with the desire for it. It thus appears that Hippocrates was correct in summarizing all their symptoms under two headings, namely fear and despondency. It is, indeed, a kind of 191 despondency which leads to ǀ hostility towards all people whom they encounter;

and there is a constant state of gloom and fear, similar to the terror that children or uneducated adults have of the dark. For, just as external darkness makes
almost all human beings fearful, except for those who are either particularly
bold by nature, or well educated, so too the colour of the black bile, in a way
similar to darkness, casts a shadow in the place responsible for intelligence and
produces fear. The fact that fluids and, in general, the mixture of the body, alter
the activities of the soul is agreed upon by the best doctors and philosophers,
and has been demonstrated by me in one particular work, in which I demonstrated that the capacities of the soul depend on the mixtures of the body.[26]

This is the reason why those who do not acknowledge the power of the
fluids—which includes the followers of Erasistratus—have not ventured to
write anything about melancholy. The common conceptions of human beings
are worthy of admiration here, as is the case also with many other doctrines of
which a considerable number of philosophers and doctors are ignorant. The
ailment is universally termed 'melancholy', I the name itself indicating the fluid   192
which is responsible. Now, if symptoms in the stomach begin first, if the melancholic ailments follow from an intensification of such symptoms, and if the
person is lightened by excretions, vomiting, flatulence and belching, we then
term the disease hypochondriacal and gassy, and we state that despondency
and fear are symptoms of it. When, however, the specific symptoms of melancholy are observed to be great, but nothing, or very little, is observed in the
gastric cavity, in these cases the brain must be thought to be suffering the protopathy, through a large accumulation of black bile within it.

The basis on which one must decide whether such a fluid is contained in the
brain itself alone or in the whole of the body was laid out a little earlier. I would
remind my students that they have seen me treat such melancholy with plentiful baths and with a daily regime involving good, wet fluid, without any other
remedy, provided that the fluid causing the trouble had not been present for so
long that it had become difficult to dislodge. When, on the other hand, the disease is already established over a period of time, it requires other, more substantial I remedies in addition to those stated. Such melancholy may also   193
supervene upon a preceding hot state of the head, resulting either from burning
heat or from an inflammatory ailment arising within it, or also from phrenitis;
it also supervenes on phrenitis itself, and on distress when accompanied by
sleeplessness. This, then, is enough on melancholy.

11. Turning to epileptic ailments, we should make careful distinctions here too,
since these also arise sometimes from the head being affected itself, and sometimes when it is affected by sympathy with other parts. Epilepsy also has three
distinct types; but here too, as with melancholy, the threefold distinction has

[26] These last thirteen words form the full title of the work which appears in this volume as *The
Soul's Dependence on the Body.*

been ignored by most doctors. The fact that the brain is affected is common to all, whether this ailment arises in the brain itself, which is true of most cases of epilepsy, or ascends from the mouth of the stomach (which doctors usually call the *stomachos*) to the brain. This is similar to the phenomenon of cataract-like symptoms arising in the eyes from an origin in the mouth of the stomach. There 194 is also | another, rare kind—or class, or distinct type, if you prefer—of epilepsy, in which the ailment begins in some part of the body or the other, and then makes its ascent to the head in a way perceptible to the patient himself. The first time I observed this was in a child of about thirteen years, when I was myself a youth, and was accompanying the best doctors of my home city, who had attended together to investigate the boy's treatment. I heard the boy recount that the state had originated in his lower leg, and had then ascended from there, straight up through the thigh, the part of the abdomen above that and the chest; then on through the neck, as far as the head; and that as soon as it had reached that point, he had lost consciousness. He was asked about the quality of this stuff that had risen to his head, but was unable to describe it. There was, however, another youth, who did not lose his senses and was able to perceive well what was happening to him, and was more capable than the other of expressing himself. He said that what rose up was like a kind of cold breeze.

My teacher Pelops concluded that what was happening was one of two 195 things: either the transmission of a quality, by means of the alteration of | contiguous parts, or the transmission of some actual airy substance. It was, he said, not surprising that a fluid generated in the affected part might have a powerful capacity, of a kind similar to that of the venom in poisonous animals. Who would believe—if it were not for the fact that we have observed the phenomenon on many occasions—that as a result of the sting of a scorpion, or of the bite of a very small spider, the whole body could undergo a great and extraordinary change, although the quantity of substance that has been emitted by the animal is very small indeed? Now, in the case of the spider bite, in spite of the very small size of the animal, we can nevertheless conceive that there is some venom moving from its mouth into the bitten body. The sting of the ray, on the other hand, like that of the terrestrial scorpion, is clearly observed to end in a very sharp point, which however has no perforation in it through which it might emit the venom. Yet we are compelled to conceive that there exists there some airy or moist substance which is extremely small in amount but very great in its capacity. Someone who was recently stung by a scorpion stated that it felt 196 as though he had been struck by hailstones; and he was completely cold, | and in a cold sweat, and was scarcely saved through medical intervention.

Pelops' claim was that it was not impossible, then, that such a substance might also be produced within the body, even without such an external cause; and that this substance, once formed within a nerve-like part, might transmit its capacity into the source of the nerves, either, as already stated, through alteration or through the upward movement of some airy substance, like a breeze. When a scorpion pierces a nerve, artery or vein with its sting, it is often clearly observed that the victim in these cases is affected by extremely powerful symptoms. Now, the sting of a scorpion may even penetrate deep within the body, having passed through the skin completely, whereas the bite of small spiders remains on the surface of the skin; and from this it is evident that the capacity of the venom can on occasion be conveyed over the whole body through the skin alone. The skin as a whole is self-continuous and it contains nerves; it is therefore by no means impossible for the capacity due to the injected venom to be transmitted quickly through the whole of it, before then being moved on into each of the parts below the skin, by contact with it; | and   197 then on from these into others, by contiguity, and from these affected parts to yet others, so that, when it reaches one of the centrally important parts, there is a risk of death.

It is here especially that the application of ligatures to the upper parts is appropriate, and shows a very clear benefit. We have had personal experience of such applications in the case of vipers and scorpions, and even of cobras— something which may seem incredible, given the speed of death in the case of this animal. Nevertheless, it once happened, when I was in Alexandria, that someone who lived on the land not far outside the city was bitten on his finger, bound it tightly at the base, and then ran to a doctor of his acquaintance in the city, so that the latter might cut off the entire finger at the metacarpal joint, in the hope that after that he would suffer no ill effect. His hope was justified: the man was saved without any further distress. I know of another case, too, where someone was restored to health after drinking the drug made from vipers as well as having his finger amputated; | and I observed another country-dweller   198 whose whole finger had been bitten by a viper, and who used a sickle that he had with him (the man was a vineyard worker) to cut off the part which had been bitten at the lowest joint. In this case the person was saved without drink-ing any drug, the wound to the finger being cicatrized by the usual drugs for that purpose.

In the case of the boy whose epilepsy began in the lower leg, too, the doctors who had gathered to investigate its cure, though they had decided to purge the entire body before applying the drug made with deadly carrot or mustard, in the meantime bound the limb at a point above the part which underwent the protopathy, and so prevented the onset of an attack, even though this had been taking place daily. All this is presented simply as a further reason for thinking that it is not remarkable that such a significant ailment should have its origin in an unimportant part. It remains, however, to enquire into the cause of the epi-leptic spasms which arise from such cases of sympathy; for here neither Pelops nor any of the other doctors with whom I associated succeeded in giving a plausible account.

Through the observation that I once made of the collapse of a patient, in
199 such a case of sympathy, | without vehement spasms, but with small, intermit-
tent motions similar to palpitation, it seems plausible that what is occurring
here is something similar to what happens very frequently at the mouth of the
stomach in hiccups. Indeed, I myself immediately start to hiccup whenever
I have taken too much pepper, and I have observed the same thing happen to
many others, if the mouth of their stomach is very sensitive. (As previously
mentioned, this part is habitually referred to, not just by doctors but by people
in general, as *stomachos*.) So, too, I have observed, in cases of collapse in those
suffering from epilepsy not through idiopathy of the brain but through sympathy, that an intermittent disturbance occurs, of a kind similar to palpitation,
rather than a continuous spasm; and this leads me to infer that a motion is taking place within the brain which is similar to that which sometimes occurs in
the mouth of the stomach as a result of substances which cause it distress. For
clearly hiccups occur when this part is burdened by a great quantity of nutrition, or when it suffers biting pains through the decay of that nutrition.
Moreover, I have quite frequently seen not just hiccups but also spasm arising
200 in the whole body, as a result of acrid fluid; | once the stuff causing the biting
pain was vomited, however, this ceased immediately.

It is, then, unsurprising that the source of the nerves, too, reaches a state
where it performs this kind of motion in its effort to eject whatever it is that has
been brought to it by the part which is undergoing protopathy. It is in the same
way too, I believe, that all the other symptoms arise which disturb the parts of
the body consisting of nerves. Those which lead to a collapse of sensation without a spasmodic or palpitating motion, however, arise from a very intense cooling; to this class belongs also lethargy. Apoplexy, through its sudden onset,
indicates that a cold, thick or viscous fluid is flooding in to fill the most important ventricles in the brain. It is not through a bad-mixture of the brain's substance as a whole that this arises, as it is in the case of lethargy, phrenitis, or
forms of *mania*, melancholy or stupefaction, or of memory loss, indistinct sensory activity and dissolution of motor function.

In all ailments of this sort—including apoplexy—you may infer the degree of
danger from the degree of impairment of respiration. In sleep, respiration takes
201 place without the presence of any | other deliberate motion, the subject lying
supine and motionless on a bed; and it is so too in ailments of the *karos* type:
the body neither moves nor has sensation, yet respiration alone is preserved.
This activity is the task of the muscles which move the chest area: we have
secure knowledge of this, acquired in a demonstrative manner, as also of the
fact that the source of motion in muscles comes from the nerves which grow
into them. Anatomy has taught us that the primary source of all nerves is the
brain. Here I say 'primary source' rather than simply 'source' because of the
spinal cord. A very large number of nerves are seen to grow out from the spinal

cord; but the control of the capacities which it possesses is provided to it by the brain. Whenever you observe that respiration is seriously impeded, and that it is being performed with difficulty, you must infer that there is a significant morbid state within the brain, which is the case in all diseases involving *karos*.

12. All these ailments, then, clearly involve the brain. So too does that known as 'darkening'[27]— I from which name, indeed, the nature of the ailment is quite   202 obvious. Its sufferers are plunged into darkness by the slightest cause, and sometimes even fall down. It happens especially when, for example, they spin in a circle; but this outcome, which in others would result from many revolutions, in their case takes place after one. It can happen also as a result of seeing someone else spin round, or indeed as a result of the rotation of a wheel or some such object, or even whirlpools in a river. The effect on them is greater when they have been in the sun, or in some other way heated the head. It seems, then, that they experience what others experience as a result of repeated circular motion, without such motion. It is generally agreed that what is happening to people in the course of such repeated motion is an uneven, disturbed and disorderly movement of the fluids and the breath; and so it seems reasonable to suppose that sufferers from this 'darkening' are experiencing something of this sort.

For this reason, some of them even benefit from the cutting of arteries, specifically from the division of the arteries behind the ears, all the way down, so that a scar is made between the two parts. I Of course, not all are healed by this   203 remedy; for there are other, much larger arteries, which rise to the brain at its base, through what is known as the 'net-like web';[28] and it is evident that the impairment arises from these. A vaporous, hot breath is carried up through these and fills the brain; and it is possible that some uneven bad-mixture arises in the brain itself which gives rise to this kind of breath. The fact that this is an ailment of the head, however, is evident from the actual sensation experienced by its sufferers; and it manifests itself sometimes through a protopathy of the head, sometimes through a sympathetic ailment of the mouth of the digestive cavity.

Archigenes, too, concedes this, writing as follows about this 'darkening' impairment in the first book of his *Signs of Chronic Ailments*:

> This state, too, has a twofold origin, either from the head or from the region of the lower abdomen.

He even attempts to make a distinction between the types, stating that in the case of protopathy of the head the condition is preceded by ringing in the ears

---

[27] I render the Greek word *skotōma* literally, as indeed required by the context; the term is also associated with dizziness or vertigo.

[28] See *The Doctrines of Hippocrates and Plato* VII.3, with n. 58.

204 and aching and heaviness of the head, or even of ⎮ impairment of the sense of
smell or of some other internal faculty of sensation (the term 'internal' here is
his own, and I take it that what he meant to refer to here was those faculties of
sensation which arise from the head), whereas in cases where it comes from the
mouth of the digestive cavity, it is preceded by heartburn and nausea. As has
now been stated many times, however, even if the head is suffering through
sympathy with another part, the resultant ailments must be considered its own.

13. In the case of what is known by doctors as *kephalaia*,[29] equally, no one would
deny that it is a disease of the head. This ailment is—to summarize in a few
words—a chronic pain in the head, difficult to dislodge, and involving large paroxysms arising from small causes, whereby the subject is unable to tolerate noises,
loud voices, bright lights or motion, and wishes to lie at rest in darkness because
of the level of the pain. Some feel that they are being struck by a hammer, others
205 have the sensation of either compression or distention ⎮ within the head; and in a
considerable number the pain penetrates to the sockets of the eyes. There are
intervals between such paroxysms, too, as there are with epileptics, and some
time may pass without any pain at all. Obviously, then, this disease involves a
susceptibility, on the part of the head, similar to that found in *kephalagia*; but the
parts affected in *kephalaia* reach an even weaker state. There is also a distinction
within *kephalagia* sufferers: in some the head is readily filled, and the condition of
the body as a whole is such as to be apt to fill it; in others, it is the parts of the head
itself that are by their nature easily affected. In the latter cases, if they have a bad
daily regime, they are likely also to succumb to the ailment of *kephalaia*.

Plausibly enough, then, some of these patients suffer pain in the meninges
enveloping the brain, others in the pericranium: the distinction here is whether
the pain does or does not penetrate to the sockets of the eyes. It is reasonable to
suppose that in those cases where the state is within the cranium the pain
206 reaches the base of the eyes, since there are outgrowths which reach these ⎮ from
the brain and from both the meninges, as well as from the vessels in them. Of
those who suffer this pain in one half of the head, however, who are usually
called 'hemicranics', some experience the pain as taking place outside the cranium, others as penetrating deep within the head. The two parts of the head,
left and right, are divided by the suture which extends the whole length of it,
within which is the line which demarcates the middle of the brain; and the division between the two anterior ventricles comes up to meet this. Those bodies
which are naturally prone to fill the head are the ones in which a vaporous, hot
breath is produced, or in which bilious residues accumulate in the mouth of the
gastric cavity. The pains which arise from the breaths are 'tensed'—this is the

---

[29] I leave *kephalaia* here and *kephalgia* below untranslated; both are clearly complaints involving
serious headaches, the former apparently similar to migraine, in current terms.

name given to those accompanied by a sensation of tension—while those which arise from bilious residues are biting; and those which arise from fulness give a sensation of heaviness, accompanied by redness and by heat in the case of hot fluids, but without these features when the fluids are not hot. Some, also, experience constant head pain after ⏐ the drinking of slightly too much wine, or of   207 wine which has been insufficiently mixed, and even more so if that wine is hot in its nature. [The pains] arise also from all hot smells—those from the fumes of styrax, incense, or in general from the fumes of all hot spices. Some cannot even tolerate the smell of rosemary.

It is natural that in some the pains arise through an excessive capacity for sensation. This is quite a frequent experience in the context of the mouth of the gastric cavity: in some people this part is so sensitive that it is unable to tolerate acrid vinegar, mustard, or other things of this kind. In others there is an almost complete absence of sensitivity; in some such cases people have been known to belch substances so remarkably foul that we ordinary bystanders are unable to bear the smell, but they experience no serious biting sensation. It may be, then, that there are such differences between different persons' heads that the same smells are tolerated without distress by some, just as if they were not even in their proximity, but are completely intolerable to others. In any case, the fact that the above are, indeed, ailments of the head, is quite clear.

BOOK IV

[In the context of his discussion of pathologies and treatments of the eyes, Galen digresses again to a discussion of types of phrenitis.]

2. ... There are two simple kinds, and a third which is a composite of the two.   225 Some phrenitics undergo loss of rationality with no confusion whatever of their powers of sensory discernment, while others, conversely, are completely undisturbed in their reason but experience sensory aberrations. And there are others who ⏐ experience both kinds of impairment. The manner of each kind of   226 impairment is exemplified as follows.

A man was left behind in a house in Rome with a boy whose job it was to work the loom. The man got up from his bed and came to the window, from which he could both see and be seen by the passers-by. He then pointed to the pieces of furniture in the room, one by one, and asked the passers-by if they wanted him to throw them down. They laughed and clapped their hands, egging him on; and he proceeded to pick up every piece and throw it out of the window, to the accompaniment of laughter and cheering. After a while he asked them if he should also throw out the loom-worker; they said yes, and he did so.

When however they saw the boy cast down from that height their laughter stopped, and they ran to lift up the broken body.

I am aware of the converse phenomenon, too, not just from a number of other cases but also from an experience of my own during my youth.[30]

I was suffering from a continuous fever in the summer, and I thought that some sort of fabric was coming out of the bed, dark in colour, which seemed to me like the threads of a garment. I attempted to remove these threads, and
227   when I found that I was not taking hold of anything in my fingers, I tried to do so ever more insistently and more vigorously. At this point I heard two companions who were present say that I was now 'plucking threads and pulling at fabric',[31] and realized that I was doing exactly what they described. I made a great effort of concentration to avoid becoming delirious, and said to them: 'You are right; help me, so that I do not become phrenitic.' They busied themselves to produce the appropriate embrocations for the head; and the whole day and the following night I experienced disturbed dreams, in response to which I shouted and at times jumped up; but on the following day the symptoms subsided.

It is obvious, then, that the origin of the symptoms involves the same cause, in generic terms, but arises from a different primarily affected place from that of those who, as discussed, suffer in the brain and the stomach through sympathy. When some bilious fluid accumulates in the brain in conjunction with continuous fever, the person suffers something similar to what someone suffers when overheated by a fire; and as a result of that a sort of smoke is naturally
228   produced, like that of an oil lamp, and this smoke travels to the I vessels which lead to the eyes, and gives rise to hallucinations within them. You have observed in our dissections that there are arteries and veins which travel to the eye from those that form the network of the choroid membrane.

BOOK VI

413   5. We do not need here to decide between the terminology of 'uterus' [*hustera*] or 'womb' [*mētra*] for the part given to women by nature for gestation, nor

---

[30] Another such case of the 'converse phenomenon', that is of visual hallucinations with unimpaired rational capacity, apart from that which Galen proceeds to recount here, is described in *The Distinct Types of Symptom*, ch. 3. A friend of his, the doctor Theophilus, 'was in other respects rational in his conversation and his ability to recognize those around him, but believed that some *aulos* players had taken up residence in one part of his house, and that they were constantly playing their *auloi* and banging. He believed that he could see them, some standing, some sitting, and playing constantly, all night and all day, without a moment's let-up. And he kept shouting at them to leave the house.'

[31] It seems that such activities were associated with delirium, and possibly even that these phrases were used to refer to it.

between the use of the plural and that of the singular noun in either case. | It is 414
better to expend one's time on matters which are actually useful—those from
which we will derive some benefit for diagnosis, prognosis or treatment.

So too, indeed, with the ailment which is called by some 'hysterical suffocation'[32] and by others 'hysterical breathlessness'; one may understand both
appellations in use by doctors as indicating a single ailment. I have observed
many 'hysterical' women—the term which they use themselves and which was
used by previous doctors, from whom, presumably, they heard it. Some I have
observed lying devoid of either sensation or motion, with an extremely small,
faint pulse, or indeed appearing to have no pulse at all, others enjoying the faculties of both sensation and motion, and unimpaired in their reason, but failing
in strength and scarcely breathing, and still others suffering convulsions of the
limbs. On this basis I take it that there are many different kinds of hysterical
ailment, the differences lying both in the severity of the effective cause and in
the distinctions between individual types.

Now, the first individual type, according to the book by Heraclides of Pontus,
involves considerable uncertainty as to its aetiology. | For there it is stated that 415
the person in question is devoid of both respiration and pulse, and differs from
a corpse only in one respect, namely that she retains a small degree of heat in
the middle parts of the body. The book, indeed, is entitled Heraclides' *Woman
Without Respiration*; and he states that there was an enquiry on the part of the
doctors present, as to whether the patient had not in fact already died....

[*Some details follow on later doctors, and on the possibility of discerning an
extremely faint but nevertheless existent breath.*]

...It is possible that in the case of hysterical lack of respiration, since the 416
whole body has been completely cooled down, breathing through the mouth
ceases altogether, while that through the arteries continues; it is also possible
that the former does continue, but is so small as to be imperceptible. It remains,
then, to enquire (in the interests of removing | any remaining uncertainty 417
regarding this ailment) as to the cause of this cooling of the body; and the
answer may be discovered by a consideration of the preceding causes, which are
as follows. As is generally agreed, it is mainly widows who are affected, and in
particular those who have previously experienced good evacuation,[33] as well

---

[32] *Husterikē pnix* or *pnixis*, literally choking or suffocation of the uterus; Galen uses this form,
rather than the straightforward noun *husteria* ('hysteria'), to refer to the condition. In what follows,
the adjective 'hysterical' could also have been rendered 'of the uterus': this is the literal sense of the
adjective, and Galen's account is of what he clearly believes to be a disease localized in this organ.
Such a translation, however, would perhaps not do justice to the extent to which 'hysterical ailments' were already established as a distinct diagnostic category, independent of the precise causal
account given.

[33] 'Evacuation' here and in several cases below translates the verb *kathairein* or cognate noun
katharsis, which are often also rendered 'cleansing' or 'purging'.

as childbirth, and who engaged in sexual intercourse with men, but have subsequently been completely deprived of all these. What more plausible inference might one make from this than that those states known as 'hysterical' arise in women because of the retention of the menses or of the seed, whether these states consist in absence of respiration, in suffocation or in convulsions? Retention of the seed is, indeed, the preferable explanation, since seed possesses very great power and is, in women, both moist and cold; and it needs to be discharged in those who are endowed with it in large quantity—just as it does in males.

In the case of males, too, indeed, I have encountered considerable diversity: some, from their youth onwards, become weak when they engage in sexual 418 intercourse, while others suffer pressure in the head, and become ⎸liable to nausea and fever, as well as to loss of appetite and deterioration in their digestion, if they do not engage in it constantly. (Plato compared the bodies of such people to trees endowed with an excess of fruit.)[34] Indeed, I have observed that some men of such a nature, if they subsequently, through a sense of shame, achieve control of their sexual impulses, are rendered sluggish and apathetic. Some even become irrationally gloomy and pessimistic, in a way similar to melancholics, and suffer impaired appetite and digestion. I know of one person who as a result of grief abstained from sexual contact with his wife, whereas he had previously indulged in it regularly. He lost his appetite and indeed became unable to digest the smallest amount of food offered; if he then forced himself, and took slightly more, he vomited immediately; and he suffered low spirits, not only as a result of this, but also without any observable cause, just as melancholics do. All this ceased very quickly once he resumed his previous habits. Indeed, it appears to me on the basis of my own consideration of the evidence that the retention of seed has a greater capacity to damage the body than does 419 the retention of menses, in bodies where the seed is itself is of poor fluid ⎸and excessive in quantity, where the lifestyle is inactive, and where there is very substantial previous sexual activity followed by sudden abstention.

I have noticed in such cases that the natural desire for discharge tends actually to cause discharge: when the seed is of this kind and amount it universally compels people to expel it. Even Diogenes the Cynic, who is generally agreed to have been the most steadfast of all human beings, in any action requiring self-restraint and endurance, nonetheless had recourse to sexual activity; this was because he wished to remove the occlusion[35] arising from retention of seed, not because he approached the pleasure attached to its evacuation as a good.

---

[34] The reference is to *Timaeus* 86c.

[35] The term, *ochlēsis*, seems here to encompass both a purely physical sense, that of the build-up of a fluid and the discomfort caused by that, and a mental or emotional one; it could also be rendered 'disturbance' or 'confusion'; it may not be irrelevant that a negative form of the word, *aochlēsia*, was used by Epicureans to refer to their desired state of 'untroubledness'.

Indeed, it is said that he once made an agreement with a prostitute that she would come to him, but that when she failed to appear at the appointed time, he ejected the seed by touching his genitals with his hand; when she did subsequently arrive, he sent her away with the words: 'My hand has already celebrated the nuptials.' It is, in fact, quite evident that people of self-control do not indulge in sexual intercourse for pleasure, but because they want to cure the occlusion, independently of whether there is any pleasure involved. | 420

I believe that other animals, too, are impelled towards sexual congress not because they have arrived at the doctrine that pleasure is a good, but moving to discharge the seed because it causes discomfort if retained. The natural tendencies to defaecate and urinate are, surely, similar. I was contemplating this situation once, when something of the kind happened to a woman who had been widowed a long time previously. She was suffering in general from disturbing tension in the nerves. Her nurse stated that her womb had become retracted; and it was decided that she should resort to the usual remedies for such conditions. When she did so, as a result both of the heat of these remedies themselves and of that arising from the contact with her feminine parts that took place in the course of the treatment, she underwent convulsions similar to those experienced in sexual intercourse, accompanied by a combination of pain and pleasure, followed by the expulsion of a large quantity of thick seed, and the woman was thus relieved of the disturbance that had afflicted her. I thus concluded that [retention of] seed which has poor fluid has a greater capacity to damage the whole body than does [that of] the menses; thus, even if the latter does sometimes arise in widows, it is the retention of seed that is both painful and harmful | to them.   421

And anyone who thinks it implausible that a small amount of fluid can be held accountable for major symptoms in the body as a whole fails, it seems to me, to take into account the facts of everyday experience. The bites of venomous spiders, for example, can be observed to affect the entire body, even though only a tiny quantity of venom has been inserted, through a very small opening. The case of scorpions is even more remarkable, both because they give rise to the most severe symptoms in the shortest possible time, and because the substance injected on contact is either extremely small in quantity or in fact nonexistent; certainly the animal's sting itself seems to lack any perforation. Yet it seems necessarily the case that either some breath, or some very fine moist substance, has been injected: people who have been stung by scorpions feel as though they have been pierced by a dart; or have the sensation that that their whole body is being assailed by a hailstorm, and simultaneously by loss of consciousness. There are those who think that some substances have the capacity to alter those things with which they come into contact, through the touch alone, by means of the capacity inhering in the quality; and that this nature is to be observed in the case of sting-rays, which have such a powerful capacity that the

422 alteration may be transmitted even through a fisherman's trident | into his hand, immediately rendering the whole hand numb.

These phenomena, then, provide sufficient evidence of the fact that a small amount of substance brings about very large alterations, through touch alone; and no less so the phenomenon of the 'Heraclean stone', which is also known as the 'magnet'. For not only does it happen that a piece of iron which has been in contact with the magnet is suspended without being attached to it; but also that a second piece is held up in the same way, after contact with that first piece, and a third after contact with the second. Since, then, it is clearly apparent that certain substances have extremely powerful capacities, it remains to enquire whether a form of corruption may arise within animals which is of such a magnitude as to have a comparable quality and capacity to that of the beast's venom. The question has, indeed, been investigated by those doctors who have addressed the topic, 'are there or are there not signs specific to poisoning?'; and those who appear to give the best account of the matter agree that the same ailments come about in the case of the administration of deadly poisons and in that of corruption arising from our own bodies. This does not, however, mean that those who have taken poison cannot be distinguished from those who have

423 not. | When a sudden death of the sort associated with deadly poison occurs in someone of naturally good fluid, who has followed an entirely healthy daily regime, and the body then becomes livid, black, mixed or diffuse, or smells badly of putrefaction, then it is stated that poison has been taken.

If it is accepted that we may succumb to similar ailments to those arising from the deadly poison, which however have their origin in our own bodies, it should be no cause for surprise that either seed of bad fluid, or menses in a similar condition, when retained and allowed to putrefy, will bring about serious symptoms in bodies which are susceptible. The importance of such susceptibility may be seen in the case of dogs: they, alone of all animals, are prone to madness, and such corruption of the fluid takes place in them that their saliva alone, when it comes into contact with a human body, brings about madness. What happens in such a case is that a bodily state gradually intensifies in the body, starting from the very small source represented by the quality within that saliva; and it may be recognized when it reaches a certain level of severity, six

424 months later, | having, in some cases, given no previous indicator. In the same way, some bad fluid produced within the animal body may lead in a short time to the co-affection of one of the major parts, from which the entire body is then swiftly altered.

The ancient belief was that those symptoms known as 'hysterical' had their root, as one may put it, in the womb; and there is substantial evidence for the likelihood of this account in the fact that such ailments arise only in widows and in those women who have experienced retention of their menstrual evacuation. The fact that, within these subjects, it is retained seed, as opposed to retained menses, that has the greater capacity, may be gathered from the case of those whose evacuation is withheld, but who are not widows: these experience different ailments (as will be discussed a little later), which do not however extend to absence of respiration, nor to violent episodes of fainting, nor to the other presentations mentioned above. It may also be gathered from the fact that some of those who have been widowed, and who experience evacuation which is either perfect or at least not significantly less than before, nonetheless experience symptoms. Consistent with this, too, | are the signs in the womb which are   425 apparent to female medical practitioners who make a thorough tactile investigation: for the mouth of the womb appears to those making this investigation to be bent inwards, in some cases as though the entire womb has been retracted, in others as though it has been moved to the side. It is for this reason that some have taken the womb to be, as it were, an animal endowed with the desire for child-production, which, when deprived of the object of its appetites, causes harm to the whole body.

Thus, Plato writes:

> The uterus or womb, as it is known, in women is an animal endowed with the desire for child-production; for these same reasons, when it remains without fruit for a long time beyond its season, it reacts angrily, wandering all over the body, blocking the paths of exit of the breath, preventing respiration and causing the body extreme confusion and all kinds of other illnesses.[36]

This is Plato's statement, to which some have added that when the womb, in its wanderings through the body, comes into contact with the diaphragm, it impedes breathing. Others, while denying that it wanders about like an animal, do still claim that, when dried out as a result of the retention of menses, it retreats up towards the main internal organs in its desire for | moisture; and that   426 when, on this upward path, it comes into contact with the diaphragm, the animal is deprived of breath.

Now, those who are ignorant of the findings of anatomy, and have made no investigation into natural and voluntary activities, may, although they have heard no demonstrative proof of such statements, consider some part of them to be possible. Anyone who has been schooled in both, however, will discern the unreliability of this account, without any assistance from me. Even if some part of the womb may appear to be drawn upwards, this will be a small part, and certainly not sufficient to indicate that its whole bulk might be drawn up all the way to the stomach, let alone that it could somehow move past this and come into contact with the diaphragm. Moreover, even if it did so, what effect would this this have in relation to absence of breath, fainting, tension in the

---

[36] The quotation is from *Timaeus* 91c.

limbs or total *karos*? In persons who are over-filled, the bulk of the stomach quite manifestly presses upon the diaphragm; and as a result of this breathing becomes more frequent, but the animal does not succumb to any other symp-
427   tom. In pregnancy, too, the womb becomes extended and | gives rise to more rapid breathing, but causes no other harm.

The very notion, furthermore, that the womb if dried out would move up towards the main internal organs through a desire for moisture is also completely absurd. If the womb were ever in need simply of moisture, it has both the bladder and the entire lower part of the intestine in close proximity to it; if the requirement were not just for moisture, but for moisture endowed with the substance of blood, then you would expect it to be drawn towards the liver, not the diaphragm.

And why in any case should it require to move its position in order to come into contact with other parts, when it is enclosed by a thick protection, in the form of its membranous covering? For all those parts which draw the moisture of the intestines to them do so through a large number of openings; and there are many openings of veins leading into the womb, through which it is possible for it to draw in blood from the vena cava, which itself contains the blood which flows from the liver. What better carrier of blood from the liver to the womb could one find than this? Indeed, by what other carrier could anything be drawn to it from that source? It is not just that this is the largest carrier; it is in
428   fact the only one that there is. This | one vein alone carries blood from the liver to all the parts below the diaphragm. Their argument is thus completely absurd—quite apart from the fact that it makes the womb into an animal. Even if this latter proposition were conceded, it might then follow that this animal would suffer distress when deprived of the proper objects of its appetite, and it might even suffer lack of nutrition—as some say happens to date-palms when they are in love[37]—but it would still not move to the diaphragm, or to any other place. Apart from any other consideration, the diaphragm is extremely dry in its mixture, and, if one accepts the claim that it has become dried, then it would require contact with some wet part.

What, then, is the reason, I will be asked, for the frequently observed retraction or sideways movement of the womb, which is reported by women's attendants[38] (although they also, incidentally, report that it frequently remains in its proper place, while women still experience hysterical symptoms)? I shall attempt to tell them the cause, following the statements of Hippocrates. My view is

---

[37] It seems that there was an ancient tradition ascribing erotic emotions to male and female date palms.

[38] The term, *maieutria*, refers to a woman with a specific role in the care of women. It is usually translated 'midwife', but, as the context here indicates, such a translation is too narrow. It seems in Galen's usage equivalent to *maia*, here translated 'nurse' (and another term which may also include midwives).

that it is tensions within the uterus that are responsible for the appearance, during palpation by a nurse, of its neck as retracted or moved to the side. I When the womb undergoes such a motion, its neck will necessarily undergo it 429 simultaneously. It remains, then, to state the cause of this retraction or sideways movement of the womb itself. The answer is the filling of the vessels which connect to it, along with their connectors. We have demonstrated, in our exposition of the aphorism in which Hippocrates states that spasm arises from voiding and filling, that the bodies of parts filled become extended, both laterally and in terms of depth, but are made shorter in length; and the part is retracted towards its source to precisely the same extent to which it becomes shorter. Indeed, even Erasistratus states that the muscles, through being filled with breath, become increased in width but reduced in length, and that retraction takes place for this reason. How, then, does this filling of the veins and the connectors come about? Obviously through retention of the menses. The blood reaches as far as the womb, but does not enter it, sometimes because it has become too thick to enter the mouths of the vessels, sometimes because they themselves become shut, so that it fills and distends the veins, and floods the connectors adjacent to them; I and by the tension of these parts the womb is, 430 through its contiguity to them, retracted.

Now, if the traction upon the womb is equal from all sides, the change it undergoes will not involve movement out of its place; but if this is not the case, it will be extended in the direction of the greater traction. The womb in women does not, then, travel from place to place like an animal; rather, it is pulled as a result of contraction. It is also correct to state that the body of the womb remains unaffected in such cases; what is in question is a distortion of its shape. Similar impressions that a particular part is affected arise elsewhere in the body too; and they often cause confusion amongst doctors, who take it that the part thus distorted is itself the part affected, since they do not believe it capable of being curved or extended.

[*The point is elaborated further, with a reference to Hippocrates' work on* Joints.]

Distortion of the womb, of the sort described above, results from the reten- 432 tion of menses; it is not itself the cause of the symptoms in the body of the living being. Rather, it shares a common cause with those symptoms, namely the build-up of retained menses which need to be cleared out. Harm also arises, in widows, through the retention of seed, even without such distortion, or indeed even without the retention of the menses.

There are different types of symptom that arise, as a function of the quantity as well as the quality of the menses and of the seed. When, for example the substance which is the underlying cause of the distress is such as to cause cooling of the entire body, the patient becomes severely and thoroughly cooled, so that she loses both breath and pulse. When on the other hand this substance is

433 thick or acrid, there are spasms; I when it contains black bile, there are low spirits; and fainting follows in cases of very severe tension, as well as in those of thorough cooling and of damage to the mouth of the stomach....I shall now give an account of those symptoms which arise from retention of menses in need of clearing out, as I previously promised to make some statement on this subject. I shall take as my starting-point Hippocrates' writings in the *Aphorisms*, one of which runs as follows:

> If a woman who is not pregnant, and has not given birth, has milk, then her menses have ceased.[39]

There are, however, also the following signs of the retention of menses, even when milk does not appear in the breasts: a sensation of heaviness throughout the whole body; nausea; lack of appetite; an anomalous sensation accompanied by shivering. If, on the other hand, there is some sort of anomalous sensation *without* shivering, and if there is also nausea, and desire for some bizarre substances, then instruct the nurse to make a tactile examination of the neck of the womb: if it has become closed without hardness, such signs indicate pregnancy.

434 I Some women also vomit their food, and eat earth, or burnt-out coals, or something of this sort. Closure of the mouth of the womb when accompanied by hardness tells us that there is some ailment of the womb, and then the woman's attendant must investigate in which direction the womb has been moved or retracted, for that will lead them to the place within the womb itself where it is affected. In some cases this is made even clearer by the presence of some pain, accompanied by heaviness, in that part; and sometimes the pain moves to the hip, and the relevant leg suffers a limp when walking.

If the menses do not appear for a long time, and the doctor administers no evacuants to the woman, then there sometimes appears an abnormal lump on the abdomen, which indicates some internal inflammation; while in some cases a tumorous lump rises at the lower extremity of the abdomen, of the kind which arises in that place also in men; in some cases this becomes purulent and requires cutting. Indeed, I have also known the colon to become purulent and to have been cut in this area, sometimes by inexperienced doctors who were unaware of what it

435 is that they are cutting, and sometimes by doctors who were aware. I In the latter cases the colon which was thus purulent was always easily cured; cuts to the womb, by contrast, are more problematic in terms of the healing of the wound.

These, then, are the kinds of symptom which follow upon the retention of menses; and, besides these, pain in the lower back, neck, forehead and bases of the eyes, as well as burning fevers and urine which is turning black and contains some red fluid, rather as if you were to add soot to the water used to wash

---

[39] *Aphorisms* 5.39.

freshly slaughtered meat. In some cases there is also abnormal weakness or strength in urination. Whenever you observe anything of this kind in women, you should suspect that it has its root, as it were, in the womb. If there is an emission of blood, or an inflammation, or *erysipelas*, in some other part of the body, one should enquire about the evacuation of the menses in these cases too; for none of these things occurs when this is properly performed. Such symptoms in general arise from the retention of menses in need of evacuation. From excessive voiding, on the other hand, there arise: lack of colour, swellings of the feet, a tendency to swelling throughout the body, bad digestion of food, as well as poor appetite, and all symptoms which typically follow as a result of the immoderate voiding of blood, | whether that voiding takes place through haem- 436 orrhoids or through some other blood-flow.

Even without the womb being affected, women sometimes experience what is known as 'the female flux', whereby the whole body is evacuated and voided through the womb (as it is sometimes also through the kidneys). This occurs mostly in the case of smooth-fleshed, phlegmatic women; and these we have healed, even without tactile contact with the womb, by medicaments for the whole body. What is voided here is sometimes a red fluid, sometimes a watery, light yellow one; if clear blood appears, as in venesection, one must pay careful attention, in case there has been some erosion in the womb. It suffers such erosions more often in its neck than elsewhere. When they are located more deeply, this will be discerned on the basis the fluid brought forth; when they are at the opening of the neck, this will be detected on this same basis, but also by touch. There is sometimes an emission of blood during pregnancy, when the veins in the neck of the womb are opened. And if the breasts of a pregnant woman suddenly become small, you should anticipate | that she is about to miscarry. 437

In a woman pregnant with twins, reduction in the size of one breast tells you that one of the embryos will be aborted. In general, too, the right breast indicates the male and the left the female, since males in general are carried on the right side of the womb and females on the left. The opposite case is rare, as it is also in other species which are by nature capable of bearing twins. (This includes many kinds of goats; sheep; and many other tetrapods.) If a woman conceives easily, but miscarries in the second, third or fourth month, then some phlegmatic moisture is collecting in the cotyledons of the womb, as a result of which the fusion of the veins and arteries arising in that place with the mouths of the vessels connecting to the womb is lacking in strength, and thus unable to bear the weight of the foetus, which tends readily to break away.

6. What is expelled through the anus gives few signs relevant to affected places near that, most being indicators which relate rather to the intestines, stomach, | 438 spleen or liver, and quite often also to the fluids of the body as a whole. Similarly, what is eliminated through the genitals does not generally indicate a specific

ailment in that area, but usually provides signs relating to the bladder, kidneys, liver, spleen, lung and chest area, as well as to the state of the fluids of the body as a whole body. Such signs are distinguished in line with the factors already stated as accompanying the ailment of each part.

When the genitals themselves have been affected, however, this may be discerned as follows. In the case of ulceration, a clear indicator is the smell in the part, as well as the elimination in the urine of some matter associated with the ulcer. Such matter is distinguished from that which comes from the bladder by the fact that it appears in the very first emission, while the matter from the bladder is mixed with the urine. Ulcerations in the genitals also cause a continuous biting pain during urination, especially when they are freeing themselves of a detached scab or accumulated matter.

It may be worthwhile to give a fuller account of *gonorrhoia*[40] and priapism.
439 The former I is an emission of seed against one's will. One may also, more clearly, term this an involuntary emission of seed, which takes place continually, without erection of the penis. Priapism, on the other hand, is an extension of the penis both in length and in diameter, without the desire for sex or increase in heat, as happens to some people when they sleep on their backs. This is the characterization of it given by some; one may also, more concisely, refer to it as permanent erection of the penis, or permanent swelling. It is named, obviously, after Priapus, who is traditionally shown in statues and paintings as having his genitals naturally in this state. The term *gonorrhoia*, clearly, is a composite of *gonē* (another term for seed) and *rhein*, to flow. The situation is the same with seed as with all other substances which are voided from our bodies, namely that such voiding takes place in one of two ways, either through expulsion from the bodies which contain them, or through a spontaneous outflow resulting from some weakness in those same bodies, which are therefore unable to hold them in.

440 It is a task of nature, in I all such cases, not just to expel, but also to retain, at the appropriate times. Expulsion takes place when the channel of outflow is opened, while the rest of the containing organ is contracted and pushes all the substance contained within the hollow towards the open channel; retention takes place when the channel remains closed and there is no pressure from the container upon what is contained, but only the opposite: contraction and holding. So, in people in a normal state, both expulsions and retentions of the moist substances contained take place within the hollow organs; in abnormal states retention takes place through weakness of the expulsive capacity, and expulsion

---

[40] I give this term (the etymology of which Galen proceeds to explain) in transliteration; the sense is clearly quite different from that it has in modern medicine, where it is applied to a specific sexually transmitted disease, although the latter involves a discharge from the genitals, which Galen could have mistaken for 'emission of seed'.

through weakness of the retentive capacity, or through some state which moves the parts in a way similar to the normal expulsive capacity, as happens in the channels of seed themselves, in violent instances of epilepsy and in other spasms. In other parts, too, such as the hands, feet or fingers, we sometimes see spasms occurring in conjunction with spasm of the whole body, and sometimes on their own; | and it is not unreasonable to suppose that such a state some-   441 times comes about in the channels of seed alone, as in the case of *gonorrhoia*, in a way similar to the non-voluntary expulsion of urine, when the capacity which holds it in is dissipated.

Now, *gonorrhoia* is an ailment of the organs of seed alone, not of the genitals, which are used by the seed as a path of outflow. Priapism, on the other hand, appears clearly to be a symptom of the genitals, although it may also be that it is an ailment specific to the arteries alone, the genitals themselves remaining unaffected. The arteries have in this case acquired, in an abnormal way, the same state which affects them in cases of the normal tension of the penis. The fact that it is breath which causes the swelling is obvious from the speed of the expansion and contraction: no moist substance is capable of bringing about such a fast change in either direction. This being so, and since it is observed in dissection that large arteries are connected to the small part which is the penis, and since it is also observed that the substance of the penis is unlike | any other   442 part—it is a body which is nerve-like[41] in its form, and its overall shape that of a pipe, except for the part known as the *glans*[42]—what other conception can one arrive at than of its being filled by vaporous breath which flows into it from the arteries, and that this is the cause of its growth in size during erection? This, too, is why the *glans* remains always the same size, because it does not have in it the pipe-shaped nerve.

What, then, is the reason that the extension of the penis takes place in the context of sexual impulse? Or that it takes place in sleep, when a person lying on his back undergoes heating in the lower back? If we can discover this, we will have a good hope of discovering the cause of the state of priapism, too. It is immediately obvious that the filling must come about either from the arteries, or from the pipe-like nerve, as its primary cause, or indeed through both of these undergoing a change with respect to its previous state. We must now investigate which of these causes is to be preferred, or whether both of them.

Let us begin that discussion here. Nature, which both shapes and brings to perfection the parts of the body, has brought it about that each moves towards its proper function, without ever being taught to do so. I myself had the clearest possible proof of this, when I reared a kid goat | which had never even seen its   443

---

[41] *Neurōdēs*: Galen means that the bodily part in question has the same kind of physical compos-ition as that of the *neura* or nerves.
[42] In Greek, literally 'acorn'.

mother. I was carrying out dissections of pregnant goats, during my enquiry into the matters that had been investigated by the anatomists regarding the development of the embryo. Finding in this case that the embryo was already at an advanced stage, I cut it free of the womb, in the usual way, then took it away, before it had seen its mother, to a house which had a large number of jars full wine, oil, honey, milk, and of other liquids, as well as many full of cereal grains, and of the fruits of trees. We observed, first of all that the newborn animal walked upon its feet, as if it has been told that its legs were for walking; secondly, that it shook off the moisture that it had from the womb; thirdly, that it scratched its side with one of its feet. We also watched it smell all the supplies in the house, and after smelling them, start to sip on the milk. At this we all cried out, as we saw a clear proof of what Hippocrates says: 'the natures of animals are untaught....'[43]

446   ...There is, then, nothing remarkable in the fact that the parts involved in generation, too, recognize, right from the outset, the activities for the sake of which they have been brought about by nature. Why is it, after all, that the womb when it has captured the seed remains perfectly closed until the completion of the foetus' growth, at which point it opens up to an extremely wide extent, and having done so for this very purpose, expels the foetus?

Here matters which are the subject of our constant observation are ignored by most people; they tend to wonder rather at very rarely seen phenomena, rather than things which are genuinely a source of wonder. What could be more wonderful than the fact that the mouth of the womb remains so perfectly closed, for nine whole months, that not even the head of a probe may be inserted, but that on the completion of its growth it achieves such a great distention that the whole living being can pass through it?

One will not, then, doubt that the capacity of the genitals, too, is self-taught,
447   so that that pipe-like | body, which is nerve-like in its form, when the animal has an impulse for sexual intercourse, becomes erect immediately, since it has a natural capacity which distends it, just like those of the heart and the arteries. The only difference is that these latter are in motion constantly, because we always require their activity, whereas the pipe-like nerve does not move constantly, but only when called upon by need. When it is expanded, the breath from the arteries then follows, just as the lung follows the chest, by virtue of procession towards the void. One might also possibly attribute to the arteries the capacity of the breath that fills the pipe-like nerve, when the animal has the impulse for intercourse; but it is far preferable to state that this activity is that of the nerve, not of the arteries. For it is reasonable to suppose that the activities arise not from the position of the parts but from their own proper substance,

---

[43] *Nutrition* 39, where the precise quotation, according to our texts of 'Hippocrates', is rather 'the natures of all are untaught'.

and that the heart would have the same activity even if it were situated in some other part, and similarly the liver, the spleen and all the others.

So, too, it is reasonable to suppose that the arteries have the same activity in every part of the body, as indeed is evident. The arteries throughout the whole body become expanded in the same way at one and the same moment; it is therefore not likely | that the arteries that connect to the penis possess 448 some other capacity apart from that which originally belongs to them elsewhere throughout the body, although naturally enough the openings of these are wider than those of other arteries, since they have been made ready for the speed with which the procession towards the void will take place (for it is evident that Nature provides what is of use for each of the activities in every location), but that they have no other special capacity for a different activity when they reach the penis. When, however, the lower back is heated, it is reasonable to suppose that the arteries both become hotter and have their openings opened wider, so that in this way too a considerable amount of substance is poured forth into the pipe-like nerve, by which the penis is soon filled and extended, the whole of this substance now being in the pipe-like nerve.

Now that this has been understood, let us turn to the priapic state. It is obvious from what has been said so far that this ailment comes about either through the widening of the mouths of the arteries, or through the production of vaporous breath by the pipe-like nerve; we must enquire which of the two should rather be considered responsible. My view is that it may come about through both causes, but that it more often | results from the widening of the mouths of 449 the arteries; for this is found more readily than the production of gassy breath in the pipe-like nerve. Moreover, I believe that I have observed such a state of the nerve on one occasion, but such a state of the arteries on many occasions: this I inferred on the basis of the preceding symptoms and the mode of treatment. In cases which were preceded by constant palpitation, gassy breath was the cause, and I healed the patient with a treatment wholly based on that assumption. Where there had been widening of the mouths of the arteries, no such symptom preceded; rather, there had been, in the different cases: unaccustomed abstention from sexual activity; consumption of foods which were acrid and of poor humoral fluid; and the use of a belt during two months of travel by one unused to wearing it. I thus drew the conclusion that there had been an opening of the mouths of the arteries, either as a result of the acridity due to the poor humoral fluid, or as a result of the production of gassy breath in disordered and violent motion.

Moreover, drugs which extend the genitals—both those which are taken orally and those which are applied to the perineum and lower back— | are all 450 hot and breathy in nature, just as those with the opposite effect are non-gassy, and cooling rather than heating.

Here one must pay careful attention, and not read this statement with excessive haste. I said 'drugs', not 'foods', because some foods are highly productive of seed, and therefore intensify the impulse towards lustfulness. This supports the statement made above, that those who have abstained from sexual activity also sometimes succumb to priapism. This happens especially in the case of people who are endowed with a large quantity of seed and who have also had an unaccustomed abstention from sexual activity, if they do not work off the excess blood through substantial physical exercise. And it happens especially if they have not removed from themselves the conception of sexual activity, as have people who are self-controlled by nature and who have trained themselves in such self-restraint over a long period, but rather find themselves returning to the imagination of sexual activity,[44] because of sights which have the capacity to provoke the impulse and because of their memory of it.

The state of such men, as regards their genitals, is entirely opposite to that of those who do not entertain conceptions of sexual activity at all. One | friend of mine who had decided to abstain completely from sex, contrary to his previous custom, experienced such swelling and increase in size of his genitals, that he was compelled to consult me concerning this symptom. He expressed his amazement at the fact that a particular athlete had a penis which had become completely shrivelled and contracted while following such a regime, while he had experienced exactly the opposite since embarking on it. I advised him at this point to expel the accumulated seed, but from then on to keep himself entirely away from sights, accounts or memories capable of stimulating him sexually. Those athletes or singers who have always refrained from sexual experience, keeping themselves entirely free from all such thoughts and fantasies, develop genitals as small and shrivelled as those of old men.

Those who from their earliest youth indulge in a great deal of sexual activity find, apart from anything else, that as the vessels in those parts become broader, not only does the blood itself coming to the penis flow more plentifully, but also the capacity of the sexual appetite increases, according to the same principle that applies to all capacities, | and was referred to by Plato when he wrote that inactivity dissolves the strength, while exercise of the proper activities increases it. Thus, indeed, the breasts remain contracted in women who have not yet become pregnant, while they become very large in those who are feeding children after pregnancy; and they remain so as long as they are providing milk and

---

[44] The difference between 'self-control' and 'self-restraint' seems trivial, but a real distinction probably underlies the terms in Greek. The terms, respectively *sophrosunē* and *enkrateia*, are established ones in the philosophical tradition, and for Galen the latter indicates a mental or emotional state of constant effort to resist various (in this case sexual) temptations, the former one in which one is habituated in such a way that one does not even experience the temptations. (See *Affections and Errors of the Soul*, I.6, with n. 17.)

breast-feeding, whereas once they cease breast-feeding the production of milk in the breasts, too, soon ceases.

Our previous examination of all these matters will thus also provide the basis for treatment, enabling us to distinguish the causes through which ailments arise in each part. Now, however, is not the time for this: the present treatise has reached its conclusion, and I shall end the account here.

Simple Drugs (excerpts)

Galen's work on 'The Capacity of Simple Drugs' is one of his three great treatises of pharmacology, the other two being those on the compound drugs ('The Composition of Drugs according to Kind' and 'The Composition of Drugs according to Place'). There is also a shorter treatise, *Antidotes*, and some others of uncertain authorship. Those other works deal with drug recipes that use many ingredients, and they give extensive lists of such recipes. *Simple Drugs* has two main aims: to explain the theoretical principles of action of the individual substances—vegetable, mineral and animal—used as drugs; and to list and describe the main such substances. The former task occupies the first five of the eleven books, the latter the remaining six, although several of these also contain recapitulations, or further formulations, of the theoretical principles. In the last six books, Galen lays out the relevant materials in three successive lists, describing the properties and mentioning some of the uses, first of plants (books VI–VIII), then of minerals (book IX) and finally of animal products (books X and XI). These descriptions also involve a partial attempt at 'quantificational' classification of the substances' properties in terms of the level of intensity of their active qualities, understood in terms of the scheme of the hot, the cold, the wet and the dry.

The work, though diffuse and sometimes repetitive in its argument, contains discussions of great importance for the understanding not only of Galen's views on drugs and their mechanisms of action, but also of his approach to empirical testing more broadly, and the relationship between empirical inputs and the construction of a theoretical and predictive model. The text also offers us a wealth of material of social-historical and medical-historical interest regarding the substances used, the attitudes towards these, the practices employed, and the role of various kinds of herbalist or medical expert in the ancient world.

Galen's pharmacological work represents a major, and under-researched, aspect of his output. Questions of particular importance here are: the precise nature of his theoretical model of drug classification and drug action; the relationship of this theoretical model to everyday observation and clinical practice; the relationship of his work with the previous tradition; the nature and extent of his own testing of the materials in use; his attitude to magic and astrology, to the social norms of his times, and to practitioners from different social and intellectual backgrounds. The following brief extracts from the work can do no more than give some glimpses into his views and practices in this area, and into the place of these in the broader history of drug use in the Graeco-Roman world.

The text seems to be the product of two phases: an earlier one, which may in some form go back to the core phase of Galen's literary activity, in the early 170s, and a much later one; it seems that Galen devoted considerable time in his later years to the pharmacological project as a whole. As mentioned in the introduction to *Mixtures*, the theoretical material in this work is conceived as following on, conceptually, directly from book III of that work.

Greek title: Περὶ τῆς τῶν ἁπλῶν φαρμάκων δυνάμεως (*Peri tēs tōn haplōn pharmakōn dunameōs*)
Kühn: XI.379–892 and XII.1–377

BOOK I

[Galen summarizes some essentials of drug action.]

3. It is only substances that have an increasing heating effect from beginning to XI.384
end of the time of their contact with the body that should be considered to be heating in their own nature, rather than in virtue of some incidental property. So too with that which is cooling. If you do not wait, but examine a substance's power immediately after bathing, you are liable to be deceived on many counts. You may quite possibly say that it is not only cold in its capacity but also hot: cold, in that it clearly has a cooling effect throughout the time of contact, and hot because it often provokes a recall of heat. | These matters too, then, must be 385
subjected to the correct distinctions; furthermore, every drug under assessment should—as also stated in *Mixtures*—be free of any acquired cold or heat at the time of the assessment, so that its natural capacity is not contaminated by any such acquired quality. Moreover, as was also discussed there, nourishment must be distinguished from drug; and it must be borne in mind that both these categories are understood in relative terms;[1] also that both may frequently be instantiated in one and the same substance; we have shown this too. Further, that some things act on, and are acted upon by, each other in respect of their whole substances, others in respect of one or two qualities; and also that some are fine, and other dense, in their composition: the former are those which are readily broken up into fine parts, the latter the opposite of these.[2] In short, one

---

[1] i.e. the status of something as either a nourishment or a drug depends on that thing's effect on a particular human (or animal) subject.

[2] Galen distinguishes between two mechanisms of drug action, one where the drug brings about its effect in the body through its active qualities (heating, drying, etc.) and another where it acts 'through its whole substance'. The latter kind of action is associated both with certain classes of drugs, including poisons, and with the notion of the inexplicability of the effect of a particular drug. See also *My Own Doctrines*, ch. 9, *Mixtures* III.1 and below V.1, IX.2.1 and XI.24, and for discussion of the concept Singer 2020. The distinction between stuffs which are fine and those which are dense or coarse in their composition is also of considerable importance in Galen's model, especially in the context of external applications such as ointments. Fineness of composition is associated with the ability of the product in question to penetrate quickly or deeply within the body.

should bear in mind all the specifications made in the third book of *Mixtures*, and conduct one's examination of the form of all drugs on the basis of those.

[*A central theme of the work is the relationship between the effects, or 'active qualities', of substances (usually plant substances) used as drugs and the discernible properties of these substances, in particular taste, and thus the procedure of inferring the former from the latter. In the following passage, after aligning his theoretical account and linguistic usage with those of his predecessors, especially Plato and Theophrastus, Galen attempts to characterize the perceptual experiences involved in each of the fundamental tastes themselves.*

Galen divides fundamental tastes into four pairs; that is, each taste may appear in a more or less intense form, so that the grand total is eight. (Neither the pairings nor the identification of these particular items as fundamental tastes accord with our contemporary classifications.) The pairs, going from milder to more intense in each case, are as follows: austēros *('tart') and* struphnos *('sour'), which represent different levels of intensity of* stuphōn *('astringent');[3]* halukos *('salty') and* pikros *('bitter');* oxus *('sharp' or 'acidic') and* drimus *('acrid');* liparos *('smooth' or 'oily') and* glukus *('sweet').*]

XI.452 39. It is not possible to communicate these precisely, any more than it is for any other perceptual experience; but it is possible to bring it to the mind of one who has shared the same sensation.

Anyone who has ever tasted quinces, apples, myrtle-berries or medlars is fully aware that there is one sort of sensation that arises in the tongue from these and another from sour things.[4] Those which are sour or cooling seem to press inwards from all sides evenly upon the part of the body which touches them, as though pushing upon, compacting and compressing it; those which are tart, on the other hand, seem to seep deep down and to induce a sort of harsh, uneven sensation, as though drying out and completely consuming the moisture of our sensory parts. There is thus a different specific experience, which is impossible to express precisely, in the two cases, that of bodies with an astringent [*or* sour] effect on us and that those with a tart flavour. Yet every
453 person of intelligence will understand | what I am saying. When the body in contact with the tongue has a vehement drying effect, and compresses and hardens it to a considerable depth, as do unripe wild pears and cherries, all such things are referred to as sour; and they differ from those which are tart in intensity....

Those things on the other hand which in contact with the tongue do not compress it, nor bind it, as do the sour ones, but have a manifestly opposite

---

[3] But, confusingly, Galen seems sometimes—including in this passage—to use *stuphōn* in place of *struphnos*.

[4] Galen here uses the word *stuphōn*, usually translated 'astringent'; see previous note.

effect, washing and cleansing it, are all—even if the effect is in some way close to that of the astringents—termed salty. Those which cleanse even more than these, to the point of painful harshness, are termed bitter. Those which bite and corrode, with a strong heat, are acrid. Those which bite without such heat are known as sharp; in these latter there is present also some fermentation. Those which seem to anoint, replenish and restore the parts of the tongue that have been made harsh and corroded ⏐ are termed sweet when the contact is accom-   454 panied by manifest pleasure, or smooth when such pleasure is absent. So, I have tried as best I can to give a verbal account of things which are difficult to communicate.

BOOK III

[Galen addresses the question of the different kinds of change or alteration in the body, in particular those caused by the action of drugs.]

4. There are two classes of alteration: those which create [new] forms,[5] and   545 those which involve the fine division, or bringing-together, of the parts within our bodies. The former class is primarily and properly termed 'alteration', while the latter is so termed in a looser sense. The capacities of drugs, we say, fall within the former class. For no change from one form to another is possible without the body being subjected to heating, cooling, moistening or ⏐ drying. By   546 'from one form to another' I mean, for example, what happens when from bread, barley or lentils there come into being blood, phlegm and yellow and black bile, and from these again bone, gristle, nerve, flesh, artery, vein, and all the other parts of the animal. Something which cuts us, such as a piece of glass or a sword, or compresses us, like a stone or piece of lead, or indeed something which binds together parts which have been divided, for example a ligature, does in a sense alter the parts in question, but is not a drug; and such alteration is not one in which those parts are transformed from their own proper nature. If you divide a loaf of bread up and crumble it into very small fragments, or again if you gather a large number of tiny pieces into one, the bread does not depart from its own proper form; nor will flesh come into being through the crumbling nor bone from its compaction. It is through coction in the stomach

---

[5] *Eidopoios*, 'form-making', an Aristotelian term (which through its Latin calque gives us the word 'specific'), more usually applied to a characteristic or differentia which is *constitutive* of a particular 'form', or species, rather than to processes of change that give rise to different forms. I here preserve the traditional translation 'form' for the Aristotelian term *eidos*, which is elsewhere sometimes translated 'type'. For the distinction between the true alteration that takes place through the agency of the active qualities and changes that merely involve breaking up or combining quantities of an unchanged substance, we may compare *The Elements according to Hippocrates*, esp. chs. 1 and 3.

and veins that it is changed into blood and phlegm, and then from these into bone, flesh and all the other parts, in a process whereby it is altered in its whole substance, and departs from its previous nature and turns into a different form.

547   As has been shown, it is only from the hot, the cold, the dry | and the wet that bodies may become subject to alteration or change into a different form of substance.

[*In the following passage Galen considers further aspects of the methodology by which drug properties are to be assessed, and introduces an element of quantificational analysis: the four-level schema according to which each of the active qualities is to be evaluated.*]

571   13. … Let us, then, take such a body [sc. one with the best possible mixture] as the standard[6] in relation to the capacities of drugs. Thus, a drug which gives rise to the same level of heat as that present in such a mixture should be termed 'well-mixed', even though it will very definitely produce a noticeable heating in an older person whose mixture is cold. Those drugs, then, which heat this chosen type of body will be termed 'hot', while those which cool it will be 'cold'. There should, furthermore, be an ordering of the levels, too. The first level of cold would be represented by rose oil; the second by rose itself; and there will
572   then be a third and a fourth, bringing us | in our account to those which are coldest of all, hemlock, opium, mandragora and wolfsbane. Similarly with the hot drugs: we should place dill and fenugreek on the first level, on the second those which manifestly have the relevant property, and so on through the third and fourth, going up to those drugs with a burning capacity. The same will apply, too, to moistening drugs: we should begin from the middle position, then place them in order, up to those with the extreme version of the quality. The value of such knowledge for the method of healing is very considerable. In reality, indeed, if someone does *not* make such distinctions, he will harm rather than help the reader. Amid all the errors made by the majority of doctors in their expositions of the capacities of drugs, the most dangerous that one comes across is the following: that in an account of, say, heating drugs they will place alongside each other dill, fenugreek, copper ore and gypsum, and in one of cooling drugs rose oil, mandragora and hemlock, as though these substances were close to each other in capacity (I mean, for example, fenugreek to gypsum, or rose oil to hemlock) and not, in fact, separated by many intervening levels of drugs.
573   I, however, | shall attempt, to the best of my ability, this very considerable and difficult task of arranging them in some order and writing down which are close and which far from each other in their capacities. And here we should not rely for their assessment on plausible accounts, but on differentiated experience:

---

[6] *Kanōn*, 'standard' or 'yardstick'; see also *Mixtures*, nn. 6 and 9.

this, too, has been explained many times previously.[7] It is surely quite evident that such a method of assessment is reliable. It is true, too, that it is very time-consuming, and extremely laborious for one who intends, as I do, to proceed by that method to the end of the task in question. For potential readers of this work, however, this method is the only one capable of furnishing them with a specialized skill, and of providing, as it were, an eye able to discern the truth.

BOOK IV

1. The meaning of 'cold', 'hot', 'dry' and 'wet', when applied to the capacity of a 619
drug, as well as the method by which these properties are to be tested, has already been clarified. Yet we also refer to drugs as emollient or constrictive, thinning or densifying, adhesive or dispersive, and by many other such terms. We should therefore give an account of these too, and also of the subject which precedes this, that is I the substance and capacity of all the fluids.[8] This subject 620
was already discussed towards the end of book I, with reference to a passage of Plato's *Timaeus*; but at that point my focus was on the perceptual experience of the tongue in each case, whereas here my focus will be on the substance and capacity which underlie these experiences.

[*Galen proceeds to discuss the effects of various qualities on the body, and in particular the similarities and differences between the 'biting' effects caused by heat and cold; and the important distinction as to whether substances are fine or dense in their composition. He then considers the effects arising from the complex nature of particular products; and returns to the question of the rational and empirical procedure by which one may infer active qualities from tastes.*]

3. ... We must bear these things in mind in our consideration of all drugs; and 628
first of all we must avoid falling into the trap of most of those who have made such enquiries. I They proceed in their account as though each substance were 629
uniform in nature, not realizing that wine, olive oil and all the rest are composed of different parts. In the case of vinegar, in particular, they are amazed if

---

[7] The precise sense of 'differentiated experience' (*diōrismenē peira*) has been a topic of scholarly discussion; essentially, Galen mean a process of testing carried out according to well-defined parameters, with a firm theoretical understanding of the possible relationships between the perceived properties of drugs and their active powers in the body, and with 'accidental' factors which will interfere with the experiment excluded; he may also be referring to the quantificational element of analysis just mentioned.

[8] The word *chumos* can refer both to fluids (especially the 'humours', blood, phlegm, etc., but also the fluids found in the biological world more generally) and to flavours or tastes; and, as Galen clarifies in book I, in the passage just before that excerpted above, I.39, in the present work he generally uses it in the latter sense. In the present case both senses seem to be included: what is at issue is precisely the connection between particular sensory experiences and particular underlying 'substances and capacities'.

we venture to state that it has lost the innate heat of wine, and possesses rather a heat due to fermentation, as indeed was the opinion of both Aristotle and Theophrastus. The vinous parts of wine are cooled down in the process of its change to vinegar, while the watery residue has a particular heat that it acquires in the fermentation, as happens also in the case of all other substances that undergo fermentation.

Thus, vinegar turns out to be a composite of parts that are very different in their capacities, some of which have undergone cooling, while others are hot. The situation is similar to that of the ash of wood that has been burnt; here too there remains some kind of internal flame, which is dispersed through the small parts; and this is quite markedly hot, while the rest of the substance is earthy and cold. Thus, when the ash is put in water, and then passed through
630   some fairly porous body, the hot, acrid parts are entirely removed, | and what remains is no longer hot; the fiery parts have been deposited in the water.... We experience something similar in the case of vinegar, where however we are unable to observe with our senses the nature of its production, and therefore mistrust the account [of its properties].

Yet through consideration of the difference between vinegar and unripe grapes, we will be justified in believing that some other flavour, which is not just sour but also acrid, has been mixed with it, and that for this reason the juice of the unripe grape is wholly cooling, so that it is appropriate for cases of over-heating, when placed in contact with the mouth of the stomach or with the whole upper abdominal region, as well as for any state where we wish to
631   bring about cooling, | whereas vinegar is not appropriate in the same way. For vinegar is not entirely one thing; nor is it only sharp, but also acrid. That which is *only* sharp is in all cases cold—for example pear, apple, the juice of black-berry, mulberry or pomegranate.... If, when you taste it, the sharpness appears strong and clear, with no apparent acridity, you will find that this fluid is defin-itely cooling; and in that case you may use it freely, for example for over-heating...or any other hot ailments. Similarly, you will find that all cold illnesses are clearly damaged by it. When, however, the quality appears to you to be combined, if that combination is with acridity, then you should infer the presence of some heat; if with astringency, that of another kind of coldness. For sharp coldness is fine in its composition, while that which is astringent is dense.

632   4. ...One should not undergo a theoretical training only—of the sort which I am constantly encouraging people to engage in, namely a training in logical method, as laid out in my work on *Demonstration*—but should also train one's sense of taste carefully in relation to each of the flavours,[9] beginning with those which most clearly manifest a single quality. If, for example, you wish to have a

---

[9] *Chumos*: see previous note.

clear conception of acridity, you should repeatedly taste garlic, onion and similar plants, chewing them for a long time, and attempting to consign your perception of that particular experience to the memory. If you wish to do the same for astringency, you should do the same with castor oil, sumac and the like; for bitterness, natron and bile; for sweetness, *siraion*[10] or honey; and also, if you wish to conceive of something without quality, or in the middle in terms of its tastable quality, | you should taste water.... 633

5. If you detect the same taste in any dry substance as you do in water which is devoid of any other quality, then that substance is evidently without any significant heat or cold, and has essentially a middle position, | albeit with a slight 634 possible inclination towards the cold. If, then, you have a substance in this position on the scale between heat and cold, which is also dry in its consistency, this substance will necessarily be earth-like, and will dry without biting. All such drugs are called by the doctors adhesive....

7. Now, there are many qualities that are present in drugs, qualities which 640 are not only different but even in conflict with, or sometimes completely opposed to, each other.... If the same drug seems to you when you taste it to be simultaneously sour and biting, I advise you to put this drug aside, turning to one which is sour without the biting. If, moreover, it appears neither sharp, nor sweet, nor bitter, but, as nearly as possible, endowed with the uncombined property of astringency[11] alone, you should then subject it to trial in the manner which I have laid down to you frequently in the past. If on the other hand it has the qualities of astringency and biting, or some other manifest quality or capacity mixed with the astringency, then it is superfluous and pointless to bring such a drug to trial, when your testing is concerned with the action of astringency.... | It is better, then, to abandon them [sc. drugs with more than 641 one perceptible property] and to taste many others in turn, investigating as far as possible pure astringency, specifically and in itself; and when you find this, then to assess the drug according to the methods which you have heard many times before. For example, if on tasting it appears to you that wild pomegranate, or castor oil...is completely sour, and that it has no other manifest quality, then conduct an examination of such substances and conduct a thorough test on the active properties of astringency. Such an examination, as has been stated frequently, must be carried out upon people enjoying perfect health and an optimal bodily constitution; and the test should have in view only ailments that are simple—that is, ones that are only hot, only cold, only dry or only wet. If the healthy | body itself appears obviously cooled, then the item in question 642 is suited to hot ailments, and if further the impact of the cold quality is

---

[10] A sweet wine; see *The Thinning Diet*, ch. 12.

[11] Again, the terminology of 'sour' (*struphnos*) and 'astringent' (*stuphōn*) is used interchangeably in this passage; see nn. 3 and 4 above.

manifest to the patient himself, then you may now venture to declare that astringency is cooling. If the converse is found, namely that bodies in health are heated by it and hot diseases are intensified, while cold ones are benefited, then one must consider that such a drug does not cool but heats.

One should conduct the trial of drugs which are acrid in the same way, on the basis of those which are so in themselves, for example garlic, onion, pepper. . . . One who mixes pepper with the juice of winter cherry will not be able to assess the effect of either; no more will one who [tries with] those things which have been mixed by nature. I encourage you to conduct the investigation of the sharp quality, the bitter quality and the sweet quality in the same manner, by bringing them to trial in their strong and, as far as possible, single forms, and so finding out their capacities by testing.

BOOK V

[*Galen lays out again the essentials of his theoretical model, then proceeds to consider the relationship between the fundamental active qualities, those understood in terms of hot, cold, wet and dry, and the higher-level ones, understood in relation to specific operations or particular diseases in the body.*]

704 1. As I embark upon this fifth book on the capacities of simple drugs, let me first remind the reader of those demonstrations made earlier which are of value for present purposes; and I shall begin with the elements. These are water, fire, air and earth, which some call rather by the terms belonging to the qualities: wet, dry, hot and cold. These, however, are the qualities, moisture and dryness,
705 | heat and cold. Bodies to which the names of these qualities are applied are: the elements common to all; those which possess some predominance, which are thus also called wet, dry, cold or hot; those so called by comparison with the midpoint within a genus or species; and those so called by comparison with some particular object. These distinctions have been made frequently; and the manner in which nourishment differs from drug has been stated too. A nourishment is dominated and mastered by that by which it is nourished, while a drug, by contrast, itself masters and dominates the body for which it is a drug. (The relational nature is essential to our understanding in both cases.) It has also been shown that a drug is by nature capable of producing an alteration either in virtue of one specific quality (that is, heating, cooling, drying or moistening), or in virtue of some pairing of these, or in virtue of its whole substance. Some of the 'destructive' drugs, a considerable number of the protective ones, all the purgatives and many of those known as *epispastic* belong to this last cat-
706 egory. I will | complete the discussion of these later on. Those which act on the whole of our bodies in virtue of one or two qualities I shall discuss in this book.

Here, again, let me take as a starting-point something that has been demonstrated above, namely that most of the 'simple' drugs are non-uniform and composite in reality, but are called simple because of the fact that they are as they are by nature, without any contribution from human technology. I shall also assume for the purposes of this discussion the distinction between drugs which are thick-bodied and earthy in their substance, those which are fine-bodied and air-like, and those, between those two categories, which are as it were watery in their quality. We take these propositions as read; and let us now begin the discussion.

2. The function of drugs in relation to human beings is accomplished sometimes by straightforwardly heating, cooling, moistening or drying the body, or by some pairing of these actions; sometimes, on the other hand, by, for example, contracting and drawing together that which has become excessively relaxed or relaxing that which is constricted, thinning out what is too dense or dens- 707 ening what is too loose in texture, softening what is hard or hardening excessive softness, evacuating what is full or filling what is empty, or other similar operations. One who has been chilled has the desire to find a heating drug, and one suffering from a burning fever has the desire to find a cooling one: in such cases this desire arises automatically from the very nature of the complaint, even if that person has no medical expertise at all. Similarly, any lay person with a moist ulceration will instruct the doctor to dry it, whereas if it is dry and lacking in moisture he will instruct the doctor to moisten it. People will also become aware of a combination of dryness and heat affecting the whole body, as happens, for example, through over-heating or fatigue. At this point they desire to bathe, they drink cold water and they make every possible effort to discover anything that will simultaneously moisten and cool—and indeed, non-doctors frequently do succeed in providing themselves with the relevant cures, instructed by nature itself. On the other hand, in such cases as inflammation, induration, swellings, erysipelas, putrefaction, shingles or gangrene, no person ever attempts to find his own cure. Such cases exceed the understanding of the 708 layperson, requiring a more exalted kind of knowledge. And this knowledge is known as medicine, its practitioner as a doctor. Here, too, the layperson's understanding will extend to the fact that a hollow wound requires fleshening up, that a dirty one requires cleansing and a uniform one cicatrization; but not to the identification of the drugs specific to fleshening-up, cleansing or cicatrizing. So, too, in the case of a muscle or tendon which is hard, tight or relaxed; such people will know perfectly well that the hard one requires softening drugs, the tight one relaxants and the relaxed one contractive drugs, but they will not know the identity of any of these. The discovery of these is the task of the doctor.

Provided that we remain within the realm of the heating, the cooling, the moistening and the drying, we will find that the knowledge of drugs is in some cases shared not just by doctors but also by laypeople; but the latter will be

completely inexpert in relation to the kinds of drug just mentioned. Now, as
709 previously shown, | discovery is not always equally straightforward, even in the
case of these heating, cooling, moistening and drying drugs. The heating power
of mustard and pellitory, or the cooling power of purslane or sleepy nightshade,
or indeed the moistening power of water and oil, or the drying power of vinegar
or sea water, is something on which practically everyone—doctor or layperson—
agrees. But whether rose oil should be said to heat or to cool, on the other hand,
is a question which provokes considerable dispute—so too for vinegar and oil,
and indeed many other such substances. Well, I have discussed these in the first
four books... in the third, distancing myself from the sophists, I went in detail,
from the beginning, through all the logical enquiries that are necessary, and
through which one will become, as one might put it, skilled or specialized, in
order to have the capacity to discover the capacities of all the drugs. In the
710 fourth, I gave | an exposition of those substances with properties specifically
perceptible to the tongue—those known as tastes [*chumoi*]—showing how one
who takes these as his starting-point may discover the primary qualities and
capacities. At the end of the book I also touched, as far as relevant, upon qualities perceptible by smell, showing how these too may be taken as a starting-
point for the discovery of the primary capacities. In this fifth book, it was my
task to give a different kind of account of capacities, namely of those which may
be termed secondary or tertiary, following on from those primary ones which
are common to all.

It is, surely, because each individual substance does not have the same mixture of those primaries that they come to be, variously, relaxant, constrictive,
emollient, hardening, loosening or densening. Further, on the basis of the
actions that each naturally performs, they have been stated to have within them
capacities which are, say, loosening or densening, emollient or hardening; causing to adhere and removing; attracting or repelling; then, in addition to these,
slackening, astringent, opening, closing, thickening, thinning, relieving or
711 inducing pain, coctive, bringing to suppuration, | dispersive, sudorific,
inducing *karos*, unconsciousness or sleep, exciting, putrefactive, burning,
corrosive, caustic, dissolving, contracting, provoking poor fluid, tempering
the fluid, purgative, staunching, roughening, smoothening, obstructing or
relieving obstruction. It is, then, possible to proceed further, and to speak in
particular terms of each action—diuretic, emetic, downward-drawing, laxative,
sternutatory, causing discharge of phlegm, inducing or restraining menstrual
flow; so, too, those which generate or extinguish the production of milk and of
seed, or which either provoke or inhibit their flow. We reach a still greater focus
on the individual capacities when we talk of certain capacities which are
hepatic, splenetic, otic, ophthalmic, odontic, ischiadic, nephritic, podagric,
arthritic, pleuritic, bechic or of those which crush stones. One may also speak
of the capacity which is fleshening, cicatrizing, agglutinating or cleansing of a

wound; indeed, it is scarcely possible to enumerate all the individual capacities, if one were to attempt to apply to them the names of the outcomes produced.

Instead, | it will surely be better and more methodical to avoid an account   712
which is both long and disorganized, and to distinguish the composite capacities of drugs according to useful distinct types. Thus, we shall not speak of wheat-bread plaster as containing a capacity which is promotive of suppuration, soothing, relieving of pain, dispersive or relaxant, but rather of one which is moderately wet and hot. (The relevant meaning of these terms in this context has already been discussed.) So, too, with iris: we should not state that it is a drug which encourages menstrual flow, or expectoration, or that it is appropriate for those suffering from pleurisy, peripneumonia or abscesses, or that it is beneficial in cases of epilepsy, spasm, palpitation and tremor, rupture or sprains, nor that it fleshens and cleanses wounds or cavities, or stops pain of the ribs, sides, liver and spleen, nor that it disperses swellings nor that it draws flesh off the bones. Equally, we should not state that it is appropriate for *gonorrhoia*,[12] or is beneficial as part of a fomentation of the womb, softening and opening it; nor, indeed, that it clears up moles or freckles, | or that it cures   713
chronic headache or that it naturally destroys and expels embryos. It should suffice to state that its mixture is hot to such-and-such an extent, dry to such-and-such an extent and fine-parted to this degree: then all the effects mentioned have been indicated, and many besides. In different terms, it would also be sufficient to state of it that it is bitter, but not to an extreme degree, containing rather the admixture of some sweetness. The first manner of instruction is proper to Empirics, while the second is especially appropriate for one concerned with rational enquiry. It is the latter which it is my present purpose to expound.

BOOK VI

[*Galen begins by summarizing the content and methodology of the work so far, before turning to a consideration of the works of his predecessors. He has particular praise for the work of Dioscorides, also mentions positively a number other less comprehensive pharmacological works, for example those of Heraclides of Tarentum, Mantias and Apollonius, as well as pharmacological material in broader works of clinical medicine, and comments that 'there is no danger of running out of useful books, even if one were to spend one's whole life reading about nothing but drugs'. He then turns to criticism of a different kind of writer.*]

---

[12] See *Affected Places*, n. 40.

Preface

797   If one does require a book, then who would be so wretched as to ignore those of Dioscorides, Niger, Heraclides and Crateuas, as well as of countless other veterans of the Art, and to exalt instead the literary productions of one who writes of incantations, or metamorphoses, of plants sacred to decans and to daimons? The authors of such works are sorcerers, whose aim is to impress the general mass of people, as you may gather from an examination of the actual books of Pamphilus. He starts his account of herbs with wormwood [(h)abroto-non], which is well known to all, then proceeds to chaste [agnos], again a very well-known shrub, then dog's-tooth grass [agrōstis], which is familiar even to the lay person, and then alkanet [anchousa], which is also universally known, as

798   is maidenhair [adiantos], which he puts next. I Thus far he has mentioned nothing beyond the plants that we know; but he then goes on to speak of one which he claims is called the 'eagle' [aetos]; this, as he admits, is not mentioned by any of the Greeks, but has been recorded in one of the books attributed to Hermes the Egyptian, which contains the thirty-six plants sacred to the celestial signs. These plants are quite evidently fictitious, and an invention of the compiler of those books, as are the Ophionikoi of Cochlas.[13] There was of course no such person as Cochlas, the name itself being invented for comic effect, as are the contents of the book itself. Similarly, these thirty-six plants themselves exist only in name, and have no underlying reality. It seems that Pamphilus, in company with a number of others, had the leisure to fill his books with such useless fictions. For my part, I consider that I have already wasted too much time in mentioning them. Let us proceed then to those which are of use.

[In the course of his own account of the first item in the alphabetical sequence, wormwood—(h)abrotonon—Galen again turns to some more theoretical considerations.]

803   1.1. We should, then, write in this manner [sc. with appropriate attention to all the relevant diagnostic differences and effects in individual cases] not just about wormwood but about all the others; those whose capacity to act arises through heating, cooling, moistening or drying are to be discovered through the methods which I have stated many times, those which accomplish their effect through the specific nature of the whole substance, through experience alone. It has also been shown that the latter include lethal drugs, antidotes for lethal drugs, and purgatives. It is not possible discover these on a rational basis; at

---

[13] This was a well-known work of comic fiction. In this passage Hermes the Egyptian is Hermes Trismegistus, a Hellenized version of the Egyptian god Thoth, under whose name was transmitted a corpus of esoteric, astrological and theological writings; it seems clear that the principles underlying the system here criticized are astrological ones.

most one may discover plausible grounds for suspecting such an effect in some cases, but certainly not in all—as has been shown earlier on. But I shall produce an account of the capacities which are discovered in this way later on,[14] after first I discussing those which act through heating, cooling, moistening and 804 drying, and through the effects consequent on these, according to each class of drug.

[*Some examples are excerpted here of the accounts Galen gives in the alphabetical section.*]

1.6. Pot-marjoram [*agēraton*]. Pot-marjoram has a dispersive capacity and one 814 which definitely relieves inflammation.

1.7. Maidenhair [*adiantos*]. Maidenhair is well balanced in terms of heat and coldness, but dries, thins and disperses. It both increases hair in balding people and disperses scrofulous swellings and abscesses; when drunk it crushes stones, has a considerable beneficial effect in drawing up viscous and thick fluids from the chest and lungs, I and stops flux in the gastric cavity. It does not present any 815 discernible heat or cooling; one should place it in the middle rank as regards that opposition and mixture.

1.8. Houseleek [*aeizōon*]. Both kinds of houseleek, small and large, dry to a small degree, because they are also astringent to a moderate degree; they are devoid of any other strong quality, the watery substance being the predominant in them. They cool to a considerable degree: they are at the third level and rank of cooling substances. They are appropriate for cases of erysipelas, but also for *herpēs* and for inflammations arising from flux.

1.9. Haver grass [*aigilōps*]. Haver grass has a dispersive capacity. This is evident from the taste—for it is slightly acrid—but also from the fact that it cures indured inflammations.

1.10. Darnel [*aira*]. Darnel dries and heats actively, so much so that it is closer 816 to the acrid drugs than is iris. It is not, however, fine in its composition like iris, but considerably deficient in that respect. It should be placed at the beginning of the third rank of heating drugs, and at the end of the second rank of drying ones.

BOOK IX

[*Book IX deals with minerals. One excerpt follows, in which Galen again returns to the problem of apparently inexplicable effects of some substances, here of particular kinds of stone which stopped bleeding.*]

---

[14] This promise appears not to be fulfilled: there is no work, or section of a work, devoted specifically to this category of drugs.

XII.192 2.1. ... Some of their capacities lie in the specific nature of the whole substance, some in their active qualities. The nature of the difference between these has been stated above. Now, then, we should discuss those which act through their active qualities, to which belongs also the method of their employment. For it has been shown that those capacities within the specific nature of the whole substance are without method or reason, and are discovered by experience alone. We do not know why this particular stone in contact with a bleeding wound stops the flow; but we do know why the stone known as haematic is applied to the capacities of the eyes, for this kind of thing is a discovery of reason.

BOOK X

[*In this first section of the tenth book, before turning to his individual account of a range of animal products, Galen gives a further recapitulation of the theoretical model, and offers a personal and ethical response to some of the more revolting animal—and human—substances used by some of his predecessors, as well as to some of the ethically dubious purposes of some of their pharmacological productions.*]

245 1. None of the materials that I am about to discuss will be of any great value to one ignorant of the statements in the earlier part of the treatise, in the first five books; and some may indeed cause positive harm, if a person engages in their use without the appropriate method. I shall continue, then, on the understanding that I am speaking to one who has learnt those earlier statements, after first offering a summary reminder of the treatise as a whole.

246 It was shown that drugs have their effect by virtue of what are | known as their 'active qualities', namely heat, coldness, dryness and wetness, and that it is through the mixture of these that they acquire the further qualities, sour, tart, salty, briny, bitter, acrid, sweet, and that some are cleansing, some repulsive, some attractive, some softening, some burning, some putrefactive, some caustic; and that some moreover acquire more specific properties, for example to promote the growth of flesh, to assist cicatrization, to agglutinate fistulae or ulcers, to purge flesh that is excessive.

It was also shown that the general capacity of a drug may be discovered indicatively, on the basis of one test,[15] and that this should not be just any old test, but one carried out with the specifications stated. Once the general capacity has been discovered, there is then no further need of tests in relation to the individual capacities, except for the purpose of further confirmation of what reason has discovered.

---

[15] *Peira*, also sometimes translated 'experience' or 'trial'.

It is the same way here, then, that we may carry out our assessment of the materials now before us, namely those derived from animals. In the books following book V, that is the sixth, seventh and eighth, we went through the plant materials—not, to be sure, all of these that are found in the whole of | the 247 inhabited world, but those which we have tested for ourselves—and in the book preceding this one, that is the ninth, we went through the minerals.[16] It remains to deal with animal materials; and then, finally, those which are found in lakes or in the sea, or in water generally, which are neither plants nor minerals nor animals. (These last are very few in number, and with be discussed last, after our exposition of materials from animal bodies.)

Here, too, our order of exposition will follow the alphabetical order of the first letters of their names. And just as, with the plants, I discussed also the fluids derived from them, so here too I will give instruction not just on the capacities of the solid parts of animals, but also on the fluids contained within them: phlegm, bile, blood, urine, faeces and so on. Now, in the context of those previous statements, there were few things amongst the materials described by other doctors of which I did not have personal knowledge. | In fact, I made it 248 my business to learn their capacities through my own test, and if I did not have such knowledge, I did not write about the material in question either, not considering it appropriate to trust the authority of another, even in a single case. For I was aware that there are some who have written much that is false. In the case of animal parts and fluids, on the other hand, I admit that there are a very large number of which I have no personal experience, of the sort communicated by some in their writings. For some of them are abominable and disgusting, others moreover actually forbidden by law. It seems extraordinary, in this context, that Xenocrates, a man who lived not in the distant past, but around the time of our grandfathers, in spite of the fact that the Roman Empire forbids the eating of humans, writes, in an extremely believable manner, about which particular ailments human brain, flesh or liver, when eaten, will heal; or which a potion made from the bones of the head, shin or fingers, whether burnt or not; or indeed blood itself.

Now those things, though certainly | against the law, are not actually abom- 249 inable; to drink sweat, urine or menstrual fluid, on the other hand, is both abominable and disgusting; and even more so faeces, the effects of which he describes when smeared onto areas within the mouth and the throat, or drunk down in the stomach. He also describes the effects of the drinking of earwax. Well, I would not subject myself to that, even if it meant I should never be sick again; and faeces seems to be far more disgusting still. It is a greater source of shame to a right-thinking person to be known as an eater of faeces than as one who commits shameful sexual acts, or a catamite; but amongst shameful sexual

---

[16] Literally, 'earthy and stone-like bodies'.

acts we are more disgusted by those who perform fellatio than those who perform cunnilingus—which seems to me a similar thing to drinking menstrual
fluid. No person in their right mind would endure a personal trial of these
things; nor even of those which are not as extreme as these, but still disgusting,
such as to have human faeces, or semen, smeared over some part of the body
because of some local ailment. Xenocrates customarily refers to the latter as
250 'seed',[17] I and he distinguishes with great care those ailments cured by the application of seed alone and those cured by the application of seed after sexual
intercourse between a man and a woman, when it is expelled from the vagina.
There would have to be a very great shortage of medicaments for someone to
treat a chillblain by the application of male semen which has not remained
inside the female but has flowed out after intercourse. Yet there is a great deal of
material of this kind in his writings on the benefits derived from animals. He
does not confine himself to the effects of drinking human urine, or the application of human faeces in the mouth, but goes through the effects of those of
every other animal too, not least of animals which are extremely inaccessible,
such as the elephant or the hippopotamus. As for the basilisk, I have never so
much as seen it; and if what is said of it is true it is dangerous even to come
near to it.

There are others, too, who have written about animals in a vein similar to
251 Xenocrates; and it is indeed from these sources that I Xenocrates himself has
excerpted most of his material. Where, indeed, would he have had the opportunity to make personal trial of such a large number and wide range of such
products? It may be observed that that previous king of our own country,
Attalus, seems to have written about many fewer, even though he was extremely
keen to try such things. And someone once praised and gave me a copy of the
treatise on the same subject by Ateuristos, which was also produced without the
personal experience of the author.

Well, I shall not mention basilisks, nor elephants, nor hippopotamuses, nor
any other animal which I have not actually made a test of; as for love-charms, or
potions to bring loves, to cause dreams or to provoke hatred—here I deliberately give the terms actually used[18]—I would, first of all, not mention them in
writing, even if I did have substantial experience of them, any more than
I would lethal drugs, or those which are known as the 'makers of affection'. Here
some of the properties in question are ridiculous, for example that of constraining your enemy so that he will be unable to speak in court, causing a woman to
252 miscarry, or preventing her from ever I conceiving, and similar such effects.
Most of these are empirically impossible; others, even if possible, are harmful to
the lives of human beings. I thus cannot help wondering what on earth these

---

[17] *Gonos*: compare *The Shaping of the Embryo*, ch. 1, with n. 3.
[18] The Greek technical terms are *philtron, agōgimos, oneiropompos* and *misētron*.

people had in their minds when they wrote them down. A form of knowledge that brings ill repute to the living could hardly be thought to be a likely source of post-humous fame. If a king made such a test upon a person who had been condemned to death, that would not be such a terrible thing. But when ordinary citizens, out of all the things available to them throughout their life, choose to write of these, one must conclude either that they are writing of things of which they know nothing, having made no test of them or, if they have made such a test, that they are the most immoral of individuals, who experiment with deadly drugs on people who have done no wrong—sometimes indeed on people of excellent character.

[*A couple of examples from later in the book, and from the last book, indicate further Galen's attitude to the imputation of magic, as well as to the problem of effects which are not easily explained.*]

2.6. I had no desire to test whether the blood of the land crocodile conduces to 263 sharp-sightedness, since I had well-established drugs for sharp sight. The same applies to the question whether the blood of chariot horses is caustic and septic, or whether that of house mice removes *akrochordones* [a kind of wart]. I had plenty of other drugs for that ailment, and indeed even for the wart known as *murmēkia* ['ant-hill'], which is harder to cure; and I was concerned not to incur a reputation for sorcery, since I was already the victim of slander from doctors who claimed that my predictions of outcomes in patients were derived not from the study of medicine but from some kind of divination....

2.21. There was one who used to administer a potion of wolf faeces to those 295 suffering from colic, not just during the acute onsets, but also in the intervals between these, in cases where the patient was free from inflammation. And I observed that some of these patients ceased to be affected by the ailment, and that even those who were still affected suffered less severely, and after a while not at all. The person in question used to prefer the whiter sort of wolf's faeces, which is excreted when the animal has eaten bones. What amazed me, here, was that it was often also beneficial even when worn [as an amulet]. The practitioner in this case would take faeces which had not yet fallen upon the ground, which is not in fact difficult; for the animal has the habit, rather similar to that of dogs, of raising one of its back legs when urinating or defaecating, and doing so upon some object which protrudes from the earth....

His instruction was that the object worn, which contained the faeces, be 296 attached to the abdomen of the patient by a cord, and this cord should preferably be made from the wool, not of any sheep, but of one that has been savaged by a wolf; this will be much more suited to this purpose. If this is not available, then the instruction was that both the strap connecting it to the abdomen and the container of the faeces itself should be made of the hide of a deer. I myself placed the faeces in a small pot, about the size of the largest kind of broad bean,

and attached it to some persons, for the sake of experiment, and I was amazed
297 | to see that most of them clearly experienced a benefit. What I did was make
two ears, as it were, in the container, by which the strap was attached. I mention
this just in case there are those who put their trust in such amulets themselves;
the point I would make is that what matters is the *substance* which is suspended,
not some foreign words, as is the practice of some of the sorcerers, for I made
the test also with other substances which have an effect on other ailments.

BOOK XI

356 24. The ash of river crabs is drying in a similar way to the substances previously mentioned, but it acts, through the specific nature of its whole substance,
wonderfully, in the case of dog-bites.... I have used them seldom in other cases,
but mainly in the way that Aeschrion the Empiric used them; this was an old
man extremely experienced in drugs, a fellow citizen and teacher of ours. He
357 had a vessel made out of red | bronze, in which he would place the crabs while
still alive, and roast them until they turned to ash, and could easily be ground
up. Aeschrion would always keep a supply of the drug in this form ready in his
house, having roasted them in summer, after the rise of the Dogstar, when the
sun was in Leo and the moon eighteen days old. He would give this drug to
victims of the bite of mad dog, every day for forty days, sprinkling a large
spoonful of it in water. In cases where the bite was not brought to his attention
at the outset, but only after some days, he would administer two spoonfuls a
day. He also administered an adhesive, consisting of Brutian pitch, gum of
opopanax and vinegar, to the wound itself—in the proportions of a pound of
the pitch, a pint of highly acrid vinegar and three ounces of the gum. This is not
strictly relevant to the matter in hand, but I have added it because of my great
confidence in the drug, no one having ever died who used it in the manner
mentioned.

358   I shall write another treatise separately on | drugs that act through the spe-
cific nature of their whole substance—to which all such things as these belong.[19]
I may be forgiven, though, for mentioning some of these out of their proper
place, both here and at other points in the present work, since the benefit from
the items mentioned is very great indeed, and I should like to save the lives of
some of my fellow human beings, even if death prevents me from writing the
treatises that should follow this one.

My teacher, Pelops, wished to give an account of the causes of all such effects;
and he reasonably enough stated that the crab, being a water animal, is of

---

[19] See n. 14 above.

benefit to those bitten by mad dogs, because their fear is of falling victim to an extremely dry ailment, namely the mad frenzy—which is, indeed, why they also fear water. The reason, he claimed, why river crabs rather than sea crabs were suitable, was that sea animals, being very dry because of the admixture of salt, would not retain a complete opposition to the mad frenzy. When asked by someone why then not all fresh-water animals were of equal benefit to the crabs, his response was that it was not possible to subject them to the same preparation ǀ as the crabs. For when these are incinerated, their ash, which is   359 extremely dry, will absorb and disperse the venom of the dog.

Well, this was the account that Pelops used to give: he claimed to be able to understand the causes of all these things, and prided himself on that. For my part, I do not try to persuade people of the truth of something of which I am not already personally convinced. I do not, then, accept even Pelops' account as true, since it is vulnerable to many counter-arguments; rather, my view is that the crabs also provide their benefit through the specific nature of their whole substance. It is because no one who used them has died that I earnestly wished to reveal this information, even if it did not strictly belong to the matter of the present discussion.

VI

SOUL AND BODY

The Soul's Dependence on the Body

One of Galen's most important and best-known philosophical works, this short treatise is constructed as a polemic against those philosophers—above all, contemporary Platonists—who refuse to acknowledge the importance of the body for the functioning of the soul, its wellbeing and its pathology. In the process it marshals as wide a range of authority as possible, from Hippocratic medical texts to the philosophical works and views of Plato, Aristotle and the Stoics, in support of its fundamental proposition. It is a rhetorical showpiece, probably aimed at a fairly wide audience of educated readers.

The philosophical significance of the work has been analysed from two perspectives in particular. First, the text espouses a striking physicalist or materialist view, namely that the soul (or its 'substance') is identical to a mixture of the body. Secondly, it sheds light on related views within the Aristotelian tradition. It attributes to Andronicus, the first-century-BC Aristotelian commentator, a view that foreshadows Galen's own: that 'the substance of the soul is either a mixture or a capacity dependent on that mixture', while preferring the former one of those two options. The latter formulation, meanwhile, has been connected with the theory of Galen's near contemporary Alexander of Aphrodisias, which in turn has been seen as a forerunner or close relative of the modern view known as 'epiphenomenalism'.

How clearly or definitively Galen adopts that materialist or physicalist view—whether it represents his final view on the matter—has been a subject of debate. On the one hand Galen's argument in this work is strongly physicalist in its thrust, and he expresses scepticism, at the very least, regarding what he at times presents as the only viable alternative, the Platonic view of the immortal, incorporeal soul. On the other it seems doubtful whether such a reductionist view can be harmonized with his conception of the soul as it appears in the round, on the basis of his other works. The medical concept of mixture, *krasis*, surely cannot do all the work that Galen would need it to do to explain the full range of psychological functions and pathologies and to provide a structural and functional account of the 'soul' or psyche. A particular problem that presents itself is the relationship between the 'bottom-up' account apparently presented here and the strong insistence on teleological explanation elsewhere. There is a further question as to whether this concept of mixture can simultaneously give an account both of the soul's permanent physical composition and of its temporary or occurrent states.

Moreover, Galen repeatedly expresses his ultimate agnosticism over the question of the 'substance of the soul', and continues to do so in works that seem clearly to post-date this one.[1] This consideration seems to undermine at least one version of the 'final view' theory, that which sees the present work as written at the end of Galen's career and

---

[1] e.g. *My Own Doctrines*, chs. 3, 7 and 14.

representing the culmination of his thinking on the matter. In fact, a number of works engaging with psychological or soul issues seem to have been written later, and arguably present more nuanced or developed thinking in this area.[2] Indeed, there seem no strong external grounds which establish the work's date with any precision, although the 'fact' that it is one of Galen's last works seems now to have irrevocably entered the scholarly discourse.[3]

An alternative to the 'final view' interpretation is one which sees the strongest physicalist statement of the work—the identity statement—as arising in the particular dialectical context of this text, rather than as representing Galen's mature view. More specifically, he may be presenting this as the view to which Aristotelians ought to be committed, on the basis of their equation of soul with form (*eidos*). Whether or not one accepts that interpretation, it is undoubtedly the case that it is the *dependence* of soul on body that is the demonstrandum throughout most of the work, not the identity of the two; and that the work—a literary and argumentative tour de force—aims to establish this dependence view on the basis of agreement between a wide range of textual sources, as well as through independent arguments.[4]

Greek title: Ὅτι ταῖς τοῦ σώματος κράσεσιν αἱ τῆς ψυχῆς δυνάμεις ἕπονται (*Hoti tais tou sōmatos krasesin hai tēs psuchēs dunameis hepontai*). (The full Greek title translates into English as 'That the Capacities of the Soul Depend upon the Mixtures of the Body'.)
Kühn: IV.766–822
Editions: Müller 1891; Bazou 2011
Translation with introduction and commentary: Singer 2013

K IV.767   1. The capacities of the soul depend on the mixtures of the body. This proposition I have put to the test and investigated on many occasions, in many different ways; and I have done so not just independently, on my own resources, but also from my earliest education, in conjunction with my teachers, and later through contact with the greatest of philosophers. It has been consistently found, not only to be the case, but also to be of practical value for those whose desire is to improve the condition of their soul. The reason for this—as I discussed in my
768   *Customary Practices*[5]— | is that we derive good-mixture of the body from our

---

[2] In addition to *My Own Doctrines*, see *Affected Places* III.9, which offers an account of the distinction between solid structures, fluids and ventricles in the brain, and their relationship to soul function, that is far more sophisticated than the simple model of 'mixture of the brain' given in the present text. Both *Affected Places* and the commentary on Hippocrates *The Nature of the Human Being* contain references back to the present work.

[3] See further n. 5 below.

[4] On these interpretive issues see Lloyd 1988; Singer 2013 (esp. 343–59, arguing for the dialectical interpretation); Havrda 2017; Vinkestejn 2022.

[5] I translate the text of this title given by the Greek manuscripts, *Peri ethōn*, while the Arabic version suggests that the mention is rather of *Character Traits*, *Peri ēthōn*—a difference just of the length of one vowel, in terms of the Greek word forms. If the Arabic version is correct, this would provide our only clear external evidence related to the date of the present work, since *Character*

food and drink and other daily activities, and may then use this mixture to contribute to the virtue of the soul. The accounts of the followers of Pythagoras and Plato,[6] and others of the ancients, show this to have been the case with them.

2. The starting-point for the whole of the following argument is an understanding of the differences of behaviour and affection of the soul in small children: these differences give clear evidence of the capacities of the soul. Some small children manifest great timidity, others an undauntable spirit; some are insatiable and gluttonous, while others are quite the opposite; some are completely lacking in shame and others have an acute sense of it. There are, moreover, many other such evident differences besides these. I have discussed them thoroughly elsewhere;[7] for present purposes the above should suffice as indicative examples of the fact that there exist innately, in infants, opposite kinds of capacity of each of the three forms or parts of the soul. From this one may deduce that the nature of the soul is not the same in each case. | And it is obvious that 769 the word 'nature' has the same sense in a discussion of this kind as the word 'substance'. For if the substance of each soul were indistinguishable, then the activities and affections would be identical also, given the same causal conditions. So evidently the substances of the children's souls differ from each other to the same extent as their actions and affections; and if the substances, then so also the capacities.

On this point many of the philosophers appear to be in some confusion, lacking a clearly articulated notion of 'capacity'. They seem to conceive of capacities as things which inhabit substances in much the same way as we inhabit our houses, and not to realize that every event has an effective cause, conceived in relational terms; and that while there is a way of speaking of that cause as a particular kind of object in itself, a capacity consists in the relation to that which arises from it; and therefore we attribute as many capacities to a substance as activities. So, for example, we state that aloe has a cleansing | and 770 toning capacity in relation to the mouth of the stomach, an agglutinating one in relation to bleeding wounds, a cicatrizing one in relation to grazes and a drying one in relation to the moisture of eyelids. But there is no other object apart from the aloe carrying out all these actions. It is the aloe that performs them all; and it is because of its ability to perform them that it is said to have these capacities—as many capacities, in fact, as the actions in question. When we say that

Traits is reliably thought to have been written after AD 192. Even on that hypothesis, however (and the content of the text of Character Traits as we know it does not clearly support it), this would not necessarily place the work at the very last phase of Galen's life—and indeed a number of later works contain references back to it; see nn. 1 and 2 above.

  [6] The relevance of the references here seems to be that Pythagoras was associated with a particular lifestyle which involved both ethical purity and certain specific dietary restrictions; he was also often regarded, in Platonist tradition, as a philosophical forerunner of Plato.

  [7] This reference very probably is to the work Character Traits (Peri ēthōn).

aloe is able to cleanse and strengthen the stomach mouth, to agglutinate wounds, to cicatrize grazes, or to dry moist eyes, there is no difference between the statement that it *is able to cleanse* and the statement that it *has a cleansing capacity*; similarly, 'being able to dry moist eye' means the same as 'having a drying capacity for the eyes'.

In the same way, when we say: 'the rational soul, seated in the brain, is able to perceive through the organs of perception, in itself to remember the objects of that perception and to discern contradiction and consistency between things, and their *analysis* and *synthesis*',[8] this statement means exactly the same as: 'the rational soul has several capacities: those of perception, memory and understanding, as well as all the others.' But since we do not merely affirm that it is able to perceive, but specifically that it is able to hear, smell, taste and touch, we state further that it has the following capacities: visual, acoustic, olfactory, gustatory, tactile. Plato attributes to it also the capacity of desire, using that term in its generic rather than in its specific sense. For he states that the rational soul has a number of desires, as does the spirited part, while the third part has far more still, and a much greater variety; and it is for this reason that he called this last part desiderative par excellence.[9] This is in fact a quite frequent usage, that whereby the pre-eminent member of a class is given the name belonging to that class as a whole. For example, it is commonly said that such-and-such a verse is by 'the Poet', or such-and-such another by 'the Poetess'; and here everyone understands 'Homer' for 'Poet' and 'Sappho' for 'Poetess'. (People use the word 'beast', too, to refer especially to the lion; and there are other similar usages.)

So, that part of the soul which we customarily call the rational is desiderative in the generic sense of that term: it desires truth, knowledge, learning, understanding and recollection—in short, all fine things. Similarly, the spirited is desiderative of freedom, victory, power, authority, reputation and honour. The part which Plato calls desiderative par excellence has the desire for sexual pleasure, and for the enjoyment of all kinds of food and drink. This part can no more have an appetite for fine things than the rational can for food or drink—or indeed for victory, authority, fame or honour. Nor, of course, can the spirited have the same appetites as either the rational or the desiderative.

---

[8] Technical terms in logical and geometrical procedure; see *The Art of Medicine*, Preface, with n. 1, and *Affections and Errors of the Soul* II.4–5, pp. 488–91 below.

[9] The main texts of Plato from which Galen derives the doctrine of the tripartite soul—central not just to his views here and in his ethical works but also to his physiology, as elaborated in *The Doctrines of Hippocrates and Plato*—are the *Republic* (book IV) and the *Timaeus*. Plato does indeed attribute specific desires, *epithumiai*, also to the rational soul, in *Republic* X, 580d ff., in spite of his identification of another part of the soul (that responsible for the desires for food and sex) as specifically 'desiderative' (*epithumētikon*).

3. Now, the fact that there are three forms of the soul, and that this is Plato's view, has been demonstrated elsewhere. So have their respective locations: the liver, the heart and the brain. There is, however, a further belief, that of these three forms or ǀ parts of the whole soul one is immortal; and of this Plato seems 773 convinced. For my part, I am unable to make a confident assertion one way or the other. Let us, then, first consider the forms which reside in the heart and the liver—the forms which both Plato and I agree cease to exist at death.[10] Now each of these organs has its individual substance. Let us not immediately enquire into the precise identity of these substances; let us rather recall that the common substance of all bodies is (as we have shown) comprised of two principles, matter and form. Matter is itself conceptually lacking in quality, but contains within it a mixture of four qualities: heat, cold, dryness and wetness; and these qualities give rise to bronze, iron, gold; and also to flesh, nerve, cartilage, fat and all such entities—those which Plato calls 'first-born' and Aristotle 'uniform'. When, therefore, Aristotle also says that the soul is [the] 'form' of the body,[11] we must ask him—or at least his followers—whether 'form', in this usage, is to be conceived as synonymous with 'shape', ǀ as in that of the organic 774 bodies, or in the sense of the other principle of natural bodies, that which crafts those bodies which are uniform and simple in terms of our perception of them, and devoid of any organic composition. And the Aristotelian response must surely be that it is this latter kind of principle of natural bodies, since indeed it is to these bodies that activities primarily belong.[12] (We have demonstrated this point elsewhere, and if necessary will demonstrate it again.)

Now, if such bodies are composed of matter and form, and Aristotle himself believes that the natural body comes about through the presence of the four

[10] In the *Timaeus* (69c) Plato explicitly refers to the non-rational 'form' of the soul as mortal—a text referred to by Galen elsewhere, in *The Doctrines of Hippocrates and Plato*, IX.9, p. 286 above, where, however, he raises a doubt as to whether this was meant literally by Plato.

[11] Aristotle defined the soul as 'substance in the sense of form of a natural body which potentially has life', *De anima* II.1, 412a19–21. 'Form' (*eidos*) is a technical term in Aristotle, especially used in the context (as in the passage cited) of the form–matter distinction; here *eidos* corresponds to the structure and essential nature of the item in question, understood also in relation to its type or species, as opposed to the matter in which that nature is realized. The term was also the focus of considerable (re)-interpretation in the Aristotelian tradition, including along the lines that Galen here goes on to suggest.

[12] The rather dense argument here is based on a number of Aristotelian texts and a particular interpretation of them. The division into levels of biological composition—elements or fundamental qualities, uniform parts and organic parts—is derived from Aristotle's *Parts of Animals* and is fundamental to Galen's biology. Closely relevant is also the *De anima*, especially the passage cited in the previous note. Galen elsewhere states that it is to the uniform (or 'homoiomerous') parts that the activities primarily belong (*Affected Parts*, III.6, p. 371); and this is in line with his theory of the fundamental 'natural capacities' in plants and animals (e.g. attraction, repulsion) which are properties of such uniform parts as flesh, bone, etc. While the view expressed seems consistent with that theory, it is here complicated by the focus on the still more fundamental level, that of the 'principle which crafts' those uniform bodies, by which is apparently meant the mixture of the lower-level elements or qualities themselves.

qualities in the matter, then he must take the 'form' to be the mixture of these qualities. And so the substance of the soul, too, it seems, would be some mixture of these four qualities, heat, cold, dryness and wetness—or, if one prefers, bodies: the hot, the cold, the dry and the wet.

We have shown that the capacities of the soul depend on its substance since, indeed, its activities do so. If, then, the reasoning form of the soul is mortal, it 775 too will be | a particular mixture (that of the brain),[13] and thus all forms and parts of the soul will have capacities dependent on mixture—this being the substance of the soul. If, on the other hand, it is immortal, as Plato believes, then why does it depart when the brain undergoes excessive cooling, heating, drying or moistening? Plato would have done well to give an equally good explanation of this point as he did of the other matters relating to the soul. According to Plato's account, death takes place when the soul is separated from the body. But why does great loss of blood, or the drinking of hemlock, or a raging fever, cause such separation? If Plato were alive, I would most gladly receive instruction from him on that point. But he is no more, and none of the Platonist teachers has ever shown me the cause of the soul's being compelled to leave the body in the circumstances I have mentioned. I will venture to state, myself, then, that not every form of body is fitted to receive the rational soul. This 776 I see as consistent with Plato's doctrine of the soul, | but I am not able to give a demonstration of it because of my ignorance of the nature of the soul's substance, if we assume it to belong to the class of non-bodily things.

For in the case of bodies, I observe that there are a large number of mixtures, which differ from each other in many respects; but in the case of a non-bodily substance which is able to exist in isolation, without quality or bodily form, I can conceive of no differentiation, in spite of long consideration and investigation of the subject; nor can I see how, if this substance is no part of the body, it can extend throughout the whole body. I have been unable to form even a vague conception of this, though I have for many years desired to. I am aware, however, of the absolutely clear phenomenon that loss of blood or the drinking of hemlock cools the body, while a powerful fever causes it excessive heat. So I repeat the question. Why does the soul definitively leave a body which is excessively cooled or heated? Much research has not provided me with the 777 answer to this, nor to such questions as: why does a build-up of yellow bile | in the head lead to derangement? Or a build-up of black bile to melancholy? Why do phlegm and all the cooling substances cause lethargic complaints, which in turn lead to impairment of the memory and understanding? Why, for that

---

[13] An alternative reading, yielding a subtly but significantly different argument, is: 'If, then, the reasoning [part] is a form of the soul, it will be mortal; for indeed it too will be a particular mixture.'

matter, does the drinking of mandragora [*mōrion*][14] cause insensibility [*mōria*], its name indeed being derived from the effect which we observe it to have on the body? And of course wine relieves us of all distress and low spirits, as our daily experience shows. Zeno apparently remarked that the effect of wine on him was like that of water on lupins, which is to make them sweet. The so-called 'wine-like root' is reputed to have an even greater effect of the same kind; some say that this is the medicine of the Egyptian stranger, of which the Poet says:

> All at once into the wine she threw the herb, and they all drank it—
> Taker of sorrow, of anger, remover or all ills.[15]

Well, never mind the 'wine-like root'. It is not essential | to our argument, when   778 we can every day observe wine having exactly the effects which the poets have described.

> Sweet wine softens you, wine which has always
> Harmed men when they drink to the depths, abandoning measure.
> Wine destroyed Eurytion the great and glorious centaur
> In the high halls of Peirithous the high-spirited Lapith,
> When he was there as a guest. Wine fuddled his spirits;
> Raging he wrought all havoc in king Peirithous' palace.[16]

Elsewhere, too, Homer says:

> [Miserable thing], that causes the wisest of men to go ranting,
> To laugh like a soft-cheeked youth and set his feet dancing
> And to utter a word which best would remain unspoken.[17]

In a similar vein, Theognis:

> Excess drinking of wine is an evil; but if a person
> Drinks of it wisely, then not an evil, a good thing.

It is genuinely true that a moderate amount of wine has excellent effects on digestion, food-distribution, blood-production and nutrition, at the same time as rendering the soul both gentler | and more confident. And these effects are   779 obviously brought about through the medium of bodily mixture, which in turn is produced through the medium of the fluids. The bodily mixture does not just transform the soul's activities, as I have said, but can also cause its separation

---

[14] Here the Arabic version gives the correct reading, whereas all the Greek manuscripts mention hemlock (*kōneion*), making no sense of the etymological connection that Galen is suggesting.

[15] Homer, *Odyssey* IV.220–1. The powerful drug is placed by Helen of Troy (who has received it from a mysterious Egyptian woman) in the wine of her guest Telemachus, who is travelling in search of his father.

[16] Homer, *Odyssey* XXI.293–8.   [17] Homer, *Odyssey* XIV.464–6.

from the body. What other conclusion is possible when one sees drugs with the powers of cooling or over-heating causing the immediate demise of their takers? And the poisons of wild beasts belong in this class too. The bite of the asp is observed to cause instant death, in a way similar to hemlock, since the effect of its venom is also a cooling one.

So one is bound to admit, even if one wishes to posit a specific substance for the soul, at least that it is slave to the mixtures of the body: these have the power to separate it, to cause its derangement, to destroy its memory and understanding, and to lower its confidence and spirit and make it more prone to distress, as happens in cases of melancholy. One must also admit, conversely, that the mod-
780 erate drinker of wine has the opposite characteristics to these. |

4. Is it then the case that the capacities of the soul are so constituted as to undergo change from the hot and cold in mixtures, but not from the dry and the wet? Not at all: both drugs and daily regime provide us with a wealth of evidence of the latter kind of influence. Before turning to the enumeration of these, I should first perhaps recall Plato's account of how the soul, under the influence of the moisture of the body, reaches a state of forgetfulness of those things which it knew before being shackled to it. The following are his precise words in the *Timaeus*, in that part of the work where he describes the gods constructing man by placing the immortal soul in 'a body replete with ebb and flow'.[18] With these words he is obviously making oblique reference to the wetness of substance of the infant. Immediately after this he continues:

> but they, being set in a great river, neither prevailed nor were vanquished, but amid much struggle both were jostled about and moved themselves;

and again, a little later:

> for as the wave was great which bore down on them and flowed away, bringing
781 them nurture, | the sufferings that each one of them underwent from the events that befell them made an even greater disturbance.

And a little further on, going over the account again, he says:

> Because of all these things that befall it, the soul becomes mindless when it first arrives in the mortal body; but when the stream of growth and nurture becomes less, and the revolutions in turn become calm and proceed on their own path, becoming more firmly established as time goes on, then the periods of each of the revolutions adjust themselves to the pattern of the objects that come upon them by nature, addressing the Other and the Same correctly, and cause their possessor to become intelligent.[19]

---

[18] This and the next two quotations come from *Timaeus* 43b.   [19] *Timaeus* 44a–b.

By the phrase 'when the stream of growth and nurture becomes less', Plato obviously refers to the moisture which was mentioned previously as the cause of the mindlessness that obtains in the soul: dryness leads to understanding in the soul, wetness to mindlessness. But since wetness brings about mindlessness, and dryness understanding, the extreme of dryness brings about the extreme of understanding, and dryness which is mixed with wetness will take away from perfect understanding to precisely the degree to which it partakes of wetness. ⏐ What mortal animal has a body entirely devoid of wetness, like the stars? There   782 is none that even comes near it. And so no body of a mortal animal approaches the peak of understanding either: all have their share of mindlessness, just as of wetness. So, given that the rational part of the soul, which has a single-form substance, suffers changes in accordance with the mixture of the body, what are we to imagine becomes of the mortal form of the soul? Surely it cannot but be a complete slave to the body.

In fact, it is preferable to say, not that it is slave to the body, but rather that this is actually what the mortal part of the soul is—the mixture of the body. For it was shown previously that the mortal soul is a bodily mixture.

So, then, the mixture of the heart is the spirited form of the soul, and the mixture of the liver is what Plato calls the desiderative, and Aristotle the nutritive and vegetative. Andronicus the Peripatetic actually dared to make an outright declaration on the substance of the soul, as a free man and without beating about the bush; I have great respect for this man, and I follow his line. (I find him similarly admirable in many other fields.) ⏐ But when he states that it is   783 'either a mixture or a capacity dependent on that mixture', I disagree with the addition of this last phrase. For if it is true that soul is a substance of some kind, endowed with many capacities, and this was correctly stated by Aristotle, who rightly distinguished an ambiguity involved here (substance is used to mean both matter and form and the composite of both, and Aristotle declared that soul is substance in the sense of form), then it is illegitimate to define it as anything but the mixture, as was shown earlier.

The Stoic doctrine, too, belongs within substance under this description. For the Stoics believe soul to be a breath [*pneuma*] of some kind; they believe the same of nature, too, but that the breath of nature is wetter and colder, while that of soul is drier and hotter. Thus, this breath too is the material proper to the soul, but the *form* of the material is a certain kind of mixture which comes about through a good balance of the airy and fiery substance. For one cannot call the soul merely air nor merely fire, since the animal's body cannot become completely cold ⏐ nor completely hot, nor, indeed, completely dominated by the   784 other to a great degree. If one of these qualities is slightly in excess, the animal will have a fever, in the periods of excessive fire, and will be cooled and livid, and will lose perception or even become completely senseless, in the periods when air predominates. For air is itself cold, but in contact with the element of fire becomes well-balanced. Thus, the Stoic view should be evident to you by now: the substance of the soul arises through some mixture of air and fire. So, Chrysippus owed his intelligence to a well-balanced mixture of these elements; and the sons of Hippocrates, those bywords for stupidity among the comedians, reached that state through excessive warmth.[20] Some might conclude from this that Chrysippus should not be praised for his intelligence, nor the sons of Hippocrates blamed for their stupidity; nor, indeed, should praise and blame attach to self-restraint or the lack of it, in the context of the desiderative part of the soul; nor, similarly, to the actions and affections of the spirited part: bravery or cowardice.

785   5. We shall consider this point in what follows. | For the moment let us conclude the argument that we set ourselves at the start. At the same time we should remember that it is not possible to demonstrate every point in every treatise; that there are two fundamental schools of thought in philosophy, one of which believes that the substance of the universe is a unified one, the other that it is interrupted by an admixture of the void; and that we have shown this latter opinion to be false by refutations which can be found in *The Elements according to Hippocrates*. For the purposes of our present argument, we have taken it as an assumption that our substance does undergo alteration, and that the mixture of this substance produces the natural body at the uniform level. On the basis of this hypothesis, then, we have shown that the substance of soul is constituted according to the mixture—unless, with Plato, one assumes it to be non-bodily and able to exist without the body. But even on that assumption, we have given ample proof that its own activities are liable to impairment from the mixture of the body. And there are yet more demonstrations to come.

786 | At this stage we should add a little on the mixtures themselves. For there is a school of thought which says that the soul is the form of the body, but that it is not dryness, but good balance of the mixture, that makes it wiser; in this they differ from those who hold that the soul's intelligence increases in proportion with the dryness of mixture. <And they may even concede that dryness is the cause of intelligence, without conceding that *excessive* dryness is the cause. Now, the followers of Heraclitus—who claimed that 'the wisest soul is a dry ray'—interpret this saying to mean that dryness is the cause of a high level of intelligence, on the grounds that the word 'ray' indicates this. One must consider this view better than the former one, when we observe as grounds for it the fact that the sun and stars, which are shining-dry, have

---

[20] Galen's hostility to Chrysippus (as seen especially in *The Doctrines of Hippocrates and Plato*) is not so great as to deny the philosopher's significance or intelligence. There may be a touch of irony here, but we should remember that Galen's main point of difference with Chrysippus in that text is a specific one, and also that he engaged seriously (albeit critically) with Chrysippus' work on logic: see *My Own Books*, chs. 14 and 18. The 'sons of Hippocrates' bear no relation to the medical Hippocrates but were simply some persons who became bywords for stupidity in classical Athens.

extreme intelligence.>[21] Why, then, do many people lose their wits at the height of old age, a period of life which has been shown to be dry? This is not to be explained by dryness, but by cold: | for this quality manifestly damages all activ-   787 ities of the soul. This point may be beyond our scope here; but it does provide a further clear indication of the proposition we are considering, namely that the actions and affections of the soul depend on bodily mixture. Now if the soul is the form of a uniform body, our demonstration will be derived from its actual essence[22]—which is the most scientific kind of demonstration. If, on the other hand, we accept the Platonic hypothesis of an immortal soul with its own pecu-liar nature, the fact of its domination by and subservience to the body is never-theless conceded, even by Plato himself, in the contexts of mindlessness in infants, in the senile and in people suffering from derangement, *mania*, or forgetfulness—whether as a result of the administering of drugs or of bad fluids that have been produced in the body.

Now, loss of memory, of intelligence, of motion or of feeling resulting from the stated causes can be regarded as impairments of the soul's ability to employ its normal capacities. But cases of people seeing things which are not there, or hearing things that no one said, or making | obscene or blasphemous or indeed   788 completely meaningless utterances, seem to indicate not just a loss of capacities which the soul innately possessed, but the introduction of some opposite cap-acity. This consideration itself might in fact cast considerable doubt on the notion of the non-bodily nature of the whole substance of the soul. For if the soul were not some quality, form, affection or capacity of the body, how could it actually acquire a nature opposite to its own, just by communion with the body? I pass over this point, to avoid a digression which might be longer than our main subject of discussion. At any rate, the overwhelming effect on the soul of the ills of the body is manifestly apparent in the case of people suffering from melancholy, phrenitis or *mania*. And the pathological phenomenon of not rec-ognizing oneself or one's family, which Thucydides reported as widespread and which I too observed in the plague of a few years ago,[23] will appear similar in

[21] The text of this passage is difficult; I have followed the sense of the Arabic version, which seems here to give a better reading. The fragment of Heraclitus (22B118 Diels–Kranz) is also attested in a different version, 'a dry soul is wisest and best' (reading *auē*, 'dry', rather than *augē*, 'ray'); but the version cited here, with its implied relationship to the heavenly bodies, must be the one which Galen knew—and it may even be correct.

[22] *Ousia*, the same word also translated 'substance'. For this criterion of a scientific demonstra-tion, see *The Doctrines of Hippocrates and Plato* II.3, pp. 242–3; and further, on the term *ousia*, *The Shaping of the Embryo*, n. 12, with the cross-references there. In this case I translate 'essence', as it is the logical or definitional sense that is primary: the claim is that the best kind of premiss for a demonstration about X is one derived directly from what X is, in terms of its true essence, or definition. But it may also be possible to interpret the word here in the material or physical sense; the claim would then be rather that, on the hypothesis stated, the demonstration would be based on facts about the soul's fundamental physical nature.

[23] Further on the Antonine Plague and Galen's experience of it, see *Freedom from Distress*, sec-tion 1, with n. 3, and *My Own Books*, ch. 1, with n. 14. The historian Thucydides famously wrote a

effect to impairment of vision due to rheum or cataracts, even though the
789   capacity of sight has not itself been affected. | The most serious impairment of
this capacity is, in fact, that of seeing three images instead of one; and this
condition is paralleled by phrenitis.

6.   Plato is actually aware of the negative effects of bad bodily fluids on the soul.
This is shown by the following quotation:

> When the fluids of sharp and salty phlegm, or any other bitter and bilious
> fluids, wander about the body without finding a path of transpiration, but are
> churned around and mix their vapour with the motions of the soul and are
> blended with it, they cause, to a greater or to a lesser extent, all kinds of dis-
> eases of the soul, few or many; and these, being carried to the three places of
> the soul, multiply the varieties of ill-temper and low spirits, of bravery and
> cowardice, of forgetfulness and ignorance.[24]

In this quotation Plato clearly concedes that the soul is caused harm by the poor
fluid of the body. Another passage, similarly, has disease of the soul caused by a
bodily condition:

790   If the seed | around a person's marrow becomes thick and glutinous, just as in
the case of a tree which is more heavily laden with fruit than the norm, he is
subject to a large number of pains in each part, and of pleasures too, in the
fulfilment of his desires and in the related progeny. This person will be passionate for most of the duration of his life; his soul will be in a state of disease
and insensibility due to the body's enormous pleasures and pains; but he will
be considered not as one suffering from illness, but as one responsible for his
own wrongdoing. The truth, however, is that sexual incontinence is for the
most part a disease of the soul, arising from a particular kind of fluid, moist
condition of the body due to looseness of the bones.[25]

This quotation, too, provides ample evidence of his view that the soul's diseases
are caused by the bad condition of the body. The opinion expressed in the passage immediately following makes the philosopher's opinion equally evident.
Let us consider what he says:

> Practically all ill deeds which are usually regarded as examples of lack of self-
> restraint in relation to pleasure, and therefore as reprehensible, on the
> grounds of their supposedly voluntary nature, are wrongly so regarded, and
> the blame attached to them is unwarranted. No one is willingly bad; one
> becomes bad because of a deficient bodily constitution and uneducated

detailed account of the symptoms and effects of the plague that struck Athens in 430 BC (*History of the Peloponnesian War* II.47–54).
[24] *Timaeus* 86e–87a.   [25] Ibid. 86c–d.

forms of nurture. Such ills are by nature alien to the person and befall him against his will.[26]

All these examples, then, show Plato's | agreement with the propositions which   791
I have previously demonstrated; and many more could be found, some, like those I have just quoted, from the *Timaeus*, others from elsewhere in his work.

7. Aristotle, too, believes that the soul's capacities depend upon the mixture of the mother's blood, from which, in his opinion, our blood derives. This is shown by the following passages. First, from the second book of *Parts of Animals*:

> Thicker and hotter blood produces greater strength, finer and colder blood conduces to greater sensory and mental powers. And a similar difference obtains with the substances which perform the equivalent role to blood [in bloodless animals]. Bees, for example, and other such creatures, are by nature more intelligent than many blooded animals; and, among blooded animals, those with cold, fine blood are more intelligent than the opposite sort. The best have hot, fine and pure blood; these are well endowed with both bravery and intelligence. That is why | the upper parts of animals differ from the lower in this respect, as   792
> also the male from the female and right from left within the body.[27]

It is quite obvious from this passage that Aristotle believes that the capacities of the soul depend on the nature of the body; and later in the same treatise he expresses the same opinion with equal clarity:

> [In their blood] some animals have what are known as 'fibres', and some do not. Gazelle and deer are examples of the latter, and so this kind [of blood] does not solidify. For the watery part of the blood is cold, which prevents it from solidifying, while the earthy part of blood does solidify when the moisture is vaporized in the course of the solidification[; and the fibres are earthy in nature]. And some animals have a sharper intelligence, not because of the coldness of the blood but because of its fineness and purity: earthy natures do not have these two qualities. Animals with lighter and purer moisture have perceptive faculties which are more readily excited, and for this reason even some of the bloodless creatures have more intelligent souls than some of those with blood, as mentioned | above, for example the bee, the ant, and other   793
> similar species. Excessively moist animals, meanwhile, are more timid; for fear has a cooling effect; so those with that kind of mixture in their heart are predisposed to this affection, since water is productive of cold.[28] Thus,

---

[26] Ibid. 86d–e.   [27] *Parts of Animals* II.2, 648a.
[28] I follow here the alternative reading of some of the Greek MSS and (with an error in transcription) that of the Aldine edition, against others that agree with our received version of Aristotle's text; according to this latter group we should read rather 'water is solidified by the cold'. Water is indeed the primarily cold element for Aristotle; and an explanation of the relationship of water to

bloodless animals are, as a generalization, more timid than the blooded variety; in states of fear they tend to become immobile, to excrete, and in some cases to change colour. But those with a multitude of thick fibres are more earthy in nature, and spirited in character, and given to lively emotions because of their spirit: for spirit is productive of heat. Solid bodies when heated cause greater heat than wet ones, and fibres are solid and earthy; they become like embers in the blood, and cause boiling in cases of rage.[29] For this reason bulls and wild boars are spirited and lively: their blood is more fibrous; bulls' blood, in particular, solidifies faster than any. But if one removes these

794   fibres, | blood does not solidify. It is just as if one were to extract the earthy part from mud: the water does not solidify; and so it is with blood. For fibres are made of earth: if they are not removed it will solidify, as wet earth does under the influence of the cold. For when the hot is forced out by the cold, the wet vaporizes too, as stated above; solidification thus takes place through drying which is due not to the hot but to the cold. But, in the case of bodies, it is wet because of the warmth present in animals.[30]

After this preamble, Aristotle proceeds:

> The nature of its blood is the cause of many features of an animal's character and sensory abilities. And this is unsurprising, since blood is the matter of the whole body; for its sustenance is its matter, and the blood is the ultimate sustenance. So, whether the blood is hot, cold, fine, thick, pure or cloudy, makes a considerable difference.[31]

There are in fact many other relevant passages of Aristotle, both in the works

795   on animals and in the *Problems*.[32] It seems to me | unnecessary to set them all out here; for my intention is merely to indicate Aristotle's view on bodily mixture and the capacities of the soul. But I will add something he says in the first book of the *History of Animals*, part of which is directly relevant to mixture, and part through the medium of physiognomical indications. For his opinion here is that the shaping of the whole body is, in each kind of animal, especially fitted to the characteristics and capacities of that animal's soul. For example, in blooded animals birth comes about from the mother's blood, and the soul's characteristics are consequent on the mixture of that blood, as was declared in

---

cold—precisely what the former reading gives us—seems to be what the argument requires at this point, whereas the relevance of the undeniable fact that water freezes seems dubious. I suggest then that the alternative reading should be preferred, also for Aristotle.

[29] Or, 'in the fluids', reading *chumois* with the Greek MSS. But the Arabic and Latin versions suggest 'rage', which also seems to fit the argument better.

[30] *Parts of Animals* II.2, 650b–651a.   [31] Ibid. II.2, 651a.

[32] The *Problems*, now thought to be a work produced by later Aristotelians, contains much material on biology, including on the biological basis of animal behaviour and of mental and emotional states in humans.

the statements cited above. But the shaping of the organic parts of the body, too, comes about in a way appropriate to the soul's characteristics, in Aristotle's own view; and, as is consistent with this, there are many indications concerning both soul characteristics and bodily mixture. Some physiognomical signs indicate bodily mixture directly, without any intermediary. Among these are the characteristics of the complexion and hair, I but also the voice and the motion   796
of limbs. Let us consider Aristotle's remarks in the first book of the *History of Animals*:[33]

> The part of the face below the forehead, between the eyes, is the brow. Those with large brows have a tendency to slowness, those with small ones a quickness in motion; those with wide brows, excitability; those with rounded ones, irascibility.[34]

This is one relevant statement; another, not much further on, runs as follows:

> Below the brow are the eyebrows; straight eyebrows are a sign of softness of character; eyebrows which curve down to the nose, of harshness; those which curve toward the temples, of a tendency to mockery and irony.[35]

And a little later:

> At the meeting-point of upper and lower eyelids are two incisions by the nostril and two by the temples; if these are long, it is a sign of bad character; and if the red part of the eye has something fleshy by the side of the nostril, it is a sign of wickedness.

And then again: 'drawn-down eyebrows, of envy.'
And again, after this:

> The white of the eyes is more or less the same in everyone, but the iris varies. In some it is black, I in some quite blue-grey, in some grey, which is the sign of   797
> the best [character].[36]

And further on he adds:

> Eyes are big or small; but the medium-sized are best. Then, they are prominent or sunken or in between; the sunken ones are the most sharp-sighted in all animals, the ones in between indicate the best character. Then, they are

---

[33] In the quotations that follow there are small differences—both additions and omissions, as well as one transposition—between the text given by Galen and that we know from the MS tradition of Aristotle. Where the MS tradition of Galen is consistent in giving something different from that tradition, these differences have been preserved, rather than 'corrected' in the light of the accepted text of Aristotle.

[34] *History of Animals*, I.8, 491b11–13.

[35] This and the next two citations are from *History of Animals* I.9, 491b.

[36] Ibid. 491b–492a.

inclined to blink or to stare, or somewhere in between; those in between are the best in character, the other kinds indicate inconstancy and shamelessness respectively.[37]

And this is what he says just a little later, about the size of ears:

They are either large, small or medium-sized; and stick out either a lot, not at all, or somewhere in between. Those in between indicate the best character, the large ones and sticking-out ones indicate stupidity or talkativeness.[38]

These are Aristotle's statements in book I of the *History of Animals*. There are 798 plenty more in another work of his, on physiognomic theory,[39] | some of which I would transcribe here too, except that that would give me a reputation for long-windedness, and would use up valuable time, when we have available to us the witness of the man who discovered this science first among philosophers and doctors: the divine Hippocrates.

8. In his treatise on *Airs, Waters, Places* Hippocrates discusses first those cities which he describes as turned towards the north. These are more or less his exact words: 'their characters are wilder rather than gentler.' And with regard to those towards the east: 'they are clear-voiced and better in spirit and understanding than the northerly ones.'[40] Then, discoursing further on the same theme, he continues:

Asia I consider very far removed from Europe in terms of the natures both of the plants that grow in the soil and of the men. Everything grows bigger and better in Asia.[41] Their land is gentler and the characters of the people are kinder and better tempered. The reason for this is the mixture of the climate.[42]

799 He regards mixture | as the reason, not just for the other phenomena he has mentioned, but also for the character traits. And his view is that the mixtures of the seasons differ in terms of heat, cold, dryness and moisture. I transcribed many statements bearing witness to this in the treatise where I demonstrate that Hippocrates maintains the same opinion on the elements in *The Nature of the Human Being* and in all his other writings. And here, in the passage following the one we are considering, the doctrine is the same. This is what he has to say about the land endowed with good-mixture, which gives a good-mixture to the people's character traits, too:

---

[37] Ibid. I.10, 492a7.   [38] Ibid. I.11, 492a–492b.

[39] There is an extant work of *Physiognomics* attributed to Aristotle, although it is not now considered to be authentic.

[40] *Airs, Waters, Places* 4.

[41] Asia in Greek and Roman usage referred to the western area of the Anatolian peninsular.

[42] *Airs, Waters, Places* 12; the next two quotations are from the same chapter.

It is neither excessively burnt by the hot, nor dried out by drought and lack of moisture, nor affected by the cold.

And so, he goes on:

Bravery, endurance, vigour or spiritedness could never take hold in such natures (whether indigenous or foreign): pleasure will necessarily reign.

Further on he says:

As for lack of spirit and lack of bravery, the fact that ⎸ Asiatic men are less war-   800
like and gentler in character than Europeans is explained by the nature of the
seasons, which do not have extremes either of hot or of cold; but are more or
less the same all the time.[43]

Nevertheless, he goes on to add:

You will also observe individual differences between Asiatic people, of whom some are better and some worse. These changes too are due to the seasons, as explained above.

Later on, referring to the inhabitants of Europe, he writes:

Wildness, implacability and spiritedness belong to this kind of nature.[44]

In another passage again, he writes:

The inhabitants of mountainous, rough, high, well-watered land, where the
changes in their seasons are great, are, as one would expect, tall and well-
endowed with endurance and bravery; these natures have a considerable
degree of wild and bestial qualities. But the inhabitants of valleys, of marshy
and humid areas, those who have more warm winds than cold ones, and use
warm waters—these people ⎸ tend to be neither tall nor upright, but stout,   801
fleshy and black-haired. They will be dark rather than light [in complexion],
and more bilious than phlegmatic; and bravery and endurance will not be
constantly present in them by nature, but will have to be established by the
imposition of rule.[45]

By 'rule' Hippocrates obviously here means the way of life that comes to be 'the rule' in any given country, under which should be included nurture, education and local custom, to which I shall return a little later. For the moment, let me add a few more quotations:

---

[43] This and the next quotation are from *Airs, Waters, Places* 16.   [44] Ibid. 23.
[45] Ibid. 24; the next five quotations are from the same chapter.

> The inhabitants of high plains, where it is windy and watery, will be tall and similar to each other, and their characters will be less brave, and gentler in character....

And indeed he continues immediately with the following points about place, writing:

> The inhabitants of narrow, waterless, bare places, which do not enjoy good mixture in terms of changes of season, will tend to be hard in their figures, vigorous, fair rather than dark, and ¦ stubborn and self-willed in their characters and their passions.

802

I need not cite a whole range of Hippocrates' sayings; in the very next line he says:

> You will observe that the physical shape and the behaviour of men varies according to the nature of their country.

And he believes this country itself to differ from other countries in terms of the hot, cold, wet and dry, as is obvious from many statements in that treatise. Thus, he remarks a little further on:

> Where the land is rich, soft, well-endowed with water, with the sources of water high off the ground, so that it is hot in summer and cold in winter, and the place is well situated in relation to the seasons, the people will be fleshy, deficient in their joints, wet, incapable of endurance, and mostly of bad character. They are lazy and sluggish; and when it comes to skilled work, neither sharp nor quick, but clumsy.

Here again he indicates clearly the dependence, not just of character, but also of dullness of intellect and of intelligence, on seasonal balance. There is another similar statement closely following:

803

> Where ¦ the land is bare, dry and hard, beaten by winter weather and burnt by the sun, there you will observe the following features. They are hard, thin, with good joints, vigorous and hairy; there is a fierce industriousness in such natures, and a restlessness; their characters and passions are stubborn and self-willed, with a tendency to wildness rather than to gentleness; they are quicker and cleverer at skilled work, and better at war.

Here, not only does character follow local mixture; but different people have different aptitudes for skilled work—that is to say, some are cleverer, others slower and duller in intellect. By now there should be no need to consider all the physiognomical remarks in books II and VI of the *Epidemics*. Let this single example suffice:

The man in whom the vein in the elbow pulses is impassioned[46] and quick-tempered;[47] the man in whom it is quiet is sluggish.[48]

The sense here is as follows. Men in whom the artery in the elbow produces a I very vehement motion are impassioned. For the ancients referred to arteries 804 too as veins, as I have frequently shown; and they did not refer to every kind of pulse as 'pulse', but only to that kind which is clearly perceptible, which is of course a vehement one. Hippocrates was in fact the initiator of the usage which later came to prevail, talking of all arterial motion, of whatever kind, as 'pulse'. But in the treatise quoted he is still using the old terminology, and what he means is that a vehement motion of the artery is evidence of a passionate and quick-tempered man. This is because what causes such pulsation is an abundance of warmth in the heart. Such warmth makes people impassioned and quick-tempered, whereas a cold mixture makes people lazy, heavy and slow to move.

9. The whole of Hippocrates' discussion of the mixture of waters and the seasons is designed to show that the capacities of the soul depend on the mixtures of the body—and not just the capacities within the spirited and desiderative parts of the soul, but those I in the rational part too.[49] His testimony is more 805 trustworthy than any, if—as is the practice of certain individuals—one were to judge the truth of a doctrine by the reliability of the witness. Personally, I do not trust the man's testimony in that sense, as many do; it is because I see Hippocrates' demonstrations to be secure that I praise him. Anyone can see that the body and soul of people in northerly regions are quite opposite from those near the tropics. And anyone can see, too, that those who live in between the two, in a region that enjoys good mixture, have better bodies and characters and understanding and intelligence than those people.

But there are certain self-styled Platonists who think that the soul, though obstructed by the body in states of disease, performs its own proper activities without assistance or hindrance from the body provided that the latter is healthy. It is, then, because of these individuals that I shall set down some of Plato's remarks which show the effects, both beneficial and harmful, of local

---

[46] The term is *manikos*, related to the medical term *mania*, madness or frenzy; but the term here (and the related one *emmanēs*, which appears twice in the Platonic texts cited) seem to indicate a less extreme or specific emotional state or disposition.

[47] Literally 'sharp-spirited' (*oxuthumos*); the term *thumos*, in the Platonic context referring to a specific range of responses associated with one part of the tripartite soul, the 'spirited', can also simply mean anger or rage.

[48] *Epidemics* II.5.16.

[49] By attributing to Hippocrates, at least implicitly, a position in relation to the three parts of the soul, Galen is engaging in a subtle (and typical) massaging of his textual authorities: the Hippocratic texts are of course quite innocent of Plato's theory of the tripartite soul.

mixture on the intelligence, in cases other than that of bodily illness. In a pas-
806 sage early on in the *Timaeus* I he writes:

> When the goddess had first made provision for you, according to this overall
> arrangement and order, she chose the place for you to be born in with a view
> to the good mixture of its seasons, which would bring forth the most intelli-
> gent sort of men.[50]

And he continues:

> Being both warlike and wise, the goddess chose the place most apt to bring
> her outstanding men, and settled this place first.[51]

Now from this it is already evident that Plato assigns a major role to places, in
the sense of the habitations of the earth, in relation to the character, understanding and intelligence of the soul. But there is more, in the fifth book of
the *Laws*:

> But there is another fact, Megillus and Cleinias, which we should not ignore,
> namely that places differ in their capacity to produce better and worse
> individuals.[52]

Here too he states quite clearly that places give rise to better and worse individuals. And then, continuing this theme, he says:

> A variety of breaths and roastings can cause anomalous and shameless natures,
> as can waters, and also the nurture provided by earth itself. This last has the
> ability not just to affect the body beneficially or harmfully, but, no less, to
> produce all these sorts of effect on the soul.[53]

807 I Here we have a clear affirmation that 'breaths', that is to say winds, and 'roast-
ings', that is the heat of the sun, have the power to affect the capacities of the
soul—in case those Platonists do not believe that breaths, or the heat or coldness of the ambient air, or the nature of waters and nurture, can bring about
improvements or deterioration in men's souls, or further, that these good and
bad effects on the soul are brought about by the medium of the mixture. Such
ignorance may indeed be in keeping with the level of education and understanding that those individuals have attained. We, at any rate, know that everything eaten is first of all sucked down into the stomach, where it undergoes a
preliminary processing; then transported by the veins which lead from the liver
to the stomach; and that it then produces the humoral fluids in the body, by
which all other parts, including brain, heart and liver, are nourished. And in the
process of nutrition these parts become hotter, or colder, or wetter than they were,

---

[50] *Timaeus* 24c.   [51] Ibid. 24c–d.   [52] *Laws* V, 747d1–5.   [53] Ibid. 747d5–e2.

in accordance with the nature of the fluids which predominate. So, then, those who are unhappy at the idea that nourishment I has this power to make people 808 more prudent, more undisciplined, more or less restrained, brave, timid, soft, gentle, quarrelsome or argumentative, should even now show enough prudence to come to me and receive instruction on their diet. They would derive enormous benefit from this in the context of ethical philosophy;[54] and the improvement in their rational capacities, too, would have an effect on their virtue, as they acquired greater powers of understanding and memory. Apart from food and drink, I would teach them about winds and mixtures in the ambient air, and even about which lands they should select and which avoid.

10. And let me remind them once more—even if they don't like it—what Plato himself, from whom they take their name, wrote on these subjects, and wrote not once or twice, but on many occasions. For present purposes three passages will suffice, two on the drinking of wine, from book II of the *Laws*, one on nourishment, from the *Timaeus*. From *Laws* II: I 809

> Let us then make the following stipulations. To begin with, up to the age of eighteen, children should not touch wine at all, for our instruction should be not to not add fire to fire, in body and soul, before the individual embarks upon labours. One must take into account the impassioned nature of the young. After this, up to the age of thirty, one should drink wine in moderation; but the young man should abstain from drunkenness and excess altogether. As he reaches forty a man should, as he lies at feasts, not just invoke the other gods, but indeed call upon Dionysus too, for the sacrament and recreation of old men. It is for this that Dionysus gave men the gift of wine, as a drug to assist us against the harshness of age. It dissipates sorrow and depression, and softens the hardened character of the soul. The effect is like that of an iron placed in fire; in the same way the soul becomes malleable.[55]

I would draw to the attention of those venerable Platonists the statements in this passage about the differences due to age, as well as those about the drinking of wine. I Plato states that the age of youth is impassioned, and that of old men 810 harsh, low-spirited and hard. The basis for this is not the number of years, but the bodily mixture that belongs to each time of life. The mixture of youth is hot and full-blooded, that of old age lacking in blood and cold. Wine-drinking is therefore of use to old men; it brings the coldness due to old age back to an

---

[54] Note that the word standardly translated as ethical, *ēthikos*, is literally the adjective related to *ēthos*, character: what these people will gain by his advice, Galen is saying, is improvement in their characters. And *ēthos* in this sense is contrasted with the domain of reason or the rational soul; hence the distinction here between this and intellectual capacities. See also *Affected Places*, n. 4.

[55] *Laws* II, 666a–c.

equal balance with warmth. The effect on one who is still growing, though, is the opposite. Here the effect is that of over-heating a physique which is already boiling and liable to vehement movements, thus inflaming it to immoderate and excessive actions. In fact, Plato wrote a good deal in book II of the *Laws* on the drinking of wine, apart from what has already been quoted. It is set down there for anyone with the inclination to read something which might benefit him. I shall quote only one more passage, which comes at the end of all the discussion of wine-drinking, where he expresses a preference for the Carthaginian rule. It is as follows:

811   But even more than the Cretan or Spartan custom, I would support ⎸ the Carthaginian rule, that no soldier should partake of wine while on a tour of duty, restricting himself rather to water-drinking throughout that whole period; that, in the city, slaves, whether male or female, should never touch it; that magistrates should not do so during their year of office; that helmsmen and active jurors should not do so at all, nor anyone intending to participate in any major deliberation of the Council; nor anyone at all during the day, except for medical reasons; nor should either the man or the woman indulge at night, if they are planning to make babies. And there are many other circumstances in which right-thinking, well-ordered individuals will abstain from wine.[56]

These conditions Plato lays down not for ailing bodies but for those in perfect health—if, that is, o most venerable Platonists, you agree that it is persons in a state of good health who fight, administer a city's affairs, sit on juries or steer ships. I would ask you then to answer the following question: is it not the case that wine acts like a tyrant, commanding the soul not to think clearly as it did before, nor to perform its previous actions correctly? And is that not the reason

812   that Plato tells us to protect ourselves against it ⎸ as against an enemy? Once it arrives in the body, it prevents the helmsman from handling the rudder as he should and the soldier from behaving with discipline in the ranks; causes the juror to blunder when he has most need of correct judgement and all magistrates to administer matters badly and issue unsound instructions. Plato's view is that wine, by filling the whole body, especially the head, with hot vapours, is the cause of immoderate action on the part of the desiderative and spirited parts of the soul, and of hasty judgement on the part of the rational.

Now, if all this is so, the above-mentioned activities are clearly damaged, through the medium of mixture, by wine-drinking; and certain others are clearly assisted. If you wish, I shall give instruction on this subject on another occasion; I shall show precisely which activities are harmed and which assisted

---

[56] Ibid. 674a–b.

by wine. For now let me transcribe a statement of Plato's from the *Timaeus*, which begins as follows:

> Thus all bad men are bad because of two causes, which are completely outside their control. And for these causes one should hold the begetter responsible rather than the begotten, and I the nurturer rather than the one nurtured.[57]   813

He goes on:

> We should try wherever possible to use nurture, practices and studies in order to avoid evil and choose its opposite.[58]

For just as 'practices and studies' dispel evil, and engender virtue, so it is with 'nurture'. And, though he uses the term 'nurture'[59] to mean the whole regime of a child, not just food, this is definitely not the sense here. For the sentence, 'We should try, etc.', is not an instruction for children but for adults. By 'practices' he means physical exercises and cultural pursuits; by 'studies' he means geometry and mathematics; and 'nurture' here can only mean that which is derived from food, gruels and drinks, including wine—the subject on which Plato expatiated in such detail I in book II of the *Laws*.   814

If anyone wishes to learn more than what is said there, on the whole topic of the capacities of foods, he may read three books of mine on the subject,[60] and a fourth on *Good and Bad Humoral Fluid*, which is the most relevant to the present subject. Bad humoral fluid has a large number of adverse effects on the activities of the body, while good fluid keeps them in perfect condition.

11. Our argument is thus not destructive of the fine teachings of philosophy, but rather a source of guidance and instruction on a philosophical point which is however not recognized by philosophers themselves. For those who believe that all are receptive to virtue (which is equivalent to saying that no one is by nature bad), and those who say that none naturally chooses justice—both err, in presenting human nature from a one-sided perspective. Not all are born enemies of justice, nor all its friends; and people of each of those kinds come about through bodily mixture. How then, they say, can one be justly praised, blamed, loved or hated for good or evil qualities which are not due to oneself I but to a mixture, which obviously derives from other sources? Our reply is that   815 it is a human universal to show affection, inclination and love for the good, and to reject, despise and flee the bad, without first asking whether or not these qualities are innate, nor whether something else has made it so or whether it

---

[57] *Timaeus* 87b.   [58] Ibid.
[59] *Trophē*, 'nurture', is also translatable as 'nutrition', and may have that narrower sense as well as the broader one where it includes a range of child-care inputs; but Galen's interpretation here is tendentious.
[60] The reference is to *The Capacities of Foodstuffs*.

has brought itself to that condition. We destroy scorpions, venomous spiders, and vipers, which owe their characters to nature, not to themselves. Plato, who talks of the first and greatest god as unoriginated, also calls him good; and we all naturally love him, though he is so from eternity and has not become good by his own agency. Indeed, he did not 'become' at all, being, rather, entirely unoriginated and eternal.

It is reasonable then that we should despise the wicked, without first investigating the cause that made them so; and, conversely, that we should love and feel attachment to the good, whether their goodness derives from nature, from education and instruction, or from choice and training. We even kill the irre-
816 deemably ǀ wicked, and for three good reasons: so that they may not harm us while they live; as a deterrent to others like them, who will fear punishment for their crimes; and, thirdly, because it is actually better from their own point of view to die, when their souls have been so severely damaged that their vice is incurable, and they can no longer benefit from the education even of the Muses themselves, or be improved even by Socrates or Pythagoras.

In this context I find the position of the Stoics extraordinary: they believe that all men are naturally fitted for the acquisition of virtue but are turned away from it by the influence of those around them. Leaving aside everything else which undermines this argument, let me just ask one question, regarding the very first human beings, the ones who had no predecessors. How did their corruption come about, and at whose hands? There is no possible answer to this. And if one sees some particularly wicked child today, it is also impossible to answer the question, who taught him that wickedness—especially so when
817 there are many children who have been brought up in the same way, ǀ by the same parents, teachers or masters, but who have opposite natures. For is not generosity in a child the complete opposite of meanness, and compassion of malice, timidity of courage, extreme stupidity of extreme intelligence, honesty of mendacity? And all these differences are to be observed in children who have had exactly the same upbringing.

We should be on our guard against such statements from our present-day philosophers—or I should say, rather, not philosophers but those who profess to practise philosophy. If they were true practitioners of philosophy, they would have concerned themselves first and foremost to take manifestly observed facts as the starting-points of their demonstrations. The most ancient of the philosophers surely followed this practice more than anyone, and gained their reputation for wisdom not by writing treatises, nor by displays of dialectical theory
818 or natural philosophy, but because ǀ they founded their study of the virtues on evident facts and then cultivated these virtues in practice, not verbally. So, then, when these philosophers observed that children, even the best educated of them, who have no example of vice before them, nevertheless make mistakes right from the outset—for it is extremely rare to see a perfect child—they

arrived at two different conclusions. Some of them declared that in fact there was no such thing as a perfect child, since they had observed none such, and that human beings are all by nature bad; others, who perhaps had observed the occasional one or two such children, decided that this is true not of all, but of most, human beings.

Certainly if one observes the facts with an open mind, as the ancient philosophers did—and if one is not motivated by a desire for quarrel or competition—one will see very few children who are well endowed from the point of view of virtue, and so will cease to claim that we are in fact all so endowed, but corrupted by parents, teachers and instructors. (For those are the only contacts that children have.) And it is foolish to claim, as some do, that we are corrupted by | pleasure and pain, the one leading towards itself, the other repelling us by   819 its unattractiveness. For if we are all naturally adapted[61] to pleasure, which is not a good but, as Plato says, 'a great incitement to evil', all are then bad by nature; or, if not all of us, but only a certain group, are so adapted, then that group is the only naturally bad one. For indeed, if there were in us no other capacity, adapted to virtue rather than to pleasure, or no capacity stronger than that which leads us naturally to pleasure, we would all be bad, since the better capacity would be the weaker and the bad one the stronger. But if this better force is stronger, then who was it that persuaded the first men to be vanquished by a weaker force? This was Posidonius' criticism of the Stoics; and Posidonius deserves the highest praise precisely for those things for which the rest of the Stoics attacked him. The resolve of those other Stoics was to betray their own country before they would betray their doctrines; Posidonius, on the other hand, preferred to betray the Stoic sect rather | than the truth. For this reason,   820 both in his work on *Affections of the Soul* and in that on *Distinctions between Virtues*, he takes an opposite view to Chrysippus, and makes many criticisms of what Chrysippus wrote in his *Logical Investigations*, but still more of what he wrote in his *Distinctions between Virtues*.

So, not even Posidonius thinks that evil enters from outside, without any root in our souls, from which to germinate and grow. There is in fact a seed of evil within us; and we have a far greater need to seek out those who will cleanse us and prevent the growth of this evil, than to avoid bad people. The Stoic view, that evil comes into us from outside, is wrong: bad people derive the majority of their badness from within, while the part due to external influence is much smaller. Now, it is this part that accounts for bad habits accruing in the non-rational part of the soul, and false opinions in the rational, just as, | if we are educated   821 by good, upright individuals, we acquire correct views and good habits.

---

[61] Galen here adopts Stoic terminology, using a verb form related to *oikeiōsis*, but rather differently from the Stoic technical sense, where it refers to the child's developing sense of what *belongs* to it as an individual; see similarly *The Doctrines of Hippocrates and Plato* V.5, with n. 25.

In the rational part of the soul mental sharpness and various degrees of fool-ishness are dependent on mixture, and so, in the non-rational soul, are well- or poorly-balanced motions, these too in different degrees. And mixture itself is consequent on the original formation and on a daily regime involving good humoral fluid. So, these phenomena are mutually reinforcing. The quick-tempered become so because of the hot mixture, but then by their quick-temperedness inflame their inborn heat. Conversely, people with a well-balanced mixture enjoy well-balanced motions of the soul, and are thus assisted towards a good state of the humoral fluids.[62]

Thus, our argument accords with clearly observed facts. It explains the causes of the effects that we experience from wine and from drugs, as well as from good and bad daily regime. It explains, further, why we experience beneficial and harmful effects from certain kinds of training and education; and, last but not least, it provides an account of the natural differences between children. Those who do not agree that the soul derives benefit and harm from the mix-ture of the body have no explanation whatsoever to give of differences in chil-
822 dren, nor of the benefits derived from daily regime, | nor of those differences in character which make people spirited or otherwise, or intelligent or otherwise.

The Scythians have only ever had one philosopher,[63] while the Athenians have had many; conversely, there are many stupid people at Abdera, at Athens very few.

---

[62] Reading *euchumia* ('a good state of the fluids') with the Arabic and Latin versions, for *euthu-mia* ('good temper'). Both readings are possible, but the restoration of *euchumia* seems in accord with the *reciprocal* nature of the relationship between psychological states and bodily mixture that Galen is here asserting.

[63] The reference is to the semi-legendary Scythian philosopher-prince Anacharsis.

Affections and Errors of the Soul

Alongside *Freedom from Distress*, this is the only work surviving in Greek from Galen's twenty-odd treatises on ethical questions.[1] It shows him in the persona of philosopher rather than doctor, and engaging in a discourse which had a significant profile and gave rise to a considerable amount of literature in the Roman imperial period—that of practical ethics or the 'therapy of the soul'. He is here writing in the same vein, and addressing the same issues, as such philosophical contemporaries or near-contemporaries as Epictetus, Plutarch, Marcus Aurelius or (in Latin) Seneca.

At the same time, this form of philosophy is conceived as in a sense medical: its aims are therapeutic, though therapeutic of the soul rather than of the body—that is, aimed at one's ethical or emotional wellbeing; and medical language (e.g. diagnosis, cure, correction, excision, healing) constantly underlies this discourse, at least at the level of metaphor. For Galen as for the other writers mentioned there is a strong parallelism—which can be traced back at least to Plato—between the health of the body and the health of the soul. In the present treatise, then, it is precisely that *parallel* that is to the fore, rather than (as in certain other texts, in particular *The Soul's Dependence on the Body*, or *Health*) a direct *influence* of the health or pathology of the one upon that of the other. In this sense, the present work—along with *Freedom from Distress*—belongs to a distinct category and has a distinct project from that of the works of medicine or of scientific methodology.

Underlying this therapeutic project is the distinction, central to Galen's Platonist psychology, between the rational and non-rational parts of the soul. A mistake on the part of the former—an error of judgement or reasoning—is a *hamartēma*, 'error'. The non-rational part, meanwhile, is the domain of *pathos*—an inappropriate or excessive emotive response of any kind. The translation 'affection' has been preferred for this technical term (other translations sometimes used include 'passion', 'affect' and 'emotion').

The date of this work, and in particular its chronological relationship with *Freedom from Distress*, has been a matter of debate. The apparent conflict in evidence for this (see nn. 14, 21 and 22 below) may perhaps be accounted for by the work's particular oral–literary nature: as explained at the outset (and as we are reminded by occasional 'I said' parentheses in the course of the text), it is a written version of a talk given on an earlier occasion, and so in its final form might have elements belonging to different phases of composition.

The textual transmission of the treatise is particularly problematic, by comparison with that of most of Galen's works: we rely on a single Greek manuscript, which contains

---

[1] See *My Own Books*, ch. 15. *Character Traits* survives in an epitomized form, in Arabic (and is translated in Singer 2013).

many scribal errors and peculiarities. Alongside places where the reading or interpretation is uncertain, there are also a number of unfortunate lacunae.[2]

Greek title: Περὶ διαγνώσεως καὶ θεραπείας τῶν ἐν ἑκάστου ψυχῇ παθῶν καὶ ἁμαρτημάτων (*Peri diagnōseōs kai therapeias tōn en hekastou psuchēis pathōn kai hamartēmatōn*). (The full title of the treatise—which may regarded either as a pair or as two books of the same work—translates into English as: *The Diagnosis and Treatment of the Affections and Errors of Each Individual Soul.*)
Kühn: V.1–113
Edition: Marquardt 1884; De Boer 1937
Translation with introduction and commentary: Singer 2013

I. Affections

V.1   1. You want a written version of the answer I gave you orally to your question concerning Antonius the Epicurean's book on *The Control of the Individual Affections*; I shall now make you one, and this is its beginning.

    Antonius should himself have made clear what he means by the term 2 'control'. To judge by the statements contained in the I book, he may be using it to denote either watchfulness or diagnosis—and possibly also correction. It also turned out, as you know, that he was unclear in most of his verbal expressions, so that they are objects of conjecture rather than of clear understanding.

    Sometimes he seems to be encouraging us to contemplate that we too, like others, commit many errors; at other times how one may discern[3] each of our errors; and, then again, how to lead oneself away for the errors—which would seem to me to be the aim of the entire discussion, for none of the matters previously stated is of any value unless it is related to this.

    Above all, his exposition would have been improved by a distinction between affections and errors. Sometimes the argument seems to refer to affections only, and often to errors; at other times you have the impression that he is discussing both. I, as you know, made this very distinction at the outset; I defined error [*hamartēma*] as arising from false opinion, and affection [*pathos*] as arising 3 from some non-rational capacity I within us that is disobedient to reason. I added that through a more generic usage both may also be referred to commonly as errors: in this way, we may refer to one acting without self-discipline, one acting in rage and one being taken in by a slander all as committing an error.

---

   [2] I have not commented on all the individual problems of translation, nor mentioned every departure from Marquardt's or De Boer's edition, in the notes here. For further detail and discussion of variant readings and interpretations see Singer 2013.

   [3] *Diaginōskein*, the verb cognate with *diagnōsis*; see *The Art of Medicine*, n. 4.

Many philosophers, including Chrysippus, have written works on the treatment of the affections of the soul; and even Aristotle and his followers, and before them Plato, wrote about it. It would have been better to learn from these people, as I did. In this first part I shall set out all the main points concisely, as you request, in the order in which you already heard them when you made the enquiry about Antonius' book.

2. It is likely that we are in error even when we believe ourselves to be in no way mistaken, as may be deduced from the following line of reasoning. We observe that all human beings imagine either that they are completely free from error or that their mistakes are very few, small and infrequent; and that the people who are ∣ most strongly under this impression are those that others 4 think make the most errors. I, for one, have found that if any proposition is supported by experience it is this one. I have observed that those who submit their own personal character to the judgement of others are seldom in error, while those who assume their own superiority without relying on the assessment of other people perpetrate the greatest and most frequent mistakes.

That respect, then, which in my youth I used to think excessive, for the Pythian oracle's 'Know thyself'[4] (the injunction did not seem a difficult one), I later found to be justified. It is only the wisest of men who could be said to know himself in the exact sense; no one else knows himself in that way, although some know themselves better than others. In all aspects of life, and in every specialized skill, everyone may recognize very large distinctions and differences, but only the highly expert or skilled person will recognize the subtle ones. So it is with errors and affections.

If someone becomes so vehemently angry over trivialities ∣ that he bites and 5 kicks his household servants, he is quite obviously in a state of affection; so too one who gives himself over to drinking, whoring and wild parties. A moderate level of emotional disturbance at a great financial or reputational loss, on the other hand, is a much less clear case of affection, as is a slightly excessive indulgence in cake; yet these too become obvious to one who has previously exercised his soul[5] and wishes to find out all those affections in need of correction—even if the failure to avoid these is less reprehensible, since they are small.

Therefore whoever wishes to become a decent person[6] should bear in mind that he is necessarily unaware of many of his own errors. How to find them all

---

[4] This injunction (in Greek *gnōthi seauton*) was inscribed on the Temple of Apollo at Delphi, and came—initially through its importance for Socrates and Plato—to be considered a fundamental element of the ethical project.

[5] The text and meaning from here to the end of the sentence are somewhat uncertain.

[6] The Greek is *kalos kagathos*, literally 'fine and good'—a conventional phrase which indicates an accepted norm of civilized behaviour, as well as having some connotations of belonging to a 'gentlemanly' social elite.

out—as I did in my own case—I shall not yet say, so that any others into whose hands this pamphlet may come may first train themselves to discover the way to discover their own errors. So, just as I encouraged you to tell me, and listened
6 in silence while you disclosed your opinions, I will now l do the same, exhorting the reader to put it down and enquire how one may recognize one's own errors.

We have, as Aesop used to say, two wallets strapped around our necks—the one in front is full of other people's wrongdoings, the one behind full of ours, so that we always see other people's but are consistently unable to see our own. Everyone recognizes this to be the truth; Plato adds the reason for the phenomenon. 'The lover,' he says, 'is blind towards the object of love.'[7] Now, since each of us loves himself best of all, he must necessarily be blind with regard to himself. How, then, is he to see his own evils? How is he to realize when he goes wrong? Aesop's fable and Plato's account seem to prove the utter hopelessness of discovering our own errors: one cannot distance oneself from self-love, and the person who is subject to this love is necessarily blind with regard to its object. Well, I would not have encouraged the reader to embark upon the business of
7 examining l the path towards the discovery of his own errors, if the matter were not a difficult one, even for a person who is highly advanced in it.

Let me declare my own opinion. So, anyone who finds a different way may take mine as well, and be benefited by the abundance of two ways of salvation instead of one. Otherwise, he may continue with mine until he finds a better. It is time, then, to say what mine is; here is the beginning of my account.

3. Since errors arise from false opinion, while affections arise from irrational impulse, I judged that one should first free oneself from the affections: it is not unlikely that these may in themselves constitute another source of false opinion. There are affections of the soul that are universally acknowledged as such: rage,[8] anger, fear, distress, envy, powerful desire; and I would add excessive haste in forming love or hatred for any object as another affection. 'Moderation
8 is best' seems to me a good saying: nothing l that happens without moderation is good.

So, how should one excise these affections, when one is not aware of having them in the first place? This awareness, as we were saying, is rendered impossible by our excessive self-love. But this argument, while it prevents you from judging yourself, at the same time admits the possibility of someone else carrying out the judgement, namely a person whom you neither love nor hate. So, when you hear some citizen being praised on all sides for not indulging in flattery, make his acquaintance and judge from your own observation whether his

---

[7] Plato, *Laws* V, 731e.
[8] *Thumos*, also sometimes translated 'spirit': the word may refer both to a particular capacity or part within the soul (the middle one in Plato's tripartite scheme) and to the particular pathology or pathological state of that part, anger or rage.

character accords with his reputation. First of all, if you see him constantly visiting the houses of the rich and powerful, let alone those of kings, you may be sure that his reputation is false. Such a man cannot always tell the truth; lying is a necessary consequence of such flattery. Similarly, if you observe that he greets such people, or attends upon them, or indeed that he dines with them. Someone who has chosen that kind of life will not just be a liar; he will of necessity be involved in every kind of corruption, | being as he is obviously devoted 9 to one or all of money, power, status and reputation. If you find a man who does not greet, attend upon or dine with men of power and wealth, a man who follows an ordered lifestyle, you may hope that he speaks the truth. But you must attempt to learn his character more deeply—something which can only be done over a prolonged acquaintance. If you feel that this is his true character, take some opportunity to speak to him in private. Ask him to tell you quite openly which of the above-mentioned affections he sees in you, emphasizing the gratitude you will feel towards him: he will be your healer, even more so than the man who heals your body.

If, then, he promises that, whenever he sees you in the grip of one of these affections, he will make it known to you, but after an interval of several days has still said nothing, in spite of having spent a considerable amount of time in your company, then you should take him to task, and again ask him (even more pleasantly than before) to let you know directly of any act of yours which he observes to have been committed under the influence of affection. If he replies that his silence is due to his having observed no such action in you in the intervening period, do not readily believe him. Do not imagine that you have suddenly become perfect. | There are two possible explanations. Either 10 this friend has been lazy in his observation of you, or he is ashamed to criticize, or even afraid of your hatred, since he will be aware that men who speak the truth are almost universally despised. Or else the reason might be a reluctance to help you—or some other reason which would be reprehensible. You may believe me when I say that it is impossible that you did no wrong at all; and you will verify this later when you see that all men make countless errors every day, and succumb to countless affections, but are never themselves aware of it. You should not imagine that you are some other kind of being than a human. And that is what you are imagining, if you fool yourself into thinking that you have acted perfectly for an entire month—or even a whole day. Of course, if you are a disputatious sort (by choice, by some bad habit of character into which you have fallen, or just because of natural | quarrelsomeness), 11 you may say that, according to my account, the wise are the ones who are not human.

Take this reply, which is in two parts. First, it is only the wise man who is completely free from error. The second part has reference to this statement that if a wise man is perfect he is not human. As to that, consider the words of the most ancient philosophers, that wisdom is an 'approximation to god'.[9] But it is impossible, in your case, that you have suddenly become similar to a god. If people who have cultivated freedom from the affections throughout their lives are not reckoned to have attained perfection in it, certainly it cannot be so for you, who have never practised it at all, and thus you should not believe someone who says that he has not seen you acting under the influence of an affection. If he says this, it is because he does not wish to help you, or has not taken the trouble to watch closely for your shortcomings, or is wary of incurring your ill will. He may even have seen you at some time get angry with someone who criticized you for your errors or affections; and therefore he very reasonably says 12 nothing, out of a distrust of your sincerity | when you say you want to know all your errors. But if you first of all separate yourself from your own actions, and remain silent, you will find that after a while people will generally put you right, especially if you thank them for their blame on the grounds that they are assisting you to be free of the harm. Just the exercise of considering whether their criticism is true or not will be of great benefit to you. If you do this continually, out of a genuine resolve to become a decent human being, you will become one.

In the first phase, even if after careful examination you arrive at the judgement that you have been unjustly and falsely criticized, do not attempt to argue that you have done no wrong. This is the first rudiment of philosophy, to put up with unfair criticism. Later, as you observe a reasonable decline in your affections, you will try to justify yourself against malicious attacks—but never in a shrill or argumentative way, never from a competitive spirit or a desire to do the other person down. You will do it for your own benefit: if his reply to your self-13 justification is plausible, you will either be convinced of his | superior awareness or, on further examination, find that his accusations are unfounded. This was the formula approved by Zeno to ensure good conduct: that we shall be secure in our actions if we imagine that we shall shortly have to justify them to our tutors. That was what he called the mass of people who are ready to offer unsolicited criticism of their fellows.

And the recipient of such criticism will have to be neither rich nor possessed of political position. In the latter case fear will prevent anyone from telling him the truth, in the former monetary gain will prevent his flatterers; and even if someone did appear to tell such a man the truth, he would stand aloof from him. If, then, someone of great power or wealth desires to become a decent human being, he must first put those things from him—and especially so today. For where will he now find a Diogenes, to tell the same truth irrespective of wealth or power, even to a king? Anyway, we must let those sort of people make their own decision. You, who are neither wealthy nor influential in the affairs of

---

[9] The phrase *homoiōsis theōi* comes originally from Plato, *Theaetetus* 176b; the use of the phrase to characterize virtue, or the aim of the good life, became prominent in the Platonic tradition.

the city, should entreat everyone to tell you what they dislike in your behaviour, and in this way have the whole world— | to use Zeno's word—as your tutors.   14

Now, I do not say that you should not give equal weight to everyone's opinions: the ones to be particularly respected are those of men advanced in years, who have led the best kind of lives. (The characteristics of those who live such lives have been considered above.) As time goes on you will achieve such awareness even without their comments, and you will recognize the nature of the errors you used to commit. At that point, indeed, you will be struck by the truth of my statement, that no one is free of affections or errors, not even the person with the best natural endowments, brought up in the best of practices, and that there will always be some mistakes, especially when one is young.

4. For becoming a perfect man is a goal which requires in each of us a discipline that will continue through practically the whole of his life. One should not put aside the possibility of improving oneself even at the age of 50, if one is aware of some defect one's soul has sustained, provided that defect is not incurable or irremediable. If one's body were in a bad state at that age, one would not give oneself up to the bad condition; one would by all means attempt to improve it, | even if one   15 were not able to achieve a Heraclean sort of good condition. No more, then, should we refrain from efforts to achieve a better state of the soul. Even if that of the wise man is beyond us—though we shall have a high hope of attaining even that state, if we have taken care of our soul from early youth—then at least we should exert ourselves that our soul be not utterly disgusting, as was Thersites' body.[10]

If it had lain in our power before being born to meet the one who had foresight[11] over our birth, we would have asked him to let us have the finest type of body. If he had refused this, we would have requested of him the second, third or fourth from the first, in terms of good condition. It would be a highly desirable outcome, even if we could not get the body of a Heracles, to have at least that of an Achilles, and failing that, that of an Ajax, a Diomedes, an Agamemnon, a Patroclus; and failing those, the body of some great hero or other. It is just the same with the soul. If one is unable to attain the most perfect good condition, one should surely accept the second, third or fourth | from the top. Such a goal   16 is quite achievable for one who is prepared to exert himself over a long period in a process of constant discipline.

In my youth—when I had already been given the above advice—I once saw a man in a hurry to open a door. When he could not get it to open, he began to bite the key, to kick the door, to curse the gods; his eyes went wild like those of

---

[10] Heracles is taken as exemplary of the best possible body, while Thersites (mentioned by Homer, *Iliad* II.216–19) was the ugliest man who came to Troy, and physically deformed. Between the two there is a traditional heroic hierarchy; the characters mentioned in the next paragraph are the most outstanding Greek warriors of the *Iliad*.

[11] On 'foresight' (*pronoia*, verb *pronoeisthai*) see also *The Best Doctor is Also a Philosopher*, n. 1.

a madman, and he was all but frothing at the mouth like a wild boar. The sight caused me to hate anger so much that I would never appear thus disfigured by it. This is sufficient to begin with: that one does not curse the gods, kick or bite objects of stone or wood, or take on the appearance of a wild man, but rather that one keeps a check on one's anger, and conceals it within. To be free of anger is a goal one cannot achieve simply by wishing it; what one can do is to control the ugly manifestation of the affection. And if one does so frequently, one will actually notice one's anger becoming less than it was previously, so that one no 17 longer gets angry over either small or I large matters to a large degree, but only over large ones, and that to a small degree.

Eventually, then, one may achieve the goal of not getting angry even over large matters; important, here, is a restraint that I have observed ever since imposing it on myself in, that of never laying a hand upon a household servant. This was a discipline practised by my father too, who frequently berated friends who had bruised their hands in the act of hitting servants in the teeth. He would say that they deserved to suffer convulsions and die from the inflammations they had sustained. They could perfectly well have waited just a little and applied the number of blows they wished, with a cane or a strap, carrying out the task in accordance with their judgement. Some have even been known to use not only their fists but even their feet on their servants, or to stab them with a stilus which they happen to be holding.[12] Once I even saw a man lose his temper and strike his servant in the eye with a reed-pen. And it is related of the emperor Hadrian that he once struck one of his household staff in the eye with a stilus, causing him to lose the sight of one eye. When Hadrian realized what had happened, he summoned the servant and agreed to grant him a gift of his own 18 request in exchange for the loss he had suffered. I But the injured party was silent. Hadrian repeated his offer, encouraging the man not to be shy but to request anything he wished. At which the servant replied that he wanted nothing but his eye back. For what gift could compensate for the loss of an eye?

I should also like to remind you of something that once happened to me, even though I have spoken of it on many previous occasions. On a return home from Rome I was travelling in the company of a friend from Gortyn in Crete, who was in other respects a worthy man—straightforward, friendly, kind, generous in his daily expenditure—but whose temper was such that he would regularly use his hands on his servants, and sometimes his legs too. More frequently, though, he would attack them with a leather strap, or with any wooden object that came to hand. When we reached Corinth, he decided to send his luggage

---

[12] This and the last sentence were thought to be scribal interpolations by Marquardt. In spite of the callousness and uncongeniality of the sentiments, however, there seem no good textual grounds to suspect them: it is uncontrolled anger, causing one to lash out immediately, and with one's own hands, that is the object of Galen's criticism, not every instance of corporal punishment carried out on one's household staff.

and his servants—all but two—from Kenchreai to Athens by boat, while we proceeded with a hired carriage by land, via Megara. We had just passed Eleusis, and were in Thriasion, when he turned to the servants he had kept with him, I and enquired about a certain item of luggage. They knew nothing about it. 19 And so he flew into a rage, and, as he had nothing else with which to strike the boys, seized a great knife which was lying there in its sheath, and brought it down, sheath and all, on the heads of both of them, not striking them with the flat of the knife (which would not have been so disastrous), but with the edge. The blade cut straight through the sheath, and both servants suffered two very serious injuries—he had hit each of them twice—to the head.

When he saw the great quantity of blood that was flowing, he fled, and ran in the direction of Athens, panicking that one of his servants might die in his presence. In the event, I saved them, and brought them to Athens. My Cretan friend, meanwhile, was thoroughly disgusted with himself. He took me by the hand, led me into a house somewhere, and offered me a strap with which he asked me to beat him for what he had done under the influence of—in his own words— his accursed rage. I responded, as you would expect, with laughter; but at this he fell to his knees and begged me to do exactly as he had asked. And of course, I the more earnest his entreaties to be flogged, the more he made me laugh. So, 20 after a fair amount of time had passed in this manner, I promised to give him his blows, if only he would in turn grant me one very small favour. He agreed, and I commanded him to submit his ears to an argument that I would expound: this would be his punishment. He promised to do so, and I discoursed at some length, explaining that the spirit of anger in us must be disciplined by the word, not with whips. And he, by exercising careful foresight over himself, improved greatly in the space of a year.

As for you, even if you are not capable of a great improvement, you should be satisfied with a quite small movement in the right direction in the first year. If you continue to withstand the affection, and to soften your rage, you will make more substantial progress in the second year. And if you persevere with an ever-greater practice of foresight over yourself in the third, fourth I and fifth 21 year, and beyond, you will become aware of a great improvement in the dignity of your life. It is a shameful thing that a man will toil for year after year to become a good doctor, a good orator, scholar or geometer, but never even consider setting aside time to become a good human being.

5. What, then, is the beginning of this discipline? Let us return again to the point that one should never chastise any of one's servants with one's own hands: if a proposition is of great importance, there is no harm in repeating it twice or even three times. I have always followed what I once heard was Plato's method with regard to the servant who makes a mistake; it is a practice of which I approve, and which I recommend you to impose on yourself, too. It is this: never to strike a servant with your own hands, nor to instruct any other to do

so, so long as you are still in a state of anger, but to postpone the punishment. Once your rage has subsided you will be able to reach a better judgement as to the number of blows to be inflicted on the culprit. Surely, indeed, it is in the first

22 place better | to show leniency; to call for the whip but chasten with words, threatening not to be so forbearing in the future, if the error is repeated. For any action is much better undertaken when your spirit has ceased its ferment, and you are free from irrational raving, at which point you will rely rather on your reasoning faculty. Rage is nothing less than a madness, as may be seen from the actions of men in the grip of it. They strike out, kick, tear their clothes, and perform every act in a furious manner, to the point where—as stated earlier— they even lose their temper with doors, stones or keys, which they rattle, bite or kick.

You may argue that the above actions are those of people who actually are mad; while your own actions are those of a person of self-control. Now, I would agree that the error of those who strike servants with their own hands is less than that of the biters and kickers of stones, doors and keys; yet it is my conviction that any act of ferocity perpetrated against a human being is also a function of some kind of madness, albeit a mild one—or that of an animal that is

23 wild and devoid of reason. For is not | the power of reason the characteristic that marks out the human from the other animals? If you wish to remove this and gratify the spirit of rage, your life is the life of an animal, not a human. It should not be thought that human temperance consists merely in refraining from kicking, biting or stabbing those around us. One who only succeeds in that may avoid the epithet 'savage'; but he could hardly be called a temperate individual. His state, in fact, will be midway between savagery and temperance. Are you going to be content with such a graduation from savagery, without any ambition to become a decent human being? Is it not a preferable aim to avoid a continued state, not only of savagery, but also of imbecility and irrationality? And this will be achieved when you are no longer a slave to rage, but perform every action by reference to the considerations which govern your judgement when made outside the influence of the affection.

How, then, can this come about? By awarding yourself the greatest esteem of which it is possible to conceive. When all other men are in the grip of anger, to remain free from that passion is to demonstrate one's superiority over the whole

24 of humankind. It may, however, be that you | wish to enjoy the reputation of superiority, but not the reality. This is just the same as though one were to desire to be thought healthy, while one is in fact sick. For is not rage a sickness of the soul? Or do you deny the sense of the ancients, who gave the name of 'affections of the soul' to all these: distress, anger, rage, desire and fear?

The following appears to me much the best course of action for one who would rid himself as far as possible of the above affections. First, on rising in the morning one should pose oneself this question, before embarking on the day's tasks: is it better to live a constant slave to the affections, or to employ reason on every occasion? The man who wishes to become a decent human being must, secondly, call to himself one who will reveal to him everything that he does wrong. He must, further, keep constantly in mind, every day and every hour of the day, the desirability of counting himself amongst those decent human beings, and the impossibility of achieving this aim without the presence of one who will reveal his errors to him; he should, indeed, regard I the person 25 who will tell him of his every false step as his saviour and the greatest of his friends. It is also important, even if you sometimes think his criticisms unjust, to preserve your calm, in the first place because it is quite likely that he has a clearer perception than you of each of your errors (as, reciprocally, you would have of his); it is also the case that even a false criticism will urge you towards a closer examination of your own actions.

The greatest element of the enterprise, though, to which you should adhere constantly if you have truly resolved to enhance your self-esteem—is to keep always present to your mind the ugliness of soul of those who are angry, by contrast with the beauty of those who are not. Just as it is true that one who has become habituated to error over a long period of time will find the stain of his affections difficult to wash out, so equally one who would become fine and upright by following certain precepts must practise each of these precepts for a long time. Such precepts will tend to disappear from within our souls, and be quickly forgotten, because of the speed with which our souls become filled with affections. So the individual who desires to be healed must not let his guard up for a moment; and we must prevail upon all and sundry to accuse us, and must listen I to them in peace; and be grateful not to those who flatter but to 26 those who rebuke.

Keep the door to your dwelling constantly open and let your acquaintances enter at any time at all—if you are prepared for them in such a way as to be confident that those who enter will not find you in the powerful grip of any of the greater errors. Although it is difficult to remove all errors, the large ones are as easy to eradicate, if one truly wishes to, if one has the will. Open your door, then, constantly, and let all your acquaintances have permission to enter at any time. And in the same way that other men attempt to make all their actions fine ones when they enter public spaces, you should attempt the same in your own home. Those people act only out of shame towards others, lest they be caught in some error; you, though, must be most ashamed in front of yourself, in accordance with the saying: 'First and foremost of men have shame for your own self.'[13]

If you act in this way you will at some point succeed in taming and softening the irrational force of the spirited part of your soul, in the same way as you

---

[13] From the *Carmen Aureum* attributed to Pythagoras; see also n. 15, below.

27 would a wild beast. | It would be a poor lookout, would it not, if a horse-trainer can take a useless animal and make it tame to be handled in a very short space of time, but you, who are not taking on an animal external to yourself, but a non-rational capacity which resides within your soul—that soul with which reason perpetually coexists—cannot tame it, if not quickly, at least over a longer period.

6. We have discussed more fully in our work on *Character Traits*[14] how one may improve one's soul to the greatest extent possible; that one must not attack its natural strength, any more than one would that of a horse or dog which one wishes to employ, but that—as with these animals—one should cultivate its quality of obedience. That treatise also demonstrated particularly how the soul must in its own turn use the spirited faculty as an ally against the other capacity—called by the ancient philosophers 'desiderative'—which rushes without reason towards the pleasures of the body. And it is no less ugly a sight than the distortion of a human being through rage, if one sees one in the grip of lust, greed, drunkenness or luxuriousness, which are the particular actions and
28 affections of the desiderative capacity of the soul. | The latter resembles not a horse or dog (the analogy we used in the former case), but an insolent hog or goat, or some other wild beast incapable of being tamed.

And therefore in this latter case there is no process of education similar to that which leads to the obedience of the spirited; its place must be taken with what the ancients called 'discipline'. This discipline consists in not allowing it the enjoyment of the objects of its desires. For such enjoyment renders it great and strong, while the disciplining process renders it small and weak: it will follow reason through its weakness, not through a natural inclination to obey. In human society, too, it may be observed that the inferior follow the superior, either by compulsion, as is the case with children and servants, or, in the case of people with naturally good qualities, by persuasion. With regard to one who has not undergone this process of discipline, this is in fact precisely the term commonly used by the ancients: they would say that such-and-such a person was 'undisciplined', meaning that his desiderative soul had not been disciplined by his rational soul.

We have two non-rational capacities in our soul. The action of the first is to
29 | become immediately indignant and enraged at apparent wrongs committed against us. This capacity is also responsible for the nurturing of grudges—an affection of the spirit whose seriousness is greater to the extent that it is longer-lived. The action of our second non-rational capacity is to be violently attracted to anything which appears pleasant, without consideration as to whether it is beneficial or harmful, good or bad. The more violent manifestations of this

[14] The reference to this work, known to have been composed after 192, is one of the main pieces of evidence suggesting a late date for the present text; see also nn. 21 and 22 below.

latter faculty should be resisted before it grows to such strength that it is impossible to remove. At that point you will be unable to restrain it even if you want to, and then you will say—as I have heard someone say who was afflicted with erotic passion—that you want to stop but cannot; and you will call on me in vain, as did that person, begging for help and for the excision of his affection. The body also has affections which are incurable by virtue of their size. Perhaps you have never even realized this fact.

It would, then, be advisable for you to consider it now, and to examine my statement that the desiderative capacity frequently advances to a state of incurable lust—lust not only for beautiful bodies, nor only for sex, but also for luxuriousness, | overfeeding, drunkenness, and unnatural perversions. Do the facts 30 confirm this statement (along with the larger part of my previous remarks) or not?

And what has been said up to now in the context of anger may be taken to apply equally to the other affections. First, that one should rely on others, not oneself, for their diagnosis; secondly, that the persons appointed for this task should not be any random selection, but people of the older generation, who are well known to be decent human beings, and who have been further subjected to our own specific examination to establish their freedom from affection. Moreover, that we should display gratitude, not annoyance, to them for any statement they make of our errors; and finally that one should remind oneself of these things, preferably many times a day, or, failing that, at least at dawn before beginning one's daily activities and in the evening when one is about to take one's rest. I myself used to read the 'Counsels' attributed to Pythagoras twice a day—first reading them from the book, later reciting them aloud.[15]

For it is not sufficient to lead a life free of anger; one must purge oneself also of | luxuriousness and lasciviousness, of drunkenness, idleness and envy. And 31 therefore another person must watch over us, to ensure that we do not make the same spectacle of uncontrolled appetite as dogs do when they eat, or perform the same undignified guzzling of a cold drink as one in the throes of a constant fever. Even if one is hungry, one should not go at one's food in this violent, uncontrolled manner; nor if one is thirsty should one drink down a whole goblet in one. How much less should a luxurious appetite for everything before one lead to indulgence in an excess of cake or any other rich food. In every case the beginner should call upon others to observe and then tell him what mistakes he has made; in due course he will be able to supervise himself, even without the presence of a trainer, and to take care that he eats less than all his companions at table, and that he refrains from rich foods, confining himself to a suitable amount of the healthy ones.

---

[15] See also n. 13. The *Carmen Aureum*, an extant verse work attributed to Pythagoras and containing moral sayings, including questions addressed to oneself, was used in this way for daily recitation aimed at self-improvement; the practice is mentioned also by Epictetus.

And after a while you should not even consider the amount consumed by
32 your fellow-diners: for it is no great achievement I to exercise greater restraint
than they do. If you have learnt truly to respect yourself, you should consider
only whether your regime shows more restraint today than yesterday. Following
this practice you will find it easier each day to abstain from the foods I have
mentioned; and you will experience a great joy of the soul, if you really are a
lover of self-control. For what a person loves, he rejoices to make progress in. It
is for this reason that one may observe the drunkard take pleasure in surpassing
his fellow-drinkers, the glutton derive joy from the sheer quantity of his food
and the man of luxurious appetites from cakes, pancakes, rich foods and heavy
sauces. I have even known some set great store by the amount of their sexual
activity.

In the same way, then, that those individuals cultivate the pursuit of the
maximum in their respective fields of endeavour, just so should we exert ourselves towards the maximization of our self-control. In doing so we shall not be
comparing ourselves with the undisciplined, nor shall we be satisfied with a
level of restraint and self-control that is merely superior to theirs. Rather, we
shall strive first of all to surpass those who are engaged in the same pursuit as
33 we are I (the competition in question here is, after all, the noblest); and secondly, to surpass ourselves. And habituation will make the healthy diet both
easy and at the same time pleasant. We should keep in mind the following very
fine motto: 'Choose the best life; and habit will make it sweet.'[16]

In the context of the earlier discussion, where I encouraged you to subject
your spirit of anger to a process of training, you had a clear indicator of the
benefit to yourself—namely that you would observe yourself no longer getting
angry. It is exactly the same with self-control: the indicator is that you no longer
experience desire for the greatest sources of pleasure. And the pathway to this goal
is through restraint. The superiority of the self-controlled person to the restrained
person lies in the fact that the former no longer desires rich foods, either
because of a long-established habit, or because of restraint—which is, as the
word itself implies, a restraining and conquering of the desires.[17] The road is
laborious and rough to begin with, as are all practices which involve the cultivation of fine habits. If, however, you wish to possess virtue in place of vice, and
34 peace of soul in place of I the itching of the body, you must train yourself in the
manner described, proceeding by restraint towards self-control. If, on the other
hand, you wish to pay no attention to virtue, or to itch throughout your body,

---

[16] The saying is quoted by other ancient authors, and attributed to Pythagoras.
[17] The distinction seems a subtle one, but *sōphrosunē* ('self-control') is conceived as the healthy
end state, in which one no longer experiences inappropriate or excessive desires, while 'restraint'
(*enkrateia*) is the conscious effort to curb them; here the latter is understood as instrumental in
achieving the former.

then you should simply forget about the present discussion. For it is not one designed to convert people to virtue; rather to show those who are already converted the way in which it may be achieved.[18]

And our topic covers both the extent to which one may carry out his own diagnosis, and the correction that takes place upon diagnosis. Our project now, however, is to consider the diagnosis of an individual's errors. And since a beginner is not able to diagnose himself, we shall have to set up a situation whereby others act as monitors, and the subject himself as apprentice, with the aim in view that he will at some point be able to recognize for himself the nature of the errors of which he has rid himself, and the distance which he still has to go to achieve his goal. Let me repeat what I have already said several times: though in one sense it is very easy to know oneself, in another it is the hardest thing of all. For one whose aim is genuine esteem, true self-knowledge is extremely difficult.

7. The above considerations—in conjunction with those that follow—are laid 35 down for anyone interested in this project. It is quite possible that there is some other way of becoming a decent human being; but if so I am ignorant of it. The above is the one that I have followed throughout my life, and I share it ungrudgingly with others, while encouraging them to teach me something in return, if it so happens that they know another road to the same goal. In the meantime, while still eager to discover that other way, we should practise the way of diagnosis and treatment which is common to all affections. And that is the way already stated. For competitiveness, love of reputation and desire for power are also affections. Less than these, but still an affection [...].[19] And as for envy, this is the worst of affections. By envy I mean the experience of distress at another's good fortune. Indeed, all distress is a form of affection; but envy is the worst case—whether we regard it as a separate affection or a type or variation of distress. And the manner of cure is the same for all of them, namely that already described.

ꟾ Shameful and abhorrent practices should be condemned in those who are 36 severely addicted to them. In such cases the nature of the practice is plain to us; when, however, we are unable to detect any such thing in our own lives, we should not conclude that it is not present: the lover is blind in relation to the beloved, and there are vices which are small enough to elude us, though these same vices would be far too large to ignore in others. It is therefore necessary to find some senior person with the capacity to see these faults, and to beseech

---

[18] The adjective corresponding to 'convert' is *protreptikos*, the same word translated 'exhortation' in the title of the sixth work in this volume. The *protreptikos* was a particular genre of literary composition, and in the context of ethics it corresponded—as suggested here—to an earlier stage in the process, where people need to be convinced of the value of the ethical project itself.

[19] A word seems to be missing here.

him to tell us everything quite freely; when he has done so, we must first of all thank him immediately, and later, contemplate in solitude, applying criticism to ourselves and attempting to excise the affection—not merely to the point where it is no longer apparent to others, but in such a way that its actual root is removed from the soul. For it may grow back, nourished by the evils of those around us. So we should consider, whenever we observe an affection in our neighbour, whether there is something similar in our own soul too. It should be cut out in the early stages of growth, before it has grown so large as to be incurable.

37 | All other affections of the soul are generally held of little account, though they are condemned when observed in others; distress, however, like bodily pain, appears bad to everyone.

One of the young men in my circle, who used to suffer grief on trivial provocations, realized that this was the case one evening, and came to me early the next morning, admitting that he had been kept awake all night by this matter, and that at some point it had occurred to him that I did not suffer the same degree of grief, even on great provocations, as he did on trivial ones. He desired to know how this had come about—whether from some training I had engaged in, or from some doctrine, or simply because I had been born like that. I told him the truth, which is that nature is the major factor in achieving a good life in childhood, alongside assimilation to those with whom one lives; but that later the major factors are doctrines and training. The fact that there are great individual differences in nature can be clearly observed in the children we see about

38 us. Some are always cheerful, others sullen, | some are ready to laugh at anything, while others cry at the smallest pretext. Some are ready to share things, others are acquisitive. Some become violently angry at the smallest occasion, and will bite and kick and attack those around them with sticks and stones if they believe themselves unfairly treated; others are patient and mild, and will not get angry or cry until they are treated very badly indeed. The poet Eupolis makes Aristides give the following rather appropriate response, when asked by Nikias, 'How did you become so strikingly just?':

> Nature in me was greatest; but then I
> Took Nature's part enthusiastically.

The young, then, have a natural readiness to distress, as well as to rage and luxuriousness—the subjects which have occupied the larger part of our discussion so far.

There are other observable differences between children in addition to those already mentioned: there are shameless children as well as modest ones; children with excellent memories, with very poor memories, as well as some who are just forgetful; some are conscientious in their studies, others negligent and lazy; and among the conscientious ones, some take positive

39 pleasure in being praised, | some are ashamed of their teachers' reproof, while

some act out of fear of beating. There are opposite reasons to be observed for laziness, too.

On the basis of the qualities that all men may observe in children, they call them either modest or shameless, and similarly, either loving of honour and beauty or the opposite of these, timid or fearless of being struck—and a range of similar epithets are applied in accordance with the individual nature. We can see that some children are natural liars, while others are natural lovers of truth. There are in fact many such differences in their characters, which we need not consider now. Some are readily susceptible to good education, others receive no benefit from it. Yet this is no reason to neglect children: rather, they should be brought up in the best possible practices. If their nature is such as to be bene- fited by this attention, then they should become good men. If it is not, | at least 40 the blame will not be ours.

The training of children is in fact rather like the care of plants. In the latter case, the farmer will never make a bramble bear grapes, for its nature is from the first not susceptible to that kind of development. He may, on the other hand, by his negligence—causing them to rely on nature alone—make vines which are in themselves perfectly suitable for bearing fruit bear very poor fruit, or indeed none at all. With animals, too: if you train a horse you will get an animal which is useful for a variety of purposes. A bear, on the other hand, may appear tame, but will never adopt that characteristic in a constant, reliable manner; and such ani- mals as the viper or scorpion will never even reach the stage of appearing so.

8. As for myself, I cannot tell with what qualities I was endowed by nature: self- knowledge is difficult enough in the case of adults, let alone small children. I did have the great good fortune to have a father who was extraordinarily free from anger, as well as being extremely just, decent and generous. My mother, on the other hand, was so bad-tempered that she would sometimes bite | her 41 maids; she was perpetually shouting and fighting with my father, treating him worse than Xanthippe did Socrates.

I was thus enabled to make a direct comparison between the fine qualities of my father's deeds and the ugly affections to which my mother was subject; and this awoke in me the feelings of warmth and love for the former behaviour and hatred and avoidance for the latter. This was not the only difference I observed between my parents. My father was never distressed by any setback, while my mother would be plunged into misery by the smallest occurrence. You have probably experienced for yourself the way in which children will imi- tate those things in which they take pleasure, but avoid what they do not enjoy watching.

This, then, was the kind of training that I had from my father. After which, on completion of my fourteenth year, I began to attend the lectures of philo- sophers of my home city—mostly those of a Stoic, a pupil of Philopator, but also

for a short time those of a Platonist pupil of Gaius. This was because of the lack of leisure of my father, who was persuaded into political activity by his fellow citizens, as they considered him the only man who was upright and indifferent to money, as well as being accessible and kind. Then there was another fellow-
42 citizen, too, | who had returned from a long trip abroad, a pupil of Aspasius the Peripatetic; and after him another from Athens, an Epicurean; with each of these men, my father made an examination of their lives and doctrines on my account, accompanying me to visit them.

My father had himself received a particularly strong training in geometry, mathematics, architecture and astronomy. He favoured the model of geometrical demonstration in education, which should prevent conflict arising between teachers in one's learning of the higher arts,[20] any more than it did for the ancient practitioners of the above-mentioned specialisms, prime amongst which are geometry and mathematics.

'So,' he said, 'you should not hastily declare yourself the adherent of any one sect, but take a long time in order to learn about them and assess them; and equally you should now and throughout your life exert yourself to learn and cultivate those qualities which are universally prized. I urge you to grow in the pursuit of justice, self-control, courage and prudence. These virtues are univer-
43 sally admired, | even by those who are aware that they have none of them; they wish to appear brave, self-controlled, prudent and just to others, though the only one they desire in reality is freedom from distress. This they want to possess even if it is not apparent to those around them. And this should therefore be the first quality you should aim to cultivate, since it is sought after by all people in preference to all the other virtues.'

These, then, I said, were the precepts I took from my father; and I keep them to this day. I do not declare allegiance to any sect, rather subjecting them all to a thorough examination; and I remain calm in the face of all events that may befall me from day to day—the same quality that I observed in my father. There is no loss that has the power to cause me distress, except perhaps the loss of all my possessions—that I have not so far experienced.[21] Under my father's training I developed the habit of scorn for honour and reputation, and of respect for truth alone. I observe the distress that most people undergo at any perceived slight to their status, or at any financial loss. As I have stated, I personally have never been seen distressed at such losses; but to be sure I have not up to this

---

[20] 'Higher arts' translates *mathēmata kala*, literally 'noble lessons'.

[21] Compare the discussion in *Freedom from Distress*. It seems odd that in the context of remarks like this one Galen makes no mention of the dramatic losses recounted there, and this has been taken as evidence that this work predates that one, although there is other evidence that seems to point in the opposite direction. (Of course, in *Freedom from Distress* Galen makes this same point, that he has not, even then, suffered a loss sufficient to cause him distress. Still a mention of those experiences would seem at least relevant.)

point suffered such a severe financial loss as to have insufficient resources | left   44
to provide for my bodily health; nor any loss of status of the kind that I have
seen many undergo when stripped of honour by the Senate. If I hear harsh
words from some quarters I set these against the kind words I hear from other
quarters, considering that the desire for universal praise is analogous to the
desire to own all the world's possessions.

It may, however, appear to you (I said), as it does to me, that it has been no
great achievement on my part to remain free from distress up till now. I have
not been deprived of all my possessions, nor have I been dishonoured. I may
have lost an ox, a horse or a domestic servant; but that was not sufficient to
cause me distress, as I had always in mind the precept of my father, that one
should not be distressed by any material loss provided that what remains is
adequate for the care of one's body. This he thought the primary consideration
regarding the extent of one's possessions: that they should keep one from hunger, cold or thirst. If one happens to have more than is necessary for these purposes, one should, he believed, use it for good works. I have, indeed, up to now
had access to sufficient resources to bestow in this way too. | And I know (I said)   45
that you possess twice what I do, and that you enjoy honour in our city;[22]
so that I cannot see what cause for distress you could have, other than insatiability. So, train yourself in this argument that I have stated, and keep it constantly in mind; practise it and consider whether what I have said is true, until
you are as firmly convinced of it as of the proposition that two times two is four.

9. So (I said), let us take our time to consider what kind of affection that is. Our
enquiry will begin with the insatiable appetite for food. For immoderate consumption of food is described in this way. And the judgement as to what is
moderate is derived from the purpose of food. Its purpose is to nourish the
body; this will be accomplished if the food is well digested; and it will be well
digested if the amount is correct; great amounts, as we know, remain undigested.
And if this ever happens, then the food's purpose is necessarily lost. If, also, the
stomach evacuates everything because it has been hurt by the biting qualities of
undigested food substances, | the symptom is known as diarrhoea, and here too   46
the purpose of the food is destroyed. For we do not take food in order to pass it
through the intestines, but so that it may be added to each part of the body. And
if it is distributed through the body without having been digested properly, this
causes bad humoral fluid in the veins.

So much for the effects of insatiability on the body; turn your attention now
to the soul, and consider its effects in each of the different contexts there:

---

[22] The use of 'our' suggests that the city in question is Pergamum, and that Galen is addressing a
fellow-citizen—as also seems borne out by the discussion of city populations and relative wealth
later in the chapter. This Pergamum context again may suggest an early date, at least for the text's
earliest, oral version.

consider, first of all, the insatiable desire for material objects. Now, some of these are sought after wrongly, for example, pearls, pieces of sardonyx, and all other kinds of precious stones which women believe to be an adornment; in this category too are garments interwoven with gold, or embellished with other unnecessary kinds of work; or garments which use materials that have to be imported from far away, such as the one known as 'silk'.[23] Certain material objects, however, are of particular value for the health of the body, and for that reason are quite rightly sought after, to begin with those objects by which we are nourished, clothed or shod; houses also belong here.

47   And in this ⎮ category should also be considered objects which are of use to the sick. There are substances like olive oil, which are of value in both health and sickness; among which some are of greater benefit to our bodies in the one state than in the other. The basis for judging the correct amount of these substances should be clear enough to you. The type of shoe which is one cubit long is not useful for its purpose, any more than the pointless possession of any more than the two shoes which are perfectly adequate for our requirements. Similarly, it is sufficient to have two sets of clothes, and the same with household servants and utensils. Yet in our case, I said, there are not only more than two sets of clothes, but far more than this of servants, utensils and indeed all material possessions. We derive an income from our possessions which is several times what is necessary simply to take care of the health of the body.

Among those who adopt what is called the life of indulgence (I said), some are to be observed spending not just twice or three times as much as us, but

48   even five or ten—or thirty—times as much. ⎮ Now, I have observed that you follow a similar lifestyle to my own; and yet you suffer distress in a way quite unlike me. Although your property increases every year, you suffer if, say, a tenth of your income is lost, even though the remaining nine-tenths are added to what you already had. I also notice that you do not even dare to spend money on fine works, nor on the purchase and preparation of books, and the training of scribes, to improve either their ability at shorthand transcription, their calligraphy or their accuracy—nor even on people who can read properly. Nor can you be seen—as you frequently see me—giving your clothes to others, or assisting people with food or medical care. You have even seen me discharge other people's debts. Now, I spend all the income that my father left me, neither putting anything aside from it nor hoarding it. But you, who put aside many times what you spend, are frequently observed to be in pain over it, while—as you admit yourself—you never see me in a state of distress.

49   Can you by now see the cause of this distress, or ⎮ do you desire still to hear it from me? I can oblige you in this respect too. You should know that every type

---

[23] In Greek the word for silk, *Sērikos*, indicates a geographical location in the far east of Asia; see also *The Thinning Diet*, n. 20.

of distress has the same cause, which is known amongst the Greeks as 'insatiability', or sometimes 'acquisitiveness'. Insatiability is so called because of the desires which are impossible to satiate; acquisitiveness because insatiable people always desire to acquire more of what they already have. Thus, even if they have twice as much of something, they still desire to have three times as much, and if they have three times as much they desire to have four times as much. And they look always to those who have more than them, not to those who have less, seeking always to surpass them in the amount that they possess.

You, for example (I said), if you consider all our fellow-citizens, will not find even thirty who are richer than yourself; it follows then that you are richer than all the others—and so of course also than the same number of wives, and all their slaves. Let us suppose, then, that the number of our citizens is about 40,000; add to these the wives and slaves, and you will find that you are not content with being richer than 120,000 individuals, but still desire to surpass the others, and I are anxious to become the absolute first. Yet it would be so far 50 preferable to be first in self-sufficiency; and this is within your power. To excel in wealth is not the work of Virtue, but of Chance, who may make both slaves and freedmen richer than us, the so-called well-born.

But you will still not be satisfied even if, as you hope, you attain more than all your fellow citizens; you will at once look around in case there is someone richer in some other city; and even if Chance serves you in this enterprise too, you will then go to foreign peoples, and desire to be richer than the rich of those lands too. And you will therefore not be the richest of men, but in perpetual want, because of your boundless desires. If you were to use usefulness as the criterion by which to measure the amount of your possessions, you would long ago have numbered yourself among the rich, or at least among the pretty well-off. I count myself in this category, although I have less than you do.

If you can persuade yourself of this, then none of your losses will harm you, and you will be blessed in this, that you no longer suffer distress over money. I And if you can remove also the insatiability of your desire for honour, you will 51 free yourself of distress in that area too. As things stand, not only is the esteem of your familiars insufficient to satisfy you; you actually want the praise of everyone in the city. And yet what fraction is that of the whole population of Asia, who know nothing of you in the first place? Perhaps, then, you want to become known to them first, and then to gain their esteem. But such a desire to be universally known is the product of an insatiable love of reputation, and the desire to be universally esteemed, of a futile love of esteem. If, then, you extend your desires in this direction, you will necessarily suffer greater grief over all those who do not know or respect you than you do know with your sleepless nights over the acquisition of money—since the number of people in question is very large.

So, if we continually and steadfastly train ourselves in this, we shall be free of distress. How then is such training to be carried out, unless we first become convinced of the truth of the statement that insatiability is the most wretched affection of the soul? For it is as it were a foundation of the love of money, of the love of reputation, of the love of esteem and of the love of power and competition.

First of all, one should keep always present to one's mind the doctrine of self-52 sufficiency, | which is obviously intimately connected with that of insatiability. To hate the latter is to love the former. So, if freedom from distress is dependent on this alone, and this is something which is in our power, then freedom from distress is a matter entirely within our power. All we must do is keep the doctrines regarding insatiability and self-sufficiency constantly to hand, and commit ourselves to the daily cultivation of the particular actions which follow from these doctrines. Even those who were not fortunate enough to get this from their early training may still attain it later, in the manner described. How could anyone not desire to be free of distress throughout one's entire life? And how could anyone not prefer this aim than that of being 'richer than Cinyras and Midas'?[24]

10. Well, these are among the many arguments which I expounded to that fellow, as also to many others on subsequent occasions. In every case they were persuaded by my arguments at the moment that I delivered them, but I saw that very few of them retained any benefit from them in the long term. Most people have developed the affections in their souls over such a long period that they cannot be cured. Those, however, who are in the grip of moderate affections, 53 | and able to recognize a little of the truth of the above statements, will be able to make their soul free and noble, by the ministrations of reason, if they follow the course already outlined: that is, to appoint a monitor or trainer with the task of restraining them from the stronger affections by constant reminders, criticism, exhortation and encouragement, as well as by presenting his own personal example of these statements and exhortations. How shameful it is that men set great store by 'freedom' as defined by human laws, but make no effort to acquire that genuine freedom that exists in nature, being content rather to be slaves to such shameless, wanton and tyrannical mistresses as love of money, meanness, love of reputation, love of power, love of esteem.

But acquisitiveness is, I have little hesitation in saying, the mother of all these. No one can become a decent human being so long as this remains in his soul. Does not anyone who does not hate such a vice deserve to die a hundred deaths? And the young should hate and avoid it especially, if they wish to be saved; for if an insatiable desire for money gets in first, in their upbringing, 54 | then after the fortieth year there will no longer be any help for them. Or you

---

[24] Cinyras and Midas were legendarily wealthy kings. The quotation here seems to derive ultimately from the poet Tyrtaeus, and is also paraphrased by Plato, *Laws* II, 660e.

may say, after the fiftieth; for I should not like you to call me inhuman, as someone did once. This was an individual who was susceptible to the desires for lux-
ury, sex, reputation and esteem, but who had very little money, and therefore
suffered in his failure to fulfil any of those desires. This person, observing my
own serenity over a long period of time, and, being conscious of his own unhappiness, begged me to instruct him how to become free from this grief. When I
told him that the correction of the affections that had by now accumulated
would require a period of many years, he cried out: 'Nothing could be more
inhuman than you!'—as if I could have exerted myself to free him from distress
in a very short time, had I so wished, but begrudged him this favour. And yet
this is the one lesson which no one could begrudge his fellow man. It is to our
own advantage for those with whom we have social intercourse not to be victims of the affections—for their souls not to be disabled by a love of reputation
or any similar vice. The better our companions are, ∣ the more beneficial they 55
will be to us as friends, too.

Let me return to the subject of the man who wishes to become a decent
human being, and set out the way he must follow towards all good qualities of
the soul. To begin with he must appoint a supervisor, to remind him of everything that he fails to see. It is, for example, sometimes difficult for one to draw
the line between acts of meanness and acts of thrift; and that will be quite
impossible for one who is just beginning to rid himself of the affection of love
of money. Virtue is close to vice in this case; so too when love of esteem is being
removed, shamelessness may arise in ill-bred souls. For a young man who
wishes to be saved, then, the person to identify his mistakes must be someone
other than himself; they should be old men who have throughout their life
given ample proof of the freedom of their judgement. And their criticisms must
not be resisted or resented. Rather, these men must receive our gratitude, and
be encouraged always to tell the truth, and when they identify an affection, we
must ∣ attempt to remove it—not all at once, but to chip away little by little at the 56
extent of it, though in the early stages this will be difficult, and will be accomplished only at the cost of much evident unhappiness. We should bear in mind
that it will not continue to be so difficult as time goes on. For our rational faculty is augmented in the process of those exercises which subdue and lessen our
affections; and the whole enterprise becomes gradually easier in proportion with
that augmentation. For clearly, if the reasoning faculty succeeded, while still
untrained, in conquering the affections at their greatest, its success will be all
the greater when in due course it acquires a double advantage. Not only will its
own nature be nobler as a result of the training, but those affections, too, will
have become smaller. Either one of these circumstances would have given us
sufficient grounds for hope; and therefore one should not at the beginning of
one's course of exercise be disheartened if one perceives only very little progress
in the cure of one's affections. It will increase gradually, and become great, if

only one has sufficient genuine love of oneself to endure the account of one's own errors—if one's desire is to become, and not just to appear, a decent human being.

57 ⏐ That, then, is the manner of identification and treatment of the soul's affections. We shall turn now to its errors.

II. Errors

58 1. The previous book covered the diagnosis and treatment, in the manner described, of the affections that arise in the soul of each individual; we should now turn our attention to the soul's errors.

Let me then begin in the best way possible (which everyone agrees to be the best way, even if they do not exemplify it in practice), namely, by giving a verbal exposition of what is meant by 'error', so that there will be no scope for ambigu-
59 ity in what follows. ⏐ I shall endeavour to make clear the customary sense of this term in general Greek usage.

The term 'error' is used in both a specific sense, to indicate something which goes wrong in the process of making a judgement, and thus involving only the rational part of the soul, and a more general sense, by which it refers also to mistakes of the non-rational part. [...]

Now, it is generally agreed that false or hasty assent is an error; but that the same is true also of 'weak assent' is not so agreed.[25] Some believe that the weak assent should be placed between virtue and vice. By 'weak assent' is meant the case where we have not yet convinced ourselves of the truth of such-and-such an opinion in the same way that we have of the opinion for example that we have five fingers on each hand or that two times two equals four. For an old man who has devoted himself to the discovery of true propositions, perhaps weak assent to one which admits of a scientific demonstration would be an error. The geometer, indeed, has the same kind of knowledge of the propos-itions taught in Euclid's *Elements* as most people have of the proposition that two times two equals four. And he will have the same kind of knowledge, too, in
60 the subject area following on from that, that of the theorems of spheres, ⏐ and of all the problems solved according to those theorems; and so also of the theorems of cones and gnomons. If, then, he is in doubt in this area for a short time, and lacks a secure assent (which some also call 'grasping') to such a proposition, this would be agreed to be an error: the error of a geometer. When someone commits errors in the actual conduct of his life, on the other hand, then those bad

[25] There is an unfortunate lacuna between the last sentence translated and this one. For the epis-temological debates and terminology referred to in the following paragraphs, see also *The Best Method of Instruction*.

opinions, as well as false, hasty or weak assent, are associated with the know-ledge, attainment or avoidance of good and evil. And in this context there is an immediate danger that a small error may cause very great harm, if our false assent concerns a belief about good and evil.

Now, the opinion of the Academics and Pyrrhonists, since they deny the pos-sibility of scientific demonstration on the subject of our enquiry, is that all assent is necessarily hasty, and that it may also be false; and that the contradict-ory opinions of the philosophers who do make declarations on matters of good and evil cannot ⏐ all be correct, although it is possible that they are all incorrect. 61 If that were the case, then good would not consist in pleasure, nor in freedom from disturbance, nor in virtue or the activity in accordance with virtue—nor, indeed, in any of the candidates mooted by the philosophers.

The first task for the man interested in becoming free of error is to investigate the question, whether a non-evident matter admits of demonstration. When he finds that it does, the next step is the enquiry into the method of demonstration; and this is not something to be conducted in a casual manner, but over a long period of time, and in association with persons of the highest credentials in terms of veracity, natural intelligence and training in logical theory. Once he is con-vinced that he has discovered this too, he should still continue to subject himself to training for a considerable additional period, before embarking on the ultimate enquiry: the enquiry into the 'good' (or as some call it, the 'goal of life') which, once attained, makes us happy, or blessed—or whatever term one prefers.

2. Is it not obviously hasty to attempt to discover the truths of these ultimate questions without first being sure that one knows the method of demonstration itself? ⏐ It certainly seems so to me. Such behaviour would be analogous to the 62 audacity of offering demonstrations on arithmetical or mathematical subjects without first being confident that one has an adequate training in mathematics. In either case, one who embarks on such a course is bound to make a large number of blunders. The fact that false arguments convince people is obvious from the plurality of the sects; and it is also obvious that they would not con-vince people of their truth were it not for their similarity [to true arguments]. Nor should one imagine that such similarity is a small one. If it were, they would have been easily and quickly detected when tested by good men.

What Hippocrates said in the context of the study of medicine appears to hold for philosophy too. He said that similarities cause people to go astray and lead to confusion, ⏐ even in the minds of good doctors, so that not only ordinary 63 practitioners, but even the best, are tripped up by them. It is thus not unreason-able to suppose that in the context of philosophy, too, good philosophers are liable to confusion and to going astray. The similarity between twins is easily seen through by anyone who knows them well, but not by a stranger. By the same token, it will be impossible for one to see through verbal similarities unless one is extremely well versed in arguments, and in the habit of daily inter-course and familiarity with them, in the same way are the twins' siblings with the twins.

This, then, is one primary and very great error made by those who make hasty declarations about good and evil in human life; and the error arises from self-regard, boastfulness, the conceit of wisdom, or love of esteem. For though it may be observed that some of the people who make such statements are actu-ally convinced of the correctness of their opinions, others merely persuade others in order to gain respect or money, but remain personally dubious of their own statements. Both types are in error, the latter consciously—an evil which 64 we may regard as due to affection— | the former unconsciously, in which case the mistake is one which falls in the category of error proper.

Such people would do well to remember those wallets of Aesop, and to find other persons to give an assessment of their own opinions; the latter individuals should not, of course, be of the same stamp as they themselves—untrained in the methods of logical proof, as well as in the other subjects of (geometry, arithmetic, astronomy) by which the soul is sharpened. Some of them have not even enjoyed the schooling of an orator, or for that matter of a grammarian,[26] which is the most widely available sort of education of all; they are so com-pletely lacking in any sort of verbal training that they cannot follow the argu-ments they hear from my lips. When making an argument I sometimes notice that this is the case, and ask them to repeat what I have just said; for it is quite plain that they are—just like 'the ass with the lyre'[27]—completely unable to fol-low the sense of my words. Nonetheless their arrogance or cheek is such that 65 even when subjected to the open scorn of persons who *are* literate, for | their inability to give an account of what they have just heard, they experience no shame, but actually believe that the truth is known to them alone, and that those who have bothered to educate themselves have merely wasted their time.

But it is no part of the purpose of my argument here to attempt to help such people as those—an attempt that would in any case be futile in most such cases, even assuming that they wished to be helped. For they are not at the age which lends itself to education. This work will, I hope, be of assistance to a person of natural intelligence, who has also had that early training which gives him the abil-ity, preferably to repeat immediately whatever arguments he hears, or at least to write them down. The person must, additionally, be completely dedicated to the pursuit of truth; this last condition is entirely within his own power. The first requirement, though, is that of the right natural endowments for the pursuit of

[26] *Rhētōr* and *grammatikos*: see *My Own Books*, n. 4, *An Exhortation to Study the Arts*, n. 7. and *My Own Doctrines*, n. 5.
[27] A proverbial expression, rather like the English 'pearls before swine'; it seems to be first attested in the comic poet Menander.

truth, and the second that of a good early education. One who lacks such a natural endowment, and who has been brought up in bad, disordered habits, will never have that desire for the truth, either from his own internal impulses or from the encouragements of others. I myself would never l claim to be able to   66 assist such a one; as I have said, I can only help one who is a friend of truth. This person, indeed, I shall endeavour to the best of my ability to set upon the right path; for I have sought it throughout my own life, and am convinced that the way that I shall now describe is the only one.

3. You should (I said), learn thoroughly the teachings of our predecessors on the method of demonstration, and first of all test this method in some other context, to see if it genuinely does discover the truth of a subject under enquiry. And here the nature of the subject in question should be such that it is adequate to confirm to the discoverer that he has indeed discovered it—as in the case of the division of a given straight line into prescribed sections.

It is quite possible that the utterly ignorant will have no idea to what I am referring. I shall try to make it clearer for them (as though talking to asses). By 'a given straight line' is meant one which is displayed on a perfectly flat surface; and by 'prescribe sections' those stipulated by the setter, who may require that the given line be divided into five equal parts, or seven, or twenty, or a hundred. Whether, then, you find your own particular method for this l or employ one   67 which has been taught to you, once you have divided the given line into however many parts you wish, the fact will confirm itself to you, and it will be manifest that each of the sections of the line so divided is exactly equal. All other such problems, similarly, will be securely discovered by virtue of things manifestly apparent, as for example when we are instructed to draw a circle around a given square, or, on the same principle, to draw a square around or within a given circle, or again to draw a circle around a given equilateral and equiangular pentagon. In each of these cases, if one is immediately able to perform the task according to the method which one has learned, the fact that one has achieved the object of the enquiry will be made evident by that object itself.

Now, the question whether the universe came into being or was ungenerated, by contrast, is not one which can be answered by the confirmation provided by the fact itself; nor the question whether it is finite or infinite; nor of the number of waves in the sea. None of these latter questions can be settled on the basis of the evident nature of the fact being discovered, as happens immediately when, for example, we are asked to draw an equilateral and equiangular dodecagon around or within a circle. l The figure drawn either within or without the circle is imme-   68 diately visible, as is the circle drawn within or without a polygon of this kind.

When, therefore, we find a method of demonstration which leads us to the object under enquiry, and is manifestly confirmed by the fact itself, we have a pretty good test of the veracity of that method; and we may later venture to apply it also in cases where such evident proof is not available. It is wrong, in my opinion, for one to start to construct proofs on the greatest of subjects—we may so term those subjects which concern our attainment of happiness—without first training oneself in other areas of enquiry, in which the actual facts of the matter will refute one who wrongly believes himself to have found the answer, and confirm the truth to one who genuinely has found it.

The method we are discussing is that employed in geometry, logic, astronomy and architecture (I use the single term 'architecture' to refer also to the design of sundials and water-clocks, of water-instruments and of all mechanical

69 devices, including | pneumatic ones.) In all these areas self-confirming proofs are available to the enquirer, as also in astronomy. For here too judgement is subject to the test of what is manifestly apparent: an eclipse of the sun or moon, for example, and the observed phenomena of fixed and moving stars, must surely count as 'manifestly apparent'.

I am well aware that this argument is extremely painful to the souls of those who are already mature in years and have no time to spend testing the method of demonstration for a long period in fields where the objects are able to give manifest confirmation of it. As I have said, self-regard, the conceit of wisdom, love of esteem and reputation, boastfulness and acquisitiveness are the motives which cause people to deceive either themselves or others into believing that they have certain knowledge. It is thus no surprise that they also succeed in convincing those who frequent their lectures, some of whom are born asses,

70 while others are basically bright, but lacking an elementary | training. Of course it suits those fraudulent teachers to have pupils of this kind, as anyone who is naturally intelligent and trained in those essential preliminaries will immediately despise them. Even in early youth I held many teachers in contempt—the sort who had the nerve to make pronouncements which were in conflict with the demonstrable truths of geometry, and who themselves had not even a vague notion of the concept of a demonstration.

Remove the qualities of boastfulness, self-regard, love of esteem and reputation, the conceit of wisdom and acquisitiveness from the seeker after truth, in the way that I have suggested, and he will approach that quest with a preparation, not of months, but perhaps even of years, before making the enquiry into the doctrines which lead to happiness or unhappiness. One who is afflicted by affections, meanwhile, of the sort previously described, I would hesitate to encourage to undertake such a long journey; and as for the other camp—those who are engaged in intrigue and slander against us—they are worthy of our contempt. It is with such arguments they have always snared their own pupils,

71 to prevent them ever subjecting themselves to the experience of | listening to the arguments that I have so far advanced. For it is a highly attractive proposition to the uneducated youth when he hears a teacher with great solemnity recommend the extreme easiness of the path to wisdom laid down by the school

known as the Cynics. For this group, too, claim that their method offers a quick way to virtue. Or some of them dispute this, saying that the Cynic philosophy is not a path to virtue, but via virtue to happiness.

It would in fact be nearer the truth to say, with some others, that it is a quick way via ignorance and arrogance to conceit. Certainly all the Cynics I have come across in my life, as well as some individuals who pretend to practise philosophy, admit that they avoid any training in logical method. When out of my presence, of course, they then refuse to converse with the man in the street (with goatherds, for example, or cowherds, diggers, or reapers), on the stated grounds that these people are not equipped with a training in argument that would enable them to follow the discussion— | as though they had themselves 72 ever had an elementary training. What they have actually done is started at once with their teacher's discourses on the goal of life, on happiness and unhappiness—arguments which that teacher believed to have the status of 'demonstration', and by which they were taken in through that lack of training. As I have said, the similarities between false and true arguments are the cause of false doctrines. It is only the most experienced in any subject area who will succeed in seeing through such similarities. One who simply rushes to make such an assessment of arguments will necessarily be unable to recognize or distinguish the false from the true.

A clear proof of this is provided by what are known as 'sophisms', which are false arguments deliberately engineered to resemble true ones. Their falsity is evident from the fact that their conclusions are untrue. Now, all false arguments contain either some untruth in one of the premisses, or some mistake in the drawing of the conclusion from those premisses; but in a sophism these features are not immediately obvious. | And so they are not perceived by one who 73 has a poor training in argument. Thus it happens that an argument will be generally agreed to be false, because of the self-evident falsity of its conclusion, and yet the solution of the sophism will be a puzzle to the untrained. The safe course for these people would be to be suspicious of all argument, and to withhold their assent in every case, until they had definitely convinced themselves that they were able to tell the difference between false and true arguments. They will get people to set them sophisms as problems to be solved, encouraging those who so wish to make a practical test of their intellect.

That, surely, is no different from the advice of those who encourage their pupils to train themselves in the solution of sophisms; at any rate I see no difference. Now, since this solution consists, as I have said, in the detection of the point of similarity between the false argument and the true, it is essential first to gain an education in the nature of true arguments. One who is sufficiently well trained in that area to be able quickly and accurately to recognize the form of a true argument will have no difficulty picking out the false ones. I have demonstrated this by teaching youths who had a previous training | to recognize true 74 arguments. I encouraged members of the audience to set them sophisms for solution. And these youths would recognize the illogicality of the sophism immediately, whether this consisted in the form of the argument, which did not constitute a syllogistic proof, or in the falsity of one of the premises. This is another clear piece of evidence for those elders with their conceit of their own wisdom, who are themselves unable to solve sophisms, of the fact that this affection is due to ignorance of true arguments.

And surely such people deserve our deepest contempt, for having ended up with an unhappy life on the basis of a hasty assent. For a false opinion regarding the goal is universally agreed to lead to unhappiness. Yet some people are so untrained in the identification of true and false arguments, that sometimes, while claiming to establish the truth of some matter, they are unaware that the argument they are giving is merely a possible one, as though the matter on which they were forming their belief were one manifestly apparent; and so they ask us to follow them and believe it without demonstration. And frequently when, on the other hand, an argument requires only an indication, they try to
75 establish it by logical demonstration. Some of them I are not even aware of the difference between something which requires an indication and something which is reliable primarily and in itself, but nonetheless attempt make pronouncements on matters where no precise examination has been carried out. And this happens with many people who have already grown old in philosophy. By heavens, do you imagine there is some ready treatment for such ignorance and false conceit of one's own wisdom?

If you have had an induration for three or four years, you may find that it is already impossible to treat; do you imagine that the souls of these old gentlemen, which have suffered from an induration for thirty years, are susceptible to treatment? Well, say for the sake of argument that they were; you would still have to ask yourself the question, whether such treatment would require days, months or years.

And so you should not be surprised that among those who claim to be practitioners of philosophy there are many with whom I do not even consider it worth having a discussion. For I am quite sure that any layman with a degree of natural intelligence and a good old-fashioned Greek education is no worse a
76 philosopher. The latter will at least understand easily what plainly I follow from certain propositions and what is in contradiction with them. As for the former, I have frequently examined them and proved that they are interested only in dispute for dispute's sake, and that they claim not to recognize when propositions are in conflict with their own doctrines. I have been involved in many discussions on the question of what follows from each chosen aim in life, with many different philosophers. Those who had had the benefit of that early training were quick on the uptake, and able to state what kind of life followed in each

case, because they understood my argument.[28] The others, having (as I have said) grown old in their false conceit of wisdom, were the only ones to state the opposite. When, as a result, the entire assembly laughed at them, they turned to abuse.

But my enquiries, conducted in conjunction with many others, into this question of what follows from each chosen aim in life, are available to you in another treatise; that work naturally contains may examples of the errors which people make. The contradictions between people's different actions throughout their lives, and the contradictions between their different statements, when they are led astray by the various sects, are all a result of false judgement. | And 77 clearly all these confusions that arise from the sects are errors, whereas the true sect has discovered not only the goal in life, but the form of life which is consequent upon it.

Here too we should make it quite clear how affection differs from error. A man might, for example, lay it down as a matter of doctrine that one should help other people, on the grounds that this is a proper goal, but may fail to do so through sleepiness, laziness, love of pleasure and so on. This kind of failure is that by affection. If, on the other hand, one makes a decision in advance to provide pleasure, or freedom from trouble, for oneself only, and for that reason refrains from assisting one's fellow-citizens or family members when they are victims of some injustice, that is a failure due to poor doctrine, not to affection.

4. Now the origin of many errors is a false assumption concerning the goal of life in each individual case. The individual errors grow from this as from a root. But it is also possible for someone to be correct about the goal, but to make some mistake in some individual matter, through failure in | understanding of 78 logical consequence. Now, as I have just said, the issue of which actions follow from each goal in life is more fully discussed elsewhere. Here let me rehearse only the chief points regarding the errors; it will be as well to repeat them so that we may have an easily memorable summary of the relevant facts.

Since the main part of human happiness depends on the enquiry into the goal, it is not surprising that all persons with any self-esteem have attempted this enquiry. But all—or all but one[29]—have made hasty pronouncements. And even this one cannot be clearly identified without an assessment of his demonstration—whether they really are demonstrations or merely appear like them. If one's concern is with the examination and control of one's own faults,

---

[28] There may be some material missing here.

[29] The suggestion, albeit made tentatively, that one sect *has* established the correct answer to the question of the goal of life would point to the possibility that Galen himself does accept one of the standard formulations of this that he refers to above. If so the most likely candidate seems to be the Platonist 'approximation to god', but if he does accept this Galen is tantalizingly vague and inexplicit on the point.

one must begin with a consideration of the correctness of the following procedure: first of all, to listen conscientiously and attentively to those who claim to have provided demonstrations on the subject in question; secondly, to attempt an assessment of those demonstrations, in the latter case again referring to the speaker for clarification of the criteria on the basis of which they expect the

79   truth of their arguments to be evaluated; | here too one must consider whether the criteria in question are of the correct sort, and check that they have not proposed a criterion of assessment which is itself in need of another criterion, and so on.[30] This kind of infinite regress is particularly to be guarded against, as one investigates—with great care, over a very long period, in collaboration with those men who appear to one to be the most truthful—what is the primary criterion of all, which is evident.[31] [...] remembering also that, in every case, one must repel any attack based on the lack of a criterion. And it was agreed that this, even without assessment, is sufficient to indicate the same capacity, in all forms of demonstration; and thus, from this point on, one must refer all the individual matters to it—a procedure which is called *analysis* by some philosophers, being a kind of 'moving up' [*ana*] from the lower-level criteria to the first one.[32]

This is quite a difficult task. You will have observed the terrible fools that those people with their false conceit of wisdom make of themselves, and the general mockery they incur, through their inability to refer even the most

80   everyday enquiries to the first criterion. | Those who wish to become expert in scientific demonstration should therefore monitor their own progress, training themselves first, as I have suggested, on a number of individual questions where the correct answer has a self-confirming status which the enquirer can recognize, as is the case in mathematical and geometrical theory, which in turn provide the basis for astronomy and architecture.

5. Let me give an example from architecture, for the sake of clarity. Imagine that a city is being founded, and that the prospective inhabitants want to know, not roughly but with precision, on each and every day, how much of the time has passed [at any point], and how much is left, before sunset. According to the method of *analysis*, this problem must be referred to the first criterion, if one wishes to find it out in the manner we learned in the study [*or* treatise] of gnomons; one must then go down the same path in the opposite direction to put the solution together,[33] again as we learned in that same study. When we

---

[30] *Kritērion* in Galen's technical usage covers both the sense of the internal mental faculty by which an assessment is made and that of the means of justification, or underlying principle or premiss, referred to in an argument. See also *The Best Method of Instruction* (where it is translated 'evaluative principle'), especially n. 3.

[31] There is a lacuna at this point, and some unclarity in the following two sentences.

[32] On the technical terms *analysis* and *synthesis*, elaborated further in the next chapter, see also *The Art of Medicine*, n. 1.

[33] The verb here is *suntithenai*, cognate with *synthesis*.

have in this way found I the path that is to be followed in all cases, and once we   81
have realized that this kind of measurement of periods of time within the day
must be carried out by means of geometric lines, we must then proceed to the
materials which will receive the imprint of those lines, and the gnomon.

And first we must enquire which shapes of bodies will be suitable for the
design which we have discovered; then we must find out in each case, by *analysis* and *synthesis*, how the design should be done; then, whenever the method
of logic indicates to us that there are manifest grounds for trust in the discovery
of the matters before us, we must turn to the practical realization of the things
discovered by it, and, again, examine how we are to produce a flat surface for
the body to be drawn. And once we have found this out by *analysis* and *synthesis*, and have constructed some such body, we must find out which instruments
should be used to draw it; and when, once again, this has been discovered by
analysis and *synthesis*, we must attempt to construct them in the form taught to
us by the method. Then, we must make a series of drawings in many forms and
give them to I people to test in practice whether the task set has been accom-   82
plished. For when the first line is hit by the first ray of the sun, and in the same
manner the last by the last, and when this is apparent in the case of all the
drawn [lines of the] sundials, we will then in a way have one manifest indicator
that the [solution to the] problem set has been found out. Another consists in
the fact that the lines drawn are all in agreement with each other.

A third such manifest indicator consists in the confirmation by an even flow
of water: for the argument discovers that this, too, will be a criterion of the correctness of the drawing of the sundials. Let me explain what I mean. Make a
hole in a vessel, which may be of any material you wish, and place it in clear
water at the moment when you see the first ray of the sun. Then, when the sundial that has been drawn indicates the completion of the first hour, make a mark
in the vessel at the point to which it has been filled by the water; then empty it
immediately and put it back it in the same water. When the sundial indicates
the second hour, examine the vessel; I then, once you find that the water has   83
reached the same point within it that you marked at the end of the first hour,
again quickly empty it and put it back in in the same place in the water. Examine
it again, and see if the sundial indicates that the water has reached the same
point within the third hour that it did within the first and the second. Once you
find that it has, then empty it once more and put it back in the water for the
fourth hour; and when you see that the water has again reached the same point
in the vessel, empty it yet again and put it straight back again, and so carry out
the examination for the fifth hour too. And if you find that it is so again on the
completion of the sixth hour, and at the end of each subsequent hour up to
the twelfth, you will be convinced—unless you are completely stupid—that the
sundial has been correctly constructed; for it has made manifest the object or
our endeavour, which was the division of the day into twelve equal parts.

Now of course, the number twelve was only chosen for convenience, as being
84 divisible by three and four, as well as by six and twelve, | which is not true of any
number smaller than it—nor of any number greater, until you get to twenty-
four. The latter was ruled out a being too large, whereas the number twelve was
considered to represent a good point of balance and was therefore adopted for
the division of the day. Its usefulness has stood the test of experience, and it is
used by many peoples including the Romans, who habitually divide estates into
twelve parts when making legacies, and also use a twelve-part division for the
majority of standard weights and measures in everyday use. If you prefer, construct a sundial which divides the day into some other number of parts, for
example one greater than twelve. We shall still be able to confirm the correctness of our solution, both by the measurement of the water-level in the punc-
tured vessel and by the internal consistency of the lines drawn. A final
confirmation will be the correspondence of the first and last lines with the
beginning and end of the day.

Reason, conducting its enquiry by the method of *analysis*, has also found out
85 the design of the water-clock. Here, again, the test of its correctness is | some-
thing manifest even to the layman. The uppermost line, that which indicates the
twelfth hour of the day, is at its highest in that part of the water-clock which
measures the longest day, and at its lowest in that part which measures the
shortest; midway between these two is the marker corresponding to the equinoxes. The area between these divisions, on the lip of the water-clock, indicates
to you the days after these four. Starting from these divisions, you will find, next
after the marker which represents the longest day, that which indicates the
point on the top line which the water will reach on completion of the twelfth
hour on the following day. And again, the third along from the solstice will
indicate the third day, and the next the fourth day. Carrying on in the same way,
you will find that every day of the year is marked by this one line in the water-
clock which I have said is the uppermost. The other lines, meanwhile, which are
lower than this highest one, you will find measure out the other hours: the first
86 one down from the 'twelfth' | corresponds to the eleventh hour—at a different
point on it for each day of the year, in exactly the same way as we just explained
in the case of the uppermost line. The next after that indicates the tenth hour,
similarly, at different points along it; the one after that the ninth; then the
eighth, and so on, down to the lowest line, which points out the first hour, just
as it appears on a sundial; and as the level of the water in the water-clock rises,
the first and all following hours appear equal, right up to the twelfth; but not
equal to those on the preceding and following days.

So, my friend, if you have never evinced any desire to discover this method—
well, what can one say? You have failed to recognize the falsity of your conceit
of wisdom, and, being completely ignorant of [the solutions of] these problems,
will never discover so much as one of them in the course of a whole year,

indeed, in the course of your whole life. For they were not discovered within the lifetime of a single man. Geometrical theory underwent a gradual progression; it started with the enquiry into the theorems of the 'elements' (as they are known) within it; to these, once they were discovered, men of I later ages added 87 that most wonderful science which, as I have said, is known as *analysis*, and gave themselves and anyone else who was interested a most thorough training in it. And they have yet to produce a more wonderful product of their ingenuity than those of the sundial and the water-clock.

Those who conducted research in these areas were not hasty in their judgements, nor boastful, as are those characters who publicly announce their pursuit and discovery of wisdom; the honour which these men granted themselves was of the genuine sort, which led them to cultivate and perfect the best capacity within their souls. By this of course I mean the rational capacity; when this is well trained and achieves its own form of good condition, the person in question is far happier than those who are slaves to bodily pleasures. For there is no other capacity of our soul by virtue of which we differ from goats, dogs, pigs, sheep or donkeys. And there is no other study which can delight the soul of a man of fine natural endowments more than that of this method of *analysis*—once I he has a certain level of attainment in it. Of course, it is very 88 hard work to begin with, as is pretty much every true study. Even if it were not a source of contentment, however, its value in the context of the most important of enquiries would still make it worth training in. It has, as already mentioned, this unique feature, namely the self-confirming nature of the things discovered by it. This is not the case with the findings of philosophy.

This is what makes it possible for so much shameless, ill-considered rubbish to be spoken in the field of philosophy. One who constructs a sundial or water-clock wrongly is refuted by the clear evidence of the facts; but the refutation of philosophical propositions is not in the same way manifest. People may say whatever they wish to once they are shameless enough to abandon logical method and claim to be taught by 'the facts themselves'. If these facts had the capacity to speak, and chose to speak to those people alone, then their boastfulness would I suppose be justified. The fact is that they do not speak, either to me or to them, and therefore clearly it is only our own capacity for reason which can discover the nature of these facts. So it seems reasonable that someone should first give a proof of his capacity to discover this nature I in some 89 context where manifest confirmation of it is provided by those facts themselves. He should explain to us the method to which every problem is analytically accessible; and he should show that he has identified the points of similarity between true and false arguments in cases where the fault is possible to detect. Otherwise he will not deserve our trust in cases where it is not so obvious.

Everyone will agree with the purport of this argument except for those rash individuals, falsely convinced of their own wisdom, for whom the path to truth is neither long nor steep—as Hesiod characterized the path to virtue[34]—but swift and short, or perhaps one should rather say, non-existent. For if it is really true that the facts themselves reveal their own nature to all men, then there is no need to spend time training oneself in any logical method. You would have, would you not—you who are so convinced of your own wisdom—to accept that this fact too is perfectly obvious to us (I mean, those of us who have not yet become wise in *your* manner), that, if Nature is alone sufficient to reveal herself, then all human beings must already know the truth of all matters?

90   Faced with this question they backtrack, | saying that not everyone is able to learn from the facts. So, then, we ask: who are the people that do receive this instruction? Their reply is themselves alone. What else can they say, since they have decided from the outset to maintain their conceit at all costs?

Well, I for one am not about to believe these people who make any assertion they wish. Why on earth should it be the case that the facts reveal themselves to them alone? Perhaps because they alone are wholly ignorant of the fundamentals of education? But this is not in fact the case: there are many others equally ignorant. Or is it that they have trained the logical capacities of their souls in lessons which are able to provide their own confirmation in practice? By no means: they have in fact had no contact with such logical training whatever. They may perhaps respond that they alone have the natural intelligence to enable them to see the facts—just like Lynkeus in the underworld.[35] But if their souls are endowed with such extraordinarily acute powers of vision, why is it that they are a complete laughing-stock when it comes to such questions as we have been discussing, questions where the truth of the discovery is self-evident

91   to the person who genuinely has discovered it? | In this field not one of them ever succeeded in finding out anything at all. Indeed, when those who have found something out explains and gives instruction about it, others learn while they alone fail to because of their poor training and mental slowness. And even if they do follow—it may perhaps happen occasionally that one of them is able to follow what is said—they are still incapable of repeating it.

There could hardly be a greater blindness with regard to the recognition of one's own errors than this, whereby men who perceive their own natural inferiority to the most ordinary of people, when it comes to understanding and remembering the discoveries of mathematics, geometry, architecture and astronomy, somehow imagine that they have discovered the truths of philosophy so easily that they venture to claim that the facts reveal themselves[36] without the assistance of the logical method or demonstration. Their self-flattery, though, is quite conscious, not the result of any real quest for the truth. This is

---

[34] Hesiod, *Works and Days* 290–1.
[35] See *The Elements according to Hippocrates*, ch. 1 with n. 3.
[36] Or possibly: 'venture to claim that they can reveal the facts....'

quite obvious from the way in which they puff themselves up in front of their students while slandering all others as being mistaken. If I ever succeed in bringing these people into the same place with me, they cannot abide it, I and begin to 92 affect a shyness which prevents them from speaking in the presence of large audiences—this in spite of the fact that they have daily attendances of twenty, thirty or more at their lectures, and they experience no shyness in that context.

Sometimes I request three or four Platonists, three or four Epicureans, the same number each of Stoics and Peripatetics, and three or four Academics or Sceptics, to be present at a discussion, so that we have about twenty people from philosophy; and I also ask a similar number of persons who have trained their rational capacity in [the basic] lessons, but have no familiarity with philosophical arguments. Such a gathering is unendurable to these people. It occasionally happens that they are compelled by persons who are not in the thrall of some sect, but who have a training in rational discourse, to be present in such a company; and that then, while they are indulging in argumentative pointscoring, and standing arguments on their heads, I a geometer joins the com- 93 pany, some doctors, and some other people with a literate education—people who have a proper schooling but who are neither practitioners of any art, because they have private means, nor slaves to any philosophical sect.

On one such occasion I, as was my usual practice, proposed that our arguments should be subjected to evaluation. Someone suggested that the best criterion for evaluation in this dispute, with regard to the void which those people claim surrounds the universe, would be if we could actually go up to it and observe whether any body which was placed in it naturally stays in the same position or moves to some other place. This suggestion met with the approval of everyone except for those philosophers, who would not desist from creating pointless quarrels with each other and with us, because of their own inability to distinguish possible arguments from necessary ones. It is possible that each body remains in the same place, and it is also possible that it does not remain there; neither side of the debate has a *necessary* demonstration in this area.

6. I thought, then, that the time had come for me to make some statement—not that I cherished any great hope of denting their false conceit of wisdom, I but so as to leave nothing untried, even though I was aware that the endeavour 94 was not a trivial one.

Now (I began), it is generally agreed that any demonstration should begin with the most manifest facts. The possibility of making a transition from these to matters which are not evident, however, is not admitted by the Academics and Sceptics, but it is accepted by the rest of us; and I believe that we can find a position superior to their despair of knowledge.

Some facts are evident to reason, some to sense perception; and sometimes these two kinds of fact appear to be in conflict. Our first requirement here is someone who is trained in this very matter, and who is able to show that there is in reality never such conflict. Of great importance, secondly, is the distinguishing of evident facts from ones which are not evident. Some people make the mistake of too hastily accepting as evident things which do not really have that status. And is it any wonder (I continued) that this happens in the area of truths of reason, with people who are too quick to form judgements, when we may observe every day that some individuals have this problem even in the area

95 of things evident to the senses? For example, | someone sees a man approaching from a distance, and says, 'That is Dion', as if he is quite certain of the man's identity. But on closer inspection the man may turn out to be not Dion but Theon. If there were no difference between the images one has of people seen at a distance and those seen close to, then disagreements arising over people seen at a distance would never be settled one way or the other. What is actually the case is that there is one level of clarity in the case of objects seen close to, and another in the case of objects seen from far off; and so, naturally, mistakes occur.

You should, therefore, bear this point in mind before turning to matters which are evident to reason. Has it never happened to you that you have hastily exclaimed: Look, here comes so-and-so—Menippus, for the sake of argument— and that when he came nearer it turned out to be Theodorus? Or have you throughout your life refrained from any assent of this kind, which is known as precipitation or rashness? I may confide in you that no one can convict me of ever having made such an error. From early youth I cultivated the habit of

96 avoiding hasty assent, | both in matters apparent to the senses and in matters apparent to reason. In making the transition to the latter, I urge you in this context too not to give assent to any of them wrongly, as I observe many of my friends do every day. Some of them withhold their belief if only one person makes a given statement; but if two, three or four people say the same thing, then they do not withhold it. Others will even give their assent to one person, and will do so hastily to two, three or four. What they never stop to consider is whether there is one single cause of all these people telling the truth—or one single cause of them all telling falsehoods.

In such cases, then, it is better to take longer, as I do, even at the cost of the name-calling of those who make hasty assents, and who make fun of my suspicious nature. It has happened to me that some of my friends have heard from some source that a certain individual had returned from his travel abroad, and have come to me with the news, and then been proved liars. When I criticize such behaviour, they do not resolve to be surer of their ground next time; far

97 from it. They actually get angry | with me and say that they are not responsible for the false information; they merely believed someone who gave them that information, and therefore the error belonged to that person. They refuse to accept the blame for having gone along with any rash and hasty assent. If they had framed their statement as I habitually do, and said that so-and-so had told

them such-and-such about such-and-such a person, they would not have been guilty of lying. As things were, their trust in the giver of that information led to them being caught in a lie along with him. Instead of stating categorically that this travelling friend of mine had returned, they could quite easily have said that they had heard of his arrival from somebody.

When people refuse to stop making hasty assents in such cases as these, where the actual facts of the matter reveal them as liars just a short time later, what is likely to happen to them in cases the facts are non-evident and therefore more difficult to grasp?[37]

When I considered the cause of this kind of hasty judgement, I realized that it was, if not acquisitiveness, then at least the conceit of wisdom, that was responsible for all such behaviour. I For they have observed the praise which 98 attaches to speed in making any discovery, either by the senses or by the intellect, and thus hope to show their own superiority to their neighbour in the speed with which they can assess the facts. What they actually display is rather the speed with which they fall into ignorance. So, then (I said), let these remarks be taken as applying to all those who make rash declarations.

7. Let us return to those philosophers who make declarations of this kind regarding the question, whether bodies placed in the void remain in one place or move downwards. The architect would not have made a declaration on this issue before making a personal expedition to that part of the universe where there is a void, and then putting the matter to the test empirically and making a definite observation as to whether any object placed there does remain in one place, or whether it moves elsewhere. That is indeed the type of starting-point an architect uses in his demonstrations—matters which are evident and universally agreed upon.

I Yet you practitioners of philosophy offer demonstrations of matters regard- 99 ing which you have no clear knowledge whatever. I was recently present at a dispute between two philosophers. One claimed that water was heavier than wood, the other that wood was heavier than water. Both produced very long arguments, considering the matter from every possible angle. The chief point of the one philosopher was that any compressed substance is heavier; the other staked his claim on the notion that water has less of the void in it. And they proceeded in this way for a considerable length of time, producing arguments to reinforce their own plausibility, but without any proof—as if it were a matter incapable of being decided on the basis of observation, which, as you know, is my practice. The philosophers, who wished to continue this discussion, asked the architect in what manner it could be clearly demonstrated which of the objects were heavier. It could not, they said, be done with a pair of scales nor by

---

[37] A sentence follows which is difficult to make clear sense of, and has thus been omitted.

means of a filled vessel; for it would be possible to stand the piece of wood [on
100 the scales], [|] but not to fill a vessel with it, while conversely it would be possible
to fill a vessel with the water.

As they continued thus in their usual fashion, the architect laughed and said:

> That's you through and through, you fellows, with your conceit of your own
> wisdom. You all reckon to understand what happens beyond the universe—a
> subject which admits of conjecture, but in which there can be no scientific
> knowledge. When it comes to these kinds of problems, though—problems
> which are sometimes understood by the man in the street—you are utterly at a
> loss. And so it is with the matter before us now, how to make a relative meas-
> urement of water and wood.

And so everyone present begged the architect to tell them how the weight of the
wood could be scientifically and reliably measured against that of the water;
and he explained the matter succinctly and clearly, in such a way that it was
understood by all except the philosophers. He was in fact constrained to repeat
the explanation a second and even a third time; and finally, with great difficulty,
they managed to understand it.

101   'It is reasonable enough,' said the architect, 'that most people say of [|] these
people that they possess nothing but the conceit of wisdom. For it has been
proved that in areas which do not admit of true knowledge they understand
nothing; yet in areas which do, they maintain that false conceit.'

Taking up the argument, I added that it was not surprising that this was the
case. They had never been prepared to undergo training in the manner of making the transition from evident matters to the non-evident, nor to educate
themselves in contexts where the facts provide their own confirmation both to
the one who discovers them and similarly refutes the one who does not.

'And,' I said, 'to give you a laugh and to enable you to realize the full extent of
their blindness, I should like to give you an account of one or two matters about
which these earnest individuals make rash assertions. Let us start with this
one—especially since there is a representative of the Peripatetics now present,
who are convinced that this universe is single, and that there is no void surrounding it, nor any void spaces within it either. Well, now, each of *these* indi-
102 viduals (here I indicated the Stoic and the [|] Epicurean)—differs from him in
two respects. The Stoic denies the presence of void within but affirms its presence outside the universe. The Epicurean admits both these types of void but
differs from these other gentlemen in another particular. For he does not accept
that there is only one universe, as the Stoic asserts (in agreement, here, with the
Peripatetic); his position is that, as the void is infinite in size, thus the universes
within it must be infinite in number. I have heard what the three of them say in
defence of their own private dreams; and yet I know that none of them is able to

advance a single demonstrative argument. Their arguments are at best probable or possible ones—and sometimes do not even belong to those kinds. You will realize the truth of what I am saying if you simply call on each of them to produce a demonstration on the very subject now before us.'

And those persons then began to make speeches in accord with what we know of them from their writings. It was abundantly obvious to the whole audience that none of them was able to present a truly compelling argument, nor one with any element of geometrical demonstration. All they could come out with were arguments of a dialectical sort,[38] like those I employed by the orators.   103 But our present discussion concerns philosophers.[39] Let us then turn to consider ourselves—those of us who do not practise philosophy—and again ask one of these sages, whether it is right to declare themselves alone to have realized the truth, when they are held in contempt by the rest of the world, laymen and philosophers alike. And the most absurd thing of all (I said) is that each of these philosophers is completely without respect if he is forced to appear outside his own flock. Now, which is the more likely candidate for knowledge of the truth: one who can withstand the scrutiny of all philosophers (except these fraudulent ones), and in addition the scrutiny of the practitioners of all the logically based arts, that is, mathematicians, arithmeticians, geometers, astronomers, architects, lawyers, orators, scholars and musicians—or one who is positively assessed and garlanded by himself alone, and who, if he ever submits himself to the assessment of others, will gain not a single vote?

Let this, then, suffice for the present on the subject of errors.

[38] *Epicheirēmata*, a technical term in rhetorical theory; such arguments are considered in the Aristotelian tradition, and by Galen, as having potentially persuasive force but being of a lower level than those required for logical or scientific demonstration.

[39] The MS has 'the rich' in place of 'philosophers' here, and 'are not rich' for 'do not practise philosophy' in the next sentence; I follow Goulston's emendation. Although the MS reading has been defended on the basis that it represents an ironical reference to the motto that 'only the wise man is rich', the sudden transition to talk of the rich seems to me impossible without any context for it. Galen's distancing of himself from the profession of philosophy is consistent with the content and tone of the text so far, especially that of the last chapters.

List of People Mentioned

N.b. Greek names are generally given in their Latinized forms (e.g. Epicurus for Epikouros, Heraclitus for Herakleitos), or else in the Anglicized version (Alexander, Euclid, etc.) in common use in English.

Adrastus (of Aphrodisias, Asia Minor, second century AD): influential Aristotelian commentator whose work survives only in fragments or mentions in later authors.

Adrian (or Hadrian, of Tyre, second century AD): successful orator or sophist at Rome.

Aeficianus: medical author, pupil of Quintus and commentator on Hippocrates in the generation before Galen.

Aelius Aristides (second century AD): sophist; author of the *Sacred Tales*, an account of his own experiences as a patient and religious devotee at the Asclepieion at Pergamum.

Aeschrion: Empiricist doctor–pharmacist, active around Pergamum in the first half of the second century.

Albinus (second century AD): significant Platonist philosopher of the period known as 'Middle Platonism', author of an extant *Introduction* to Plato's dialogues which groups them thematically and gives a paedagogic order for their reading. (An outdated scholarly theory identifies him with Alcinous, another important figure in Middle Platonism.)

Alexander of Aphrodisias (Asia Minor, second–third century AD): important Aristotelian commentator and philosopher, known particularly for distinctive views on the theory of soul or mind; a younger contemporary who shows some knowledge of Galen's work.

Anacharsis (? sixth century BC): semi-legendary prince of Scythia, supposed to have immersed himself in travel and culture and attempted to introduce Greek education and customs to his own people, otherwise traditionally regarded by the Greeks as barbarous and brutal.

Anaxagoras (of Clazomenae, Asia Minor, fifth century BC): philosopher who espoused a theory of fundamental principles or elements and how they form the entities of the cosmos and biological world.

Anaximander (of Miletus, early sixth century BC): natural philosopher and astronomer, possibly responsible for the invention or Greek adoption of the gnomon or sundial pointer, and associated with a theory of constant change and interplay of elements in the explanation of cosmic processes.

Anaximenes (of Miletus, sixth century BC): natural philosopher and cosmologist, associated with the view of air as the primary element and of the constant change of substances into each other.

Andronicus of Rhodes: head of the Aristotelian school, probably in the first century BC, credited with the first major edition or paedagogic ordering of Aristotle's works; he may be responsible for the crucial introductory role assigned to the *Categories* in the subsequent curriculum (for both Aristotelians and Platonists).

Antoninus Pius (reigned AD 138–61): Roman emperor, predecessor and adoptive father of Marcus Aurelius Antoninus.

Apelles (fourth century BC): Greek painter, considered in later literature to have been pre-eminent in his field.

Archigenes (of Apamea, Syria, first–second century AD): medical author, influenced by 'Pneumatist' school of medicine; responsible for a detailed and complex theory of the diagnostics of the pulse, with which Galen engages in detail. His work does not survive except in quotations in Galen and others.

Archimedes (of Syracuse, third century BC): most important Greek mathematician, responsible for brilliant and innovative proofs especially in geometry, and credited also with a number of ingenious technical inventions.

Aristippus (fifth–fourth century BC): disciple of Socrates and founder of the Cyrenaic school of philosophy; he espoused a hedonist and non-conventional ethics, but advocated the ideal of self-control alongside the pursuit of pleasure.

Aristo of Chios (third century BC): Stoic philosopher, pupil of Zeno, who was however seen by some as departing from orthodox Stoicism in certain crucial respects.

Aristotle (fourth century BC): toweringly influential philosopher and scientist; his works and thought are of huge importance for Galen in the areas of logic, element theory, biology, philosophy of mind and ethics.

Asclepiades (of Bithynia, first century BC): an influential philosophical–medical author who subscribed to some version of a particle theory of matter, and whose physiological and pathological views were adapted by the Methodists.

Asclepius: the Greek god of medicine; his sanctuaries in the Greek and Roman world were the site of 'temple medicine', a set of practices which involved 'incubation' (sleeping within the sanctuary in the hope of receiving a divinely sent cure or instructive dream) but also consultation with medical practitioners who made recommendations for lifestyle and diet and offered medical interventions (e.g. venesection). In Galen's lifetime, and in his early career, one of the most important such sanctuaries was at Pergamum—a city which also boasted a newly built temple to the hybrid god, 'Zeus Asclepius'.

Aspasius (first half of second century AD): influential commentator on Aristotle; though his works have mainly not survived, a part of his commentary on the *Nicomachean Ethics* constitutes the earliest significant extant passage of Aristotelian commentary.

Athenaeus of Attalia (Asia Minor, first century BC/first century AD): 'Pneumatist' medical author, probably influential on Galen; he seems to have subscribed to an element theory not dissimilar to Galen's, while according a particular role to *pneuma*, under the influence of Stoicism; he also contributed important work on the pulse.

Attalus: name of three kings of Pergamum in the Hellenistic period (I: 241–197 BC; II: 159–138 BC; III: 138–133 BC), associated with a growth in the city's power and cultural prestige.

Bassus: mentioned a few times as an associate or student of Galen's; precise identity not known.

Boethus, Flavius: originally from Syria (Ptolemais), an influential member of Roman society who achieved consular rank, and ended his career as governor of Syria Palaestina; he also had serious interests in Aristotelian philosophy and in anatomy, and was one of Galen's major patrons in his early years at Rome.

Carneades (second century BC): head of the Platonic Academy during its sceptical phase and important representative of philosophical Scepticism.

Chrysippus (third century BC): third head of the Stoic school of philosophy; one of the most important and prolific philosophical authors of antiquity. None of his works survives today, although Galen (somewhat ironically in view of his almost wholly hostile view) provides us with a major source of information about his views and arguments.

Commodus (reigned AD 180–92): son of and successor to Marcus Aurelius, with whom his reign contrasted sharply, through his focus on personal interests (including promotion of favourites and addiction to the amphitheatre, where he himself appeared as Hercules) at the expense of public duty; he was also known for brutal purges of both senators and close associates.

Crates (fourth–third century BC): see Diogenes.

Damon (fifth–fourth century BC): music theorist and intellectual with political interests, possibly with a connection to the Pythagoreans; views on the ethical or character-forming effects of different kinds of music are attributed to him from Plato onwards.

Democritus (of Abdera, second half of fifth century BC): follower of Leucippus, along with whom he was one of the chief proponents of ancient Atomism; according to this theory all that exist are indivisible, unchanging atoms and the void between them, the combinations and motions of these atoms giving rise to all perceptible properties in the universe.

Demosthenes (384–322 BC): influential forensic and political orator, famous as a master of classical Greek prose and for his political campaign against Philip of Macedon.

Diocles (of Carystus, Euboea, fourth century BC): important medical author who subscribed to an element theory similar to Galen's and wrote on a wide range of medical topics, including embryology, fevers and diet; his work survives only in fragments.

Diogenes (of Sinope, on Black Sea, fourth century BC): originally a follower of Socrates, founder of the Cynic school of philosophy and teacher of both Crates and Zeno of Citium. While outraging public sensibilities with their complete rejection of social norms, the Cynics also espoused a (proto-Stoic) indifference to bodily comforts and the reversals of fortune.

Dioscorides, Pedanius (of Anarbazus, Cilicia, first century AD): author of the still extant *Materia Medica* (*Peri hulēs iatrikēs*), a compilation of information on the pharmaceutical properties of animal, mineral and (mainly) plant substances, including some derived recipes, a source drawn on by Galen.

Empedocles (of Acragas, Sicily, fifth century BC): philosopher–poet who propounded an influential theory of four elements or 'roots' (air, water, earth, fire), their interaction controlled by the principles of Love and Strife; his work has medical and also religious dimensions.

Epictetus (first–second century AD): Stoic philosopher, at one time the slave of a high-up official at the court of Nero, later running his own school at Nicopolis in north-west Greece; his work survives through the *Discourses* of Arrian, which present Stoic teaching in the form of lively lectures and imagined conversations, aimed at the ethical development or self-improvement of the pupil.

Epicurus (341–270 BC): philosopher who propounded a physical theory of atomistic materialism and the ethical view that the goal of life is pleasure, conceived as freedom from bodily pain or mental disturbance.

Erasistratus (of Ceos, third century BC, active at Alexandria): younger contemporary of Herophilus and major figure in the history of anatomy; distinguished sensory from motor nerves and accurately described the valves of the heart. Probably an important influence also on Galen's physiological theories, although the latter mentions him largely for a number of doctrines which he rejects: the view that the arteries contain only air (*pneuma*); the mechanistic model of explanation, which posits the principle of *horror vacui* (or 'the following towards what is emptied') as the main principle explaining movement of substances in the body; and the refusal of venesection in all cases.

Euclid (fourth–third century BC): mathematician whose *Elements* present a series of proofs in arithmetic and in plane and solid geometry; their method, proceeding on the basis of definitions, postulates and axioms through a process of deduction to theorems, was regarded as a model or standard for logical demonstration.

Eudemus: Peripatetic philosopher who moved in the highest echelons of Roman society, having been a family friend and possibly also teacher of Galen at Pergamum; his influence and connections were instrumental in gaining Galen advancement in his early career at Rome.

Eugenianus: follower or associate of Galen's at Rome, dedicatee of the later books of *The Therapeutic Method* as well as of *My Own Books*.

Euripides (fifth century BC): one of the three great Greek tragedians; by Roman imperial times his work had become a central literary classic, and was much drawn upon for quotations which make moral points or raise ethical issues.

Favorinus of Arles (first–second century AD): orator and philosopher who espoused Scepticism within the Academic tradition.

Gaius: 'Middle' Platonist philosopher, teacher of Albinus.

Glaucon: philosopher with medical interests and follower of Galen's at Rome.

Hadrian (reigned AD 117–38): predecessor of Antoninus Pius; associated with the promotion of Greek culture in the Roman Empire and with a number of building projects; he seems to have supported a significant renovation and rebuilding project at Pergamum.

Heracles (Roman 'Hercules'): legendary hero, taken as exemplary of the peak of strength and courage.

Heraclianus: son and follower of Numisianus, of the school of Quintus; he apparently preserved the anatomical works of Numisianus in secret and had them destroyed on his own death.

Heraclides of Erythrae (Asia Minor, late first century BC): doctor of the school of Herophilus and commentator on Hippocrates.

Heraclides of Pontus (fourth century BC): Platonist philosopher and physical theorist whose particle theory seems to have influenced Asclepiades; author of a dialogue on *The Woman without Respiration* (*Peri tēs apnou*); his work survives only in fragments and mentions in later authors.

Heraclides of Tarentum (first century BC): Empiricist doctor who wrote on a range of medical, including pharmacological, topics; his work survives only in fragments.

Heraclitus (of Ephesus, sixth–fifth century BC): notoriously obscure philosopher whose work encompasses questions of epistemology as well as cosmology and physics; he focused on fire as the fundamental physical force in the universe.

Hermes: Greek messenger god, more broadly associated with communication, writing and learning.

Herodotus (of Halicarnassus, Asia Minor, c. 485–424 BC): the 'father of history'; his *Histories* contain a wealth of ethnographical and geographical information, as well as chronological narratives which centre on the power of Persia and the Persian War.

Herophilus (of Chalcedon, late fourth–third century BC): alongside Erasistratus major figure in the development of anatomical knowledge, especially of the brain, nerves and the vascular system; gave a detailed anatomical account of a number of organs; also a major contributor to the theory of diagnosis by the pulse and to dietetics.

Hesiod (*c.* seventh century BC): early Greek epic poet, author of the *Theogony* and the didactic *Works and Days*.

Hipparchus (of Nicaea, second century BC): astronomer and geographer who made exact observations of the heavenly bodies and whose work is quoted by Ptolemy.

Hippocrates (of Cos, fifth/fourth century BC): legendary doctor who later came to be seen as the exemplar of excellence in medicine; a canon of disparate works, the so-called 'Hippocratic corpus', began to be assembled under his name from Hellenistic times onward, along with a commentary tradition and debates about authenticity; it is now impossible to attribute any work in the corpus to the historical figure with any degree of certainty.

Homer (*c.* eighth–seventh century BC): legendary poet credited with the writing of the *Iliad* and the *Odyssey*; in Galen's time the two epics were a foundational plank of Greek education, and much quoted within the literary culture to which Galen belongs.

Leucippus: see Democritus.

Lucius Verus (reigned AD 161–9): appointed by Marcus Aurelius on his accession as co-ruler, and given command during the Parthian War (161–6); he died on return from a joint expedition with Marcus to the Danube province.

Lycus (of Macedon): medical author and Hippocratic commentator in the generation before Galen; a pupil of Quintus.

Marcus Aurelius Antoninus (reigned AD 161–80): Roman emperor, philosopher and patron of Galen; he spent much of his later life, including the first few years (169–76) of Galen's 'second stay' at Rome, on military campaign on the borders of the empire in central Europe.

Marinus (of Alexandria): anatomist of the generation or two before Galen, apparently responsible for a major revival of medical research and teaching after a long period of neglect; through his pupils Quintus and Numisianus he was influential in the establishment of a loosely constituted school that continued these interests and teaching.

Martianus (or Martialius or Martialis): prominent doctor and medical theorist during Galen's early career in Rome; follower of Erasistratus.

Milo of Croton (*c.* sixth century BC): Olympic athlete of legendary strength, supposedly also a pupil of Pythagoras.

Musonius Rufus (first century AD): influential Stoic philosopher who wrote nothing but whose teaching survives through fragmentary references in later authors; teacher of Epictetus.

Numisianus: anatomist, pupil of Quintus.

Panaetius (second century BC): Stoic philosopher of 'Middle' period; influential, both personally and through his writings, on the development of Stoicism at Rome. His writings were intensively used by Cicero; he was also the teacher of Posidonius.

Pelops: Galen's second major medical teacher, at Smyrna; a pupil of Numisianus.

Pheidias (of Athens, second half of fifth century BC): pre-eminent classical sculptor, responsible for the statues of Athena Parthenos in the Parthenon and of Zeus at Olympia, the latter considered one of the seven wonders of the ancient world, and credited with work on a number of the other Parthenon sculptures.

Philistion (of Locri, fourth century BC): medical author and element theorist whose views are closely based on Empedocles' and who seems to have been influential on Plato.

Pindar (of Boeotia, sixth–fifth century BC): most famous and best preserved of the Greek lyric poets, especially known for his odes celebrating victors at various prestigious games.

Plato (*c.* 428–348 BC): foundational figure in Greek philosophy; student of Socrates; he presents his views not directly but through recounted or imagined dialogues between historical figures, most prominently Socrates; his views on metaphysics, dialectic, epistemology, politics, ethics and soul theory (psychology) conditioned the subsequent course of Greek philosophy, and his work in the latter two areas (especially in the *Republic* and the *Timaeus*) is of particular relevance for Galen.

Pliny the Elder (first century AD): Roman gentleman and author of the *Natural History*, a hugely valuable resource for ancient everyday life, including medical and dietetic practices.

Plutarch (of Chareonea, Boeotia, first–second century AD): littérateur and Platonist philosopher, author of a series of biographies of famous people and of works on literary–cultural and philosophical themes.

Polybus (of Cos, early fourth century BC): pupil and son-in-law of Hippocrates; credited, on good doxographical evidence, with the authorship of the 'Hippocratic' *The Nature of the Human Being*, a crucial text for Galen; and regarded by Galen himself as almost on a par with Hippocrates in his reliability.

Polycitus (fifth/fourth century BC): sculptor, considered pre-eminent in antiquity; author of a treatise, the *Canon* ('Standard') summarizing the ideal proportions constitutive of male beauty, using mathematical relationships; the name seems also to have been applied to his most celebrated statue, the *Doryphoros* ('Spear-Bearer'), which was thought to exemplify these ideal proportions.

Posidonius (of Apamea, Syria, first century BC): Stoic of 'Middle' period, credited by some with moving away from orthodox Stoicism (and in Galen's view of thus eliminating its most rebarbative features) under the influence of a greater engagement with Plato; known personally to Cicero, he contributed to the spread and popularity of Stoicism in the Roman elite.

Praxagoras (of Cos, second half of fourth century BC): influential medical author and anatomist, teacher of Herophilus; he may be credited with the clear distinction between veins and arteries, while apparently obscuring the difference between arteries (which he held contained only *pneuma*) and nerves.

Protagoras (of Abdera, fifth century BC): early and prominent sophist; associated with the view that 'man is the measure of all things', and with an agnostic view on the existence of the gods.

Pythagoras (sixth–fifth century BC): semi-mythical figure whose own views are difficult to recover with any certainty, but considered in the ancient Platonic tradition as a forerunner of Plato in his metaphysical theories and view of the soul, and known for his ascetic lifestyle and dietetic stipulations.

Quintus (mid-second century AD, Rome): doctor and anatomist; pupil of Marinus and teacher of a number of the most significant medical figures in the generation immediately before Galen.

Rufus (or Rouphos) of Ephesus (first/second century AD?): significant medical author; few of his works survive, but he seems to have been influential on Galen and others in a number of important areas, especially as regards diseases (including melancholy).

Sabinus (first–second century AD): medical author and Hippocratic commentator.

Sappho (seventh–sixth century BC): pre-eminent female poet of antiquity, famed for her intense and intimate lyrical poems especially of love; her work survives mainly in fragments.

Satyrus: Galen's first medical teacher, at Pergamum; a pupil of Quintus.

Septimius Severus (reigned 193–211): Roman emperor, successor of Commodus after the months-long reign of Pertinax.

Sergius Paulus, Lucius: Roman of consular rank who moved in the elite circles to which Galen was introduced.

Socrates (469–399 BC): philosopher who inspired and enraged by his ethical and intellectual challenge, engaging people in uncompromising dialogue on issues of ethics, religion and politics, while denying his own claim to knowledge. He wrote nothing but his arguments and episodes of his life are recounted by Plato and Xenophon.

Teuthras: fellow-student of Galen's from Pergamum, whom he also knew at Rome.

Thales (first half of sixth century BC): supposed founder of the Milesian school (see also Anaximander, Anaximenes), a shadowy early natural philosopher, to whom are attributed astronomical observations and predictions as well as the theoretical claim that 'all things come from water'.

Theophrastus (of Eresus, c. 371–c. 287 BC): pupil and successor of Aristotle, and continuer of his project especially in the areas of biology, botany and ethics.

Thessalus (of Tralles, first century AD; not to be confused with the Thessalus sometimes mentioned as Hippocrates' son and close disciple): prominent and successful proponent or refounder, at Rome, of the 'Methodist' school of medicine, originally due to Themison a couple of centuries earlier; central to his medical theory is a conception of the body as consisting of corpuscles and channels or pores, a reduction of all pathological conditions to the categories of 'constricted' or 'loose' states of these and (according to Galen) a widespread use of the 'diatritus' method of treatment, i.e. the imposition of a fast for two whole days from the incidence of a disease. He is attacked by Galen for all these distortions of medical reality, and for his lack of traditional education—which he seems to have vaunted, consciously championing a non-literate and non-elite model of medical education which could be assimilated in a short time.

Thucydides (second half of fifth century BC): major Greek historian, author of *Peloponnesian War*, chronicling the war between Athens and Sparta in the last third of the fifth century; gave a detailed account of the plague at Athens.

Xenophon (c. 430–354 BC): Athenian soldier and writer; author of a number of historical works as well as writings about Socrates, of whom he was a close associate.

Zeno (of Citium, 334–262 BC): founder of the Stoic school of philosophy, succeeded by Cleanthes and Chrysippus.

Bibliography

Adamson, P, Hansberger, R. and Wilberding, J. (eds) (2014). *Philosophical Themes in Galen*. Bulletin of the Institute of Classical Studies Supplement 114. London: Institute of Classical Studies.

Barigazzi, A. (1991). *Galeni De optima docendi genere, Exhortatio ad medicinam (Protrepticus)/Galeno Sull' ottima maniera d' insegnare; Esortazione all medicina*, text and translation. Corpus Medicorum Graecorum V 1.1. Berlin: Akademie Verlag.

Barnes, J, Jouanna, J. and Barras, V. (eds) (2003). *Galien et la philosophie*. Entretiens sur l'antiquité classique 49. Vandoeuvres-Geneva: Fondation Hardt.

Barton, T. S. (1994). *Power and Knowledge: Astrology, Physiognomics, and Medicine under the Roman Empire*. Ann Arbor: University of Michigan Press.

Bazou, A. (2011). Γαληνοῦ Ὅτι ταῖς τοῦ σώματος κράσεσιν αἱ τῆς ψυχῆς δυνάμεις ἕπονται. Athens: Academy of Athens.

Beck, L. (trans.) (2005). *Pedanius Dioscorides of Anarzabus: De materia medica*. Altertumswissenschaftliche Texte und Studien 38. Hildesheim: Olms-Weidmann.

Boudon, V. (2002). *Galien, Tome II: Exhortation à l' étude de la médecine; Art médical*, texte établi et traduit. Collection des Universités de France. Paris: Les Belles Lettres.

Boudon-Millot V. (2007). *Galien, Tome I: Introduction générale; Sur l' ordre de ses propres livres; Sur ses propres livres; Que l' excellent médecin est aussi philosophe*, texte établi, traduit et annoté. Collection des Universités de France. Paris: Les Belles Lettres.

Boudon-Millot, V. (2012). *Galien de Pergame: un médecin grec à Rome*. Paris: Les Belles Lettres.

Boudon-Millot, V., Jouanna, J. and Pietrobelli, A. (2010). *Galien, Tome IV: Ne pas se chagriner*, texte établi et traduit. Collection des Universités de France. Paris: Les Belles Lettres.

Boudon-Millot, V. and Pietrobelli, A. (2010). 'Galien ressuscité: édition princeps du texte grec du De propriis placitis'. *Revue des Études Grecques* 118: 168–213.

Bouras-Vallianatos, P. and Zipser, B. (2019). *Brill's Companion to the Reception of Galen*. Brill's Companions to Classical Reception 17. Leiden: Brill.

Brunschön, C. W. (2021). *Galeni De locis affectis V–VI/Über das Erkennen der erkrankter Körperteile V–VI*. Corpus Medicorum Graecorum V 6.1.3. Berlin: De Gruyter.

Das, A. (2020). *Galen and the Arabic Reception of Plato's Timaeus*. Cambridge: Cambridge University Press.

De Boer, W. (1937). *Galeni De propriorum animi cuiuslibet affectuum dignotione et curatione; De animi cuiuslibet peccatorum dignotione et curatione; De atra bile*, edidit. Corpus Medicorum Graecorum V 4.1.1. Leipzig and Berlin: Teubner.

De Lacy, P. (1978–84), *Galeni De placitis Hippocratis et Platonis/Galen On the Doctrines of Hippocrates and Plato*, edition, translation and commentary. Corpus Medicorum Graecorum V 4.1.2 (rev. edn 2005). Berlin: Akademie Verlag.

De Lacy, P. (1996). *Galeni De elementis ex Hippocratis sententia/Galen On the Elements according to Hippocrates*, edition, translation and commentary. Corpus Medicorum Graecorum V 1.2. Berlin: Akademie Verlag.

Debru, A. (1996). *Le Corps respirant. La pensée physiologique chez Galien*. Studies in Ancient Medicine 13. Leiden: Brill.

Devinant, J. (2020). *Les Troubles psychiques selon Galien. Étude d' un système de pensée*. Études Anciennes 159. Paris: Les Belles Lettres.

Duckworth, W. L. H., Lyons, M. C. and Towers, B. (1962). *Galen on Anatomical Procedures: The Later Books*. Cambridge: Cambridge University Press.

Garofalo, I. (1991). *Galeno: Procedimenti anatomici*. Milan: Rizzoli.

Garofalo, I. and Lami, A. (2012). *L'anima e il dolore: De indolentia; De propriis placitis*, testo greco a fronte. Milan: Rizzoli.

Garofalo, I. and Vegetti, M. (1978). *Opere scelte di Galeno*. Turin: Unione Tipografica-Editrice Torino.

Gärtner, F. (2015). *Galeni De locis affectis I–II/Über das Erkennen der erkrankter Körperteile I–II*. Corpus Medicorum Graecorum V 6.1.1. Berlin: De Gruyter.

Gill, C. (2010). *Naturalistic Philosophy in Galen and Stoicism*. Oxford: Oxford University Press.

Gill, C., Whitmarsh, T. and Wilkins, J. (eds) (2009). *Galen and the World of Knowledge*. Cambridge: Cambridge University Press.

Haase, W. and Temporini, H. (eds) (1994). *Aufstieg und Niedergang der römischen Welt* II.37.2. Berlin: De Gruyter.

Haars, M. (2018). *Die allgemeinen Wirkungspotentiale der einfachen Arzneimittel bei Galen: Oribasius, Collectiones Medicae XV*, introduction, translation and pharmaceutical commentary. Quellen und Studien zur Geschichte der Pharmazie 116. Stuttgart: Wissenschaftliche Verlaggesellschaft.

Hankinson, R. J. (ed.) (2008). *The Cambridge Companion to Galen*. Cambridge: Cambridge University Press.

Hankinson, R. J. and Havrda, M. (eds) (2022). *Galen's Epistemology: Experience, Reason, and Method in Ancient Medicine*. Cambridge: Cambridge University Press.

Havrda, M. (2017). 'Body and cosmos in Galen's account of the soul'. *Phronesis* 62: 69–89.

Helmreich, G. (1893). *Claudii Galeni Pergameni Scripta Minora*, vol. III. Leipzig: Teubner.

Helmreich, G. (1901). *Galenus de optima corporis constitutione; Idem de bono habitu*. Erlangen: K. b. Hof- und Univ.-Buchdruckerei von Fr. Junge.

Helmreich, G. (1904). *Galeni De temperamentis libri III*. Leipzig: Teubner.

Helmreich, G. (1907/1909). *Galeni De usu partium libri XVII*, 2 vols. Leipzig: Teubner.

Janick, J., Paris, H. S. and Parrish, D. C. (2007). 'The cucurbits of Mediterranean antiquity: identification of taxa from ancient images and descriptions'. *Annals of Botany* 100(7): 1441–57, published online 10.10.2007, doi: 10.1093/aob/mcm242.

Johnston, I. and Papavramidou, N. (2024). *Galen on the Pulses: Medico-Historical Analysis, Textual Tradition, Translation*. Berlin: De Gruyter.

Kalbfleisch, K. (1923). *Galeni De victu attenuante*. Corpus Medicorum Graecorum V 4.2 (pp. 431–51). Leipzig and Berlin: Teubner.

Koch, K. (1923). *Galeni De sanitate tuenda*. Corpus Medicorum Graecorum V 4.2 (pp. 1–198). Leipzig and Berlin: Teubner.

Kühn, K. G. (1821–33). *Galeni Opera Omnia*. Leipzig: Knobloch.

Lami, A. (2010). 'Sul testo del *De propriis placitis* di Galeno'. *Galenos* 4: 81–126.

Lloyd, G. E. R. (1988). 'Scholarship, authority and argument in Galen's *Quod animi mores*', in Manuli and Vegetti (eds), 11–42.

Manetti, D. (ed.) (2012). *Studi sul De indolentia di Galeno*. Rome: Fabrizio Serra Editore.

Manuli, P. and Vegetti, M. (eds) (1988). *Le opere psicologiche di Galeno. Atti del terzo Colloquio Galenico internazionale, Pavia, 10–12 settembre 1986*. Naples: Bibliopolis.

Marquardt, J. (1884). *Claudii Galeni Pergameni Scripta Minora*, vol. I. Leipzig: Teubner.

Mattern, S. M. (2008). *Galen and the Rhetoric of Healing*. Baltimore: Johns Hopkins University Press.

Mattern, S. M. (2013). *The Prince of Medicine: Galen in the Roman Empire*. Oxford: Oxford University Press.

May, M. T. (1968). *Galen: On the Usefulness of the Parts of the Body*, 2 vols. Ithaca: Cornell University Press.

Müller, I. von (1891). *Claudii Galeni Pergameni Scripta Minora*, vol. II. Leipzig: Teubner.

Nickel, D. (2001). *Galeni De foetuum formatione/Galen Über die Ausformung der Keimlinge*, edition, translation and commentary. Corpus Medicorum Graecorum V 3.3. Berlin: Akademie Verlag.

Nutton, V. (1979). *Galeni De praecognitione/Galen On Prognosis*, edition, translation and commentary. Corpus Medicorum Graecorum V 8.1. Berlin: Akademie Verlag.

Nutton, V. (1999). *Galeni De propriis placitis/Galen On My Own Opinions*, edition, translation and commentary. Corpus Medicorum Graecorum V 3.2. Berlin: Akademie Verlag.

Nutton, V. (2015). 'What's in a nomen? Vlatadon 14 and an old theory resurrected', in B. Holmes and K.-D. Fischer (eds), *The Frontiers of Ancient Science: Essays in Honor of Heinrich von Staden*, 451–62. Berlin: De Gruyter.

Nutton, V. (2020). *Galen: A Thinking Doctor in Imperial Rome*. Abingdon/New York: Routledge.

Petit, C. (ed.) (2019). *Galen's Treatise Περὶ Ἀλυπίας (De indolentia) in Context: A Tale of Resilience*. Studies in Ancient Medicine 52. Leiden: Brill.

Polemis, I. and Xenophontos, S. (2023). *On Avoiding Distress and On My Own Opinions*, critical edition with translation. Trends in Classics. Supplementary Volumes 151. Berlin: De Gruyter.

Rocca, J. (2003). *Galen on the Brain: Anatomical Knowledge and Physical Speculation in the Second Century AD*. Studies in Ancient Medicine 26. Leiden: Brill.

Salas, L. A. (2020). *Cutting Words: Polemical Dimensions of Galen's Anatomical Experiments*. Studies in Ancient Medicine 55. Leiden: Brill.

Schäfer, W. (1908). *De Galeni qui fertur De parvae pilae exercitio libello*. Diss. Bonn.

Siegel, R. E. (1976). *Galen on the Affected Parts*, translation from the Greek; text with explanatory notes. Basle: Karger.

Singer, C. (1956). *Galen on Anatomical Procedures (De anatomicis administrationibus)*, translation of the surviving books with introduction and notes. London and Oxford: Wellcome Institute for the History of Medicine and Oxford University Press.

Singer, P. N. (1997a). *Galen: Selected Works*. Oxford World's Classics. Oxford: Oxford University Press.

Singer, P. N. (1997b). 'Levels of explanation in Galen'. *Classical Quarterly* 47: 525–42.

Singer, P. N. (2013). *Galen: Psychological Writings: Avoiding Distress, Character Traits, The Diagnosis and Treatment of the Affections and Errors Peculiar to Each Person's Soul, The Capacities of the Soul Depend on the Mixtures of the Body*, translation with introductions and notes by V. Nutton, D. Davies and P. N. Singer, with the collaboration of P. Tassinari. Cambridge: Cambridge University Press.

Singer, P. N. (2016/2021). 'Galen', in *Stanford Encyclopedia of Philosophy* (Fall 2024 Edition), Edward N. Zalta and Uri Nodelman (eds.), forthcoming URL = < https://plato.stanford.edu/archives/fall2024/entries/galen/>.

Singer, P. N. (2017). 'The essence of rage: Galen on emotional disturbances and their physical correlates', in R. Seaford, J. Wilkins and M. Wright (eds), *Selfhood and the*

Soul: Essays on Ancient Thought and Literature in Honour of Christopher Gill, 161–96. Oxford: Oxford University Press.

Singer, P. N. (2019a). 'Galen and the culture of Pergamum: a view of Greek medical–intellectual life in Roman Asia', in B. Türkmen, F. Kurunaz, N. Ermiş and Y. Ekinci Danısan (eds), *II. Uluslararası Bergama Sempozyumu, 9–10 Mayıs 2013*, 131–69. Izmir: Kültür ve Sosyal İşler Müdürlüğü, Bergama Belediyesi.

Singer, P. N. (2019b). 'New light and old texts: Galen on his own books', in Petit (ed.), 91–131.

Singer, P. N. (2019c). 'Note on MS Vlatadon 14: a summary of the main findings and problems', in Petit (ed.), 10–37.

Singer, P. N. (2019d). 'A new distress: Galen's ethics in Περὶ Ἀλυπίας and beyond', in Petit (ed.), 180–98.

Singer, P. N. (2020). 'A change in the substance: theory and its limits in Galen's *Simples*', in M. Martelli, C. Petit and L. Raggetti (eds). *Galen's Treatise* On Simple Drugs. *Interpretation and Transmission. Archives Internationales d' Histoire des Sciences* 70, 16–53. Turnhout: Brepols.

Singer, P. N. (2023). *Galen: Writings on Health: Thrasybulus and Health*, translated with introduction and notes. Cambridge: Cambridge University Press.

Singer, P. N. and Rosen, R. M. (eds.) (2024). *The Oxford Handbook of Galen*. Oxford: Oxford University Press.

Singer, P. N. and van der Eijk, P. J. (2018). *Galen: Works on Human Nature*, Vol. 1: *Mixtures (De temperamentis)*, translated with introduction and notes. Cambridge: Cambridge University Press.

Smith, W. D. (1979). *The Hippocratic Tradition*. Ithaca: Cornell University Press.

Tieleman, T. (1996). *Galen and Chrysippus on the Soul: Argument and Refutation in the De Placitis books II–III*. Philosophia Antiqua 68. Leiden: Brill.

van der Eijk, P. J. (2015). 'On "Hippocratic" and "non-Hippocratic" medical writings', in L. Dean-Jones and R. M. Rosen (eds), *Ancient Concepts of the Hippocratic: Papers Presented at the XIIIth International Hippocrates Colloquium, Austin, Texas, August 2008*. Studies in Ancient Medicine 48, 15–47. Leiden: Brill.

Vinkestejn, R. (2022). *Philosophical Perspective on Galen of Pergamum: Four Case-Studies on Human Nature and the Relation between Body and Soul*. Philosophia Antiqua 166. Leiden: Brill.

Von Staden, H. (1989). *Herophilus: The Art of Medicine in Early Alexandria*. Cambridge: Cambridge University Press.

Index